Topics In Environmental Physiology And Medicine

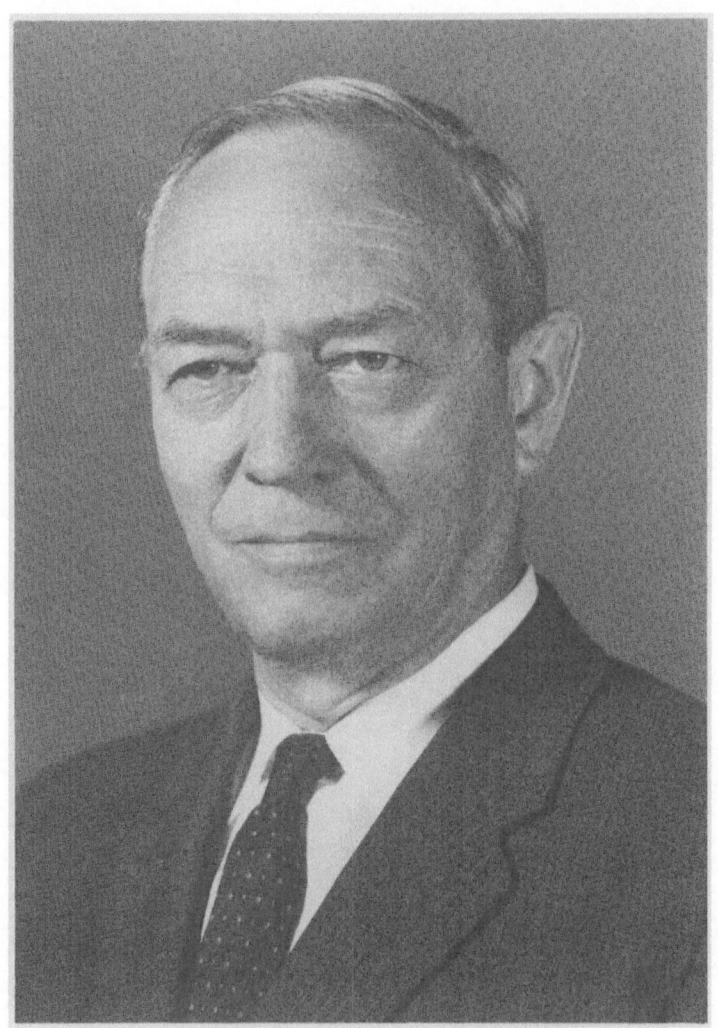

WALLACE OSGOOD FENN
1893 - 1971

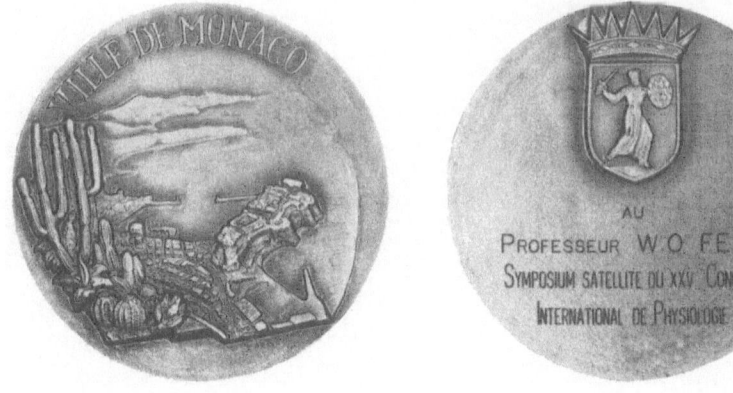

Dr. Fenn's last award, The Honor Medal of the City of Monaco (July, 1971)

Carbon Dioxide
and
Metabolic Regulations

Edited by

Gabriel Nahas

and

Karl E. Schaefer

Satellite Symposium of the
XXV INTERNATIONAL CONGRESS
OF PHYSIOLOGY
July 20 - 21 - 22 1971
International Conference Center
Monte-Carlo, Monaco

Springer-Verlag New York · Heidelberg · Berlin

1974

Library of Congress Cataloging in Publication Data

Schaefer, Karl Ernst, 1912-   comp.
 Carbon dioxide and metabolic regulations.

 (Topics in environmental physiology and medicine)
 1. Carbon dioxide in the body—Addresses, essays,
lectures. 2. Carbon dioxide—Physiological effect—
Addresses, essays, lectures. 3. Metabolic regulation—
Addresses, essays, lectures. I. Nahas, Gabriel G.,
1920-   joint comp. II. Title. [DNLM: 1. Carbon
dioxide—Metabolism. QV314 S294c 1974]
QP535.C1S3   574.1'9212   74-6247
ISBN-13:978-1-4612-9833-5

© 1974 by Springer-Verlag New York Inc.
Softcover reprint of the hardcover 1st edition 1974

ISBN-13:978-1-4612-9833-5   e-ISBN-13:978-1-4612-9831-1
DOI: 10.1007/978-1-4612-9831-1

Preface

Wallace O. Fenn (1893–1971)

The proceedings of the satellite symposium of the XXV International Congress of Physiology on "CO_2 and Metabolic Regulations" are dedicated to Wallace Osgood Fenn. Dr. Fenn had agreed to be honorary conference chairman of this meeting, but was unable to attend because of the illness from which he died two months later on September 20, 1971.

Wallace O. Fenn was born of an old New England family in Lanesboro, Massachusetts on August 27, 1893. His father was dean of the Divinity School at Harvard University. It was at Harvard that Fenn received his A.B. (1914) and his M.S. (1916). He then started his Ph.D. thesis there under the plant physiologist W. J. V. Osterhout, took a year out to serve as a nutrition officer in the U.S. Army, and finished his degree in May 1919.

From 1919 to 1922 he was instructor in applied physiology under Cecil K. Drinker at Harvard, and from 1922 to 1924 was a Traveling Fellow of the Rockefeller Institute, with A. V. Hill and Sir Henry Dale, in England. In 1924, at the age of 31, he was appointed professor of physiology at the newly formed School of Medicine and Dentistry at the University of Rochester and remained there as chairman for 35 years. In 1959 he became Distinguished University Professor of Physiology, and in 1962, director of the Space Science Center of the University.

Wallace Fenn was truly a universal physiologist—one of the few who could still encompass the whole of physiology. His contributions over 50 years covered four main eras in the development of physiology: muscle, electrolyte, respiratory, and hyperbaric study.

The study of muscle contraction started in 1922 when Fenn became the first American to work in A. V. Hill's laboratory. Fenn concluded this work by saying, ". . . There is a fairly good quantitative relation between the heat production of muscles and the work which they perform; and a muscle which does work liberates, *ipso facto*, an extra supply of energy which does not appear in an isometric contraction." (Fenn [1923]). A. V. Hill referred to this as the "Fenn effect," and so it has been known ever since.

Fenn's data showed first that if a muscle shortens it produces more heat than during an isometric contraction over the same time period. He then showed that this extra heat production was proportional to the external work done by the muscle. It was clearly not determined by the load alone, nor by the change in length. This was the first evidence that shortening is an active process and that muscle is not simply a prestretched spring shortening passively.

At the University of Rochester Fenn began working on the relationship between the force exerted by muscle and the velocity with which it shortens. He first described the now familiar force-velocity curve under the title "Muscular force at different speeds of shortening." (Fenn [1935]). Fenn and Marsh fitted the observed curve to an exponential relationship, which present-day kinetic theory would predict. Andrew Huxley and, later, Richard Podolsky justified the model of contraction (based on making and breaking of cross-bridges between interdigitating sliding filaments) on the grounds that it would reproduce the force-velocity curve discovered by Fenn and Marsh.

Fenn next studied gas exchange by nerve and by muscle. In 1927 he measured for the first time the quantitative amount of oxygen required by a nerve to conduct an impulse. Similar studies on the metabolism of contracting muscles led him to consider the role of potassium in nerve and muscle activity. At the time, although it was known that muscle fibers were rich in potassium, almost nothing was known of the mechanisms by which cells accumulated and maintained a high potassium content.

In the 1930s Fenn pioneered the field of potassium metabolism. He made the first measurements of potassium, sodium, magnesium, and calcium in nerve. He was the first to measure intracellular pH in muscle and nerve by the CO_2 titration method, which still is the most acceptable one today. He showed that intracellular potassium was mobile and that muscle potassium shifted in response to various environmental factors.

Fenn showed that during contraction, potassium was lost from muscle in exchange for sodium and that the process was reversed in recovery. For the first time he showed that sodium could penetrate muscle. All of these observations, performed in the pre-flame photometry era of electrolytes, established the necessary foundation for the Hodgkin–Huxley hypotheses concerning initiation and propagation of nerve and muscle impulses and the magnitude and polarity of electrical potential differences across cell membranes.

Fenn showed that potassium escaped from muscle during contraction *in situ* and that a large part of this potassium appeared in the liver. He demonstrated that potassium uptake was linked with carbohydrate metabolism, particularly with glycogen deposition,

and developed the concept that potassium tends to follow the Cori cycle. He was always quick to seize new opportunities. When radioactive potassium became available to him in 1939, Fenn ingested a sample. He was thus the first not only to study the kinetics of potassium metabolism, but also to demonstrate potassium incorporation into blood cells, which were previously thought to be impermeable. He showed that nearly all muscle potassium in the body is exchangeable, proving that high intracellular potassium content is not maintained by binding or sequestration of potassium, but rather by an active process.

Thus, by 1940 Fenn had discovered that contracting muscle produces extra heat proportional to work; he had described the force-velocity` relationships; he had discovered the potassium-sodium exchange during muscle contraction, and in addition, the mechanism for concentrating potassium in cells.

In 1941, at the onset of America's entry into World War II, he pioneered a completely new field, that of respiratory physiology. He focused his attention on the use and application of pressure-breathing devices to extend the aviator's altitude tolerance in nonpressurized planes. To simulate these conditions he installed a low-pressure chamber that was even more primitive than the one used 70 years before by Paul Bert in Paris. Exhibiting his usual thriftiness, he purchased for $500 a tank originally designed to transport beer. This device stood on its end in his laboratory, had a hatch on top, and could barely accommodate two subjects in the sitting position. To enter, one had to climb a homemade wooden ladder, crawl in through the two-foot-wide hatch, and then lower himself like an acrobat to a stool six feet below. The second man entered on the shoulder of the first. In this chamber Fenn and his group of young collaborators "flew" nearly impossible missions to altitudes which on occasion reached 50,000 feet (87 mm Hg). Fenn passed out so many times that the dean, George Whipple, forbade him to enter the chamber. The dean of the Medical School of the University of Rochester could ill afford to lose his most brilliant professor, even for the war effort. With his young collaborators (Chadwick, Otis, and Rahn), Fenn developed theory and assembled facts which today form basic cornerstones in pulmonary physiology. His previous interest in muscle physiology contributed to the new attention he directed to the mechanics of breathing. His pressure-volume diagram of the thorax and lung (Fenn [1946a]) is now a classical concept. This, combined with the measurements of airway resistance, allowed him to describe for the first time the mechanics and work of breathing (Fenn [1951]), and laid the foundations for the more recent developments in this area.

The other problem that intrigued him was the behavior of the alveolar gas exchange. An article entitled "A theoretical study of the composition of the alveolar air at altitude" set forth the equations that describe the relationships and interactions between O_2, CO_2, and N_2. These equations are today the tool of every respiratory physiologist, and Fenn's graphic display of these on the O_2–CO_2 diagram were extended many years later in the form of a book. This analysis also led to the theoretical description of the ventilation-perfusion relationships.

In the postwar years Fenn's department, with Hermann Rahn and Arthur Otis as anchor men, became the training ground for respiratory physiologists from the United States and abroad: Arthur Dubois, Marsh Tenney, Gaby Nahas, Dan Proctor, the late Bob Clark, Leon Farhi, Don Gilbert, Pierre Dejours, Hilding Bjurstedt, Paul Sadoul, Tulio Velasquez, Carl Magnus Hesser, Emilio Agostoni, Sue H. Rodgers, Hugh Van Liew, Al B. Craig, Al Soffer, John Knowles, Harold Bitter, Richard Ament, Einar Aksnes, John Chapin, Mike Lategola, Walter Massion, Ben Ross, Jim Drorbaugh, Bob Stroud, and many others. Life-long associations which extended beyond purely scientific endeavors were sealed among many of the pupils in Fenn's department.

During this period he wrote with Hermann Rahn the "O_2–CO_2 diagram," which was published by the American Physiology Society and has become the slide rule of the respiratory physiologist (Fenn, [1946b]).

In recent years he turned his attention to the basic problems of the effects of hydrostatic pressure *per se* upon biological processes, an area that he liked to call barophysiology. Bacterial cultures became a favorite organism since they can be pressurized without a gas phase and also because with them the predicted volume changes during metabolic reactions can be modified by the effects of external pressures. Furthermore, bacterial cultures are very inexpensive to raise and maintain.

In addition to his long and productive research career he was an outstanding teacher. Like all great teachers, he could make difficult subjects appear quite simple, always, however, leaving the listener with the feeling that many exciting aspects were yet to be explored.

He also felt it his duty to serve scientific societies and scientific advisory bodies whenever he was asked. Over the years he chaired innumerable committees as adviser for the National Academy of Science, the National Research Council, the National Institute of Health, the United States Army, Navy and Air Force, and the National Space Agency.

He served the American Physiological Society in every capacity, as treasurer (1937–40), secretary (1943–46) and president (1946–48). Under his presidency the APS was reorganized and an appointed position of executive secretary–treasurer was created.

Also during Fenn's presidency the APS Fall Meetings were instituted. The purpose of this was to draw some papers away from the overcrowded program of the Federation Meeting and to provide a smaller meeting that was more conducive to friendly social gatherings. The first Fall Meeting was held in Minneapolis in September 1948. At this meeting the custom of having a past-president address was instituted by Dr. Visscher, then President. Fenn's "Physiology on Horseback" (Fenn [1949]), the first of these addresses, should be required reading for all students in biology.

In this piece Fenn humorously emphasizes the importance of basic research with the following anecdote:

> A man called up a veterinarian about his sick cat, and described its symptoms. The veterinarian understood calf for cat and prescribed a pint of castor oil which was duly administered (more or less). Some days later the veterinarian met his client and inquired about the welfare of the patient. The man threw up his hands in despair and said that the cat had had a hard time and had enlisted the assistance of three other cats. One was digging holes for him, the second was covering them up and the third was way out in front opening up new territory. We probably need and should have two applied researchers for every one in basic research, but we cannot do without the latter, the fellows who are out in front opening up new fields, developing new interpretations, new products, new ideas and new methods. How few of the papers in our scientific journals are really original and new, in the sense that the theory of relativity, for example, is new? Yet one such good new idea is worth a thousand others because it stimulates a flood of new work.

He also cautioned the "foot soldier" physiologists not to follow exclusively "men on horseback" who wished to lead scientists into large, expensive applied research programs:

> In these days of easy money for grants-in-aid there is a danger of setting up so large a team of inexpert workers that the accumulated data exceed the digestive powers of the responsible investigator. The result is one type bad research. The investigator over-busies himself to such an extent that he leaves himself no time to think. He is a victim of the project complex. He is an empire builder. He should get off his horse and go back to his knitting in the Ivory Tower.
>
> I do not say that all extensive projects are bad. Most are necessarily large and very good. But the danger does exist. Another danger of easy money is the one-more-technician complex, the idea that any problem can be worked out by adding one more technician without additional allowance for time to think. Easy money and the empire-building complex is partly responsible also for the manpower shortage. In one famous case A helped B to obtain a fat grant. Then B in his affluence tried to take two skilled electrophysiologists away from A's laboratory to help him on his project. One government agency creates so many new jobs by grants that other government agencies are unable to secure needed personnel. Salary levels rise, which is good, but the overall quality and quantity of good research does not. Thus we have a rising tide of diversion from true scientific work.

Fenn was instrumental in developing the publications of the American Physiological Society to their present level of universal excellence. He was a member of the Board of Publication Trustees of the American Physiological Society from its inception in 1933, serving as chairman from 1950 to 1955. He was chairman of the Board when it provided the means to purchase Beaumont House, insisting that Beaumont be the home of the Federation. The APS Handbook series was suggested and implemented during his last year as chairman and he co-edited the respiration section of the *Handbooks of Physiology* with Dr. Rahn. Also during his term on the Board he was instrumental in the founding of the *Journal of Applied Physiology* in 1948. He and others felt that much of the applied physiology done during World War II, particularly that on human physiology which emphasized man and his environment, should be published in the scientific literature. APS was the organization to do it; thus the birth of the *Journal of Applied Physiology*, so valuable to all respiration physiologists.

Fenn's interests and energies were not confined to APS. He helped Dr. Bronk revitalize the Union of American Biological Societies, which became the American Institute of Biological Sciences, and succeeded in getting the APS to be the first charter member of AIBS in 1948. Fenn was always a champion of AIBS and served as its president from 1957 to 1958.

His interests were also international in scope. He served as a member of the Council of the International Union of Physiological Sciences in 1956; was secretary general from 1959 to 1965; presided over the XXIV Congress in Washington in 1968, and at that time, on the occasion of his 75th birthday, was unanimously elected the president of IUPS. After the Leiden Congress in 1962 he started the *IUPS Newsletter*, which today reaches physiologists all over the world. He compiled and edited the "History of the International Congresses of Physiological Sciences, 1889–1968" and arranged to have a copy for everyone attending the 1968 Washington congress. He also promoted the inclusion of satellite symposia as an official activity of the international congresses.

The Dutch composer Jurriaan Andriessen dedicated Fenn his "Respiration Suite" (written for double wind quintet), first performed at the First International Respiration Dinner Group meeting at Alphen aan de Rijn, Holland, on September 12, 1962, during the time of the Leiden Congress. On the jacket of the recording is the statement, "An understanding of the musical performance of these artists, in a physiological sense, rests to a large extent on the work of Dr. Wallace O. Fenn and his associates on pressure-volume relationship of the lungs and chest, on the composition of alveolar air during breath holding, and on physiological effects of pressure breathing."

Finally, Dr. Fenn was more than a great scientist. He was a humanist and a dedicated family man.

In 1919, a few months after obtaining his Ph.D. degree, Wallace O. Fenn married Clara Bryce Comstock. They had four children, two sons and two daughters, and thirteen grandchildren. It was a true family, which many members of the department came to know when visiting the Fenns at Highland Avenue or at Canandaigua Lake.

In the Fenn household there was a simplicity, a genuine quality of life that one rarely encounters. His son William said it very simply:

It was always surprising to us children, and I'm sure to his grandchildren too, that Pop was so honored among men, because he never acted at home the way it seemed that such a man should act. He mowed lawns, washed dishes, played games with his children, played tricks on them, taught me how to throw an outside curve and an inside curve, cut bushes, felled trees, built docks, rowed and sailed boats, paddled canoes, roamed through the woods, picked wild berries, skated remarkably well, and did all the things that fathers do with their families.

A little extra measure of energy was present in Pop, or else he was more ready than most to use it. When things seemed too quiet at home, he was apt to jump up and say, "Let's go cut down a tree," or tackle some other difficult task that needed doing, or go off on a picnic. Then there would be a great bustling about, rounding up equipment, figuring how to attack the project, and then going at it.

We had several memorable tree-cutting operations at our place in Canandaigua, one of which was particularly so because almost all of the family, including grandchildren, were in on it. A large old tree had died in the winter and was leaning slightly over a neighbor's property and in danger of falling. We rigged a strong restraining line to another tree to help control its fall and commenced to cut. My brother, David, did most of the chain sawing, and notched it properly. Finally, it was evident that the tree was about to come down. All the grandchildren and their mothers got a safe distance away and Dave began the last sawing operation while the rest of us put all the force we could on the rope. Then the tree cracked and tilted about 30 degrees off vertical. Dave jumped clear and the rest of us took up slack and tugged away. But no matter how we pulled and got it swaying, the tree refused to come any further. After a couple of minutes of this effort, Pop walked up to have a closer look at the cut. Then he picked up an axe, gave one mighty blow in the right spot, and down she came with a great majestic crash while the whole gang yelled "Timber" as loud as we could. All the grandchildren charged to the tree and climbed into its branches in triumph, and Pop was the hero of the day.

Dr. and Mrs. Fenn, a most gracious and kind "grande dame," informally entertained in their home the various members of his large department, giving special attention to foreign visitors isolated from their homeland.

The annual departmental Christmas parties were special occasions never to be forgotten. The highlight was the reading of a poem Dr. Fenn had composed a few hours before and typed himself, such as one entitled "The Brownies in the Laboratory."

The passing away of Wallace O. Fenn marks the end of the era, started by Claude Bernard over a century ago, when a man of genius could encompass and explain all of physiology.

But above all, Dr. Fenn will be remembered by those who knew him well as a truly dedicated man who added a universal dimension to his scientific endeavors.

G.G.N.
K.S.
N.C.

Dr. Fenn's Last Manuscript:
An Exchange of Correspondence

Gabriel Nahas

In July 1970, Karl Schaefer and I asked Dr. Fenn to be honorary conference chairman of a satellite symposium of the XXV International Congress of Physiology, to be devoted to "CO_2 and metabolic regulations." From then on, the following correspondence was exchanged between us. This correspondence appears to be the most fitting preface to the talk which Dr. Fenn wrote for the symposium, but was unable to deliver. We are privileged to print this last paper of Wallace O. Fenn as an introduction to this monograph.

September 14, 1970
Dear Gabriel:

I have your letter about the Symposium on CO_2 scheduled for July 20–21, 1971 where you have named me as "Honorary Conference Chairman." I think I have already consented over the phone to allow the use of my name in that capacity although I do not much like the honorary roles. Anyhow it would be a pleasure to visit Monaco again and I shall have to be in Europe anyway at about that time so I cannot think of any good reason for refusing if you think that it would be helpful to you.

We have just returned from two weeks in Brasov, Rumania and are about to leave for three weeks in Spain for the ICSU meeting in Madrid plus a week of vacation.

With many thanks for the "honor" which you are giving me in this affair.

Sincerely yours,
Wallace O. Fenn

September 17, 1970
Dear Dr. Fenn:

Thank you for your letter of September 14. It was never my intention to place you in a dusty honorary niche, and I expect you will be a most effective and active participant in the CO_2 symposium. I believe, therefore, that it would be most fitting to appoint you President of this gathering. As you know, in France you will be addressed as "Monsieur le President." I would also like to ask you if you could be the speaker after the dinner which will be offered by Prince Rainier and lecture on "CO_2 and the Sea."

Bon voyage to Spain, and best personal regards to you and Mrs. Fenn.

Sincerely yours,
GGN:jo   Gabriel G. Nahas

October 8, 1970
Dear Gabriel:

I must have expressed myself badly. I am quite content with the title "honorary chairman" and I decline the Presidency of the gathering. The title "CO_2 and the Sea" is an interesting and challenging idea but I must give that one some further consideration. It would take me into many dusty (or wet) corners of knowledge with which I am perhaps not very well acquainted and I must be sure that I could manage it well enough to make a good story.

I could consider giving one of the brief regular papers on "Partial molar volumes of CO_2 in different media." There may be nothing really new in this, but I do not think that the subject has ever been brought up in exactly that way before. I have a fair amount of data to offer which I am about to put into print. That also is just a tentative thought.

Anyhow thanks for your letter and I look forward to your symposium with much pleasant anticipation.

Sincerely,
WOF/ek   Wallace O. Fenn
CC: Dr. K. E. Schaefer

November 3, 1970
Dear Gabriel:

I do not seem to find the exact dates of your proposed symposium on CO_2 for next summer. This is important for me because I have to get to Munich for a meeting of the Executive Committee Saturday, July 24th and should perhaps arrive the night before. How will that interfere with your symposium and also with serving as after dinner speaker at the end of the symposium? Please let me know because I am also applying for rooms in Munich and am asked to state date of arrival. I suppose I could take my wife to your symposium and she could entertain herself somehow during the meetings.

Sincerely,
WOF/ek   Wallace O. Fenn

November 5, 1970
Dear Dr. Fenn:

The CO_2 Satellite Symposium of the XXV International Congress of Physiology will be held in Monaco Tuesday and Wednesday, next July 20 and 21. This will give you ample time to be in Munich on the 24th as there are good air communications between Nice and Munich.

Everyone will be delighted to see Mrs. Fenn at this meeting, and I hope that since Prince Rainier has accepted to sponsor the meeting there might be some entertainment for the ladies.

With best personal regards.

Sincerely yours,
GGN:jo   Gabriel G. Nahas

November 16, 1970
Dear Gabriel:

I am sorry that I had to bother you with the dates of your Monaco symposium. Later I found them in the Congress announcement in fine print on the map. Anyhow I am relieved to know that there will be time for me to get to Munich. It also tells me that I cannot attend the diving symposium in Marseille.

You have complimented me by asking me to talk at the banquet and I should like to do it if I can persuade myself that I have anything to say. The only original work I have is the measurement of the volume occupied by CO_2 in water, serum and blood and bicarbonate solutions. The volumes are per mole of CO_2, 33 cc in water, about 22 in bicarbonate and 15 in blood. I am not sure how well I can explain these interesting results, but I can try. I do not see that this has any real physiological significance, but it may tell us something of the condition of the CO_2 in these different media. What about the rest of your program? The effect of CO_2 tension on metabolic rate seems pertinent. Also the CO_2 tension in different animals. I suppose I should also be interested in preparing a discussion of the CO_2 in the atmosphere and its ups and downs. All of these topics may well be already well covered in your program and I am not particularly well equipped to deal with any of them. You do not want anything very heavy for an after dinner speech anyway—perhaps a half hour at best. I was once much interested in the life of Joseph Black and his contribution to the history of CO_2. So I suppose that I might refer to the history of the subject very briefly. I am not however a very witty or entertaining speaker and if I am really wise, I shall refuse your kind invitation altogether and take my pleasure in listening to someone else. I do not know whether the partial molar volume of CO_2 would fit into your program anywhere but if you have 5 minutes free at any time where you think it would not be too much out of place, I could present my findings very briefly and that would be enough to make me feel respectable in a scientific way and not have to content myself with being just an "honorary." Then I could refuse your banquet invitation with a clear conscience.

Let me hear from you while I try to find some better inspiration.

Sincerely,
WOF/ek   Wallace O. Fenn

December 9, 1970
Dear Dr. Fenn:

Enclosed is a tentative program of the CO_2 symposium. You will note that you are chairman of Session II, CO_2 and pH Regulation of Cellular Functions. You are also scheduled for an evening lecture which is concerned with a topic of such a magnitude that you might discuss just about any topic without digressing from your subject. You certainly could discuss, under this heading, the data concerning the volume occupied by CO_2 in water and other solutions. However, I do not want to ask you to discuss any topic which you wouldn't like to; therefore, the final decision will be up to you. I am sure that I express the feeling of everyone by saying that we would like very much to hear you give a talk on CO_2—at your own pace.

With best personal regards.

Sincerely yours,

GGN:jo   Gabriel G. Nahas

December 21, 1970
Dear Gabriel:

I can, of course, put together everything that is known about CO_2 and the Sea and make a scientific talk, lasting either 10 minutes or an hour. It won't be a very new and exciting discourse I fear, but just a lot of known facts strung together. I cannot make out of it any very thrilling view of the future or clue to the cure of cancer. You said previously, however, that you wanted this at the banquet. For that you want something light and somewhat frivolous perhaps. It would be better to ask Cousteau to do that. Which do you really want now or would you be satisfied if I merely talked for 10 minutes at one of the sessions on my own work—for 10 minutes. That would show that I am still doing something and would satisfy me. I guess I will do whatever you want me to attempt, but I am not sure what it is at present. Is it an evening lecture or a post prandial patter? Either way I am immensely complimented by the invitation.

We wish you and yours a very Merry Christmas and a happy New Year as always. With this opportunity to greet you I shall probably "forget" to send you a customary Christmas card in the interests of relieving the Post Office.

Sincerely,

WOF/ek   Wallace O. Fenn

January 11, 1971
Dear Dr. Fenn:

Thank you for your letter of December 21, and let me extend to you and Mrs. Fenn my very best wishes for this year.

As things stand now, your contribution to the CO_2 symposium consists of a ten-minute talk, which you could give in opening the session which you are chairing. Furthermore, I would be most grateful if you could also give an informal talk on CO_2 following the evening banquet; the exact nature and length of the address would be left to your own desire. Many people still remember your address to the Philadelphia Philosophical Society on "CO_2 adaptation" and your talk to the American Physiological Society on "Physiology on horseback" and your prefatory remarks to an *Annual Review of Physiology* volume on "Born 50 years too late."

With best personal regards.

Sincerely yours,

GGN:jo   Gabriel G. Nahas

January 25, 1971
Dear Gabriel:

Very well then, if you insist! I will try to give an address on CO_2 and the Sea. I believe that a half-hour would be more than enough and all I can do is to try to cover some of the high points of present knowledge of the subject. I do not see a paper by me listed in the program where I am Chairman and for that I am grateful. I will try to work in my little bit about the volume occupied by CO_2 either in some introductory remarks or, better, in the evening address. It is only an interesting little theoretical point with no obvious practical consequences.

I shall have to go to Munich immediately after the close of your symposium so I will be unable to attend the other symposium at Marseille which I would otherwise like very much to do.

Many thanks. I still think it would be better if you asked Cousteau to make that speech or one like it.

Yours sincerely,

WOF/ek   Wallace O. Fenn

During the spring of 1971, I spoke several times with Dr. Fenn over the telephone to discuss the program of the symposium. One of these conversations took place when he was in the hospital. In July, a week before the symposium, Dr. Fenn called me; he had had a relapse and would not be able to travel to Europe. His voice was strained and sad. I was shocked, and a few days later conveyed the news to Hermann Rahn in Monaco. Hermann tried with Kurt Kramer to charter a Lufthansa plane so that Dr. Fenn could at least attend the Munich meeting.

From Monaco we sent a wire to Dr. Fenn: "Your friends and pupils assembled in this meeting are discussing your findings and send you every best wish for a prompt recovery."

Karl Schaefer and I also wrote Dr. Fenn asking him for the manuscripts he had prepared for delivery at the meeting. We did not know whether Dr. Fenn, who had been ill for several months before the symposium, had been able to write any of them.

August 16, 1971

Dear Gabriel:

Your request for manuscripts represents a rather large order for me. I have been almost flat on my back in bed ever since you last telephoned me. It was lucky I cancelled out because the night I was supposed to fly out from New York, I developed a good second case of thrombophlebitis in my other leg and since then I have had at intervals two more probable pulmonary embolisms. So I have been in the depths of despair and am still confined to my home with much limited activities. It is hard to find references and get manuscripts into final shape under these conditions and indeed I can hardly think physiology any more. I will give the possibility some serious thought, however, and I hope you will send me your deadline. I

suppose it has already passed. I had thought that the Molar volume of CO_2 might be included in the evening paper. I have a lot of rather good data, but I do not yet know how to interpret the figures and would like to withhold actual publication perhaps a little longer. I could, of course, send you typical data without suitable interpretation.

I hear that your symposium went very well and I wish very much that I could have been there.

Sincerely,

WOF/ek   Wallace O. Fenn

In spite of his illness, Dr. Fenn had been busy preparing the talks he was to deliver in Monaco. He was especially eager to complete one which described some of his later work on the "Partial pressure of gases dissolved in deep water." He sent a copy of this manuscript to some of us.

August 17, 1971

Dear Friends:

I am sending a copy of this manuscript to a few friends in the hope of eliciting some helpful comments before I actually try to publish this paper. Perhaps it should be accompanied by another strictly thermodynamics version. Anyhow I hope that some of you may be interested in this effort of mine.

Sincerely,

WOF/ek   Wallace O. Fenn

Enc: "Partial pressure of gases dissolved in deep water"

CC:

Prof. Hermann Rahn

Dr. T. Enns

Dr. G. Nahas

Dr. R. Forster

Dr. A. DuBois

Dr. R. Margaria

August 27, 1971

Dear Dr. Fenn:

Under separate mail I am sending you the medal (Figure 1) which was awarded to you by the City of Monaco. We all missed you at the symposium on CO_2 but so many of your pupils were there that your ideas and impetus were still present throughout our debates.

I thank you very much for the draft of your manuscript on the molar volume of CO_2, which I would like very much to publish in the forthcoming monograph; but I will wait for further instructions from you. Since this talk was intended as an after-dinner lecture, the lack of precise references doesn't matter, and you should not worry about this small matter. I spoke with Hermann Rahn a few days ago and he informed me that you still had to limit your activities. I am sure that this is only temporary and that when fall comes you will feel much better.

I am looking forward to visiting you in Rochester, but I have to postpone my visit until the end of the third week of September. I will let you know exactly when I will come.

Again, I want to tell you how much all of your pupils and colleagues in respiratory physiology did miss you this summer in Europe. All those I met asked me to convey to you their warmest wishes and best greetings.

With best personal regards.

Sincerely yours,

GGN:jo　　　　　Gabriel G. Nahas

cc: Dr. Karl Schaefer

September 9, 1971

Dear Gabriel:

You did send me a letter about the medal and I think I read it, perhaps somewhat hastily. Now I cannot find the letter. I hope you can send me a duplicate. Bedroom confusion is terrible. Anyhow I recall that no mention was made of the person to whom I should address my letter of thanks. I should guess that a letter to Prince Rainier himself is appropriate. If so, will you please send me the exact name, title and method of address. It is very difficult to look up these details from home. Anyhow it is a very beautiful medal of which I am very proud

although I seem to have done nothing to earn it.

Sincerely yours,

WOF/ek　　　　Wallace O. Fenn

This was Dr. Fenn's last letter to me.

Wallace O. Fenn died on September 20, 1971, concerned until the end that all of his last scientific commitments be fulfilled. He entrusted to Hermann Rahn the care of publishing his last two manuscripts. His manuscript on "Partial pressure of gases dissolved in deep water" appeared in *Science* (Fenn [1972]). His talk on "Carbon Dioxide and the Sea" was forwarded to me by Hermann Rahn:

November 30, 1971

Dear Gabriel:

I am enclosing the manuscript of Wallace Fenn for inclusion in the CO_2 Symposium Proceedings. Arthur DuBois and I have made the minor corrections indicated.

I consider this a fascinating story, beautifully and simply told, and most fitting for the Proceedings.

Sincerely yours,

Hermann Rahn

Bibliography

Fenn, W. O. *J. Physiol.* (London), 58:175–203 (1923).

———, "Muscular force at different speeds of shortening." *J. Physiol.* (London), 85:277–97 (1935).

———. *Am. J. Physiol.*, 146:161–78 (1946*a*).

———, "A theoretical study of the composition of the alveolar air at altitude." *Am. J. Physiol.*, 146:637–53 (1946*b*).

———, "Physiology on Horseback." *Am. J. Physiol.*, 159:551–55 (1949).

———. *Am. J. Med.*, 10:77–90 (1951).

———, "Partial pressure of gases dissolved in deep water." *Science*, 176–1011 (1972).

Carbon Dioxide and the Sea

Wallace O. Fenn

I am scheduled to talk on CO_2 and the sea or, by the program, "50 Years of CO_2." This is not a subject of my own choosing, but it was thrust upon me and accepted only after offering some much better suggestions for this task. It is a very deep subject, 10 km in fact. The subject is also hypercapnic and decidedly perhaps hyperoxic and hyperbaric —up to at least 1000 atm. By the time I finish I suspect that you will all be thoroughly compressed or depressed and gasping for air. Neither of these conditions is good for the digestion of a dinner like the one we have just had. On the other hand, the subject is a rather wet one and is therefore conducive to good drinking. So if you sip a bit while I am talking, you may possibly survive. I guarantee that I won't take more than 30 minutes to exhaust my eloquence and to impress you or depress you with my message that does contain one new item which tempted me to run down the street shouting "Eureka" for sheer joy. The rest is probably rather dull, however, and I must at the outset confess my own disqualification as a speaker on this subject. I have never really been underwater, except twice in a submarine and some breath-hold diving and all I know of the underwater world is what I have learned from Dr. Cousteau's wonderful moving pictures. So I probably have a very dry presentation of a very wet subject.

The origins of CO_2 and the sea seem to be the subject of much controversy and speculation. It is, however, a very earthy subject because in all our solar system only the earth has both CO_2 and water in any quantity. The rings of Saturn are said to be water and there is perhaps a little on Mars, but none on Venus in spite of a very dense atmosphere. There all the water appears to have been dissociated into H and O_2. The H escaped the gravitational field and the O_2 was used to oxidize C to CO_2 which now forms the bulk of the atmosphere. There seems to be no CO_2 in the outer planets but only CH_4. Perhaps, *when* all the water in our oceans has lost its H to outer space, we shall be left with an atmosphere of CO_2 like Venus. That, however, is a long time ahead; and probably on the very day he was fatally stricken with a heart attack, my late friend Lloyd Berkner told me during a coffee break at the National Academy of Sciences that he had found the dissociation of H_2O by short wave lengths in the upper atmosphere to be proceeding very slowly, if at all, at the present time.

Be that as it may, I am not much alarmed by the prophets of doom who keep telling us that the excessive burning of fossil fuels is going to raise the CO_2 in the atmosphere until the climate becomes warm and we will all be panting for breath or running short of O_2. However, I have little fear of this in the forseeable future for several reasons.

(1) Harrison Brown estimates that in the last 70 years enough CO_2 has been produced from burning fossil fuels to raise the CO_2 percentage in the atmosphere 12%, i.e. from 0.03% to 0.0336%. However, records show only a 2% increase. Thus, 5/6 of the CO_2 produced in 70 years was deposited in the sea

or used in photosynthesis. I must admit, however, that others have estimated that 40% of the CO_2 remains in the atmosphere, but the time for this is not included in the estimate.

(2) Roger Revelle also estimates that in the period since the origin of the earth the amount of CO_2 liberated from volcanoes, etc. was 40,000 times as much as exists now in the atmosphere. At least over long periods only 1/40,000 of the CO_2 liberated from fossil fuels might be expected to remain in the atmosphere.

(3) The total amount of C in all the fossil fuels known to exist, if burned to CO_2, would raise the CO_2 in the atmosphere to a concentration of 3.4% if it all were to remain in the atmosphere. In 70 years, however, 5/6 of it would be in the oceans or sediments and in a longer period even more of it would be thus disposed of. At most, therefore, one might expect a concentration in the atmosphere of 0.6%.

(4) If the CO_2 concentration in the atmosphere is regarded as a balance between the rate of uptake for photosynthesis and the rate of production by animals, then an increase in CO_2 would increase photosynthesis. Likewise a lowered PO_2 increases photosynthesis so there is a built-in biological control for the CO_2 concentration in the atmosphere. Just how effective this control may be I do not know.

(5) It seems more likely, however, that the level of CO_2 in the atmosphere is controlled mainly by the reaction of silicates with CO_2. Urey has calculated the equilibrium in this reaction which produces $MgCO_2$ and SiO_2 and has found that it gives a P_{CO_2} concentration not far from that actually existing in the atmosphere.

(6) The actual total amount of CO_2 in the ocean as CO_2, bicarbonate and carbonate is 60 times the amount in the atmosphere, and it seems more likely that this vast store of CO_2 actually controls the level of P_{CO_2} in the atmosphere, rather than the biological activity of animals and plants.

There are many other aspects of CO_2 in the sea that I might discuss. I will mention one of them just to show that I am not unaware of these facts. Rahn has shown why the partial pressure of CO_2 should always be so very much lower in water breathing animals than it is in man or other air breathers. This, of course, is because the solubility of O_2 in water is very low compared to that of CO_2. For this reason the gills must process a lot of water to get enough O_2. This very much over-ventilates the blood for CO_2. In emerging from the sea the ancestors of man had to adapt to a P_{CO_2} concentration some 10 times higher than they were accustomed to. So it can be done. And perhaps it is due to higher P_{CO_2} that man's brain is superior to that of the fish. It might even be that the necessity of adapting to a still slightly higher P_{CO_2} due to fossil fuels might result in still further improvement.

I have been interested for some years now in the effects of hydrostatic pressure on physiological reactions. Pressure may indeed be the limiting factor in the depth of dives that are possible for man. Pressure does tend to inhibit any reaction that runs with an increase of volume, i.e. where the volume occupied by the products of the reaction is greater than the volume occupied by the reactants and vice versa. From this point of view the study of pressure becomes a tool of some importance in elucidating the processes involved in complex physiological reactions. It is for this reason that I have been interested in pressure and it is only under the sea that one encounters really high pressures in nature. So I have been studying various reactions to determine first, the effects of pressure and second, the volume change which the reaction produces.

Pressure inhibits the growth of *Streptococcus faecalis* because it inhibits glycolysis, which causes an increase in volume and glycolysis represents the main source of energy for this organism. The reason pressure enhances the tension produced in a muscle twitch may be that it increases the breakdown of ATP, which results in a decrease in volume. Pressure enhances hemolysis of rbc and hemolysis results in a decrease in volume. All these findings are in accord with the general rule that pressure inhibits reactions that cause an increase in volume, and vice versa.

I have studied another reaction that

appears to be contrary to this rule and this leads me into the main problem which I wish to put before you. Morgan Wells at LaJolla showed in his Ph.D. thesis (1969) that pressure moves the oxygen dissociation curve to the right. This might be interpreted as a decreased affinity of Hb for O_2 under pressure. So I thought that if pressure inhibits the combination of O_2 and Hb, then this reaction should cause an increase in volume. I have, however, now measured this volume change in scores of experiments by three different methods. In two methods I measured the actual change in volume when a given weight of rbc was oxygenated and in the other method I have measured the increasing weight of a given volume of rbc that results from oxygenation. I have never found an increase of volume in such a reaction, but I have found a decrease when the experiment is so set up that during the actual measurement O_2 moves from physical solution into the Hb. In such a case there is always a decrease in volume just about equal to the volume that was occupied by the O_2 in the ambient solution before it had access to the Hb molecule. So it turns out that the volume occupied by O_2 when in the Hb molecule is just about zero. Either it goes into a void in the Hb molecule or it changes the conformation of the molecule in such a way that the Hb decreases in volume just about enough to compensate for the volume that the O_2 occupies in the Hb molecule. When dissolved in water, one mole of O_2 occupies 31 ml to 32 ml per mole, but that final average of all my measurements gives a partial molar volume of 0.4 ml to 3.5 ml per mole. This, I think, may become a point of some consequence in the study of the Hb molecule.

I have also studied the pmv of CO and CO_2 in the Hb molecule. CO behaves much like O_2. The effect of CO_2 is perhaps more pertinent to my present topic. In water 1 mole of CO_2 occupies about 33 ml and increases the volume of the water in which it dissolves by just that amount. If dissolved in dilute NaOH, its pmv is only about 24 ml/mole. The increased ionization of the CO_2, as

HCO_3^-: I suppose, causes some electrostriction that packs the water very tightly around it and so reduces the total volume. Of even more interest, however, is the fact that the volume occupied by CO_2 in blood for the partial molar volume is only about 15 ml, even though most of the CO_2 absorbed is in the form of bicarbonate. Correcting for the amount of CO_2 still in the form of H_2CO_3, the partial molar volume of the remainder in blood is only about 5 ml to 10 ml per mole, which is very different from the 33 ml/mole occupied by the CO_2 in water. These figures are still a little tentative, but they are based on many careful measurements. The exact significance of this discovery is beyond me at the moment, but I think that it will play its role in the future. I hope that it's a finding of some interest to this audience.

In trying to understand these facts I have been led to another finding that represents the chief message of my talk tonight. Morgan Wells, in studying the effects of a pressure of 100 atm on HbO_2, found that when measured by an O_2 electrode, pressure increased the Po_2 about 14%. I at first thought that this was due to a dissociation of HbO_2, but he found that the Po_2 of plasma or water under 100 atm of pressure was increased by the same 14%. Actually, in the same laboratory some years before, Enns, Scholander and Bradstreet (1965) had found by a very ingenious method that 100 atm of hydrostatic pressure increases the partial pressure of O_2 and nitrogen by about the same 14% and that helium and CO_2 were not very different. From these results they predicted that at 10,000 m of depth or at 1000 atm the Po_2 would be increased fourfold over that at the surface! Cogitating on this rather remarkable result, I thought I saw a chance for a fine perpetual motion machine.

I imagined a column of distilled water 10,000 m high, all at constant temperature and all saturated with O_2 at 1 atm. Then I fitted a teflon membrane to the bottom of a tube full of oxygen gas that reached from the surface of this water column nearly to the bottom. The teflon membrane was supposed to be a permeable only to O_2 and to nothing else. Then I left the whole system, for a few centuries if necessary, until complete equilibrium had been established and then I exposed the teflon membrane to the water. I thought that the O_2 in the water at 4 atm partial pressure would promptly diffuse into the teflon tube exposed to 1 atm at the surface. O_2 would then be forced out of the teflon tube at the top and would redissolve in the water to replenish what the water had lost, and this then would establish perpetual motion. But when I calculated what the barometric pressure would be at a depth of 10,000 m in the O_2 tube, I discovered to my delight that it would be just about 4 atm. So once again there would be no diffusion either way and perpetual motion is impossible. I consulted experts in thermodynamics about this and found that this was right indeed. At complete equilibrium the molecular free energy must be the same at the top and the bottom of the water column at equilibrium because this is the very definition of equilibrium. The same must be true in the column of O_2 gas. Since then the molecular free energy of 100% O_2 at the surface must be equal to that in the water saturated with 100% O_2 at 1 atm, it must also be true that the partial molar free energy (or the chemical potential) must be equal at the bottom of the teflon tube and in the adjacent water.

Now 1000 atm raises the partial pressure of the O_2 about fourfold, depending on temperatures and other factors. This means that it takes 4 times the pressure of O_2 to keep the same amount of O_2 in solution in the water when it is under a pressure of 1000 atm hydrostatic pressure. But how does the water know how hard it must squeeze the O_2 in order to bring it into equilibrium with the barometric pressure in a teflon tube that I might put down there?

The problem becomes even more challenging when one considers other gases such as He and CO_2. These behave rather differently and turn out to be a special case. Calculations show that with the teflon tube full of He the barometric pressure at a depth

of 10,000 m would be about 1.2 atm instead of 4 atm and for CO_2 the pressure would be about 6.2 atm. If the water were then saturated throughout at the start with 1 atm of He or CO_2, how would it react to this situation at a depth of 10,000 feet? Here we come back to the partial molar volume of these gases in water. One mole of He weighs only 4 g, but it occupies about 30 ml when dissolved in water. So with a density of 4/30 it should float to the surface like a cork. It does indeed tend to do so, but this is balanced by the tendency of diffusion to maintain equal concentrations. Equilibrium is reached when these opposing effects are balanced. Now CO_2 has the opposite effect. It has a molecular weight of 44 and a partial molar volume of only 33. So its density is about 1.33 and it should tend to sink. These effects have been calculated by equations of thermodynamics by I. Klotz with whom I have had the pleasure of consulting. One of these equations states that

$$\log \frac{m_s}{m_d} = 1.7 \times 10^{-8} \text{mol wt}(1 - V\rho)d$$

where d is the depth in cm, mol wt is the molecular weight, V is the volume occupied by 1 g of the gas in solution, and m_s and m_d are concentrations of the gas at surface (s) and depth (d). In effect, when the density of the water is equal to 1.0, the gas would float up if V were greater than 1.0 and sink if V were less than 1.0. Indeed, this equation applies not only to gases but to salts in solution as well. Therefore, it becomes a very interesting equation for oceanography. Using this equation it turns out that at equilibrium the concentrations at a depth of 10,000 m, relative to the concentration at the surface, would be 0.35 for He and 1.43 for CO_2. Helium floats up and CO_2 sinks. Oxygen is a special case because its molecular weight is 32 and its partial molar volume is 32 ml/mole so that the difference is zero. That is why my first calculation in the teflon tube came out just equal to the predicted partial pressure of O_2 in the water. It was a lucky break. Actually the barometric pressure of oxygen at 10,000 m and 27°C would be nearer 3.5 than 4.0. Using this figure the partial pressure of He in the water should be $0.35 \times 4 = 1.4$ and for CO_2 would be $1.43 \times 4 = 5.72$ atm. These figures agree rather well with the barometric pressures calculated for the teflon tube full of these two gases.

So for gases dissolved in any fluid and saturated with any gas at the surface at 1 atm, we conclude that the partial pressure at any depth at complete diffusion equilibrium will necessarily be adjusted so that at true equilibrium it will be equal to the barometric pressure in a teflon tube (permeable only to that gas) at the same depth. This, then, becomes a very easy way to calculate the partial pressure of any gas at any depth in an ideal column when it is at constant temperature and left long enough to attain complete equilibrium. It cannot, of course, be applied directly to the ocean where there are so many currents and, for the respiratory gases at least, so much uptake and output at different levels. For a given O_2 content and temperature, however, the partial pressure of O_2 would be about four times as great as it would be at the surface for the same O_2 content. In this respect the whole concept seems to me to be of great practical usefulness.

Klotz has pointed out that this same principle applies to other substances, including most electrolytes which have partial molar volumes that are less than their molecular weights. So the weight of the displaced water is less than their own weight and they tend to sink until this settling is balanced by diffusion pressure upwards. The differences are not great and, of course, they are upset by ocean currents. So Edmond and Gieskes (1970) have shown that in the Brazil Basin in the South Atlantic the salinity at great depths is actually somewhat less, rather than more, than it is at the surface. Surface evaporation probably had a lot to do with the rapid decrease found near the surface.

This also raises a number of intriguing physiological questions. Piccard in the Trieste claims he saw a fish at the bottom of the Mariana Trench in the Pacific Ocean at a depth of about 10,000 m. The fish looked at him, so he wrote, and then swam away. He may have looked, but I doubt if he saw anything because no light had ever entered his eye before. But he did manage to swim unless he was an optical illusion. How did he adapt to such a pressure of 1000 atm? Frogs develop muscle contractures or rigor mortis at 200 atm and surface fish do likewise. Pressure tends to liquefy protoplasm from a gel to a sol, breaks down ATP and phosphocreatine, inhibits glycolysis, hemolyzes red blood corpuscles, denatures enzymes and shifts the O_2 dissociation curve far to the right. Most of these effects have been seen only at very high pressures of thousands of atmospheres. If O_2 poisoning depends on the partial pressure of O_2 rather than O_2 concentration, then the fish seen by Piccard would need some special protection against O_2. The effects of a high partial pressure of O_2 without a corresponding increase in concentration has never to my knowledge been tried. But the only way to try it is to combine a high hydrostatic pressure with a 1 atm concentration of O_2, and this complicates the interpretation. Zobell (1967) has shown in bacteria that O_2 is more poisonous at high hydrostatic pressures. This could mean either that pressure raises the partial pressure of the O_2, as we know it does, or that it might cause some other change in the system that enhances the poisonous effect of a 1 atm concentration of O_2. Certainly the O_2 electrode responds to the partial pressure of O_2 rather than to the concentration. The best proof of this may be that it predicted quite accurately the pressure of O_2 with which O_2 saturated-water at high hydrostatic pressure would be in equilibrium. Whether the biological response to O_2 depends on its partial pressure remains an open question and a very interesting one.

Another problem faced by Piccard's fish at the bottom of the Mariana Trench relates to the transport of O_2 from the gills to the tissues. The data of Morgan Wells suggest that the O_2 dissociation curve is shifted to the right in proportion to the increase in hydrostatic pressure. Also Johnson and Schlegel

(1948) reported years ago that hydrostatic pressure up to 1000 atm caused no measurable change in the O_2 saturation of the Hb. From these data one can tentatively conclude that an O_2 dissociation curve plotted against concentration of O_2 rather than partial pressure of O_2 would give the same values at all hydrostatic pressures.

To show this I have measured the values of Po_2 for 50% saturation at hydrostatic pressures up to 1000 atm. When these are plotted against the hydrostatic pressure, the points parallel the calculated total partial pressure of O_2 at the same depths. So when the Po_2 goes up 4 times at 10 km, the Po_2 for 50% saturation also goes up about 4 times. So in a sense we ought to plot our O_2 dissociation curves not against the partial pressure of O_2, but against the concentrations of the O_2 in physical solution. Of course, partial pressure and concentrations ordinarily are proportional quantities, but *not* under high hydrostatic pressure.

This is a new and rather remarkable feature of this extraordinary molecule of Hb. In combining with O_2 or with CO there is no volume change and therefore the saturation is independent of pressure. O_2 concentration in the ocean reaches a minimum at intermediate depths because of the O_2 uptake by marine organisms. In most parts of the ocean cold polar currents containing O_2 saturated at the Po_2 of the air surface serve to replenish the O_2 concentration at greater depths, so the average concentration is about half that at the surface. This would certainly be enough to saturate the arterial blood to an extent adequate for the survival of a fish at low temperature.

The next question concerns the effect of pressure on the diffusion of O_2 for the same concentration gradient. It seems to be *the concentration gradient, not the partial pressure gradient, that determines diffusion*. In the case of O_2, where there is no buoyancy factor, the concentration is the same at all depths, but a partial pressure gradient remains from 4 atm to 1 atm between the surface and 10 km. This does not tend to equalize because the

solubility of O_2 is diminished in proportion to the rise in partial pressure of O_2. The partial pressure of O_2, incidentally, does not increase linearly with pressure, but rather logarithmically as it does in the atmosphere. But diffusion should be proportional to the product of the partial pressure gradient and the solubility. It seems likely, therefore, that diffusion rates of CO_2 and O_2 in both the gills and the tissues of the fish would be little affected by 1000 atm of pressure. Actually, diffusion might be slightly accelerated under pressure because the viscosity of water actually decreases slightly over the first 1000 atm but increases at still higher pressure. (Weale, Chemical Reactions at High Pressures, London, 1967, p. 24). High pressure might accelerate some rate-limiting reaction causing volume decreases, so diffusion or some volume-increasing reaction might take over as the rate-limiting process in some physiological functions. This is one of the ways in which pressure might affect physiology.

I must consider now the effect of O_2 and CO_2 transport under high pressures. Pressure increases the dissociation of water and the dissociation of H_2CO_3 so that at 1000 atm the pH would be about 0.34 pH units lower than the normal surface value of 8.1 in sea water. The total CO_2 content certainly increases with depth, as Esmond and Gieskes (1970) have found in the Brazil Basin that at about 5 km of depth the total CO_2 has gone up from 2.0 to 2.3. Most of this is probably due to metabolism of living organisms at intermediate depths; part, however, may also be due to the tendency of CO_2 to settle out, although this must occur very slowly. If the partial pressure of CO_2 at the surface is 0.03% of an atmosphere, it might be 0.1% at 10,000 m and the calculated partial pressure would then be perhaps 6 times as great, or 0.6% = 4.5 mm. It does not seem likely that a change of this sort would pose any serious problem for Piccard's fish. In pure water a pressure of 1000 atm lowers the pH about 0.17 pH units from a pH of 7.0.

So for CO_2 and the sea, I think I have somewhat expanded our ideas of how the partial pressure of a gas increases at depth, although I do not myself entirely understand the mechanism of this thermodynamic necessity. Anyway, there are many physiological problems for life at great depths, but they do not seem to be especially related to CO_2 or to O_2.

For 50 years of CO_2—I think I have discovered that CO_2 tends to sink in water, but I would like a good experiment to prove it.

* The answer to Fenn's question is given by Frank C. Andrews in his paper: "Gravitational effects or concentrations and partial pressures in solutions; a thermodynamic analysis," published in *Science*, 178:1199–1201 [1972].

Acknowledgment

The organizing committee,* on behalf of all the participants of this Symposium, wish to express their deep appreciation to the government of S.A.S. Prince Rainier, Sovereign of the Monaco Principality, which made this meeting possible.

The members of the Symposium wish also to thank the Scientific Center of Monaco and its president, his Excellency A. Crovetto, for their generous support.

Finally, the hospitality provided by the honorable Mayor of Monaco and by Captain Jacques-Yves Cousteau, Director of the Oceanographic Institute, and his staff, is acknowledged with thanks.

*Nicolas Chalozinitis
 Gabriel Nahas
 Karl Schaefer

Note to the Reader

For an easier understanding of this book, we suggest that before reading any chapter, you first look at all the illustrations and read the accompanying captions. Then read the text.

Participants

C. ALBERS, Universität Regensburg, Regensburg, Germany

A. ARVANITAKI, Institut de Neurophysiologie et Psychophysiologie, Marseille, France

D. BARGETON, Universite de Paris, Faculté de Médecine, Paris, France

J. BIGGERS, Johns Hopkins University, Baltimore, Maryland

A. M. BROWN, Department of Physiology and Medicine, University of Utah College of Medicine, Salt Lake City, Utah

D. BURSAUX, Université de Paris, Faculté de Médecine, Paris, France

P. CALDWELL, College of Physicians and Surgeons, Columbia University, New York, New York

D. O. CARPENTER, National Institute of Mental Health, Bethesda, Maryland

N. CHALAZONITIS, Institut de Neurophysiologie et Psychophysiologie, Marseille, France

N. CHERNIACK, Hospital of the University of Pennsylvania, Philadelphia, Pennsylvania

A. COURNAND, College of Physicians and Surgeons, Columbia University, New York, New York

A. DuBOIS, University of Pennsylvania School of Medicine, Philadelphia, Pennsylvania

Y. ENSON, College of Physicians and Surgeons, Columbia University, New York, New York

V. FENCL, Harvard Medical School, Boston, Massachusetts

G. GURTNER, The Johns Hopkins University, Baltimore, Maryland

J. HAGEGE, Hopital Tenon, Paris, France

F. HALBERG, University of Minnesota, Minneapolis, Minnesota

R. KELLOGG, University of California School of Medicine, San Francisco, California

C. LENFANT, National Heart and Lung Institute, National Institute of Health, Bethesda, Maryland

H. LOESCHKE, University of Gottingen, Gottingen, West Germany

W. LONGMORE, St. Louis University Medical School, St. Louis, Missouri

G. LONGOBARDO, I.B.M. Corporation, Mohansic, New York

U. LUFT, Lovelace Foundation and Clinic, Albuquerque, New Mexico

A. MOYSE, Faculté des Sciences, Universite Paris—Sud, Orsay, France

G. NAHAS, College of Physicians and Surgeons, Columbia University, New York, New York

H. RAHN, State University of New York Medical School, Buffalo, New York

F. RECTOR, JR., University of Texas Southwestern Medical School, Dallas, Texas

G. RICHET, Hopital Tenon, Paris, France

B. RYBAK, Faculté des Sciences, Université de Caen, Caen, France

K. SCHAEFER, Submarine Medical Research Laboratory, Groton, Connecticut

J. SEVERINGHAUS, University of California Medical Center, San Francisco, California

R. SHIPLEY, Veterans Administration Hospital, Cleveland, Ohio

B. SIESJO, University Hospital, Lund, Sweden

M. STUPFEL, Air Pollution Research Center of the French National Institute of Health and Medical Research, Paris, France

G. TURINO, College of Physicians and Surgeons, Columbia University, New York, New York

C. VAN YPERSELE de STRIHOU, Faculte de Medecine, Université de Louvain, Louvain, Belgique

R. VAYSSIERE, Musée Oceanographique, Monaco-Ville, Monaco

Contents

Part I Carbon Dioxide and pH Regulation of Basic Metabolic Processes

Co-Chairmen: A. Moyse and Arthur DuBois

Part II Carbon Dioxide and pH Regulation of Cellular Functions

Co-Chairmen: Mme A. Arvanitaki and John D. Biggers

Part III   Carbon Dioxide and pH Effect on Oxygen and Carbon Dioxide Transport

Co-Chairmen: Hermann Rahn and Claude Lenfant

Part IV   Carbon Dioxide and Regulation of Organ Function

Co-Chairmen: A. Cournand and H. Loeschcke

Part V Adaption to Carbon Dioxide

Co-Chairmen: Karl E. Schaefer and R. Vayssiere

Part VI Mathematical Models for Carbon Dioxide Regulation

Co-Chairmen: John Severinghaus and Daniel Bargeton

Contents

Part I

Carbon Dioxide and pH Regulation of Basic Metabolic Processes

Part I

Carbon Dioxide and pH Regulation of Basic Metabolic Processes

1. Carbon Dioxide and Metabolic Regulations in Plant Photosynthesis

A. Moyse

Laboratoire de Physiologie Cellulaire Végétale,
Associé au C.N.R.S., Université Paris—Sud, 91—Orsay, France

Abbreviations

ADP, ATP: adenosine di- and triphosphate
NAD, NADP, NADH, NADPH: nicotin-
   amide adenine dinucleotides, oxidized
   form and reduced form
-oses-P: phosphorylated sugars
PEP: phosphoenolpyruvate
PGA: phosphoglycerate
Pi: inorganic phosphate
RuDP: ribulose-1, 5-diphosphate

Photosynthetic CO_2 fixation by plants is a fundamental process of the carbon cycle. It conditions the physico-chemical and biological balance of the biosphere.

The high activity of CO_2 fixation by plants in the ambient air where CO_2 level is quite low, is striking. Indeed, the maintenance of a low CO_2 concentration in the air is of prime importance for the life of animals.

Therefore, the increase of CO_2 level since the beginning of the industrial era is alarming. This increase is of nearly 10%, so the actual concentration is about 340 ppm in volume, in spite of the buffer effect of sea water and limestone.

However, the plant kingdom seems to be the main way for maintaining the CO_2 concentration at a low level.

CO_2 is used for several purposes in the life of plants, but besides photosynthesis its role is minor. Fermentation enhancement and respiration inhibition are regulated by CO_2 concentration higher than 3% or 4%.

Plants respire like animals. However, photosynthetic CO_2 fixation and the subsequent O_2 evolution by plants in the light are at least 10 times higher than their respiratory gas exchange in darkness. Under the optimal conditions of photosynthesis, the ratio of gas exchange in the light to gas exchange in darkness can reach 20 or even 50, depending on the plants.

Therefore, the regulation of photosynthesis appears to be the most important process of plant physiology regulation.

This report is an attempt to point out the specific role of CO_2 in the regulation of photosynthesis.

The Photochemical Steps of Photosynthesis

Photosynthesis in green plants brings on the reduction of CO_2 to the oxido-reduction level of sugars.

The conversion of light into chemical energy requires two light-driven reactions that are realized by two linked photochemical systems (RABINOWITCH and GOVINDJEE [1969]). They generate a reducing agent NADPH, which is the reduced form of pyridine-nucleotide, and an energy-rich phosphate compound adenosine triphosphate, ATP, by the mechanism of photophosphorylation (Figure 1). In the cell or, more exactly, in the chloroplasts (organelles in which photosynthesis takes place), the fixation of CO_2 proceeds with the assistance of NADPH,

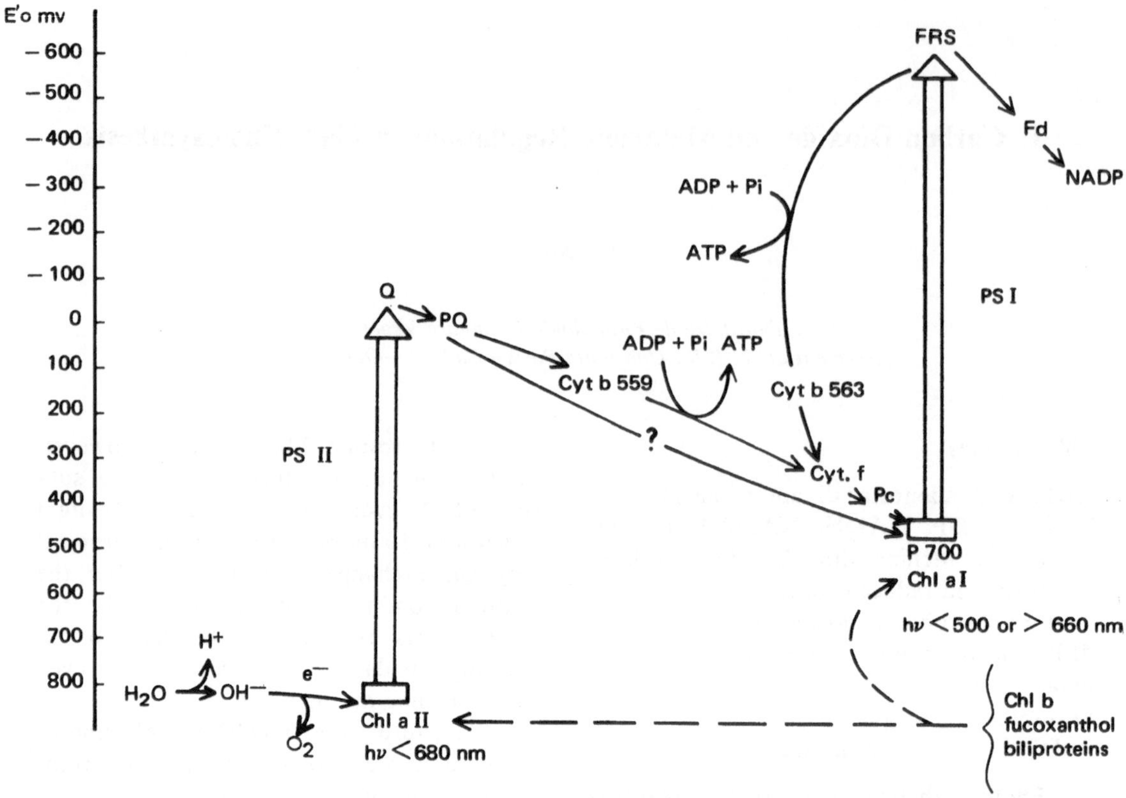

Fig. 1. Diagram of the (2) photochemical reactions of photosynthesis. Chl a I, Chl a II: holochromic proteins of chlorophyll *a* involved respectively in photosystem I (PS I) and photosystem II (PS II)

Chl b: chlorophyll b
Cyt: cytochromes
Fd: ferredoxine
FRS: ferredoxine reducing substance
Pc: plastocyanin

PQ: plastoquinone
P_{700}: electron carrier pigment, photoactive center of photochemical system I
Q: fluorescence quencher of Chl a II
?: non-phosphorylating transfer

ATP and a number of soluble enzymes. NADPH reduction and photophosphorylation involve the close association of pigments that trap and convert the energy of photons, and of molecules that transfer the electrons to the photochemical reaction while the protons migrate through the membrane systems of the chloroplasts.

The fixation and the reduction of CO_2 are nonphotochemical reactions. They are called dark reactions. They take place in the stroma of chloroplasts (Figure 2).

What problems are encountered by the processes of fixation and reduction of CO_2?

How are they regulated when external and internal conditions change?

Carbon Dioxide Concentration of the Atmosphere and the Circulation of Carbon Dioxide in the Tissues

For most plants in the light, photosynthetic absorption of CO_2 can compensate for the release of respiratory CO_2 only if the concentration of CO_2 in the ambient air is at least between 50 ppm and 150 ppm (this is true when O_2 is 21 %).

At this concentration, called the "carbon dioxide compensation point," CO_2 exchange

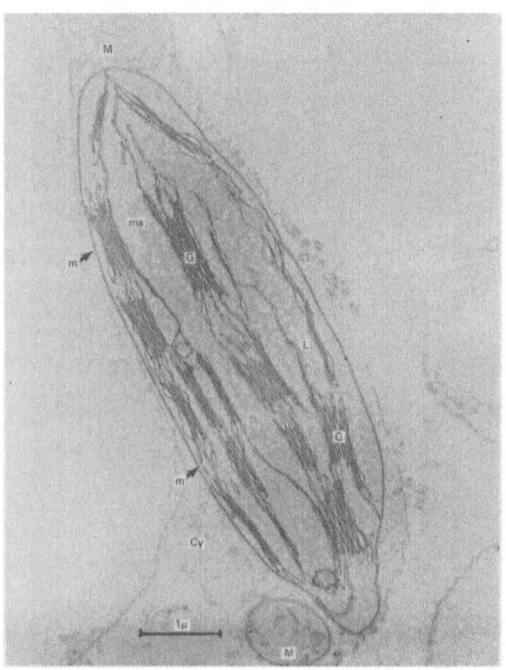

Fig. 2. (A) Electron micrograph of a cross section of a *Bryophyllum* chloroplast.

cy: cytoplasm
G: granum
L: lamella
m: outer membrane of the chloroplast envelope
m′: inner membrane of the chloroplast envelope
M: mitochondria
Ma: matrix, also called chloroplast stroma (stained with MnO_4K)

(Courtesy of Mrs. C. Sarda)

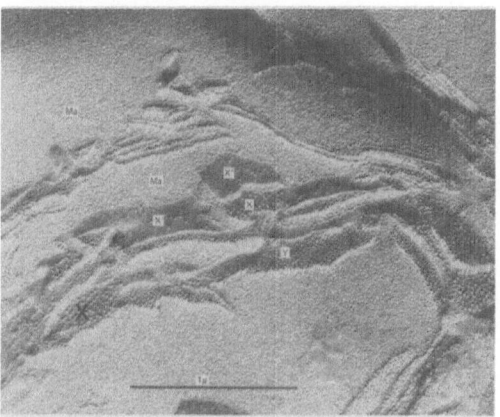

Fig. 2. (B) A deep-etched thylakoid membrane of a bean fractured chloroplast.

Ma: matrix, or chloroplast stroma which contains the Calvin cycle enzymes
X: membrane surface with large, densely packed, bound particles (about 150Å), probably involved in photoact II
X′: membrane surface with large, loosely distributed bound particles (about 150Å)
Y: membrane surface with small, densely packed bound particles (about 150Å) probably involved in photoact I

(Courtesy of Mrs. A. LaCourly)

between the surrounding atmosphere and the atmosphere inside the tissue is null.

When the concentration of O_2 is zero, the CO_2 compensation point is also nearly zero.

For some plants that originate from tropical and desert countries (corn, sugar cane, some kinds of *Amaranthus* and *Atriplex*), the CO_2 compensation point is nearly zero whatever the concentration of O_2.

At concentrations of CO_2 above the compensation point, the rate of photosynthesis first increases linearly and then reaches a plateau of saturation. For wheat leaves this plateau is reached at 400 ppm of CO_2 when light intensity is 10,000 lux and

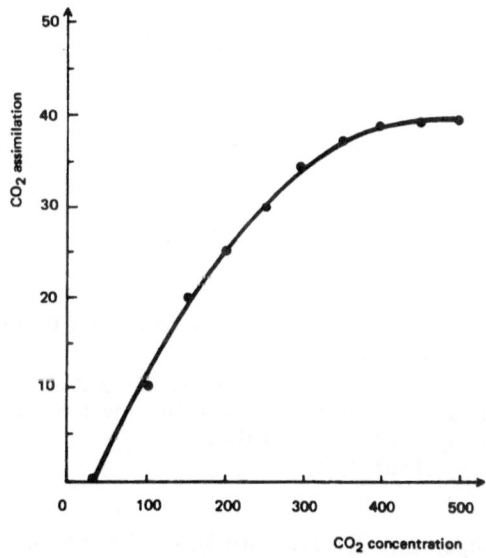

Fig. 3. Effect of CO_2 concentration (volume in ppm) on the rate of CO_2 assimilation by wheat (mg^{-1}/g^{-1} fresh wt) in 21% O_2 and 10,000 lux light, at 19.7° C

(JOLLIFE and TREGUNNA [1968]).

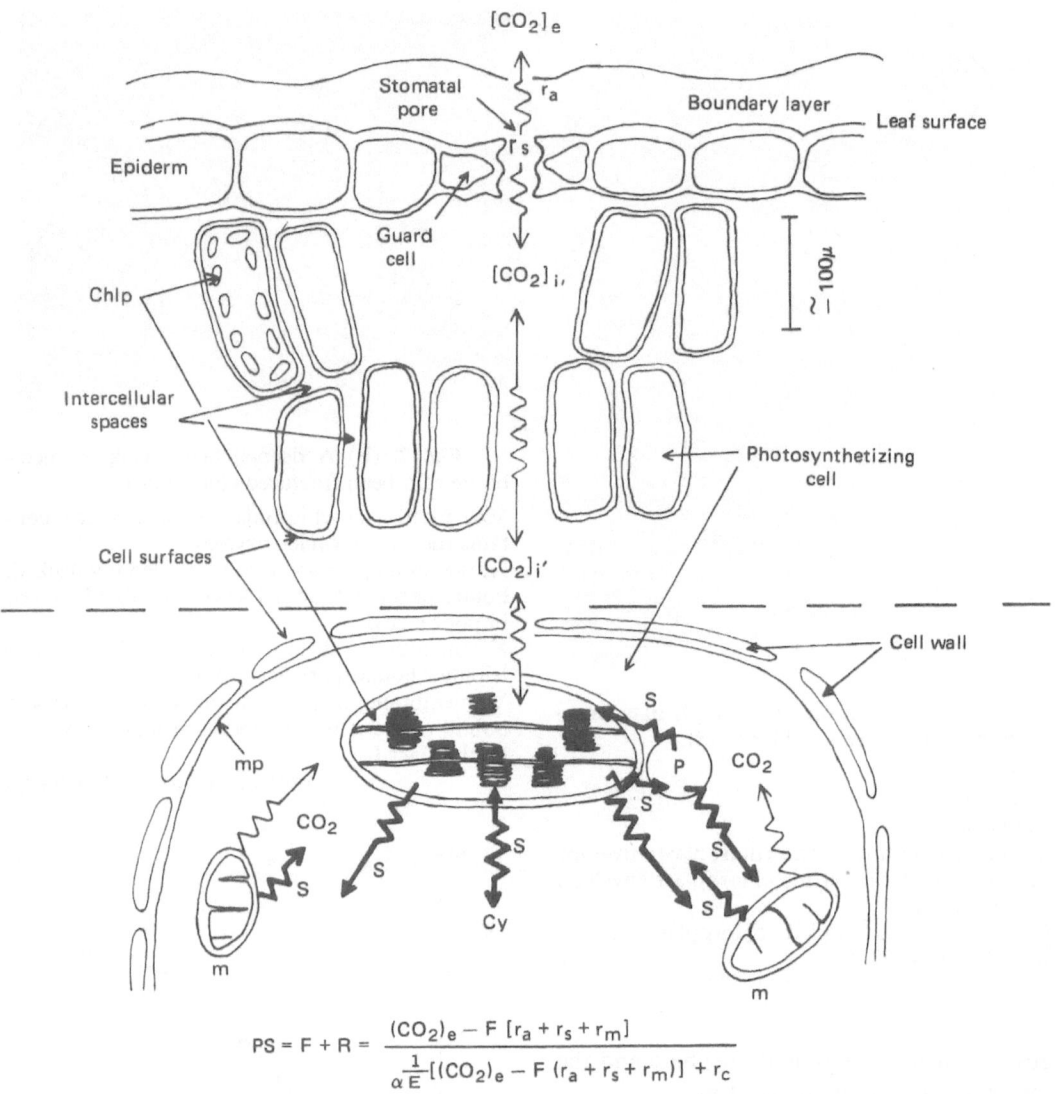

$$PS = F + R = \frac{(CO_2)_e - F\,[r_a + r_s + r_m]}{\frac{1}{\alpha E}[(CO_2)_e - F\,(r_a + r_s + r_m)] + r_c}$$

Fig. 4. A schematic representation of CO_2 fluxes and of mesophyll resistance in leaves

chlp: chloroplasts
$[CO_2]e$: CO_2 concentration in the ambient air
$[CO_2]i$: CO_2 concentration within the intercellular spaces of the plant tissue
Cy: cytoplasm

m: mitochondria
mp: cellular plasmic membrane
P: peroxisome
S: substrate which can exchange between the organelles *ra, rs*, and the equation (as in text)

temperature 20°C (Figure 3). At either higher light intensity or higher temperature the compensation point should be higher. But generally under any condition, there is always a CO_2 compensation point that makes obvious the existence of internal limiting

factors when external factors (temperature, light) are not limiting themselves.

Experiments in atmosphere containing $^{12}CO_2$ and $^{14}CO_2$ show that photosynthesis fixes indifferently respiratory CO_2 released by respiration and atmospheric CO_2; besides the carbon isotope fractionation, according to Graham's law, there is a 2% deficit for ^{14}C compared to ^{12}C. The difference in fixation rates between external CO_2 and respiratory CO_2 released into the cells is determined only by the rate of diffusion of the molecules of CO_2, whatever their source, to chloroplasts. It is to be noted that, at least in the light, the enzymatic reactions that take place in these organelles do not evolve CO_2, unlike the enzymatic reactions of cytoplasm and mitochondria.

When CO_2 from the ambient air is absorbed, the first step concerns its entry through the epidermis of the leaf. It enters mainly through the stomata, orifices that exert an important effect on the diffusion of gas and water vapor between the intercellular spaces and the external atmosphere.

Opening and closure of the stomata controls the exchange of gases. When open, orifices have a $5\,\mu$ to $15\,\mu$ diameter (Figure 4).

At the surface of leaves, there is a boundary layer of air that strongly limits the rate of CO_2 diffusion. According to Fick's law, the rate of CO_2 influx F can be expressed by the following equation:

$$F = \frac{(CO_2)e - (CO_2)i}{ra + rs} \text{ moles cm}^{-2}\text{ min}^{-1}$$

where $(CO_2)e$ and $(CO_2)i$ are CO_2 concentrations in the ambient air and around the sites of carboxylation.

The notations ra and rs represent the diffusion resistance to CO_2 transfer in the boundary layer and in the stomata.

The first process that regulates photosynthesis is linked to the effects of CO_2 and other external factors on the opening and the closure of stomata.

The absorption of light by chlorophyll induces the opening of stomata. They shut in darkness. In very dry air plants encounter a stress. The stomata close, so that the water-loss of the leaves is lowered. As long as the plants do not undergo any water stress, a rise in temperature is favorable for the opening of stomata.

The importance of the concentration

effect of the atmospheric CO_2 is obvious; the stomata which remain open in the light and under low CO_2 concentration tend to close when the CO_2 concentration increases to 1000 ppm or 2000 ppm.

It is likely that the opening process of the stomata is linked with the photosynthetic metabolism that produces a turgor increase of the two stomata cells positioned around the orifice (guard cells). A mechanical water uptake occurs. Because of the asymmetrical thickness of the cellulosic wall of the guard cells, the orifice opens.

The classical hypothesis is that the removal of CO_2 by the photosynthetic carboxylation results in the enhancement of the pH in the guard cells. Phosphorylases would be stimulated as the pH increases, starch hydrolysed into glucose-1-phosphate, and the osmotic force elevated. Unfortunately, this mechanism would be too low to account for the rate of stomatal movements. Therefore, another very clever suggestion has been proposed (ZELITCH [1969]).

It is known that low CO_2 concentrations induce an important accumulation of glycolate in the tissues. The further metabolism of glycolate brings about the oxidation of NADPH into NADP. Consequently, the increased NADP level would result in a stimulation of the rate of electron transfer as well as an enhancement of the photophosphorylation activity in the stomatal cells. This overall acceleration may result in an efficient "pumping" of solutes or ions, especially of K^+. Indeed, guard cells of several species contain large concentrations of potassium when they are open in the light. The increase in potassium ions in these cells may be related to the functioning of an energetically "active pump."

After entering the cell, CO_2 is dissolved and is transferred only in the liquid phase. Respiratory CO_2 joins CO_2 coming from the ambient air. The rate of photosynthesis is determined by the sum of CO_2 from both sources.

There is no problem for the penetration of CO_2 through the cellulosic cell wall, as the pores allow a free diffusion. However, extracellular CO_2 influx must be transferred through the plasmic membranes of the foliar parenchyma cells, called mesophyll. Dissolved CO_2 and bicarbonate must also diffuse through the membranes of chloroplasts in order to reach the sites of carboxylation. Respiratory CO_2 (or bicarbonate) must be in addition diffuse through the outer membranes of the mitochondria.

The sum of resistances which limit the free diffusion of CO_2 to the carboxylation sites is called "mesophyll resistance."

The rate of net photosynthesis *PS* can be expressed by the following equation (CHARTIER et al., [1970]).

$$PS = F + R =$$

$$\frac{(CO_2)e - F(ra + rs + rm)}{\frac{I}{\alpha E}[(CO_2)e - F(ra + rs + rm)] + rc}$$

$$(g\ cm^{-2}\ sec^{-1})$$

where

$(CO_2)e$ = CO_2 concentration in the ambient air $(g\ ml^{-1})$;

F = rate of CO_2 influx per unit leaf area $(g\ cm^{-2}\ sec^{-1})$;

R = rate of CO_2 flux from respiration sites to sites of carboxylation $(g\ cm^{-2}\ sec^{-1})$;

ra = diffusion resistance to CO_2 transfer in the boundary layer of air $(cm^{-1}\ sec)$;

rs = diffusion resistance for CO_2 in the stomata and the cuticle of epidermis $(cm^{-1}\ sec)$;

rm = diffusion resistance for CO_2 in the mesophyll to the sites of carboxylation in the chloroplasts $(cm^{-1}\ sec)$;

rc = carboxylation resistance $(cm^{-1}\ sec)$;

α = maximum efficiency of light radiation conversion;

E = flux density of light irradiation incident on the leaf $(W\ cm^{-2})$.

The above equation describes a rectangular hyperbola. It fits well with the expression of the rate of photosynthesis as a function of light intensity or as a function of CO_2 concentration in the ambient air, shown on Figure 3. (Graphs representing photosynthetic intensity have the same shape whether the independent variable is light or CO_2 concentration).

Every parameter of the equation can be either directly or indirectly determined from experimental results except *rm* and *rc*, which are calculated by means of a set of linear equations $y = ax + b$, after substituting *rm* with *y*, *rc* with *x*, *a* and *b* with the relevant experimental values.

The carboxylation resistance *rc* depends upon the rate of biochemical processes described below.

Carbon Dioxide Fixation and Reduction

Photosynthesis can be formulated by the following equations. The first reaction only is light-dependent. The three others are dark chemical exergonic reactions; they summarize the CO_2 cycle, called the Calvin cycle (Figure 5).

(1) $H_2O + NADP + ADP + P_i \xrightarrow{h\nu} NADPH + ATP + \frac{1}{2}O_2$

(2) $CO_2 + RuDP \longrightarrow 2\ PGA$

(3) $PGA + NADPH + ATP \longrightarrow$ Trioses P $+ NADP + ADP + P_i$

(4) Trioses P $+ ATP \longrightarrow ADP + RuDP$ and other sugars $+ P_i$

Resistance to carboxylation depends directly upon reaction (2) and indirectly upon the three other reactions which allow the RuDP regeneration.

If reactions (1), (3), and (4) are not rate-limiting, for example under high incident radiation (NADPH and ATP are in sufficient amounts), the photosynthesis rate depends only on CO_2 concentrations at the sites of carboxylation and on the affinity for CO_2 of the enzyme RuDP-carboxylase, which mediates CO_2 fixation. This affinity is rather low (Michaelis constant $Km = 4.5 \times 10^{-4}$ M

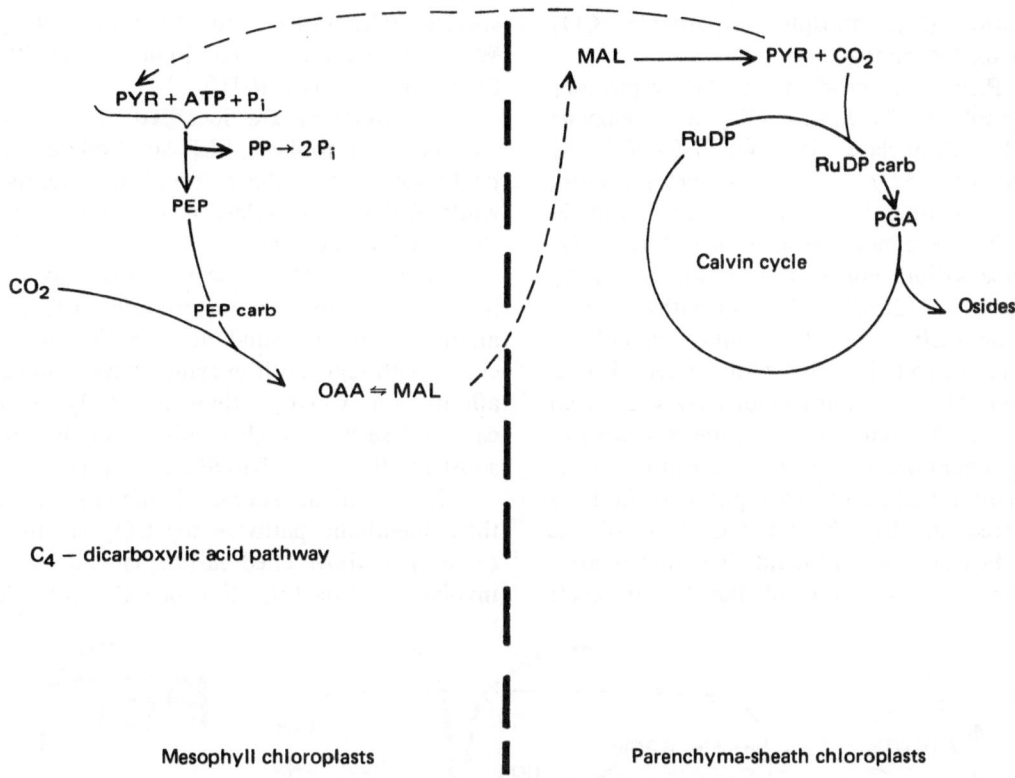

Fig. 5. A schematic representation of the metabolic pathways in chloroplasts, persoxisomes and mitochondria, and of the substrate exchanges between these organelles. Left: Calvin cycle in chloroplasts CH (BASSHAM and KIRK [1967]). In the upper portion of the diagram, the substrates remain in the chloroplasts; in the lower portion, they migrate more or less easily in the cytoplasm.
Upper right: glycolate oxidation in peroxisomes PER. Lower right: serine synthesis in mitochondria M

AA: amino acids
cat: catalase
G2PP: glycolaldehyde thiamine pyrophosphate
DHAP: dihydroxycetone-phosphate
DPase: fructose-1, 6-diphosphate and sedoheptulose-1.7-diphosphate phosphatases
E4P: erythrose-phosphate
Fac: fatty acids
F6P: fructose-6-phosphate
FDP: fructose-1.6-diphosphate
GAP: glyceraldehyde-phosphate
G6P: glucose-6-phosphate
gly: glycine
glyc: glycolate
glycer: glycerate
glyox: glycoxylate

PGA: phosphoglycerate
6PGlu: 6-phosphate-gluconate
R5P: ribose-5-phosphate
Ru5P: ribulose-5-phosphate
RuDP: ribulose- 1.5-diphosphate
RuDPcarb: ribulose-1.5-diphosphate carboxylase
S7P: seduheptulose-7-phosphate
SDP: sedoheptulose-1.7-diphosphate
Ser: serine
tal: transaldolase
tc: transcetolase
TCA: tricarboxylic acids cycle
TPP: thiamine pyrophosphate
UTP: uridine triphosphate
Xu5P: xylulose-5-phosphate

according to COOPER et al. [1969]) in plants which fix C by the above cited pathway (Calvin cycle species; see CALVIN [1955]). This may be the cause of their high CO_2 compensation point.

In plants with a low CO_2 compensation point, an alternative pathway of carboxylation occurs: the C4–dicarboxylic acid pathway of carboxylation (HATCH and SLACK [1970]), which is described by the following equation (2′): phosphoenolpyruvate + CO_2 ⟶ oxaloacetate + P_i.

PEP is a product of the respiratory metabolism. The *Km* for CO_2 of the enzyme PEP carboxylase is low: 7.5×10^{-6} M (WAYGOOD, MACHE, and TAN [1969]). Indeed, it is the cooperation of reactions (2′) and (2) which determines the lowering of the CO_2 compensation point (Figure 6). In plants with the C4–dicarboxylic acid pathway, cells having PEP carboxylase-containing chloroplasts surround cells with active RuDP carboxylase-containing chloroplasts. Such an anatomical arrangement is quite favorable to CO_2 retention. Moreover, the isotopic fractionation associated with photosynthesis is lowered so that the $^{13}C/^{12}C$ ratio of the C4–dicarboxylic acid plants is higher relative to the $^{13}C/^{12}C$ ratio of the Calvin cycle

species (OESCHGER and LERMAN [1970]; WHELAN, SACKETT, and BENEDICT [1970]; SMITH and EPSTEIN [1971]).

Carboxylases are localized within the stroma of chloroplasts. PEP carboxylase may be located beside the chloroplast envelope, while RuDP carboxylase is associated with the thylakoid lamellae.

Within the chloroplasts the stroma pH is about 7.7 to 8.4. Accordingly, CO_3H^- anions are more abundant than CO_2 molecules. Although both enzymes have a lower affinity for CO_3H^- than for CO_2, PEP carboxylase has a higher affinity for the first substrate than does RuDP carboxylase.

In succulent species (*Crassulaceae*) a third metabolic pathway for CO_2 is implicated. The above cited carboxylases are also involved, but dark fixation of CO_2 and PEP

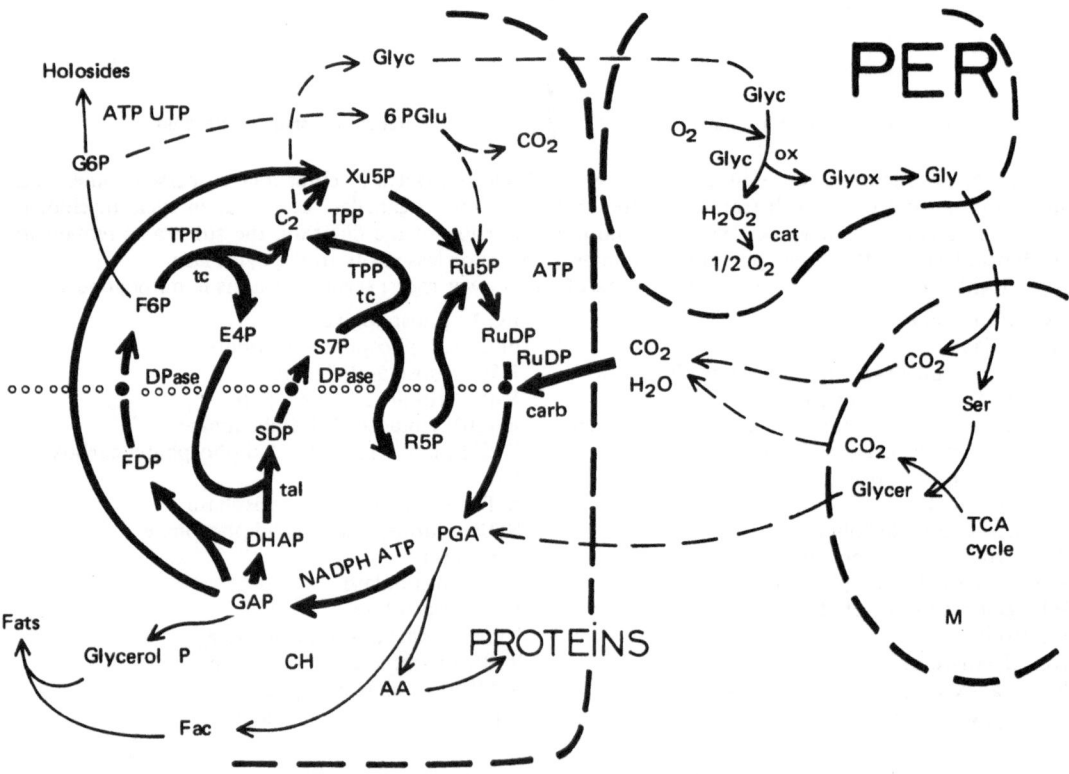

Fig. 6. Relations between mesophyll cells chloroplasts and bundle sheets cells chloroplasts in C_4 plant metabolism (after HATCH and SLACK [1970]).

carb: carboxylases   OAA: oxaloacetate
MAL: malate   PYR: pyruvate

synthesis after RuDP carboxylation can be much more active than the light-dependent CO_2 metabolism (MOYSE [1965]).

Steady-state Equilibrium of Carbon Dioxide Molecules and Bicarbonate Anions; Bicarbonate and Carbon Dioxide Activating Mechanism

CO_2 molecules and bicarbonate anions rapidly reach a steady-state equilibrium, especially in the carbonic anhydrase-containing chloroplasts of the Calvin cycle species. This enzyme plays a role in photosynthesis as it facilitates the supply of CO_2 to RuDP carboxylase.

In the C4–dicarboxylic acid plants, carbonic anhydrase is one to ten times less active than in the Calvin cycle species (EVERSON and SLACK [1968]). It is located within the cytoplasm. However, at pH 8.0, PEP carboxylase activity in the presence of CO_3H^- is higher than RuDP carboxylase activity in the presence of CO_2.

In cells, activities of the carboxylases are far from being saturated. CO_2 concentration, if it were the same in the cell medium as in a solution in equilibrium with air (8 μmole at temperatures between 20°C and 30°C), would be only 1/100 of the concentration required to saturate RuDP carboxylase *in vitro*.

The CO_2-fixing capacities of ruptured chloroplasts or of isolated enzymes are always lower than the *in vivo* capacities, whether calculated per unit chlorophyll or per unit protein. However, intact isolated chloroplasts, still surrounded by their external envelopes, exhibit CO_2-fixing capacities similar to the *in vivo* observed capacities (MOYSE [1969]).

The apparent *Km* of intact carboxylating chloroplasts for the substrate is much lower than the isolated RuDP carboxylase *Km*. This discrepancy could be explained by the operation of a process for concentrating CO_2 or CO_3H^- in the chloroplasts (LATZKO and GIBBS [1968]). It has been suggested that this process would be an active transport for CO_2

or bicarbonate, dependent on the energy released by photophosphorylation (CHAMPIGNY and MIGINIAC–MASLOW [1971]).

Metabolite Movements to and from Chloroplasts and the Mechanism for Regulating the Rate of Carbon Dioxide Fixation

Information about the movement of phosphorylated sugars within the cell has been obtained with *Chlorella* exposed to $^{14}CO_2$. There is undoubtedly a rapid exchange of PGA and dihydroxyacetone-phosphate between chloroplastic and cytoplasmic pools. In addition, glycolate and malate can readily diffuse from chloroplasts. The diffusion of these compounds from intact isolated chloroplasts to the suspension medium is also rapid. But fructose diphosphate and sedoheptulose diphosphate permeate more slowly through the outer membrane of the chloroplast. The chloroplast envelope appears to be only slightly permeable to fructose-1-phosphate, sedoheptulose-1-phosphate, and RuDP, so the major part remains in the chloroplast stroma.

Calvin cycle intermediates, especially phosphorylated sugars that are retained in the chloroplasts, have a potential role in the regulation of the light-activated enzymes, as discussed below. They allow the maintenance of pools of substrates at the level of the sites for regulation of the enzymes.

Light Activation of the Photosynthetic Enzymes; Dark Inhibition of the Respiratory Enzymes

RuDP carboxylase activity in the *Chlorella*, or isolated chloroplast, is strongly enhanced upon exposure of the algal cells (or organelles) to light for a very short time. Likewise, diphosphatases that catalyze the conversion of fructose-1,6-diphosphate into fructose-6-phosphate and of sedoheptulose-1, 7-diphosphate into sedoheptulose-7-phosphate are light stimulated.

Diphosphatases play a role in the regulation of the regeneration of the CO_2 acceptor,

RuDP, by controlling the synthesis of sugars, substrates of the Calvin cycle transketolization reaction.

Pyruvate-phosphate-dikinase, which has a potential role in the C4–dicarboxylic acid pathway of CO_2 fixation, is also light stimulated (HATCH and SLACK [1970]).

At present, the mechanism of light stimulation of these enzymes is unknown. On the other hand, the mechanism of stimulation of the glyceraldehyde-3-phosphate dehydrogenase can be better explained. This enzyme is involved in the reduction of PGA to phosphoglyceraldehyde in the presence of NADPH in chloroplasts. A light-mediated inter-conversion of the NADH-linked glyceraldehyde P dehydrogenase, into the NADPH form is likely. NADPH and ATP activate the conversion which can be very rapid (MULLER, ZIEGLER, and ZIEGLER [1969]; MULLER [1970]).

On the other hand, isotopic studies of the respiratory metabolites during light-dark or dark-light transients have shown that several oxidation activities are lowered by illumination in the Calvin cycle plants (CALVIN and MASSINI [1952]). Such is the case for the tricarboxylic acid reactions, probably due firstly to a NADPH and ATP excess in the cells, and secondly to the exhaustion of the acetyl-CoA as PGA is used up for sugar synthesis.

This is the case for the synthesis of 6-phosphate-gluconate, the first step in glucose oxidation by the pentose-phosphate pathway (BASSHAM and KIRK [1967]).

Light stimulation of the Calvin cycle pathway on the one hand and light inhibition of the respiratory metabolism on the other enhance the mechanism of reductive photosynthetic CO_2 metabolism.

Photorespiration and Carbon Dioxide Evolution during Photosynthesis

Part of photosynthetic CO_2 can be evolved and lost from the plant. During the last 10 years it has been demonstrated that light enhances a CO_2-evolving process that is distinct from the dark respiration. This process is directly related to the photosynthetic mechanism and to the participation of peroxisomal respiration, as opposed to mitochondrial respiration[1] (JACKSON and VOLK [1970]).

Photorespiration is a typical feature of the Calvin cycle plants. The rate of photorespiration is much higher than the rate of dark respiration. It has been estimated that from 10% to 20% of CO_2 fixed by photosynthetic carboxylation can be released by photorespiration. This process involves glycolate that is derived from sugar phosphate intermediates of the photosynthetic carbon reduction cycle. The formation of glycolate is explained as an oxidation of a glycolaldehyde thiamine pyrophosphate addition compound formed during the transketolase reactions of the cycle (Figure 5). Then glycolate would be formed from disruption of 2 ketose: fructose-1-phosphate and sedoheptulose-1-phosphate (BASSHAM [1964]).

Although formed in the chloroplasts, glycolate is oxidized to glyoxylate in peroxisomes. In the leaf cells, these organelles are frequently appressed to the surfaces of chloroplasts. During the oxidation of glycolate, the H_2O_2 produced is immediately decomposed by the catalase which is located in the peroxisomes (TOLBERT and YAMAZAKI [1969]).

Isolated peroxisomes fail to oxidize glyoxylate to CO_2. The reaction could occur to some extent in the chloroplast, provided glyoxylate be transfered back to the chloroplast. But the dominant process appears to be the amination to glycine within peroxisomes (Figure 5). Then it is assumed that in mitochondria the conversion of glycine to serine, according to the following equation, constitutes the biggest proportion of the total photorespiratory CO_2 release.

Indeed, serine-hydroxymethyltransferase, the enzyme which mediates this conversion, has been found to be located in mitochondria.

---

[1] It is to be noted that (a) in the dark, the nonmitochondrial oxidative pentose-phosphate pathway can represent up to 50% of the plant cellular oxidative activity, and (b) the role of mitochondria in photorespiration is dealt with below.

$$\begin{array}{c} ^+\text{COOH} \\ | \\ \text{CHNH}_2 \\ \text{glycine} \end{array} + \begin{array}{c} ^+\text{COOH} \\ | \\ \text{CHNH}_2 \end{array} + 2\text{H}_2\text{O} \rightarrow$$

$$\begin{array}{c} ^+\text{COOH} \\ | \\ \text{CHNH}_2 \\ | \\ \text{CH}_2\text{OH} \\ \text{serine} \end{array} + \text{NH}_4\text{OH} + {}^+\text{CO}_2$$

It is proposed that in peroxisomes, serine would be converted into glycerate, the first intermediate metabolite to sugars, and that subsequently it would be converted into PGA and trioses-phosphate in the chloroplasts.

The major fate of the glycolate metabolism is determined by the existence of a metabolite shuttle between chloroplasts, peroxisomes and mitochondria. The balance of the exchange results in the release of 1 CO_2 mole for 2 glycolate derived from the photosynthetic Calvin cycle. This shuttle would provide a means for oxidizing the excess photosynthetic NADPH when glyoxylate, after its return to the chloroplast, is reduced to glycolate.

One may think that phytophysiologists' imaginations go beyond reality. However, one has reason to believe that reality is much more complicated than most would imagine.

Sunlight powers the green plant physiology. It supplies the required energy for the reduction of CO_2 in chloroplasts as it sustains CO_2 diffusion into tissues, cells and chloroplasts. Its role also includes the opening of stomata and the regulation of CO_2 concentration at the sites of carboxylation. Light stimulation of the reductive pentose-phosphate pathway and light inhibition of the respiratory metabolism make its field of influence still wider.

The role of solar energy can be best appreciated by considering the reduction of pyridine nucleotides and ATP synthesis.

On the other hand, CO_2 and carbonates participate in the regulation of photosynthesis by controlling carbon diffusion and fixation. Carbon dioxide and organic substrate exchanges between chloroplasts, cytoplasm, peroxisomes, and mitochondria determine the overall balance of C assimilation.

In plants with the highest capacity of CO_2 fixation (C4–dicarboxylic acid plants), the cooperation of two active carboxylases makes it possible to suggest a pattern for inorganic carbon fixation and accumulation which would allow a better regulation of CO_2 level in the atmosphere.

Acknowledgments   I gratefully acknowledge Mrs. J. Brangeon, Dr. M. L. Champigny, and F. Maury for their assistance in translating the text and preparing the manuscript.

Bibliography

Bassham, J. A. *Ann. Rev. Plant Physiol.*, 15:101–20 (1964).

———, and Kirk, M. In Shibata, K., Takamiya, A., Jagendorf, A. T., and Fuller, R. C., eds., *Comparative Biochemistry and Biophysics of Photosynthesis* (Tokyo, 1967 and New York, 1968), pp. 365–78.

Calvin, M. *Proc. Third Intern. Cong. Biochem.*, *Brussels, 1955*, C. Liebecq, ed. New York: Academic Press, 1956, pp. 211–25.

———, and Massini, P. *Experientia*, 8:445–57 (1952).

Champigny, M. L. and Miginiac-Maslow, M. *Biochim. Biophys. Acta*, 234:(3):335–44 (1971).

Chartier, P., Chartier, M., and Čatský, J. *Photosynthetica*, 4:48–57 (1970).

Cooper, T. G., Filmer, D., Wishnick, M., and Lane, M. D. *J. Biol. Chem.*, 244:1081–83 (1969).

Everson, R. G. and Slack, C. R. *Phytochemistry*, 7:581–84 (1968).

Hatch, M. D. and Slack, C. R. In Reinhold, L. and Liwschitz, Y., eds. *Progress in Phytochemistry*, Vol. II. New York, 1970, pp. 35–106.

Jackson, W. A. and Volk, R. J. *Ann. Rev. Plant Physiol.*, 21:385–432 (1970).

Joliffe, P. A. and Tregunna, E. B. *Plant Physiol.*, 43:902–06 (1968).

Latzko, E. and Gibbs, M. *Zeits. Pflanzenphysiol.*, 59:184–94 (1968).

Moyse, A. In *Travaux Dédiés à Lucien Plantefol* Masson et Cie Éd. (Paris, 1965), pp. 21–44.

———. *Physiol. Vég.*, 7:43–56 (1969), *Biochimie Fonctionnelle des Structures Cellulaires* (in Russian), Acad. Sc. SSSR ed., 87–96 (1970).

Müller, B. *Biochim. Biophys. Acta*, 205:102–09 (1970).

———, Ziegler, I. and Ziegler, H. *Europ. J. Biochem.*, 9:101–06 (1969).

Oeschger, H. and Lerman, J. C. *Chemische Rundschau*, 25:585–88 (1970).

Rabinowitch, E. and Govindjee, —. *Photosynthesis*. New York: John Wiley, 1969.

Smith, B. N. and Epstein, S. *Plant Physiol.*, 47:380–84 (1971).

Tolbert, N. E. and Yamazaki, R. K. *Annals N.Y. Acad. Sci.*, 168:325–41 (1969).

Waygood, E. R., Mache, R. and Tan, C. K. *Can. J. Bot.*, 47:1455–58 (1969).

Whelan, T., Sackett, W. M. and Benedict, C. R. *Biochem. Biophys. Res. Comm.*, 41:1205–10 (1970).

Zelitch, I. *Ann. Rev. Plant Physiol.*, 20:329–50 (1969).

Moyse Discussion

NAHAS: You showed a slide, where CO_2 fixation was plotted against CO_2 concentration in the atmosphere. This dose response curve had an exponential form indicating that all active sites are saturated. Is there some autoinhibition?

MOYSE: Indeed, the plateau indicates that all active sites of CO_2 fixation may be saturated. CO_2 at high concentrations brings on autoinhibition, but only after a few hours.

RAHN: Comparing diffusion pathways in different organisms, perhaps you can say something about the length of the diffusion pathway from the external surface of the cells to the inside. Can you compute the boundary layer?

MOYSE: The diffusion pathway from the external surface of leaves to the sites of CO_2 fixation is from about 10μ for cells near the surface to 1 mm in length for furthest cells. The boundary layer thickness depends on the movement of air and on the hairs of the plant. It is from a few microns to 1 mm thickness.

LONGMORE: Does citrate play a role? I noticed that you omit citrate from the picture?

MOYSE: There is no citrate in chloroplasts. Citrate forms in the mitochondria.

BARGETON: What is the overall efficiency, the ratio of energy used-energy stored in chemical form?

MOYSE: The best efficiency is conversion of one molecule of CO_2 into phosphorylated sugar for 8 photons absorbed. Then, 2 quanta are necessary for the transfer of 1 electron and 4 quanta allow the reduction of 1 molecule of NADP and the synthesis of 2 or 3 molecules of ATP. The fixation of 1 CO_2 yields 2 PGA, the reduction of which requires 2 NADPH and 2 ATP. In calories, the maximum efficiency is 25% in blue light, 35% in red light. But under natural conditions, it is not over 1% or 2%.

CHALAZONITIS: Well I am, of course, ignorant, but I would like to ask you if in darkness the diffusion of CO_2 from the outside of the tissue to inside, to the chloroplasts inside, is primarily related to the differences in partial pressure of CO_2 between the outside and inside. In other words, is the Fick law followed or is it a nonlinear relation?

MOYSE: CO_2 fixation follows Fick's law as long as no ions or membranes interfere. Otherwise there is a more complicated relation which depends on the membrane potential.

NAHAS: Is there any carbonic anhydrase in plants? And is most of the CO_2 fixation in the form of CO_2 or in the form of bicarbonate?

MOYSE: Yes, there is some carbonic anhydrase in plants. The fixation is mainly in the form of CO_2. As a matter of fact, there are two kinds of plants: the plants of the Calvin's cycle type that have carbonic anhydrase in the chloroplasts; and sugar cane and other tropical plants that are poor in carbonic anhydrase and likely may fix bicarbonate directly.

2. The Regulation by Carbon Dioxide of Carbohydrate and Lipid Metabolism in Isolated Perfused Tissue [1]

William J. Longmore, Amy M. Liang, and Michael L. McDaniel

Department of Biochemistry
St. Louis University School of Medicine
St. Louis, Missouri 63104

In 1960 Hastings and Dowdle reported that increasing medium bicarbonate concentration in the physiological range from approximately 10 mM to 40 mM, while maintaining pH at 7.40, caused glycogen synthesis from glucose in rat liver slices to increase 60% (HASTINGS and DOUDLE [1960]). In further studies it was found that fructose (HASTINGS and LONGMORE [1965]) and especially glycerol (LONGMORE, HASTINGS, and MAHOWALD [1964]) also served as substrates to produce the rise in glycogen synthesis as total CO_2 concentration of the medium was increased, while pyruvate did not (HASTINGS and LONGMORE [1965]). In addition to the effect of CO_2 on glycogen synthesis, it was observed that acetate-1-^{14}C and pyruvate-2-^{14}C incorporation into triglyceride and phospholipid fatty acids was increased an average of fourfold in rat liver slices when medium total CO_2 concentration was increased from 10 mM to 40 mM at pH 7.40 (LONGMORE, et al. [1967]; LONGMORE [1968]). Bicarbonate has been shown by various workers to affect the activity of several enzymes *in vitro*, including glucose-6-phosphate dehydrogenase, glucose-6-phosphate phosphohydrolase, phosphoenolpyruvate carboxykinase, glyceraldehyde phosphate dehydrogenase, and aconitase (BANDURSKI and LIPMANN [1956]; CHANCE and PARKE [1967]; DICKMAN and CLOUTIER [1951]; DYSON, ANDERSON, and NORDLIE [1969]; LEVY [1963]; ANDERSON and NORDLIE [1968]; ANDERSON, HORNE, and NORDLIE [1968]; McDANIEL and LONGMORE [1971]). The last two, glyceraldehyde phosphate dehydrogenase and aconitase, assume importance in the present report.

To establish the physiological importance of the results obtained with liver slices and enzyme preparations, studies on the effect of change in total CO_2 concentration at constant pH on carbohydrate and lipid metabolism in isolated perfused rat liver and lung have been carried out.

Glycogen synthesis from glucose and glycerol has been shown to be increased in the isolated rat liver perfused with a medium in which the total CO_2 concentration was increased from 8 to 40 mM at pH 7.4 (LONGMORE, NIETHE, and McDANIEL [1969]). As an integral part of those studies, it was shown that intracellular pH remained constant while intracellular bicarbonate concentration followed rather closely the extracellular bicarbonate concentration. Thus, the effect of changes in extracellular total CO_2 concentration on liver metabolism at constant extracellular pH may be assumed to be due to

[1] The work herein was supported in part by Grants AM 10602, 11113, GM 446, HE 13405 and the Missouri Heart Association.

15

intracellular changes in total CO_2 concentration and not change in intracellular pH.

To establish whether incorporation of acetate into lipids of the perfused liver was affected by the total CO_2 concentration of the medium perfusing the liver, as were liver slices, the incorporation of acetate-1-^{14}C into triglyceride and phospholipid fatty acids and cholesterol was studied using perfusion and

experiments (Figure 2) showed a similar result in that acetate-1-^{14}C incorporation into triglyceride and phospholipid fatty acids was greater the first hour, during exposure to medium containing 34 mM bicarbonate, than the second hour of perfusion with medium containing 10 mM bicarbonate. Once again, acetate-1-^{14}C incorporation into cholesterol was essentially unaffected

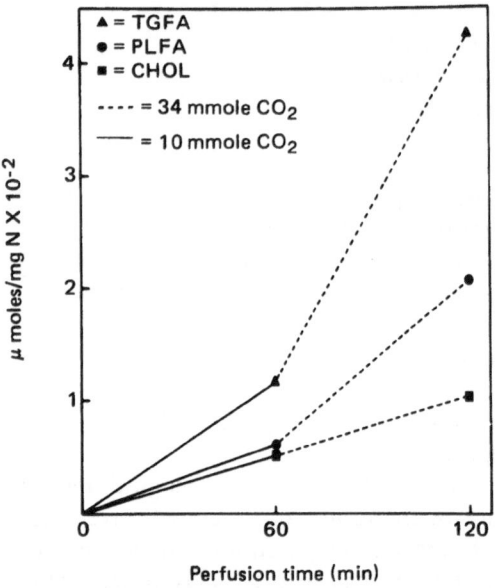

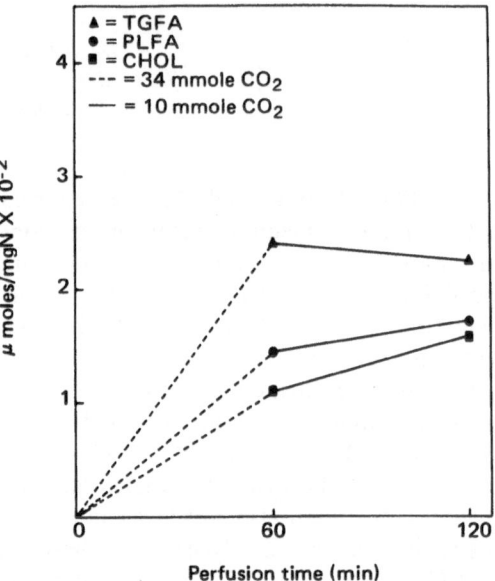

Fig. 1. Incorporation of acetate-1-^{14}C into tryglyceried fatty acids (TGFA), pospholoid fatty acids (PLFA), and cholesterol (Chol) of livers perfused with medium containing 10 mmole total CO_2 the first hour and 34 mmole total CO_2 the second hour of perfusion. pH = 7.4. Methods are as previously described. LONGMORE, *et al.* [1967]; MCDANIEL, LIANG, and LONGMORE [in press].

Fig. 2. Incorporation of acetate-1-^{14}C into triglyceride fatty acids (TGFA), pospholoid fatty acids (PLFA), and cholestorel (Chol) of livers perfused with medium containing 34 mmole total CO_2 the first hour and 10 mmole total CO_2 the second hour of perfusion. pH = 7.4. Methods are as previously described. LONGMORE, *et al.* [1967]; MCDANIEL, LIANG, and LONGMORE [in press].

assay methods previously described (LONGMORE, et al. [1967]; LONGMORE, NIETHE, and MCDANIEL [1969]) (Figure 1). While a marked rise in the incorporation of acetate-1-^{14}C into triglyceride and phospholipid fatty acids occurred when the liver was perfused with medium containing 34 mM bicarbonate (hour 2) as compared to perfusion with medium containing 10 mM bicarbonate (hour 1), no rise in incorporation into cholerestol was observed. The companion livers of these

by the bicarbonate concentration of the medium perfusing the liver.

Recently we have become interested in lung lipid metabolism and have developed a satisfactory isolated rat lung perfusion system. As part of that study, the effect of bicarbonate concentration on the incorporation of acetate-2-^{14}C into lung phospholipids has been determined. The perfusions were carried out for 2 hours with medium containing either 15.6 mM or 42.0 mM bicarbonate at pH 7.40.

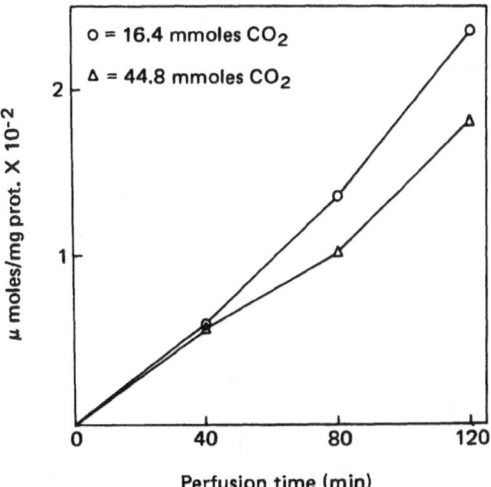

Fig. 3. Incorporation of acetate-2-^{14}C into phospholipids of isolated rat lung perfused for 2 hours with medium containing either 15.6 mmole bicarbonate or 42.0 mmole bicarbonate. pH = 7.4.

Lung samples were obtained at 40, 80 and 120 minutes. The results (Figure 3), unlike those obtained with the liver, show that increased bicarbonate concentration of the medium perfusing the lung actually caused little or no change in the incorporation of acetate-2-^{14}C into phospholipids. If the permeability of lung tissue is considered to be more like that of muscle than liver, the fact that a change of CO_2 concentration did not affect incorporation of acetate into lung phospholipids may be attributed to the lack of permeability of the cell to bicarbonate. Accompanying the change in medium bicarbonate concentration, in order to maintain a constant pH, is a change in P_{CO_2}, and thus in dissolved CO_2. Even in muscle tissue, it would be expected that such a change might alter intracellular pH. However, if intracellular pH of the perfused lung was altered, the change did not produce a marked effect on fatty acid synthesis.

In order to determine the biochemical basis for the CO_2 effect on metabolism observed in liver, it was of interest to ascertain which enzymatic activities are responsive to CO_2 concentration in the isolated perfused

liver Measurements have therefore been made of concentrations of several key intermediates of the Embden–Meyerhof pathway and citric acid cycle in liver perfused with medium containing approximately 10 mM and 33 mM bicarbonate. The perfusions were of the cross-perfusion type (LONGMORE, NIETHE, and McDANIEL [1969]) and the data is displayed so that the 100% line is the concentration of each metabolic intermediate in liver perfused with medium containing 10 mmole bicarbonate, and the deviation from 100% is the result of change produced by perfusion with 33 mmole bicarbonate. The percent changes are an average of the effect produced in livers perfused with medium containing 10 mmole bicarbonate the first hour and 33 mmole the second hour, and 33 mmole bicarbonate the first hour and 10 mmole bicarbonate the second hour. The results (Figure 4) are from livers which had available in the perfusate 14 mmole glycerol and 17 mmole glucose. It is observed that glucose-6-phosphate, fructose-6-phosphate, fructose-1,6-diphosphate and citrate concentrations in the liver were elevated, while 3-phosphoglycerate, phosphoenolpyruvate and aspartate were decreased. A second series of experiments was performed in a similar manner, except that the only substrate added to the perfusate was glucose at a physiological concentration of 5.8 mmole. The results (Figure 5) are somewhat similar to those presented in Figure 4, with the exception that pyruvate and citrate concentrations are markedly elevated and malate concentration is depressed.

Interpretation of the cross-over plots is complicated by the fact that although the net flux of carbon flow in the liver is toward glucose (that is, the liver is normally a gluconeogenic organ), it is possible that the flow of carbon is being regulated in the glycolytic direction. If so, the synthesis of 3-phosphoglycerate would appear to be inhibited. The changes in metabolite concentrations surrounding phosphoenolpyruvate, pyruvate, malate, and asparate are difficult to interpret due to the multiplicity

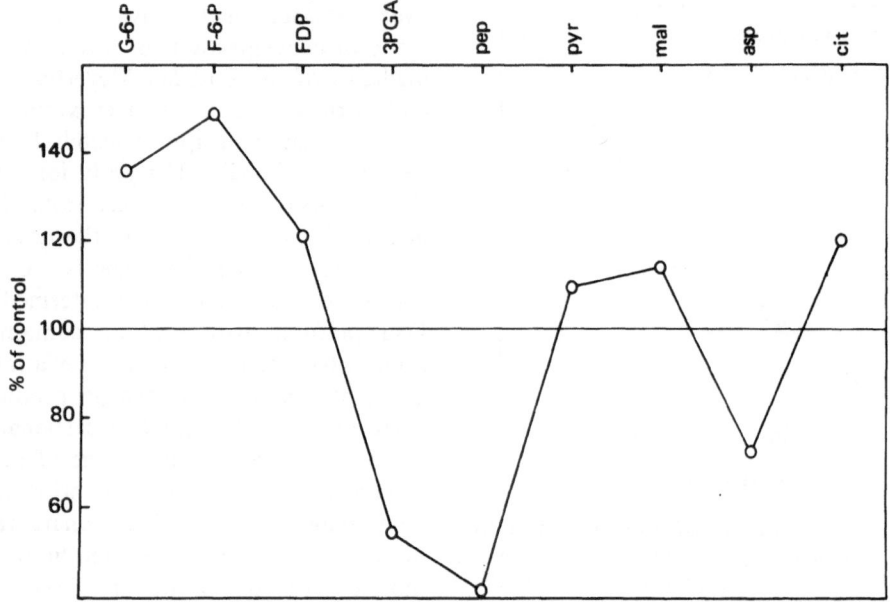

Fig. 4. Comparison of metabolite concentrations in liver perfused 1 hour with medium containing 33 mmole total CO_2 to liver perfused with medium containing 10 mmole total CO_2 (100% level). Substrate: 14 mmole glycerol and 17 mmole glucose. Methods are as previously described (MᴄDᴀɴɪᴇʟ, Lɪᴀɴɢ, and Lᴏɴɢᴍᴏʀᴇ [in press]).

G-6-P: glucose-6-phosphate   pyr: pyruvate;
F-6-P: fructose-6-phosphate   mal: malate;
FDP: fructose-1, 6-diphosphate   asp: asparate;
3PGA: 3-phosphoglycerate   cit: citrate
PEP: phosphoenolpyruvate

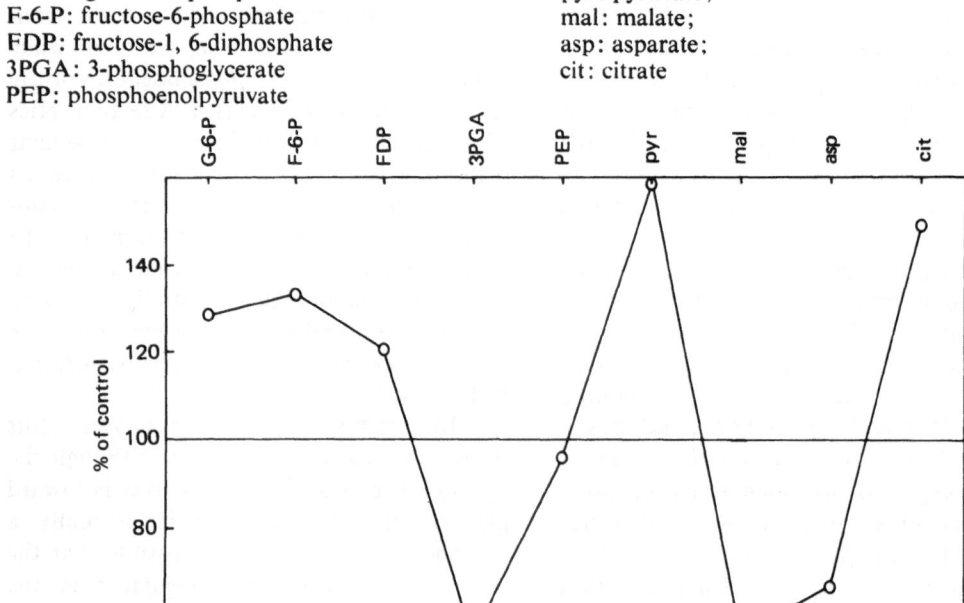

Fig. 5. Comparison of metabolite concentrations in liver perfused 1 hour with medium containing 34 mmole total CO_2 to liver perfused 1 hour with medium containing 11 mmole total CO_2 (100% level) Substrate: 5.8 mmole glucose. Methods are as previously described (MᴄDᴀɴɪᴇʟ, Lɪᴀɴɢ, and Lᴏɴɢᴍᴏʀᴇ [in press]). For abbreviations, see Figure 4.

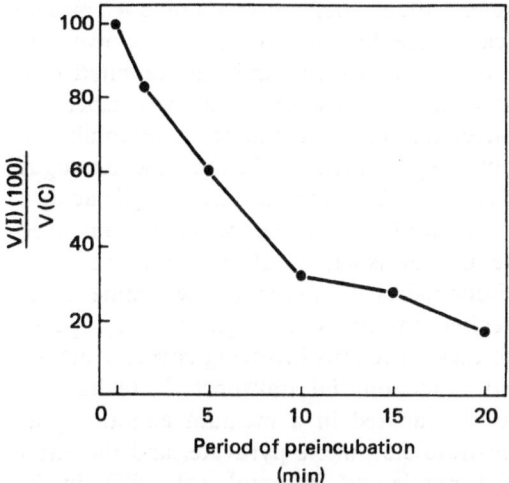

Fig. 6. Inhibition of the conversion of citrate to *cis*-aconitate by preincubation of aconitase with bicarbonate. $V(I)$ is the initial reaction rate after preincubation in assay medium containing 47 mmole HCO_3^-. $V(C)$ is the initial reaction rate after preincubation in assay medium containing 47 mmole NaCl. Methods are as previously described. MCDANIEL and LONGMORE [in press].

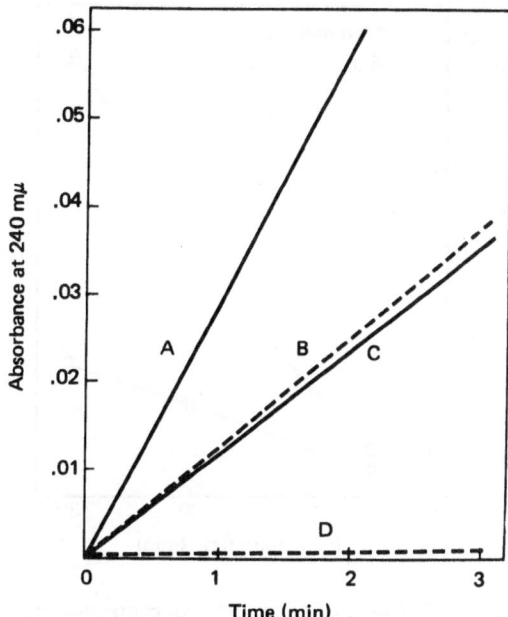

Fig. 7. Inhibition of the conversion of isocitrate to *cis*-aconitate and citrate to *cis*-aconitate by preincubation of aconitase with bicarbonate. The conversion by aconitase, preincubated 28 minutes in the presence of assay medium containing 47 mmole NaCl or in the presence of assay medium containing 47 mmole NaHCO₃, of isocitrate to *cis*-aconitate (curves A and C, respectively) and of citrate to *cis*-aconitate (curves B and D, respectively) is shown. Methods are as previously described. MCDANIEL and LONGMORE [in press].

of reactions, both intra- and extramitochondrially, surrounding pyruvate metabolism.

The marked decrease of 3-phosphoglycerate with increased total CO_2 concentration is of special interest. In studies of the NAD^+ binding site of 3-phosphoglyceraldehyde dehydrogenase, Chance and Park (CHANCE and PARK [1967]) observed that NAD^+ binding was inhibited by CO_2. No evidence was presented to indicate specifically that the presence of CO_2 would alter preferentially the formation of 3-phosphoglycerate from 3-phosphoglyceraldehyde as opposed to the reverse reaction. Inhibition of this enzyme could produce the observed increase in fructose-1,6-diphosphate, fructose-6-phosphate, glucose-6-phosphate, and glycogen since both glycerol and glucose enter into the pathway before this enzymatic step. If the reverse reaction was not inhibited by CO_2, gluconeogenesis from endogenous substrates could continue.

The observed accumulation of citrate is of interest in that citrate accumulation as a result of increased total CO_2 concentration, and independent of pH change, has also been reported by Adler [1970] in rat diaphragm, and by Simpson [1967] in rat kidney. Enhanced cytoplasmic citrate levels could increase fatty acid synthesis by providing increased acetyl CoA availability (SPENCER and LOWENSTEIN [1962]) as well as by stimulating acetyl-CoA carboxylase (MARTIN and VAGELOS [1962]), the first committed step in fatty acid synthesis. It must be remembered that citrate is made in the mitochondria but may be utilized either in the mitochondria or cytosol. In order to determine the enzymatic basis for the "CO_2 effect," we undertook *in*

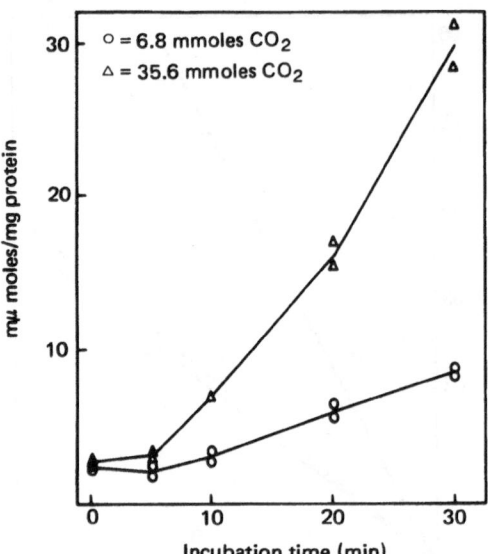

Fig. 8. Effect of total CO_2 concentration on citrate production by isolated rat liver mitochondria. Mitochondria (5 mg protein/ml) were incubated in the presence of either 6.8 mmole or 35.6 mmole total CO_2 at pH 7.3 and 5.5 mmole pyruvate, 2 mmole ATP, 2 mmole phosphate, 1 mmole MgCl₂, 250 mmole sucrose, 20 mmole Tris and bovine serum albumin, 1 mg/mg motichondrial protein at 37°C. Citrate was assayed as previously described. McDaniel, Liang, and Longmore [in press].

vitro studies of the effect of CO_2 on reactions related to citrate synthesis, utilization and mitochondrial transport. The results of these studies have suggested that the effect is not one or the other, but may involve at least two of the three possibilities.

Studies using a purified bovine liver aconitase preparation have demonstrated that bicarbonate inhibits the activity of this enzyme (McDaniel and Longmore [1971]). Figure 6 shows the inhibition of the conversion of citrate to *cis*-aconitate by preincubation of the enzyme in 47 mmole bicarbonate. Twenty-minute preincubation produces an 80% inhibition of this activity. Further studies have shown many interesting features of bovine liver aconitase, including differential inhibition of the activities of aconitase (Figure 7). Upon preincubation of

the enzyme in medium containing 47 mmole bicarbonate for 28 minutes, the conversion of citrate to cis-aconitate was inhibited to a more marked extent than was isocitrate conversion to *cis*-aconitate. The inhibition could be prevented by addition of an analogue of citrate, 1,2,3-propane tricarboxylic acid.

Other *in vitro* experiments have involved the use of isolated rat liver and rat lung mitochondria in order to determine more precisely the role CO_2 might play in regulating these reactions involving citrate synthesis and mitochondrial transport. Mitochondria were incubated in a medium containing as substrate 5.5 mmole pyruvate, and the effect of 7 mmole and 36 mmole total CO_2 in the medium at pH 7.3 on citrate levels was measured. The citrate measured was that amount present in the total incubation mixture, both intra- and extramitochondrial. As shown in Figure 8, when mitochondria were incubated for 20 minutes, three times more citrate was present in the medium containing 35.6 mmole CO_2 than in the medium containing 6.8 mmole CO_2. As lung tissue had not shown an increased acetate

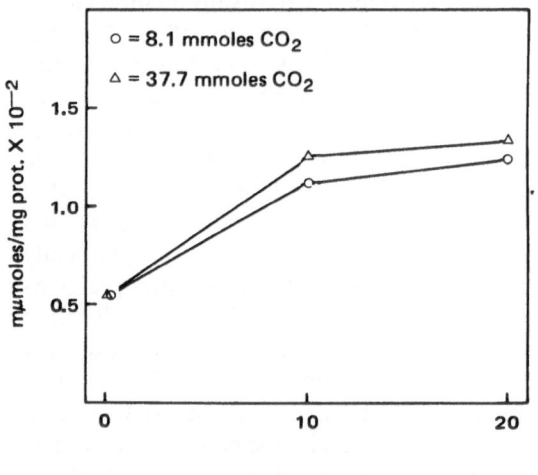

Fig. 9. Effect of total CO_2 concentration on citrate production by isolated rat lung mitochondria. Mitochondria (4 mg protein/ml) were incubated in the presence of either 8.1 mmole or 37.7 mmole total CO_2 at pH 7.3 and 5.0 mmole pyruvate. Other conditions were as given in caption to Figure 8.

conversion to fatty acids in the presence of increased CO_2 concentration, rat lung mitochondria were incubated under essentially the same conditions as liver mitochondria. No effect on citrate accumulation was observed upon raising the CO_2 from 8.1 mmole to 37.7 mmole (Figure 9). Incubation of the *liver* mitochondria in the presence of fluorocitrate, which is known to inhibit citrate oxidation, gave evidence that about 70% of the increase in citrate content was due to inhibition of citrate oxidation.

Experiments were then performed, using rat liver mitochondria, to determine the effect

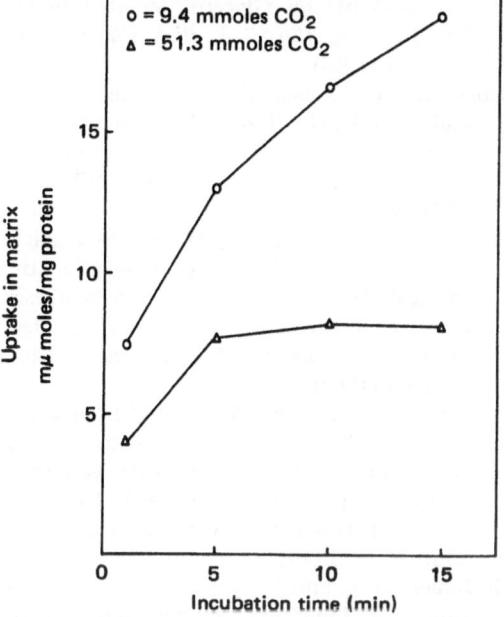

Fig. 10. Effect of total CO_2 concentration on ATP-supported citrate uptake by isolated rat liver mitochondria. Mitochondria (5 mg protein/ml) were incubated in the presence of either 9.4 mmole or 51.3 mmole total CO_2 at pH 7.3 and in the presence of 1 mmole citrate-1, 5-^{14}C, 2 mmole ATP, 30 mmole fluorocitrate, 1 μg/mg protein rotenone and 20 mmole Tris. Separate incubations were carried out in the presence of sucrose-U-^{14}C to determine non-matrix space. Mitochondria were isolated after incubation by a modification of the method of Harris and van Dam [1968] and citrate assayed as previously reported. MCDANIEL, LIANG, and LONGMORE [in press].

of CO_2 on citrate uptake during *in vitro* incubation. Mitochondria were incubated with 1,5-^{14}C-citrate under appropriate conditions, and citrate uptake into the mitochondrial matrix was determined. Matrix space was determined by use of sucrose-UL-^{14}C. Oxidation was inhibited by addition of fluorocitrate and rotenone. Intramitochondrial citrate concentrations were found to be markedly less in the presence of increased medium CO_2 concentration (Figure 10). These results indicate a decrease in citrate uptake of the mitochondria in the presence of higher CO_2 levels. Further evidence for an effect of CO_2 on citrate transport has been obtained through the addition of nigericin to the mitochondrial incubation mixture. Nigericin catalyzes K^+/H^+ exchange, thereby collapsing the pH gradient across the mitochondrial inner membrane, and inhibits anion uptake. The results of these experiments suggest that CO_2 either dissipates the pH gradient responsible for citrate or that CO_2 competes with citrate for uptake into the mitochondria.

In conclusion, increased total CO_2 concentration within the physiological range has been found to regulate both carbohydrate and lipid metabolism in the isolated perfused liver. This regulation may be produced by the effect of increased CO_2 concentration upon glyceraldehyde-3-phosphate dehydrogenase, producing decreased glycolysis, and upon citrate metabolism and mitochondrial transport, which leads to an increased extramitochondrial citrate concentration and hence increased fatty acid synthesis. This increase in fatty acid synthesis may be produced by providing greater quantities of acetyl-CoA as substrate for fatty acid synthesis and by stimulation of acetyl-CoA carboxylase. Similar effects on fatty acid synthesis and citrate metabolism have not been observed in lung tissue. This presentation does not report data which suggest that carbohydrate and lipid metabolism in kidney, another tissue capable of gluconeogenesis, may also be regulated by bicarbonate concentrations.

CO_2, the most terminal of all end

products of biochemical oxidation, may play an important role in the normal regulation of metabolism in certain tissues. Abnormal changes in acid-base balance may also markedly alter metabolism through changes in CO_2 concentration.

Acknowledgments   The authors wish to thank Miss Carolyn Niethe for her excellent technical assistance.

Bibliography

Adler, S., "The Role of pH, P_{CO_2}, and Bicarbonate in Regulating Rat Diaphragm Citrate Content." *J. Clin. Invest.*, 49:1647–55 (1970).

Anderson, W. B., Horne, R. N. and Nordlie, R. C., "Glucose Dehydrogenase Activity of Yeast Glucose 6-Phosphate Dehydrogenase. II. Kinetic Studies of the Mode of Activation of Bicarbonate, Phosphate and Sulfate." *Biochemistry*, 7:3997–4004 (1968).

Anderson, W. B. and Nordlie, R. C., "Glucose Dehydrogenase Activity of Yeast Glucose 6-Phosphate Dehydrogenase. I. Selective Stimulation by Bicarbonate, Phosphate and Sulfate." *Biochemistry*, 7:1479–85 (1968).

Bandurski, R. S. and Lipmann, F., "Studies on an Oxalacetic Carboxylase From Liver Mitochondria." *J. Biol. Chem.*, 219: 741–52 (1956).

Chance, B. and Park, J., "The Properties and Enzymatic Significance of the Enzyme-Diphosphopyridine Nucleotide Compound of 3-Phosphoglyceraldehyde Dehydrogenase." *J. Biol. Chem.*, 242:5093–5105 (1967).

Dickman, S. R. and Cloutier, A. A., "Factors Affecting the Activity of Aconitase." *J. Biol. Chem.*, 188:379–88 (1951).

Dyson, J., Anderson, W. B., and Nordlie, R. C., "Inhibitory Effect of Physiological Bicarbonate Levels on the Activities of Glucose-6-Phosphate." *J. Biol. Chem.*, 244:560–66 (1969).

Harris, E. J. and van Dam, K., "Changes of Total Water and Sucrose Space Accompanying Induced Ion Uptake or Phosphate Swelling of Rat Liver Mitochondria." *Biochem. J.*, 106: 759–66 (1968).

Hastings, A. B. and Dowdle, E. B., "Effect of Carbon Dioxide Tension on Synthesis of Liver Glycogen *In Vitro*" (trans.). *Assoc. Am. Physicians*, 73: 240–46 (1960).

Hastings, A. B. and Longmore, W. J., "Carbon Dioxide and pH as Regulatory Factors in Metabolism". *Advan. Enzyme Regul.*, 3: 147–59 (1965).

Levy, H. R., "The Interaction of Mammary Glucose-6-Phosphate Dehydrogenase with Pyridine Nucleotides and 3β-Hydroxyandrost-5-en-17-one." *J. Biol. Chem.*, 238: 775–84 (1963).

Longmore, W. J., "The Effect of Variation of CO_2 Concentration on Pyruvate Metabolism *In Vitro*." *Biochemistry*, 7:3227–31 (1968).

Longmore, W. J., Hastings, A. B., and Mahowald, T. A., "Effect of Environmental CO_2 and pH on Glycerol Metabolism by Rat Liver *In Vitro*." *J. Biol. Chem.*, 239: 1700–04 (1964).

Longmore, W. J., Hastings, A. B., Harrison, E., and Liem, H. H., "Effect of CO_2 and Cations on Fatty Acid and Cholesterol Synthesis by Liver *In Vitro*." *Amer. J. Physiol.*, 212: 221–27 (1967).

Longmore, W. J., Niethe, C. M., and McDaniel, M. L., "Effect of CO_2 Concentration on Intracellular pH and on Glycogen Synthesis from Glycerol and Glucose in Isolated Perfused Rat Liver." *J. Biol. Chem.*, 244: 6451–57 (1969).

McDaniel, M. L., Liang, A. M., and Longmore, W. J., "Effect of CO_2 Concentration on Intermediates of the Embden–Meyerhof Pathway and the Citric Acid Cycle in Isolated Perfused Rat Liver." *J. Biol. Chem.* 246: 4813–17 (1971).

McDaniel, M. L. and Longmore, W. J., "Activation and Inhibition of the Activities of Bovine Liver Aconitase." *J. Biol. Chem.* 246: 4818–24 (1971).

Martin, D. B. and Vagelos, P. R., "The Mechanism of Tricarboxylic Acid Regulation of Fatty Acid Synthesis." *J. Biol. Chem.*, 237: 1787–92 (1962).

Simpson, D. P., "Regulation of Renal Citrate Metabolism by Bicarbonate Ion and pH: Observations in Tissue Slices and Mitochondria." *J. Clin. Invest.*, 46:225–38 (1967).

Spencer, A. F. and Lowenstein, J. M., "The Supply of Precursors for the Synthesis of Fatty Acids." *J. Biol. Chem.*, 237: 3640–48 (1962).

Longmore Discussion

SIESJÖ: I was very much interested by your statement that variations in the extracellular bicarbonate concentrations were followed by corresponding changes in the intracellular bicarbonate. Is this the case with the intact liver too?

LONGMORE: We have not carried out experiments to determine such changes in the intact animal. Indeed, such experiments would be very difficult to perform. In our perfusion experiments we are maintaining a constant extracellular pH by varying in a constant ratio P_{CO_2} and $[HCO_3^-]$.

SIESJÖ: Do you consider the effect to be due to the bicarbonate concentration and not to the CO_2 concentration as such?

LONGMORE: Generally it has been found that enzymatic carboxylation reactions requiring biotin utilize the ionic species of CO_2 (HCO_3^-), while those reactions not requiring biotin use CO_2. However, this has little bearing on our study as we do not believe that the effects of change in total CO_2 concentration on metabolism that we observe necessarily involve CO_2 fixing reactions.

SIESJÖ: You have not studied the effect of an intracellular acidosis?

LONGMORE: We have shown that limited extracellular pH changes does not alter the incorporation of acetate into liver lipids while glycogen synthesis from a variety of substrates is markedly affected. However, we have not measured intracellular pH under such conditions.

SIESJÖ: Have you or anyone else studied the effect of pH changes or bicarbonate changes on the redox state of different tissues?

LONGMORE: We have not and I don't know of any such studies.

BARGETON: I would like to ask Dr. Longmore if he thinks that the regulating effect of CO_2 on the metabolism of the liver has something to do with the different blood supplies of the liver? The liver receives blood from the hepatic artery with a lower CO_2 concentration compared to blood supplied by the portal vein which contains a higher tension of CO_2.

LONGMORE: That is a very intriguing question to which I have no answer. In our system, the livers are perfused through the portal vein, which is normally the major supplier.

BARGETON: Can you tell me something about the potassium-sodium exchange in your system and whether there was any sign of anoxia?

LONGMORE: We have not studied the potassium-sodium exchange in the perfused liver. Anoxia is not a problem with our liver perfusion system as erythrocytes are present in the medium perfusing the liver to provide an adequate O_2 supply.

RAHN: Dr. Longmore, I'm very impressed with the nice data that you have brought and I'm also impressed with the large difference in CO_2 content. And now I would like to ask a more general question. How do you apply these findings, or would you be willing to speculate for what this process is normally?

LONGMORE: Prior study has demonstrated the stimulating effect of increasing CO_2 concentration on fatty acid synthesis to be linear from 10 mM to 33 mM total CO_2. We use the extreme ranges of CO_2 concentration seen clinically to make our changes greater and easier to measure. As in any control system, only small changes actually occur in the system before regulation occurs to correct for the change. Only under abnormal conditions would extracellular bicarbonate concentration be at such levels, but intracellular and mitochondrial total CO_2 concentrations may vary greatly, dependent upon the rate of cellular respiration and thus the energy needs of the cell.

RAHN: So I should turn my question around and say that your data provide a beautiful proof of our concept . . . that the pH regulating processes retain the constant bicarbonate!

LONGMORE: That would be better.

RAHN: Thank you very much. I'm happier too.

SIESJÖ: I wonder if you have any data on the rate of glycolysis in your system?

LONGMORE: We do, but I am not able to quote you figures from memory.

3. The Nature of Dynamics of Cellular Carbon Dioxide

Arthur B. DuBois

University of Pennsylvania School of Medicine
Philadelphia, Pennsylvania (19104)

My assignment was to discuss the paper by Dr. Chinard. Unfortunately, Dr. Chinard is not here. But for the last month I have been traveling through France and looking at monuments such as cathedrals, limestone caves, and bones, and began to suspect that they might have something to do with CO_2. The cathedral looked too smooth and white to be granite. I determined by scratching it with my fingernail that the cathedral was a soft material more likely to be calcium carbonate. The limestone caves had been eroded by water with CO_2 dissolved in it, and the bones were obviously composed largely of CO_2, the sole remains of our ancestors of long ago. So I have really been looking at a large pool of CO_2 in France. We have been standing, sitting, walking, or living within structures built of CO_2. This gets us back to "The nature of dynamics of cellular CO_2."

We've talked about nature; but how dynamic can a cathedral or bones be? Yet they represent the end product of a dynamic process and are still dynamic in that they are still being built up or torn down with time. So we return to the idea of CO_2 in a steady state in the cell, or in a dynamic state entering or leaving.

Now we're back to the paper that Dr. Chinard might have given. His approach is to inject a substance such as bicarbonate and study the changes in concentration down-stream over the next few seconds in the blood leaving the tissue. By this means he can determine how fast the CO_2 exchanges with the pools in the tissue. This dynamic process lasts one second, rather than a million years, as did the dynamic process of the bones, or a hundred million years as did the dynamic process of the deposition of silicates and calcium carbonate in fossils.

The steady-state concentrations, and the input and output of substances to and from that steady-state concentration, would be studied with the type of isotopes which Dr. Chinard has used. In this, the cell puts out as much CO_2 as it produces, as CO_2 dissolved in water. CO_2 combines with water as H_2CO_3; the latter dissociates into H^+ and HCO_3^- ions. In this steady state, concentrations are neither rising nor falling in the cell as a whole, although substances are moving back and forth across the membrane. But some cells do seem to separate the hydrogen ion, putting it out at one side, perhaps in exchange for sodium and potassium ions, while bicarbonate ions are put out on the other side of the cell, perhaps in exchange for chloride ions. In these cells, the CO_2 excreted lowers the P_{CO_2} and the cell accepts CO_2 from the blood to continue the process, provided carbonic anhydrase is present. Such cells can pump ions, and examples of this are in the production of gastric acid, cerebro-spinal fluid, the aqueous humor in the eye,

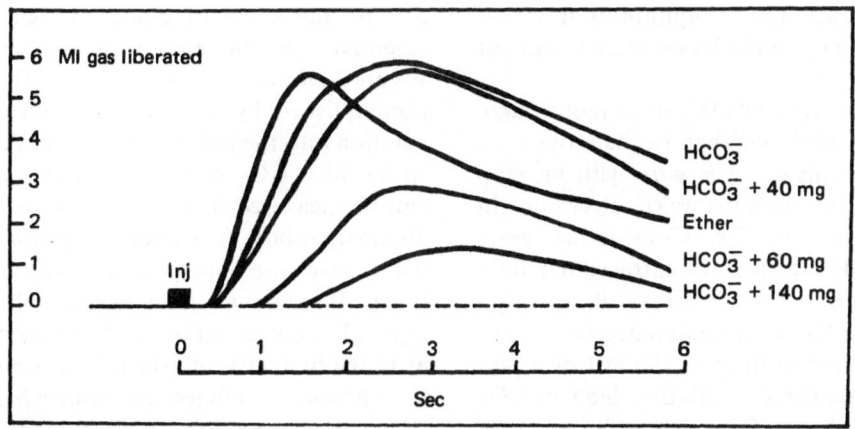

Fig. 1. Measurement of the evolution of gas in the alveoli after injection into the pulmonary artery of a solution of ether (left curve) or bicarbonate (second curve), or of bicarbonate after different doses of acetazolamide.

Figure 1. reprinted with permission from K. A. Feisal, M. A. Sackner, and A. B. DuBois, *J. Clin. Invest.*, 42:24 (1963).

the production of gas in the swim bladder, and the acidification of urine in the renal tubule.

So much for the steady state. In the unsteady state, which is the topic assigned in this period, we ought to talk about a transient increase or decrease of total CO_2. If there were an increase of CO_2 this would produce a rapid increase of hydrogen ion and bicarbonate ion concentration, particularly if carbonic anhydrase were present in the cells. This increase would exceed the cell's ability to diffuse or exchange hydrogen ion and/or bicarbonate ion. If the cells in a steady state were just able to diffuse enough hydrogen ion through the membrane to maintain a given pH, then extra hydrogen ion would accumulate in the cell with the transient rise in CO_2, and this could not pass through the membrane sufficiently fast. Since only the red cell is well buffered, by hemoglobin, only the blood really accepts CO_2 as if there were an *in vivo* titration or dissociation curve. The other tissues in the body do not seem to be able to buffer this so fast and therefore do not seem to be able to accept as much CO_2 because the hydrogen ion cannot be fully buffered within the cell, and it cannot diffuse out of the cell within the first few

seconds. Then as a new steady state is reached, after more than 10 or 20 minutes, hydrogen and bicarbonate ions diffuse out of the ordinary cells and body tissues. These then take part in buffering, giving an *in vivo* titration curve, or dissociation curve of the body, that is different from the one that occurs during the first few minutes. Examples of these states are found in rebreathing expired air. For example, if you breathe for 10 minutes in a bag that contains O_2 but let the CO_2 build up in the body, the CO_2 space in the body seems to be that of the blood and not that of the whole body. Even though the CO_2 is produced in the body tissues, it is poorly buffered there; the increases of intracellular hydrogen ion stimulate respiratory efforts, a result found when rebreathing in a bag. This hydrogen ion accumulation also prevents the building up of CO_2 as bicarbonate inside the tissue cells, except in the red blood cells and plasma. Another example of this would be as follows: If a single breath of CO_2-enriched air were inspired, the CO_2 molecules that passed into the lung tissue would raise the hydrogen ion concentration in these cells and in the red cells. But the red cells would not diffuse all their hydrogen ion to the plasma by the time they had left the lung capillaries. Later, equilibration would change the P_{CO_2} in the blood after it had left the lungs.

Before I left Philadelphia a month ago, Dr. Forster told me that he had obtained evidence for this effect *in vitro* with his stop flow apparatus, using a P_{CO_2} electrode (in collaboration with Dr. Constantine years ago) or a pH electrode in extracellular fluid (in collaboration with Dr. Crandall, recently). He reported this at a conference in Scandinavia about a month ago. The gist of it was that if he combined a solution high in CO_2 with red cells low in CO_2, the resulting change in P_{CO_2} with time had a fast phase, but a slow phase as well. If he followed the change in pH of the extracellular fluid with a stop-flow apparatus and a pH electrode, the readjustment of pH was very much slower. His interpretation of the slow phase was that it was due to the CO_2 re-equilibration. In a one-second dynamic process we deal with the exchange between substances entering and leaving a pool. This can be studied not only using isotope tracers à la Chinard, but also by measurements of the gross changes as in the following figures.

As the speed of blood gas reactions is essential to the function of the lung capillary, Figure 1 shows a direct measure of that speed accomplished by injection of a bicarbonate solution into the pulmonary artery. The speed with which CO_2 comes off in the capillary can be measured if the animal is enclosed in an air-tight box. A pressure gauge on the box will register the volume of gas evolved in the lungs. If ether, an inert gas in solution, is injected, it comes off in the gas phase rapidly, as in the first curve on the left. If bicarbonate is injected, it comes off somewhat more slowly because of the time it takes to dissociate and to form CO_2. It has to go into the red cell for that purpose.

If you add a small amount of a carbonic anhydrase inhibitor, acetazolamide, you can slow up the rate at which CO_2 comes off, indicating that the red cell is a limiting factor. Yet as much comes off as did before until as you add more acetazolamide to inhibit to a greater extent; then less CO_2 comes off, stopping at a point when the blood leaves the capillary. Finally, still more acetazolamide inhibits CO_2 output still further. In other words, *in vivo* there is not enough carbonic

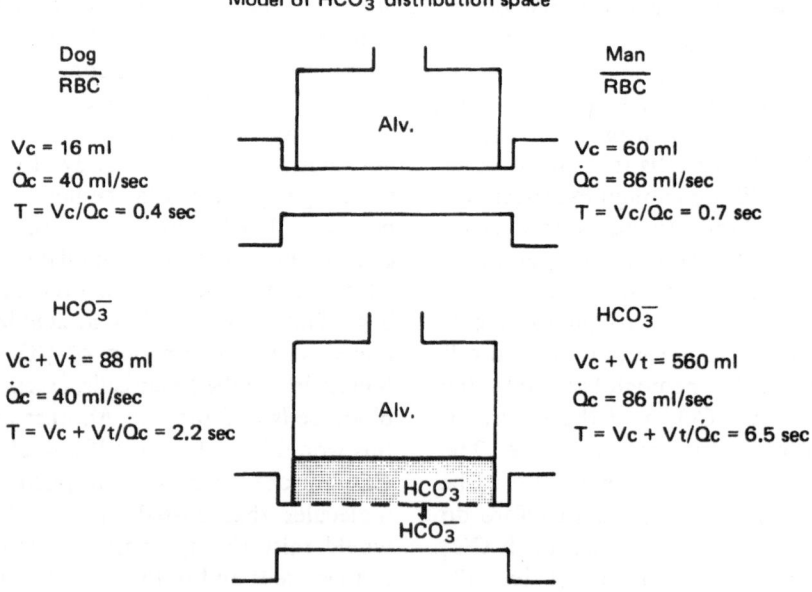

Model of HCO_3^- distribution space

Fig. 2. Tissue space for CO_2 in dogs, and values calculated for man.

anhydrase, when inhibited, to complete this reaction within the red cell as far as the evolution of CO_2 in the lung capillary. But, according to Forster, the hydrogen ion has not had enough time to diffuse out of the red cell or into the red cell to reach equilibrium, even with no inhibition of carbonic anhydrase, and so further P_{CO_2} changes will occur after the blood has left the capillary.

Figure 2 shows the capacity of the lung tissue for CO_2, i.e. its distribution space. This can be measured either by this bicarbonate injection method or by Chinard's method, both methods indicating that there is some dilution space for CO_2 in the lung tissue and that CO_2 behaves as if there is a pool with which it can equilibrate in a single passage in 1 or 2 sec. The size of this pool is given in the figures in the columns in the illustration. The volume of capillary blood in man would be about 86 cc, the volume of the tissue and capillary blood together would have the space equivalent to about $\frac{1}{2}$ kg, and the passage time, or the duration of passage, would be about 6 sec into and out of this pool, instead of about 1 sec, which is the duration that the red cell spends in its passage through the lung capillary.

I see that there will be more on the program later about tissue spaces, mathematical models, and bones, so perhaps my talk has been something of an introduction to these topics. The topic of dynamics of CO_2 in the cells is now open for discussion.

DuBois Discussion

SEVERINGHAUS: The question I would like to ask is, Are you proposing that there is a reversed gradient produced when blood passes through the lung during exchange because of this delay of hydrogen ion transfer? And is this related to the Ween effect that a number of people have been studying, in which case there is a nonexchanging lung and in which the P_{CO_2} in the nonexchanging alveolus is found to be higher than that in the blood?

DUBOIS: I wasn't suggesting a reversed gradient, but I believe the implication is that there is

simply a delay in the equilibration which would occur and that this delay produces a subsequent re-equilibration in blood after it has left the lungs. This would give an artifact in blood samples drawn from the artery in the transient, unsteady state, as when you have a sudden change in P_{CO_2} in the lung. This is Forster's conclusion, or his interpretation. I'm not sure of the term "Ween effect." Which effect is this?

SEVERINGHAUS: This is the protein charge effect on the capillary wall due to the fact that the endothelium is supposed to be negatively charged. I think there are many people here who have worked on this; I have not. Perhaps Dr. Cherniak or others would like to speak of this. Before we go to that, could you tell us in which direction the P_{CO_2} gradient would be expected to be between the arterial blood and alveolar gas during gas exchange, because of the delay of hydrogen ion exchange?

DUBOIS: If you raise the CO_2 in the lung to about the level of mixed venous P_{CO_2}, you would essentially acidify the inside of the red cell. That hydrogen ion would become buffered by hemoglobin, but perhaps not comfortably so, in that some of the hydrogen ion would prefer to leave the red cell if it could. Later on, after the blood leaves the lung capillary, the subsequent changes in plasma P_{CO_2} and pH depend on which molecules or ions move across the membrane, and this has not yet been published.

SEVERINGHAUS: But during normal gas exchange the same process should occur, shouldn't it? Because when you give up CO_2 from the red cell going through the lung, most of that CO_2 has to be generated in the red cell and thus there would be a relative tendency for hydrogen ion from the plasma to diffuse into the red cell later on.

DUBOIS: Yes, I see what you mean. I'm not sure in which direction this would be during the steady state. It would be rather a small effect. Perhaps some of the others here who have worked on these gradients could help us out.

GURTNER: It seems possible that delayed equilibration could cause these differences observed, especially if you are measuring gas in one case and comparing that with a measurement made with a CO_2 electrode in the blood made many minutes afterward. We have tried to look at this by taking a mass spectrometer and attaching a small capillary tubing covered with a membrane with which we can then measure both gas and blood, or tissue and blood, or cerebral spinal fluid and blood, and we'll talk a little bit about this tomorrow. The advantage to this is that these techniques are extremely rapid and we have had time constants on the order of a second, and when we do this (we haven't done this in the lung but we have done it between the cerebral spinal fluid and the blood), we find that these differences appear even with this rapid method of analysis, so because of this, we think the CO_2 differences observed are not due to delayed equilibration of hydrogen ion across the red blood cell membrane.

We measured in the cerebrospinal fluid, we measured in the blood coming out of the sagittal sinus and in the jugular vein. They were steady-state measurements but they were measurements made in the flowing blood in the vessel itself so that the delay from the capillary to the vein would just be the transient delay due to the flowing blood, not a delay due to someone's drawing a sample and putting it in an electrode.

DUBOIS: There are two problems to that: One problem is the steady state and the other is the time it takes the blood to get to your sampling probe. I wonder whether to do this mixed venous type of equilibration, you might pick up the difference if you went to the lung and put your probe in the left atrium and then took a breath of CO_2. This would be stressing the system to the point where you might begin to see a measurable difference if there really is a delay in equilibration, but you're still dealing with a transit time of 5 sec from the capillary to the pulmonary vein.

GURTNER: Again, we didn't do this in the lung yet. Would you say that the transit time is that long—5 sec—on that order?

DUBOIS: For the whole lung, I suppose; I'm more used to dealing with dogs and transit time in the pulmonary artery of the dog is 1 sec, in the capillaries it's about 4/10 sec, in the pulmonary veins it would be about another second. In man it's about, I suppose, two or three times as long, so you'd be dealing with a time interval on the order of 4 or 5 sec.

GURTNER: In the original measurements made by Dr. Ferrigan and myself in Dr. Rahn's department, the gradients we talk about are between alveolar gas and mixed venous blood, so I wouldn't think that we would pick up any artifact due to breathing CO_2. Other people have measured similiar gradients between arterial blood and alveolar gas, but I think that the only nonequilibration that might be pertinent in this case would be the CO_2 coming from the tissue into the blood.

DUBOIS: The question would be as follows: If you measured the pH of a sample of blood and followed it over the course of time after it had left the lung, would you find a change with time due to the re-equilibration between the inside and the outside of the red cell. That experiment might be worth doing with pH electrodes. Take a sample from the pulmonary vein and follow it. I don't know how fast you could get it. It you could get quite close to the capillary you might find some changes.

SIESJÖ: When studying acid base metabolism in a tissue like the brain, the blood parameters we are looking for are the mean capillary pH and the mean capillary CO_2 tension. And now the only thing we can do under ordinary circumstances is to measure arterial blood and venous blood and try to integrate over the capillary length. This can probably be done under normal circumstances with no inhibition of carbonic anhydrase, but when we have carbonic anhydrase in the animal, then the question is one of how the mean capillary values across tissue relate to the values which you measure in a sample which has reached a steady state?

OTIS: I believe that the change in hydrogen ion concentration would additionally give an amount of CO_2 and would be greater in the presence of carbonic anhydrase than with carbonic anhydrase absent. If the hydration of CO_2 is the rate-limiting step, if you had no hydration of CO_2, then there would be no change in hydrogen ion concentration, so the more the reaction is slowed down, the less, I believe, will be the magnitude of a transient in hydrogen ion concentration change.

SEVERINGHAUS: Could I also agree with what Dr. Otis has just said? In reference to Dr. Siesjö's question, when Diamox has been added direct to the brain, the capillary will be more alkaline than normal because there is not time for the additional CO_2 metabolized and added to the blood in the brain to be generated into hydrogen ion. Nevertheless, the extracellular fluid in the brain is more acid than normal, as seen by an electrode sitting on the surface of the brain, and this indicates that the hydrogen ion is what is generated by metabolism, not CO_2 as a gas.

LOESCHKE: Dr. DuBois, can you give me any data about the exchange of bicarbonate between interstitial fluid and the cells? Let's imagine that we can do an experiment with a rectangular increase of bicarbonate concentration in blood and that we know approximately how much time it takes until blood will exchange with extracellular fluid. What would be the half-time of exchange with cells?

DUBOIS: Dr. Loeschke, by convention I believe that in red cells the half-time is thought to be on the order of 1/10 sec or 2/10 sec and that in most other cells, including the lung cells, it is thought to be considerably longer, on the order of at least several seconds. I don't have any personal data on this, but I remember from Dr. Chinard's work that when he injected bicarbonate and followed the curve in the blood leaving the tissue, he found that ordinarily bicarbonate equilibrated with a space in the lungs, which indicated that the bicarbonate was entering the bicarbonate pool of the lung tissue. Now when he gave a carbonic anhydrase inhibitor, he abolished the pool into which the bicarbonate was passing, and subsequent experiments allowed him to interpret what we interpreted it, too, from our injections of bicarbonate—that the passage of bicarbonate from the blood into the lung tissue cells was by means of the so-called facilitated diffusion of Jacobs, wherein the CO_2 leaves the bicarbonate, passes through the cell membrane, and reacts with the lung tissue cells through the aid of carbonic anhydrase to form bicarbonate in the lung tissue cells. So the large space I pictured for bicarbonate in the lung in fact is only present when carbonic anhydrase is present in the lung tissue. Dr. Chinard called attention to some measurements of two or three different investigators

of carbonic anhydrase in the lung tissue that showed it to be present. Therefore, I can't give you the figure for the rate of passage of bicarbonate directly across the lung cell membrane, but I believe it's slow since in the absence of carbonic anhydrase he did not find participation in this pool over the course of several seconds. And I think that's the conventional view of people I've talked to who are studying the passage of ions through cell membranes—that the red cell is an exception in that the bicarbonate passes through it quickly but that in the case of other cell membranes, it doesn't seem to.

OTIS: Did I understand from Dr. Longmuir that the liver cell also might be permeable to bicarbonate?

LONGMUIR: Yes, that's our feeling.

OTIS: Then it could behave like a red cell in those terms, exchange bicarbonate for chloride, or something like that?

DUBOIS: But I think he mentioned 20 min.

LONGMUIR: That's right. It's a process that requires approximately 20 min to establish equilibrium for the concentrations we were looking at. It's slow, but it's there.

DUBOIS: Oh, yes. Well that would be the same for other ions, that they all get there eventually. It's just a matter of how long.

LONGMUIR: Well the liver is certainly a leaky organ as compared to anything else. It's much different than it would be for a muscle or plasma membrane, I'm sure.

FITZGERALD: I'm just wondering and I'd like to ask Dr. DuBois a question. Certainly CO_2 affects the permeability of the blood brain barrier—at least there's evidence to that effect—and I'm wondering whether there is any evidence to the effect that molecular CO_2 influences the permeability of the red blood cell membrane, specifically to the hydrogen ion. It seems rather odd, but I wonder if there is any evidence in that direction.

DUBOIS: I haven't heard any information about it. If somebody here has some information, it would be worth a thousand guesses. Offhand, I don't exactly see why CO_2 should affect the permeability of the red cell membrane to hydrogen ion. Does anybody know?

SEVERINGHAUS: I'd like to ask Dr. Fitzgerald what the evidence is that CO_2 affects the permeability of the blood brain barrier.

FITZGERALD: Well, there was some evidence in about mid-1950 that it did increase the incorporation of drugs, acetazolomide, some dyes and also some viruses. There were no measurements made of the arterial P_{CO_2}. These experiments were done on rats, and the exposure concentrations were rather large but the exposure durations very brief. I think they were 15% to 20% CO_2 which, of course, is very large, but the exposure times were 1/2 min or 15 sec. I believe Margaret Lavendar was one of the authors; I can give you the reference more exactly later on.

SEVERINGHAUS: Did they make any determination of what part of the blood brain barrier was more permeable? Was it just the choroid plexus, for example; did they have any way of demonstrating whether it was flow-limited?

FITZGERALD: Well, I don't think there were any flow-limitation measurements and I forget the precise details of the experimentation. With reference to the virus, however, apparently there was some central nervous, some more cortical involvement, because a much higher percentage of these animals were paralyzed than the nonexposed animals. However, as I recall, most of the effect was in the medulla.

COURNAND: In view of the complexity of the phenomena involved in the equilibrium between air and blood that you have presented us, I would like to know what your opinion is about the various methods of lung and bag system that were used in the past to reach a plateau in order to define the partial pressure of CO_2 in the incoming mixed venous blood. I would like to have your answer, and I would like to put a rider to my question later.

DUBOIS: Well, as I understand the position, there's a difference between the blood samples drawn and subsequently analyzed and the gas samples analyzed showing equilibrium, particularly when there has been a fairly large CO_2 production, as in exercise for a transient change due to breathing a breath of CO_2 to reach this equilibrium point. And I don't know the explanation for this phenomenon. The explanation that would follow from Forster's phenomenon and which he has implied to me might be the possible explanation of the phenomenon, although I don't think he's determined it quantitatively yet. If this be true—that the lack of equilibration of hydrogen ion is the cause of this effect—then that means that the blood sample is in error and that the gas bag is correct, as far as the P_{CO_2} goes. Until it's determined as to what the mechanism is, I wouldn't be able to say which is correct, the gas bag or the blood. Right now I think it's a very interesting turn of events because the question is left hanging at this point and remains to be answered.

COURNAND: You are probably very familiar with the fact that about 40 years ago the method of lung bag was used to obtain an idea of the CO_2 tension of the blood (mixed venous blood). Now the extraordinary thing is that whether you start with a high CO_2 in the bag or a low, you reach a plateau usually within about 15 sec. I think the method became popular again about five to six years ago.

I'm strongly puzzled by the fact that you did reach a plateau at a different level of CO_2 to start with in the bag, that you used a figure of P_{CO_2} that was finally obtained on the plateau and measured a blood flow for so long (using, of course, a sample from the arterial blood and CO_2 output), and that these figures coincide remarkably with those that have been obtained with more exact methods, methods more direct of defining the blood flow. I have always been tremendously puzzled by the fact that you could use these figures in a system of extraordinary complexity and yet that they would seem to correspond to the actual blood flow to the lung.

DUBOIS: Yes, I would agree with you. I remember reading those papers that you had written with Richards and Strauss, and I was very impressed by that rebreathing method. In Fenn's lab we used it, and so I entered this field through the gas phase myself and I tend to believe the gas bag, until somebody shows that the gas bag is wrong. But that would suggest that everybody who did bloods gave the wrong P_{CO_2} because they analyzed it too late; but on the other hand, the blood gas contents would be correct because the gas can neither enter nor leave, so the Fick would be correct when done by blood samples. The only question hanging, really, is whether the partial pressures measured in the blood after the blood's been drawn and has stood around for several seconds are equal to those that were present in the blood after it actually left the site of gas exchange. The implication of this delayed hydrogen ion equilibration across cell membranes would be that the blood sample measurements are incorrect, particularly in an unsteady state. But since I've been away from Philadelphia for a month, I don't know what Forster's last word is on this at the moment. I'll have to go back to find out.

OTIS: I have some difficulty in seeing how the hydrogen ion diffusibility could be limiting. If bicarbonate and chloride can exchange freely, won't the hydrogen ions take care of themselves?

DUBOIS: Initially the hydrogen ion would bind with the hemoglobin. The data that Forster had show that there was a slow phase. To explain this, one would have to say that hydrogen ion is not happy in its union with hemoglobin and would like to leave and get out of the red cell. This state of unhappiness would be reflected in the transmembrane potential as a Donnan equilibrium. This potential represents a state of disequilibrium and would like to decay if it could. If the hydrogen ions are in different concentrations across the membrane, they presumably would tend to seek the same level, and I suppose there is a tendency for them to migrate from a higher to a lower concentration.

OTIS: I'd like some comment on whether these crazy gradients that some of us have measured between lung and blood are what you might call real or apparent. That is, is there really a difference between the P_{CO_2} in the blood, the bulk of the blood, the bulk P_{CO_2} of the blood, and the bulk of the gas phase, or is this some local effect, or the result of delayed reactions and things that happened before or haven't happened yet? I think it makes some difference in one's feeling about it in terms of the thermodynamic requirement because if you think of pumping the CO_2 from one level pressure to another you can calculate the thermodynamic work required, and the thing that's going in the other direction, of course, is the

diffusion of CO_2 down this gradient, so we would have to match the pumping of CO_2 with the diffusing capacity of the lung for CO_2. I don't know the answer to all these questions. . . .

GURTNER: Could I break in here? I think it's an appropriate time. As regards the difference between gas bag and blood sample, it is our feeling that both gas bag and blood sample are right, and that there's a specific mechanism, localized, having to do with a charged membrane. In this microscopic environment ions such as hydrogen ions are attracted toward these negative charges. The pH in its microenvironment is lower (that of the hydrogen ion is higher), and if the bicarbonate is somewhat similar in a flowing system to the way it is in the blood, this bicarbonate can associate with the hydrogen ion and cause P_{CO_2} in the local environment of these capillary walls (which only extend, say, 10Å or 20Å) to be higher than in the bulk phase. It is with this local environment of P_{CO_2} that the alveolar capillary membrane and alveolus are in equilibrium. Now we further think—and we have some evidence for this—that this is a general phenomenon that occurs in tissue as well, and we have measurements of cerebrospinal fluid and blood. To turn to the thermodynamic requirements for the system: this is a reversible system; as blood passes through the blood exposed to these charges, the CO_2 goes up; after it gets away from the charges the CO_2 goes down. So it's the kind of a process that you analyze with the first law of thermodynamics, not the second law of thermodynamics. It's a reversible process, so it is, I think, thermodynamically sound to maintain that this can happen in a local environment.

DUBOIS: Dr. Gortner, various questions have been asked me about the mechanism you propose, and perhaps I don't fully understand these questions about the mechanism, but one is, Which is the prime mover? It seems here that since CO_2 is the prime mover, it would hardly be the end product also affected, unless it's in a positive feedback loop with further energy put into the system. The other question is whether, due to the fact that CO_2 is so highly diffusible, it is possible to maintain a P_{CO_2} gradient.

GURTNER: In answer to your second question, we feel that the CO_2 gradient occurs within the capillary due to a gradient of hydrogen ion caused by these charges, and also a gradient, a nonsteady state (perhaps I shouldn't say that), caused by the association of bicarbonate with the hydrogen ion and attracted by these charges, which results in the production of CO_2. We envision this as something that occurs in a manner analogous to the reaction in a fuel cell into which you continuously put in reactants, in which the reaction goes on and you are observing it. It is not an equilibrium phenomenon and we have evidence that if you stop flow, the CO_2 does come to equilibrium. So we're not trying to make a perpetual motion machine here.

SEVERINGHAUS: You say the prime mover; in that sense, is it the heart?

GURTNER: The blood flow, indeed, is keeping the reaction off equilibrium so what's limiting, us here is the transit time through the capillary (which Dr. DuBois said is 4/10 sec) which, at least in our calculations, turned out to be on an order of magnitude such that these chemical reactions, this coupling of chemical reaction and diffusion could not reach its equilibrium state.

SIESJÖ: Dr. Gurtner, your theories here remind me very much of the discussions of the surface pH. I was just wondering what sort of charge density you visualized in the capillaries.

GURTNER: For example, if there were a potential, as on the red blood cell, of 17 mv negative, the red blood cell wall would be 17 mv negative to the bulk phase of the solution. Now this would account for a pH difference of about 3/10 of a pH unit. From the Nernst equation with a 62-mv potential difference, one would get a 10-fold difference of hydrogen ion concentrations. From our calculations, all we need for this sort of gradient to exist is a difference on the order of, say, 10 mv, and there is evidence (although it isn't well known) of streaming potential in blood vessels, especially veins. Sawyer, a biophysicist and surgeon, showed that the potential difference between blood vessels, veins, between the walls and the bulk phase, is on the order of hundreds of millivolts, not just the tens of millivolts. They measured streaming potentials that were on the order of 2, 3, and 10 to 15 mv, and by the usual Smolchovsky relationship that relates streaming potential to zeta potential, they would calculate zeta potentials that would be on the order of hundreds of millivolts.

DUBOIS: One question is whether, say, 3/10 of a pH unit would produce enough CO_2 to cause the amount of CO_2 seen in blood or the lungs or account for the difference between them. The actual hydrogen ion concentration is 10^{-7} moles. It would be rather a small number of hydrogen ions, and the number of CO_2 molecules that you can get is roughly equivalent to the number of hydrogen ions which displaced them, so offhand it would seem that this would not account for the number of CO_2 molecules you need to raise the P_{CO_2} in the lungs.

GURTNER: Well, that's why Dr. Severinghaus mentioned the Ween effect. The Ween effect is the effect of an electric field on the dissociation of a protein. If you put a protein in an electric field, say an electrophoresis apparatus or something similar to that, and you turn on a voltage difference, the protein will tend to move according to its charge. Now the proteins are negatively charged and around these negative charges are counter ions—hydrogen ion, sodium, potassium, etc. When you put this in a field the counter-ions tend to move faster than the protein itself and so the electric field would pull the counter-ions away from the protein. Now some of these counter-ions are hydrogen ion, and since the proteins are weak acids the proteins tend to exhibit hydrogen ion dissociation; they act as buffers. They give off hydrogen ions and essentially this Ween effect would, because of proteins, act as a source of hydrogen ion, so when you put a protein in the vicinity of a negative charge you don't just get a couple of hydrogen ions out, you get a lot of hydrogen ions out, because the hydrogen ion acts as a buffer. So this is absolutely necessary for the working of the hypothesis and it's considered in the 1969 paper. Also, we think we did some experiments with ion exchange membranes, which are artificial charged membranes, and found CO_2 differences across ion exchange membranes when we flowed bicarbonate solution. So I think you're absolutely right, we need a source of hydrogen ion; and the source of hydrogen ion is a protein mediated by this Ween effect.

SEVERINGHAUS: Dr. Gurtner, have you measured the pH of fluids such as a mock extracellular fluid in contact with the surface of the lung to see whether that, in fact, is more acid than the venous blood entering the lung?

GURTNER: We haven't done this. If this is going on in a very, very small volume of blood, say with a thickness of the order of 25 Å, and we were measuring the bulk, say the effluent coming out . . .

SEVERINGHAUS: I mean a small pocket of fluid, perhaps a few microliters of fluid sitting on the surface of the lung, might come to hydrogen ion equilibrium with this surface rather than with the bulk of blood leaving the lung.

GURTNER: Well, hydrogen ion is in equilibrium, so the hydrogen ion would be higher near the charges, where it fell under the influence of the charge, than in the bulk phase of the solution. Now when you got away from that charge and the electric potential was less, hydrogen ion would be less—it actually is a Donnan potential—so that you have to consider in this case electrochemical equilibrium rather than just chemical concentration.

LOESCHKE: Dr. Gurtner, I have some impression that there may be some one error in play in your conclusions, and I do agree that potential of the proteins, the surface potential, would drag hydrogen ions in to the surface, but now I think there should be a difference stated between what we call hydrogen ion concentration and hydrogen ion activity. I agree that hydrogen ion concentration would increase in this spot, but in this potential, hydrogen ions are fixed by the potential, which means that they would not as easily react as in acid and give the chemical action which you postulate. Therefore, I think hydrogen ions are directed to the surface of the protein just because their activity is diminished by the potential. Would you tell me what you think about this?

GURTNER: If you look in Kocholsky and Curran's book on irreversible thermodynamics and biophysics you will see a section devoted to activities and electrochemical potentials and in that they show that chemical reactions occur proportional to concentration, so assuming that, in this case we have a Donnan equilibrium of hydrogen ion, the hydrogen ion activity is the same near the charge as in the bulk phase. The concentration is higher, and the chemical reaction will occur in proportion to the concentration rather than in proportion to the activity. This is very nicely and elegantly presented by Kocholsky in this book.

KELLOGG: I'm not sure I'm understanding very much of this, but it seems to me that if there is a negative charge on the membrane attracting an hydrogen ion, it should also be repelling bicarbonate ion. To what extent will these two effects cancel out in affecting the equilibrium of CO_2?

GURTNER: That's right. I am sorry to have taken so much time on this. It isn't my doing, but I will give you the complete model now and bore everyone to death with it. What we postulate is that when blood enters the capillary it's exposed to an electrical field due to these negative charges. This also affects the protein and the Ween effect occurs, causing the hydrogen ion to come to electro-chemical equilibrium almost instantaneously, before the bicarbonate can move away from the charges, before it can be repelled. Therefore, the concentration of hydrogen ion is higher than it is at equilibrium, but as relates to the activity of bicarbonate, let's say that the hydrogen ion can then associate with this bicarbonate that has not yet reached its equilibrium and produce CO_2. Now this all takes place in time and if we then stop the blood in the capillary we would allow everything to come to equilibrium, in which case we would have a Donnan equilibrium for hydrogen ion, a Donnan equilibrium for bicarbonate and we'd have no difference for CO_2 because it isn't charged. It's something which requires time and chemical reaction to occur. This is why we think it is thermodynamically sound.

BROWN: If there is a negative charge on the capillary wall, then how do you account for the fact that one can explain the distribution of sodium chloride, or potassium for that matter, between extracellular and intra-cellular fluid on the basis of a capillary wall that has no charge and is characterized strictly by Donnan distribution?

GURTNER: All a Donnan distribution means is that the concentration is different because there's a difference in electrical potential.

Now if you're measuring between a place of zero electrical potential and another place of zero electrical potential with a barrier that's charged in between, and the system is at chemical equilibrium, you'll measure the same concentration between the two places of zero chemical potential. You'll measure a different concentration in the places where there is an electrical potential, and throughout the whole system the electrochemical potential will be the same.

BROWN: But I think if you calculate—for example, if you plug the values for sodium outside and inside and to the nearest equation—you come out across with zero voltage for sodium between extracellular and intracellular fluids.

GURTNER: Well, what we're talking about here is fixed charge potentials, not diffusion potentials and, as a matter of fact, since you bring this up, I'm sure you're aware of the work of Gilbert Ling, who doesn't believe in active transport and who says that all of sodium and potassium differences across cells is purely passive; the action potentials are allegedly due instead to the differences in binding powers of proteins for various ions, which come about due to conformational changes in proteins, so these things have been considered. In fact, Dr. Ling's written a book about this.

SEVERINGHAUS: Perhaps another answer to Dr. Brown is that you can't measure the sodium in the place where the charge is negative, which is just at the capillary endothelium. You measure on one side or in the bulk, and there it's the same, but there is a boundary layer place where there would be a depletion of sodium. It's only because an accretion of hydrogen ion occurs that the product of hydrogen and bicarbonate are increased; therefore, there is more H_2CO_3 locally that can then diffuse as a new species. With sodium, however, you won't see any difference as a result of this local charge; it would just be repelled from that area.

BROWN: Well, it is true that you get field effects across membrane, but these field effects are usually negligible when the ionic strength of the solution on both sides of the membrane are reasonable. You can demonstrate a voltage across a membrane, but in general (at least with the membranes I am familiar with), one has to work with low ionic strength solution so that you don't saturate the sites in the membrane.

4. Relationships between Blood and Extravascular P_{CO_2}, $[H^+]$ and $[HCO_3^-]$ in Lung, Cerebrospinal Fluid, and Brain

Gail H. Gurtner, B. Burns, A. M. Sciuto, and D. G. Davies

Department of Environmental Medicine
The Johns Hopkins University
615 North Wolfe Street, Baltimore, Maryland 21205

Several investigators have observed, under conditions of little or no gas exchange, that large differences in P_{CO_2} (ΔP_{CO_2}) occur between mixed venous blood and alveolar gas (JONES, et al. [1969]; GURTNER, SONG, and FARHI [1969]; DENNISON, et al. [1969]; GUYATT, et al. [1971]. Gurtner and his colleagues have found that ΔP_{CO_2} was related to both $[H^+]$ and $[HCO_3^-]$ activity by the mixed venous blood. They developed a model explaining their results that involves a coupling of bulk flow, diffusion, and chemical reaction near a negatively charged capillary wall. This model was considered in their article that appeared in *Respiration Physiology* and will be considered only briefly at the present time. The model postulates an intra-capillary H^+ difference due to a negatively charged capillary wall. There is a large amount of evidence that walls of blood vessels carry fixed negative charges. This evidence is reviewed in the 1969 paper.

In the dynamic situation, we believe that in the vicinity of these negative charges H^+ reaches electrochemical equilibrium (a Donnan equilibrium) faster than HCO_3^-, resulting in a transient disequilibrium and production of CO_2 by the association of $[H^+]$ and $[HCO_3^-]$ ions. If the transit time of blood through the capillary is short enough, a steady-state disequilibrium state can occur between $[H^+]$ and $[HCO_3^-]$ near the capillary

wall, resulting in a higher P_{CO_2} near the wall than in the bulk phase of the capillary blood.

The rapid movement of H^+ ions is of crucial importance in this model and is thought to be due largely to the H^+ ion dissociation of large protein molecules when exposed to an electric field (Ween effect).

Large negatively charged macromolecules such as proteins, which move slowly by diffusion, tend to lose their faster moving counterions (such as H^+, Na^+, etc.) when exposed to an electrical field. Since proteins are weak acids, the loss of counterions, including H^+ ion near the charged groups on the protein molecule, causes dissociation of the acid groups. The proposed dissociation of protein causes the H^+ ion activity to approach equilibrium near the charged capillary wall faster than $[HCO_3^-]$ can escape due to electrostatic repulsion and causes a transient production of CO_2 near the wall due to the association of $[H^+]$ and $[HCO_3]^-$. If the transit time of blood through the capillary were shorter than the time for $[HCO_3^-]$ to reach equilibrium, a steady state P_{CO_2} difference could occur within the capillary, and consequently in the alveolar capillary membrane and alveolus. However, if the capillary transit time were sufficiently long, the effect of the increase of $[H]^+$ near the charged capillary wall would be balanced exactly by the effect of the decrease in

$[HCO_3]^-$ and no differences in CO_2 would result.

We believe that under certain circumstances (high pulmonary blood flow rate), nonequilibrium of $[H^+]$, $[HCO_3^-]$, and CO_2 might occur within the capillary. Arguments supporting our belief, in light of present knowledge concerning rates of chemical reaction and diffusion in blood, are given in the appendix of the paper by Gurtner, Song, and Farhi [1969].

In order to test this hypothesis, the cardiac output of five dogs was changed by hemorrhage and subsequent reinfusion of the blood. Simultaneous measurements of ΔP_{CO_2} and cardiac output were obtained. We found that when cardiac outputs falls, ΔP_{CO_2} starts to decrease and eventually disappears (GURTNER, SONG, and FARHI [1969]).

Quantitative Relationships between ΔP_{CO_2} and Blood pH

If there is a difference in H^+ ion concentration between the wall and bulk phases of capillary blood and if $[HCO_3^-]$ is assumed to be the same near the wall as in the bulk phase, the law of mass action leads to the following relationships:

$$H^+ = K_{[CO_2]} \frac{H_2CO_3}{HCO_3^-} = K_{[CO_2]} \frac{\alpha P_{CO_2}}{HCO^-_3},$$

$$\Delta H^+ = K_{[CO_2]} \frac{\Delta P_{CO_2}}{HCO_3^-}, \text{ and} \qquad (1A)$$

$$\frac{\Delta P_{CO_2}}{HCO_3^-} = \frac{\Delta H^+}{\alpha K_{[CO_2]}}$$

where α is the solubility coefficient and $K_{[CO_2]}$ is the effective equilibrium constant.

If the distribution of H^+ around a negative charge can be described by Boltzmann's distribution law, then

$$H_w = H_B e^{+f\psi/RT}$$

where w indicates concentration near the capillary wall, B indicates concentration in the bulk phase, and ψ indicates the potential difference between the wall and bulk phases.

Since $\Delta H^+ = (H^+_w - H^+_B)$, $\Delta H^+ = H_B (e^{f\psi/RT} - 1)$, ΔH^+ at constant ψ is a constant multiple of H^+_B, and therefore, ΔP_{CO_2} should be directly related to H_B and inversely related to blood pH as follows:

$$\frac{\Delta P_{CO_2}}{HCO_3^-} = \frac{H^+_B(e^{f\psi/RT} - 1)}{\alpha K_{CO_2}} \qquad (1B)$$

Gurtner, Song, and Farhi [1969] found that $\Delta P_{CO_2}/HCO_3^-$ increased in proportion to H^+ ion as predicted by equation 1B.

These results are shown in Figure 1 where $\Delta P_{CO_2}/HCO_3^-$ is plotted against the pH of mixed venous blood. The solid line gives the slope of the predicted relationship and it can be seen that the model fits the experimental results fairly well.

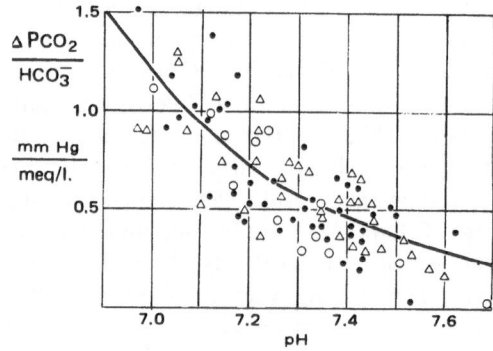

Fig. 1. Relationship between the normalized P_{CO_2} gradients ($\Delta P_{CO_2}/HCO_3^-$) and mixed venous pH. The solid line indicates the slope of the predicted relationship (see text).

However, the real situation is more complex because $[HCO_3]^-$ near the wall is decreased both by the electrostatic repulsion of the negative charges and the chemical reaction forming CO_2. Gurtner, Song, and Farhi [1969] considered the rate of change of CO_2 and HCO_3^- activity in a small volume of blood passing through a pulmonary capillary under the influence of charges on the wall. In their treatment of the problem it is assumed that at time $= 0$ the volume of blood enters the capillary and is acutely exposed to an electrical field. This assumption seems reasonable if one keeps in mind that the surface area of the pulmonary capillary bed is large compared with that of the pulmonary artery. Because of the difference in surface area, it seems unlikely that blood entering the capillary near the wall would have been exposed to an electrical field near the wall of a pulmonary artery. This acute application of an electrical field causes the H^+ ion to reach equilibrium nearly instantaneously (due to the Ween effect). The H^+ ion then associates with HCO_3^-, forming CO_2.

These more complex relationships have been expressed in terms of equations elsewhere (Gurtner, 1972; Gurtner, 1973). From these equations several factors are involved in the magnitude of ΔP_{CO_2} as follows:

(1) H^+ and HCO_3 concentration in the bulk phase,
(2) electrical potential difference between wall and bulk phase,
(3) diffusion coefficient and thickness of the charged layer,
(4) chemical reaction rate,
(5) the time the blood is exposed to the electrical field.

The reaction rate for dehydration of H_2CO_3 would have to be faster than the uncatalyzed rate for this mechanism to form significant amounts of CO_2; however, if the rates were 100 times faster than the uncatalyzed rate, the ΔP_{CO_2} would be nearly as great as if the rate were infinitely fast. Roughton [1964] has estimated that the carbonic anhydrase activity inside red cells is sufficient to speed up the reaction 10,000 times. Carbonic anhydrase is also present in the lung. We need to assume that there is enough of this enzyme to speed up the reaction 100 times. Although several other enzymes appear to be present on the wall of the pulmonary capillaries (VANE [1969]), carbonic anhydrase need not be present on the capillary wall, as carbonic acid formed by association of HCO_3^- and H^+ should be freely diffusable into the alveolar capillary membrane where the enzyme can facilitate the dehydration reaction.

In regard to the duration of electrical exposure, the time the blood is in contact with the wall depends on the type of flow through the capillary. If there were strictly laminar flow, this time might be long. However, since the red cells are about the same size as the capillary, it seems likely that some mixing might occur due to the mechanical deformation of the cells. Mixing would tend to increase the quantity of blood exposed to the electrical field in a single transit time through the capillary and decrease the time that any volume of blood was under the influence of the charged capillary wall.

The Applicability to Other Weak Acids and Bases and to Tissues other than Lung Tissue

It should be noted that this mechanism should affect other weak acids and weak bases as well. It is evident from equation 1B that for weak acids, the ratio of $\Delta HA/A^-$, all other factors remaining constant, is inversely proportional to the ratio of the equilibrium constant divided by the [H⁺] activity.

Similar relationships have been derived for weak bases that should be relatively excluded from the area near the charge (Gurtner, 1973).

The site of action of this mechanism should not be only the pulmonary capillary; it should be present in all capillaries since all vascular walls appear to bear surface charges.

We attempted to test these two predictions by measuring the distribution of a C14-labelled weak acid, Barbital (pK7.8), and a C14-labelled weak base, trishydroxymethyl amino-ethane [THAM (pK 7.77)], between a fluid-filled lobe of lung and mixed venous blood in a living dog and between cerebrospinal fluid and arterial blood in the same dogs.

We measured weak acid and base distribution between CSF and blood because the composition of CSF should reflect the composition of the extracellular fluid (ECF) of brain. This means that we could ascertain if the uncharged form of Barbital was concentrated in the ECF and if the uncharged form of THAM was partially excluded from the ECF, as predicted by the hypothesis.

The steady-state differences in uncharged Barbital and THAM normalized from the blood concentration of Barbital and THAM are shown in Figures 2(A) and (B). The degree of concentration of uncharged Barbital and the exclusion of THAM was a function of blood pH, as predicted by the model.

An even better test of the hypothesis would be a measurement of the distribution of ammonia between CSF and blood. Ammonia is a weak base (PK 9.3) which exists

as a gas. The permeability of biological membranes to ammonia is similar to water (Klocke et al, 1972). It is known that water moves very rapidly across the blood brain barrier probably at a similar rate to CO_2 (Davson, 1966). Thus since ammonia is so diffusable the distribution of this weak base would be unaffected by factors such as filtration out of freshly formed CSF, which might affect a slowly penetrating weak base such as THAM. This sort of filtration can cause exclusion of large molecules such as sucrose from the CSF (Davson, 1966).

The distribution of ammonia between CSF and blood has been measured in dogs (Stabenau et al., 1959). They found ammonia was relatively excluded from the CSF. It is possible to recalculate their published data and plot their results in the manner in which we plotted the THAM data. This is shown

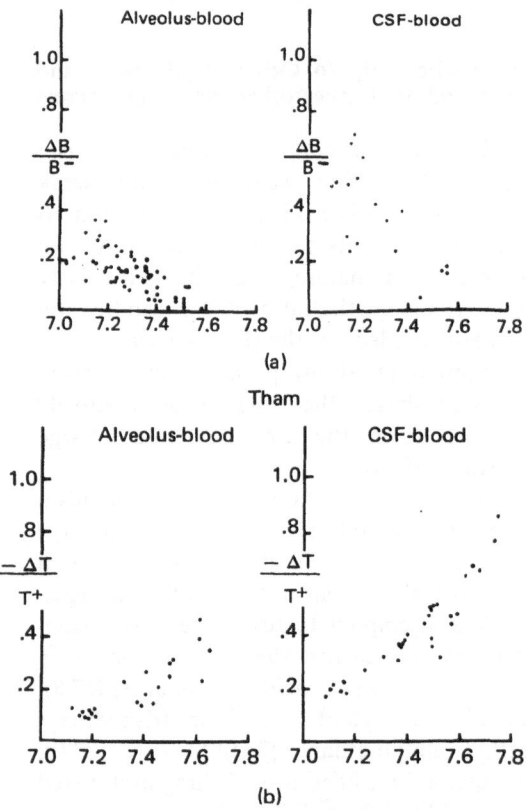

(a)

(b)

Fig. 2 (A), (B). Relationship between steady-state differences in concentration of the uncharged form of a weak acid (barbital) (A) and a weak base (THAM) (B) normalized for the blood concentration of each ($\Delta B/B^-$) and ($\Delta T/T$). Note that barbital is concentrated and THAM relatively excluded from the CSF, as predicted by the model. Also, the degree of concentration or exclusion is dependant on the pH of the blood, again as predicted by the model.

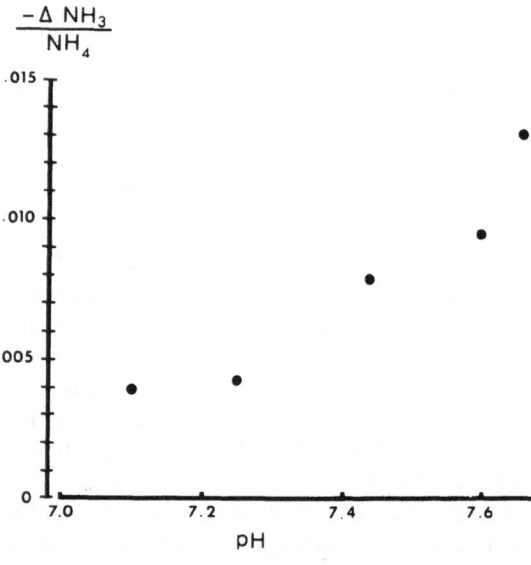

Fig. 3. The steady state concentration differences of ammonia between CSF and arterial blood divided by the concentration of ammonium ion in the arterial blood ($-\Delta NH_3/NH_4^+$) is plotted against the pH of arterial blood.

This data is recalculated from mean results of Stabenau et. al. (1959) in which the distribution of ammonia in different acid base states was presented. Ammonia is relatively excluded from the CSF and the degree of exclusion increases as the blood becomes more alkaline. These results are consistent with the charged membrane hypothesis.

in Figure 3. Note that the degree of exclusion of ammonia increases as the blood becomes more alkaline, similar to THAM and as predicted by the hypothesis.

Relationship between Cerebrospinal Fluid (CSF) and Blood, PCO₂, [HCO₃], and [H⁺]

The principal investigator of this study is Dr. Donald Davies, and reports of his work have previously been published (Davies Dissertation Abstracts, 1970; DAVIES, FITZGERALD, and GURTNER [1973]; DAVIES, GURTNER, and RILEY [1971]; DAVIES and GURTNER [1973]).

We felt that since weak acids and bases were distributed between CSF and blood as predicted by the charged membrane hypothesis, perhaps CSF and cerebral venous blood Pco₂ would also exhibit such a relationship. The experiments were performed as described below.

The Acid-base Experiments

Metabolic acidosis. In anesthetized, paralyzed, artificially ventilated dogs, arterial PA_{CO_2} was held constant before, during and after infusion of dilute HCl. pH was measured using a Radiometer pH microelectrode, CSF Pco₂ was measured using the astrup equilibration technique, blood PA_{CO_2} was measured with a CO_2 electrode, HCO₃ was calculated. We found that the acid-base relationships between CSF and blood were as described in Figure 4A. After rapid infusion of the HCl at constant PA_{CO_2}, [H⁺] activity of the CSF was found to increase and after 2 to 3 hours did not differ statistically from blood [H⁺] activity. The increase in [H⁺] was largely accounted for by an increase in CSF Pco₂ (about 75% of the increase was due to CO_2), while significant differences in steady state [HCO₃⁻] concentration occurred between CSF and blood.

Respiratory acidosis. If the paralyzed, ventilated animals were respired with CO_2 air mixtures, the acid-base relationships were described in Figure 4(B). Similar to metabolic acidosis, there were large steady-state

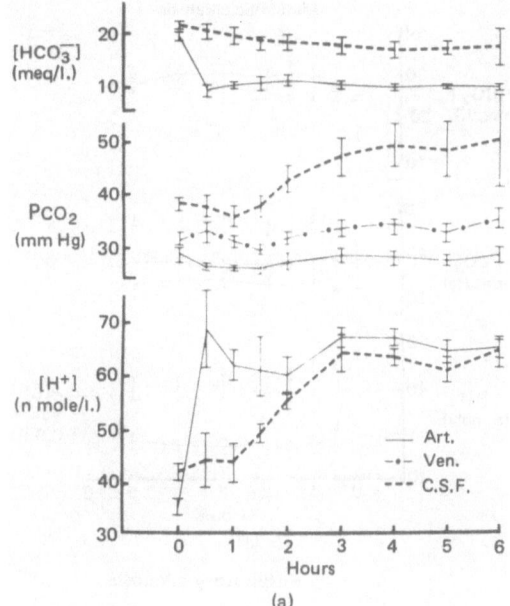

(a)

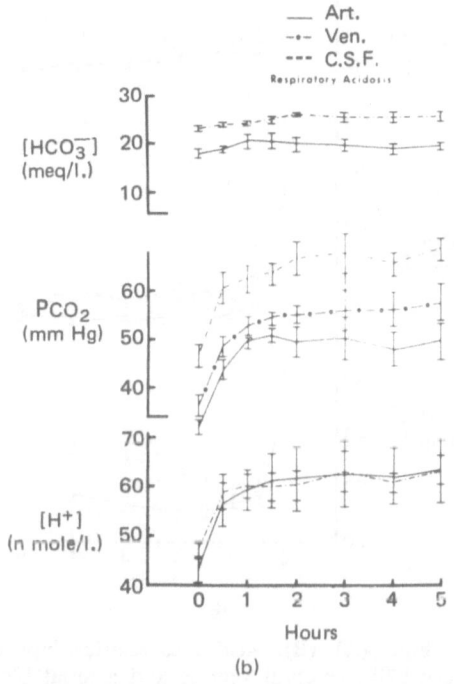

(b)

Fig. 4 (A), (B). Acid-base relationships between CSF, cerebral venous and arterial blood during pure metabolic acidosis (A) and pure respiratory acidosis (B). Note that large steady-state ΔPco₂ and HCO₃⁻ concentration differences occur between CSF and venous blood where as [H⁺] activity is not different.

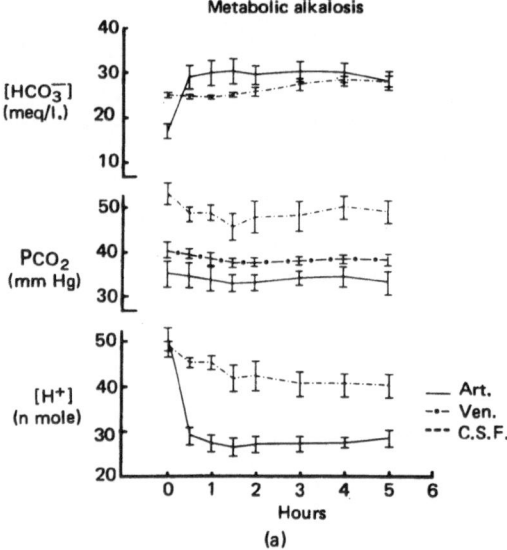

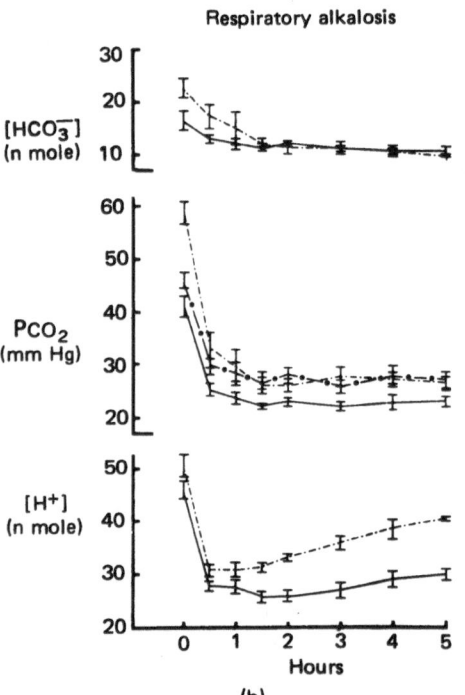

Fig. 5(A), (B). Acid-base relationships between CSF, cerebral venous and arterial blood during pure metabolic (A) and respiratory alkalosis (B). Note that HCO₃ appears to reach equality between CSF and blood in both cases.

Pco₂ and [HCO₃⁻] differences between CSF and venous blood, but H⁺ activity was not different between CSF and blood.

Metabolic alkalosis. Figure 5(A) gives the results during metabolic alkalosis. At constant PA_{CO_2}, the infusion of [NaHCO₃] caused large steady-state [H⁺] differences to occur between CSF and blood while equality for [HCO₃⁻] concentration was reached between CSF and blood in the presence of a CO_2 difference.

Respiratory alkalosis. During respiratory alkalosis the differences between CSF and venous Pco₂ disappeared, as the results reveal in Figure 5(B). We feel that this represents a confirmation of the charged membrane hypothesis. During respiratory alkalosis it is well known that cerebral blood flow decreases as PA_{CO_2} decreases. Since the mechanism predicts a Pco₂ difference which is directly proportional to blood flow, we would expect that ΔP_{CO_2} would disappear with decreasing blood flow.

In the absence of a Pco₂ difference there was no [H⁺] and [HCO₃⁻] difference between venous blood and CSF [not shown in Figure 5(B)]. This might indicate a cause and effect relationship between ΔP_{CO_2} and the regulation of brain [H⁺].

The Findings of the Experiments

The relationship between ΔP_{CO_2} and blood H⁺. The relationship we noted was also observed by Gurtner, Song, and Farhi [1969] when ΔP_{CO_2} was measured across the alveolar capillary membrane under conditions of no gas exchange. In Figure 6, ΔP_{CO_2} (CSF-V) is plotted against blood [H⁺] activity. A highly significant correlation is present, as predicted by the model.

The relationship between [HCO₃] differences across the blood brain barrier and [H⁺$_a$]. In Figure 7, the ratio of [HCO₃] CSF and [HCO₃⁻] arterial is plotted against [H⁺]$_a$. At low blood [H⁺] activity, [HCO₃] is the same in blood and CSF, while at high [H⁺] activity there are large [HCO₃] differences.

It is interesting to note that the [HCO₃]⁻ ratio changes in the same direction as the DC potential difference $P-D$ across the blood-brain barrier. At high [H⁺$_a$] activity Severing-

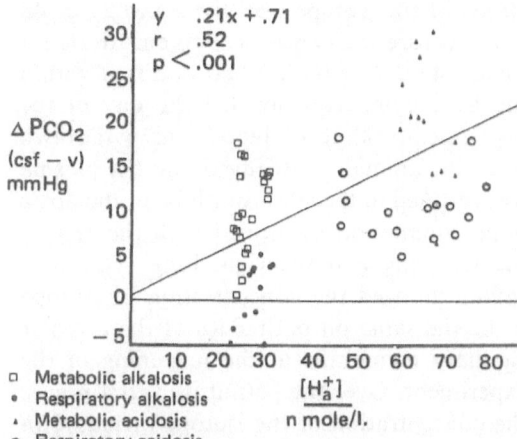

Fig. 6. Relationship between ΔPco$_2$ and H$^+$ activity of the blood. A statistically significant relationship is present, as predicted by the model.

haus, Pappenheimer, and others have measured potential differences of about 10 mV, CSF positive to the blood. According to the Nernst equation, 10 mV would represent a distribution' ratio of 1.45, which is smaller than the measured ratios. Of course, if the potential difference between CSF and blood is a diffusion potential, Goldman's equation should be used. However, if [HCO$_3$$^-$] permeability is larger than for other ions, Goldman's equation gives $P-D$ similar to the Nernst equation. We feel that [HCO$_3$] permeability may be larger than for other ions due to movement as CO$_2$.

The relationship between [HCO$_3$$^-$] *ratio and* ΔPco$_2$. In Figure 8, [HCO$_3$] CSF/ [HCO$_3$] is plotted against ΔPco$_2$. A highly significant relationship is present, even including the metabolic alkalosis data where no HCO$_3$ differences occur in the presence of a change in ΔPco$_2$.

A Theoretical Model Explaining the Acid-base Relationships between CSF and Blood

If there is a CO$_2$ difference between CSF and blood, H$^+$ and HCO$_3$$^-$ cannot be in equilibrium simultaneously between CSF and blood. Consider the case in which H$^+$ did not cross the blood-brain barrier. Under these

circumstances, HCO$_3$$^-$ could reach equilibrium and H$^+$ differences would occur. This is similar to our findings during alkalosis. If [HCO$_3$$^-$] did not cross the barrier, H$^+$ would be in equilibrium and HCO$_3$ differences would occur; this is similar to our findings during acidosis.

Although it is hard to believe that any ion would not move across the blood-brain barrier at all, quantitative changes in permeability might occur.

H$^+$-dependent permeability changes are known to occur in several biologic membranes. In frog muscle, cell membrane anion permeability increases as H$^+$ activity decreases (HUTTER and WARNER [1961].) If similar changes occur in the blood-brain barrier, we might expect that at low H$^+$ activity [HCO$_3$$^-$] permeability may be large enough relative to [H$^+$] permeability so that HCO$_3$ concentration is the same in CSF and

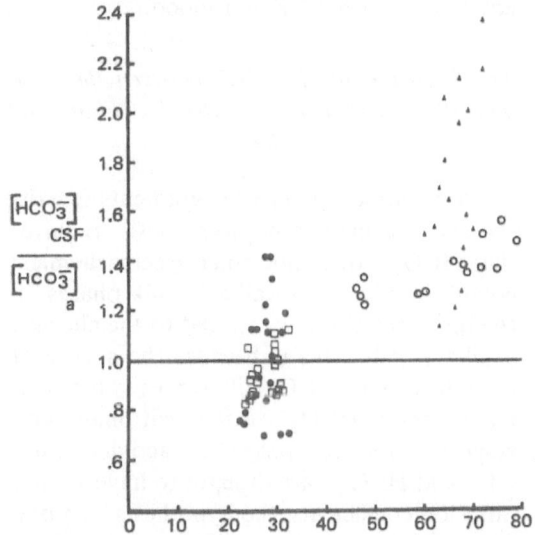

Fig. 7. Relationship between the ratio of [HCO$_3$]$^-$ concentration between CSF and blood, and between CSF and blood [H$^+$]. Note steady-state [HCO$_3$$^-$] differences during acidosis. This may be due to H$^+$-dependent permeability of the blood-brain barrier.

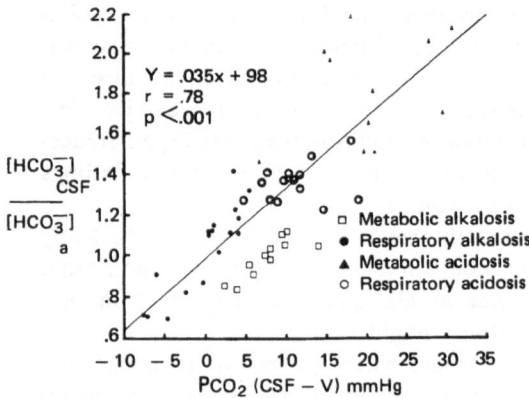

Fig. 8. Relationships between HCO_3 ratio and ΔP_{CO_2} between CSF and blood, indicating a very significant relationship. A cause and effect relationship may be present (see text).

blood. At high blood H^+ concentrations, HCO_3 permeability decreases relative to $[H^+]$ permeability and H^+ activity can approach equality between CSF and blood.

The Distribution of $^{36}CL^-$ between the CSF and Blood and between Alveolar Fluid and Blood

For intracapillary CO_2 gradients to exist the charged membrane hypothesis requires that HCO_3^- does not reach electrochemical equilibrium between wall and bulk phases, in the time that blood is exposed to the charged capillary wall. This is because the source of the intracapillary CO_2 differences is the relative excess of HCO_3^- in the wall phase with respect to the wall phase H^+ activity. Since CL^- and HCO_3^- are thought to have similar diffusion coefficients, the hypothesis also predicts that intracapillary differences for CL^- should occur and that the electrochemical potential of CL^- should be higher in alveolar fluid and CSF than in the bulk phase of capillary blood since these structures should be in equilibrium with wall phase rather than bulk phase capillary blood.

We chose to measure the steady state distribution of $^{36}CL^-$ between CSF and between alveolar fluid and blood in dogs.

$10 \ \mu C$ of the isotope was given I.M.24 or 48 hours before the experiment to ensure that a steady state distribution had occurred within the fluid compartments. On the day of the experiment 200 cc of blood was withdrawn from the animal, centrifuged and the plasma was instilled in the left lower lobe of the dog's lung. Ventilation continued with the rest of the left lung and the right lung. This procedure allowed the concentration of isotope to be the same on both sides of the alveolar capillary membrane at the beginning of the experiment. Over the period of 3 to 4 hours, the concentration of the isotope increased in the alveolar fluid with respect to blood and a steady state seemed to be present after that time. There were no significant changes in $^{36}Cl^-$ activity of the blood over the experimental period. The CSF sample was taken from the cisterna magna at the end of the experimental period. We performed the experiment at different H^+ activity of blood by changing the inspired P_{CO_2} of the paralyzed respired animals. Since the rate of exchange of $^{36}Cl^-$ was so slow, only one acid base state was investigated in each animal.

The steady state distribution of $^{36}Cl^-$ is plotted in Figure 9.

We found that the ratio of $^{36}Cl^-$ activity (CSF/blood) was highest when the H^+ activity of arterial blood was around 30 nM and that the ratio decreased as H^+ activity increased. This relationship held for both CSF and alveolar fluid. Fencl et al. (1966) had demonstrated a similar relationship between CSF and blood in goats. Their data is also plotted in Figure 9. This sort of relationship between the ratio and arterial H^+ is not predicted by the hypothesis, which predicts a constant ratio. We find the $^{36}Cl^-$ ratio largest under conditions in which the ratio for HCO_3 is smallest and vice versa. This data led us to reconsider our model for the regulation of CSF H^+ activity.

In the model discussed above, we proposed that if there is a step up in P_{CO_2} between CSF and blood, H^+ and HCO_3^- cannot be simultaneously in equilibrium between blood and CSF.

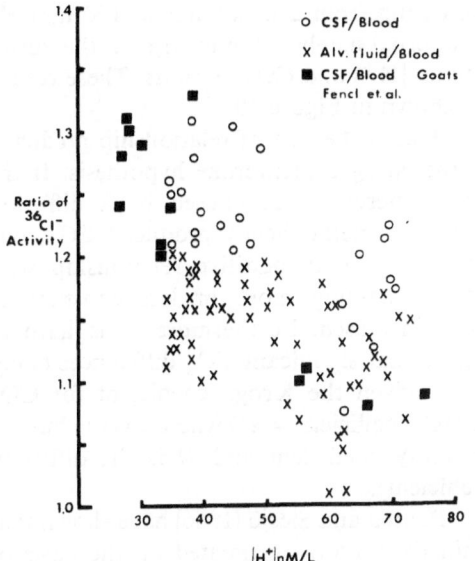

Fig. 9. The steady state ratio of ^{36}Cl$^-$ activity in alveolar fluid or CSF to the ^{36}Cl$^-$ activity of arterial blood is plotted against the H$^+$ activity of arterial blood. Data published by Fencl et al. (1966) from goats are also included. The ratio is largest at the H$^+$ activity at which the HCO$_3$ ratio is smallest and vice-versa. The charged membrane hypothesis predicts that both HCO$_3$ and Cl should be stepped up in CSF and alveolar fluid (see text).

In a steady state H$^+$ or HCO$_3^-$ could approach equilibrium more or less closely depending on the permeability of the blood brain barrier to one ion with respect to the other. We suggested that the permeability of the blood brain barrier is related to the H$^+$ activity of the blood being relatively larger for H$^+$ during acidosis and larger for HCO$_3^-$ during alkalosis. However, there is a questionable assumption in this model. For H$^+$ activity to come to equilibrium between CSF and blood, permeability to H$^+$ would have to be orders of magnitude larger than to HCO$_3$. This seems unlikely. If, however, the H$^+$ sensitive changes in permeability were different for Cl$^-$ and HCO$_3^-$, we could explain the distribution of H$^+$, HCO$_3^-$, Cl$^-$, and CO$_2$ without requiring a large permeability to H$^+$.

The charged membrane hypothesis predicts that the electrochemical potential for HCO$_3^-$, Cl$^-$, and CO$_2$ is higher in the wall phase of capillary blood than in the bulk phase. The structures in equilibrium with the wall phase should also reflect this difference in electrochemical potential. However, there are constraints on the system which are not considered by the hypothesis. These constraints are electroneutrality and osmotic equilibrium. If both HCO$_3^-$ and Cl$^-$ were stepped up to the same degree then electroneutrality would require that Na$^+$ be stepped up to the same extent. This would mean that large osmotic differences would occur between CSF and blood.

If we constrain the system so that electroneutrality and osmotic equilibrium with the bulk phase is required, both HCO$_3^-$ and Cl$^-$ cannot be stepped up simultaneously in the CSF. The ion to which the permeability of the blood brain barrier is highest would come closest to equilibrium between wall phase and CSF. Let us consider acidosis. If the permeability to HCO$_3^-$ was large relative to Cl$^-$ during acidosis, then CSF HCO$_3^-$ would come close to equilibrium with the wall phase. The H$^+$ activity of the CSF would be determined by the ratio of HCO$_3$ to CO$_2$. It can be shown that, if there is a chemical equilibrium between CO$_2$ and HCO$_3^-$ in the wall phase, the electrochemical potential of CO$_2$ and HCO$_3^-$ in the wall phase would be stepped up by the same factor. This means that if the CO$_2$ and the HCO$_3$ in the CSF are in equilibrium with the CO$_2$ and HCO$_3^-$ in the wall phase then the ratio of HCO$_3^-$/CO$_2$ and therefore the activity H$^+$ would be the same in the CSF and the bulk phase of blood.

This modification of the above hypothesis could therefore explain our experimental results during acidosis without requiring very large permeability to H$^+$. If the permeability to Cl$^-$ increased during alkalosis with respect to HCO$_3^-$ then the magnitude of the step up in HCO$_3^-$ would become less than the step up in CO$_2$ and the CSF would be relatively acid to blood. This would agree with our results during alkalosis.

Both the original hypothesis and the modified hypothesis depend upon pH sensitive changes in the permeability of the blood brain barriers and both would explain our data. We could distinguish between the two by measuring the permeability of the barrier to Cl using the ventriculo-cisternal perfusion technique described by Fencl et al. (1966). We have found that the permeability to Cl^- increases during alkalosis as predicted. We have not, however, made any measurements of HCO_3^- permeability.

Measurement of Tissue P_{CO_2}

The principal investigator of this work is Dr. Burns and reports of it have previously been published. (Burns, B., Dissertation Abstracts [1971] BURNS and GURTNER [1971]).

A membrane-tipped probe of 300 μ diameter was used by Dr. Burns. The membrane was made by layering polypropylene over teflon and pulling both over a small stainless steel capillary tubing. The flux of gas across this membrane was small and was the same in gas and in stirred and unstirred liquids. This indicates that in liquids there is no depletion of the boundary layer which would tend to indicate falsely low values for partial pressures. Additional experiments using tonometered brain tissue homogenate indicate that there is very little boundary layer depletion, even using very viscous homogenate suspensions.

In vivo brain tissue, measurements of partial pressure of CO_2, O_2, and the inert gases (argon, N_2O and N_2) were made after long equilibration with inert gases–O_2 mixtures. Tissue tensions of the inert gases were similar to blood; O_2 tensions ranged from 2 mm Hg to 40 mm Hg; tissue P_{CO_2}, however, exceeded what would have been predicted on the basis of the metabolic rate and diffusivity of CO_2 in brain tissue. Cortical P_{CO_2} at a depth of 2 mm to 3 mm averaged 90 mm Hg in the normocapnic subject. The magnitude of the difference between tissue and arterial CO_2 tension (ΔP_{CO_2}) was proportional to both arterial $[H^+]$ and $P_{A_{CO_2}}$, with ΔP_{CO_2}

decreasing from a maximum of 100 mm Hg to approximately 10 mm Hg at the lower arterial $[H^+]$ and CO_2 tensions. These results are shown in Figure 10.

This is the sort of relationship predicted by the charged membrane hypothesis. If the P_{CO_2} difference was caused by a diffusion barrier to metabolically produced CO_2, one would expect an additive relationship with P_{CO_2} remaining more or less constant as $P_{A_{CO_2}}$ increased. Furthermore, it is hard to believe that significant CO_2 differences could occur, given the Krogh coefficient for CO_2 (Krogh coefficient $= \alpha D$ where α is the bunsen solubility coefficient and D is the diffusion coefficient).

Ponten and Siesjö [1966] have shown that brain tissue P_{CO_2}, estimated on the basis of diffusivity and metabolic production, should be between arterial and venous P_{CO_2}.

It seems possible that these large P_{CO_2} differences may play a role in tissue acid-base balance similar to the one which we proposed as operating between CSF and blood. Siesjö (reporting in a personal communication) has

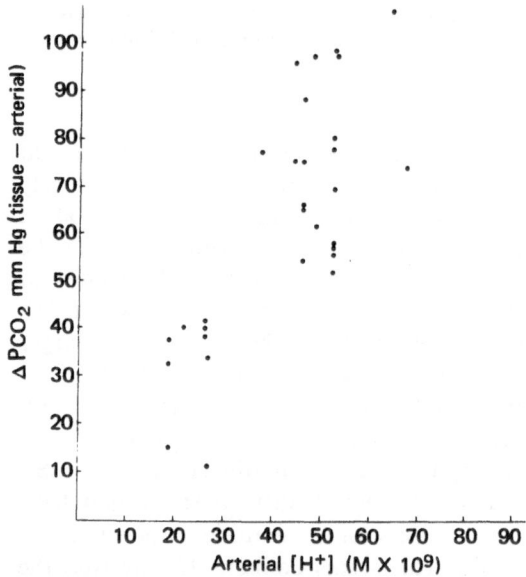

Fig. 10. Relationship between ΔP_{CO_2} (tissue-arterial blood) and arterial blood H activity. Tissue P_{CO_2} was measured with a 300μ membrane tipped probe connected to a mass spectrometer (see text.

found that CSF and intracellular HCO_3^- increase markedly during chronic hypercapnia. This is similar to our findings that large HCO_3^- differences occur between CSF and blood during hypercapnia and may indicate that the PCO_2 differences may be involved in a cause and effect manner.

Bibliography

Burns, B. and Gurtner, G. H., "Cerebral gas tensions." *Physiologist*, 14(3):116, (1971).

Davies, D. G., Gurtner, G. H., and Riley, R. L., "Relationship between CSF and blood PCO_2, [H$^+$] and [HCO_3]$^-$ during acidosis and metabolic alkalosis." *Federation Proceedings*, 3(2):249 (1971).

Davies, D., Fitzgerald, R., and Gurtner, G., "Acid-base relationships between cerebrospinal fluid and blood during metabolic acidosis." *J. Appl.Physiol.* 34:243–248 (1973).

Davies, D., and Gurtner, G., "Cerebrospinal fluid acid balance and the Ween effect." *J. Appl. Physiol.* 34:249–254 (1973).

Davies, H., "Physiology of the cerebrospinal fluid." Churchill, London (1967.

Dennison, D., Edwards, R. H., Jones, G., and Pope, H., "Direct and rebreathing estimates of the O_2 and CO_2 pressures in mixed venous blood." *Resp. Physiol.*, 7:326–34 (1969).

Fencl, V., Miller, T. B., and Pappenheimer, J. R., "Studies on the respiratory response to disturbances of acid-base balance, with deductions concerning the ionic composition of cerebral interstitial fluid." *Am. J. of Physiol.* 210:459–472 (1966).

Gurtner, G., Energy requirements for intracapillary PCO_2 gradients *J. Appl. Physiol.* 34:740 (1973).

Gurtner, G. H., "Non-equilibrium steady state differences in partial pressure of CO_2 in concentration of weak acids and bases between blood and tissue." *Biophysical Journal* 12:597–609 (1972).

Gurtner, G. H., Song, S. H., and Farhi, L. E., "Alveolar to mixed venous PCO_2 differences under conditions of no gas exchange." *Resp. Physiol.* 7:173–187 (1969).

Guyatt, A. R., Yu, C. J., Lutherer, B., and Otis, D. B., "Studies of alveolar mixed venous CO_2 and O_2 gradients in the rebreathing dog lung." *Resp. Physiol.* 17:178–194 (1973).

Hutter, O. F., and Warner, A. E., "The Effect of pH on the 36Cl$^-$ efflux from frog skeletal muscle." *J. Physiol.* (London), 189:427–43 (1967).

Jones, N. L., Campbell, E. J. M., Edwards, R. H. T., and Wilkoff, G., "Alveolar to blood PCO_2 differences during rebreathing in exercise." *J. Physiol.* (London) (1969).

Klocke, R., Anderson, K. A., Rotman, H., and Forster, R. E., "Permeability of human erythrocytes to ammonia and weak acids." *Am. J. Physiol.* 222:1004–1013 (1972).

Roughton, F. J. W., "Transport of oxygen and carbon dioxide." In W. Fenn and H. Rahn eds., *Handbook of Physiology*, Vol. 1. Washington, D.C.: American Physiological Society, 1964. pp. 810–13.

Stabenau, J. R., Warren, K., and Rall, D., "The role of pH gradients in the distribution of ammonia between blood and cerebrospinal fluid, brain muscle." *J. Clin. Invest.* 38:373–383 (1959).

Vane, J. R., "The release and fate of vaso-active hormones in the circulation." *Brit. J. Pharmacol.*, 35:209–42 (1969).

Part II

Carbon Dioxide and pH Regulation
of Cellular Functions

1. Carbon Dioxide Effects on Nerve Cell Function

David O. Carpenter,* John H. Hubbard,† Donald R. Humphrey,‡
Harry K. Thompson, and Wade H. Marshall

Laboratory of Neurophysiology
National Institutes of Mental Health
Bethesda, Maryland 20014

Introduction

In this paper we will examine the sensitivity of three distinct populations of nerve cells to CO_2. The aims of the study are threefold: first, to separate specific effects of CO_2 from pH effects; secondly, to determine the variety of nerve cell responses to CO_2 and, if possible, make some generalizations about the effects of this agent; and finally, to understand the ionic mechanisms of this response. Unfortunately, this third goal has not to date at all been achieved.

If there is a "classical" study on the effects of CO_2 on nerve cells, it is that of Lorente de Nó [1947], who studied frog sciatic fibers. He found that CO_2 had the following effects on activity: It raises threshold for stimulation; it decreases conduction velocity; it increases height and duration of the action potential; and it increases resting membrane potential. He reports that each of these effects of CO_2 increases with CO_2 concentration and that none was a result of the pH change.

In the central nervous system CO_2 has a variety of effects on gross indicators of nerve cell activity. Ivanov [1962] reports that low concentrations of CO_2 (up to 5%) cause desynchronization of EEG patterns in cortex and thalamic regions and slow wave activity in the medulla. Gellhorn [1953] reports that 10% CO_2 decreases the responsiveness of the specific sensory projection areas to auditory and visual stimuli but increases the reactivity of the hypothalamic-cortical projections. Furthermore, marked shifts in the D-C potential of the brain occur with inhalation of 6% to 20% CO_2. With the higher concentrations this is accompanied by a marked reduction of electrocorticographic activity (WOODY, MARSHALL, BESSON, THOMPSON, ALEONARD, and ALBE-FESSARD [1970]).

Krnjević, Randić, and Siesjö [1965] have studied the effects of CO_2 on excitability of single cortical cells to microiontophoretic application of L-glutamate and found a mixture of excitatory and depressive effects. They were able to record intracellularly from six cells in the post-cruciate area and reported that membrane potential of these neurons increased by a few millivolts during CO_2.

In intact mammalian preparations CO_2 in general tends to decrease excitability of neurons. Even at concentrations as low as 5%, CO_2 acts as an anesthetic agent on the

* Present address: Neurobiology Department, Armed Forces Radiobiology Research Institute, Bethesda, Md 20014

† Present address: Division of Neurosurgery, University of Pennsylvania, School of Medicine and Veterans Hospital, Philadelphia, Pennsylvania 19104

‡ Present address: Department of Physiology, Emory University, Atlanta, Georgia 30322

corneal reflex (POULSEN [1952]). CO_2 also depresses jaw reflexes (JURNA and SÖDERBERG [1963]) and it has been shown that in man 5% to 10% CO_2 produces a significant degree of analgesia (DUNDEE, BLACK, and NICHOLL [1960]).

There are a variety of observations on the effects or lack of effects of CO_2 on spinal nerve cells. The spinal monosynaptic reflex is markedly depressed by CO_2, although polysynaptic reflexes are not so dramatically affected (BROOKS and ECCLES [1947]; KIRSTEIN [1951]). Krnjević et al. [1965] report that 20% CO_2 does not have any effect on resting membrane potential of spinal motor neurons, nor on the submaximal response of Renshaw cells to ventral root stimulation. However, Gill and Kuno [1963] found that the responsiveness of phrenic motor neurons was dramatically decreased by 6% CO_2. In the isolated toad spinal cord Washizu [1960] reports that 15% CO_2 causes a marked hyperpolarization of motor neurons, but believes this to be primarily a result of the pH change. In this isolated preparation he reports that increasing acidity results in hyperpolarization.

In contrast to its effects on frog and mammalian nerve, CO_2 results in a depolarization and excitation in most neurons of *Aplysia* (CHALAZONITIS [1959, 1963]; BROWN and BERMAN [1970]). These effects of CO_2 have been studied in great detail over many years by Drs. Chalazonitis and Arvanitaki, who have developed sensitive techniques for measuring pH and P_{CO_2} in single neurons. They found that while cells tend to be excited by CO_2, there are marked differences in sensitivity among the identified cells in the ganglion. Thus, some cells are depolarized more than others and show greater changes in patterns of discharge (ARVANITAKI and CHALAZONITIS [1961]; CHALAZONITIS [1961]). Administration of CO_2 is always accompanied by changes in intracellular and extracellular pH (CHALAZONITIS [1959]), and many of the effects of CO_2 are thought to result from the pH changes.

In a recent study Brown and Berman [1970] attempted to determine the mechanism of the CO_2 effect on *Aplysia* neurons. Their observations agreed with the above conclusion that CO_2 causes a depolarization of *Aplysia* neurons, except that they found one identified neuron which was sometimes hyperpolarized and sometimes depolarized by CO_2. All cells showing a response to CO_2 showed an increased membrane conductance. They concluded that the effects of CO_2 result from the change in extracellular pH, and that CO_2 *per se*, decreased intracellular pH, or increased bicarbonate ion are without effect on *Aplysia* neurons. In a second paper Brown, Walker, and Sutton [1970] show that a fall in extracellular pH results in an increase in membrane conductances to Cl^- and K^+, and postulate that this is the mechanism of action of CO_2 on these cells.

The experiments reported in this paper were begun in parallel with the work in which this laboratory has been engaged for a number of years on the effects of CO_2 and pH on cortical DC potentials (RAPOPORT and MARSHALL [1964]; WOODY, THOMPSON, and MARSHALL [1966]; WOODY, et al. [1970]). The initial aim of the study was to compare the effects (seemingly contradictory at that time) of CO_2 on *Aplysia* neurons with those effects reported on frog and mammalian neurons. After becoming convinced that the effects of CO_2 on *Aplysia* neurons were primarily due to pH, we shifted to experiments on mammalian systems, where pH shifts were not large due to the body's buffering abilities. Here we have attempted to study the effects of CO_2 on a variety of mammalian neurons and to understand the sites of action of CO_2 on various reflexes.

Results

Carbon Dioxide on Aplysia *Neurons*

Forty-five successful experiments were performed on identified and unidentified *Aplysia* neurons. Recordings were made as previously described (CARPENTER [1967, 1970]). Ganglia were maintained under constantly flowing sea water. The recording chamber was placed in a nearly tight lucite box. For exposure to CO_2 (5% to 20%) the perfusion fluid was suddenly changed from normal sea water to sea water equilibrated with the gas for at least 30 min. Simultaneously gas was forced through the box containing the recording chamber. pH and P_{CO_2} were monitored on some samples of the seawater and measured on an Instrumentation Laboratories pH–P_{CO_2} meter.

In agreement with the previous reports we found that most *Aplysia* neurons are excited by 10% CO_2, which in unbuffered sea water gives a pH of about 5.5. The pacemaker neurons tend to show much less effects than the silent or synaptically excited neurons. However the giant neuron, cell R_2, is frequently hyperpolarized and inhibited by CO_2, in agreement with Brown and Berman [1970], who reported that about half of the cells R_2 are hyperpolarized and half depolarized by CO_2. They relate these opposing effects to two different internal Cl^- concentrations in cells from different animals.

Also in agreement with Brown and Berman, we have found that most of the effects of CO_2 application can be mimicked by exposure to sea water of the same pH made acidic by addition of HCl or H_2SO_4. In acidic solutions of pH not less than 5, all responses are reversible. Effects are frequently not reversible below pH 5 and cells sometimes depolarize markedly with an irreversible loss of normal membrane resistance.

In all cells tested, CO_2 and pH caused a fall in membrane resistance which was more pronounced at lower pH values. It seems likely that all of the effects of pH are on membrane conductances, as suggested by Brown and Berman (1970). In these neurons an electrogenic Na^+ pump is directly responsible for a considerable portion of the resting membrane potential (CARPENTER and ALVING [1968]). This pump acts as a constant current source, and therefore the potential generated varies with membrane resistance. With changes in pH the electrogenic pump showed no effects that could not be explained on the basis of the effect on membrane resistance.

In several R_2 cells, it was possible to separate what appeared to be a direct response to CO_2 from the response to pH. One such experiment is shown in Figure 1. In this experiment the preparation was being perfused by seawater containing 25 mmole Tris + buffer. The solution was not pre-incubated with CO_2, but a small reservoir was located just outside of the chamber into which CO_2 could be bubbled during perfusion. This allowed a short time of perfusion with a solution with a rising P_{CO_2} but without large pH changes. When the buffering capacity was saturated, the pH fell.

Parts 1 and 2 of Figure 1 show the intracellular recording from cell R_2 and the pH of the seawater monitored from an area adjacent to the ganglion. CO_2 was applied at the first arrow and the solution changed to normal seawater at the second arrow. The dashed line represents a membrane potential of 70 mv. The first effect of CO_2 was a small but clear hyperpolarization occurring with a latency of about 1 min. However, when pH fell below 7.0, the membrane depolarized relative to the control; although synaptic input was also clearly increased, the depolarization was not a result only of this synaptic input.

In part 3 membrane potential is plotted against pH. Voltages are averages taken from three repeated applications of CO_2 to this cell. The initial membrane potential was taken as zero and is indicated by the thin horizontal line. On exposure to CO_2 the membrane potential increased by about 2 mv on every test, then depolarized by an average of 8 mv as pH fell. On return to normal seawater, membrane potential returned to control values.

Although this transient response would appear to be a true response to CO_2, it was not always evident. The transient hyperpolarization was never observed in any cell except R_2 and could be separated from a pH response only in those neurons which were depolarized by pH alone. Certainly the most dramatic effects of CO_2 application are the results of pH changes. Because of the transient

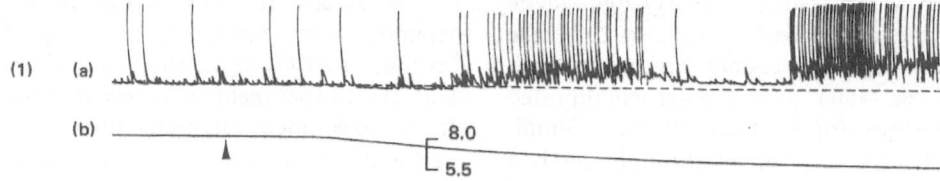

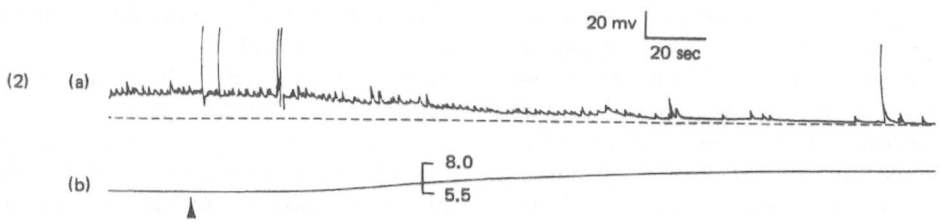

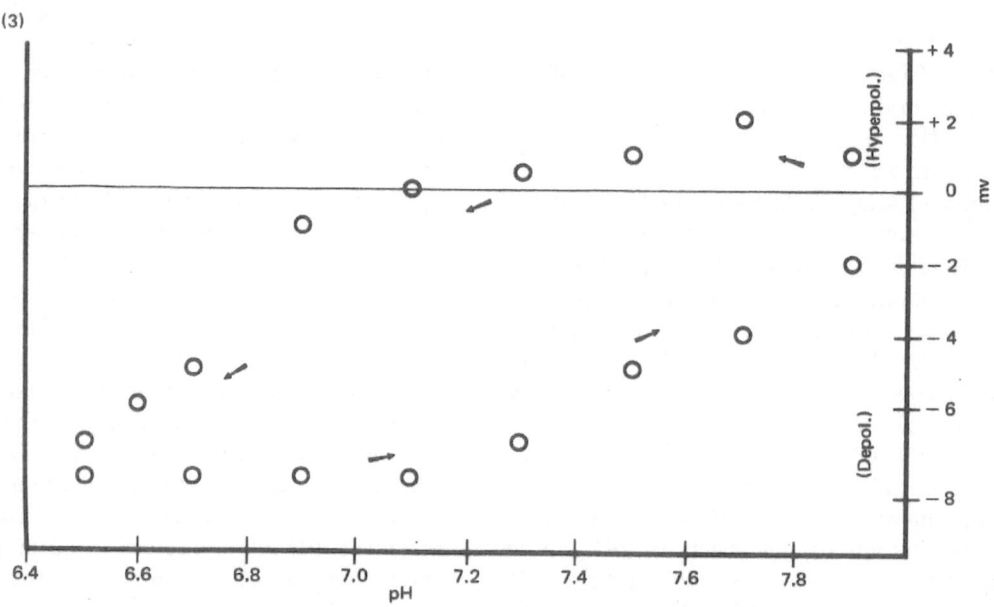

Fig. 1. The effect of 10% CO_2 on membrane potential of cell R_2. Traces 1 and 2a are penwriter records of intracelluar potential from R_2, while 1 and 2b are pH recorded from a pH electrode placed in the recording chamber adjacent to the ganglion. At the arrow in 1, equilibration of a small reservoir with 10% CO_2 was begun. At the arrow in 2, the perfusion fluid was returned to normal seawater. In 3, membrane potential is plotted against pH from the above record and 2 other runs of CO_2 applications on this cell. The dashed line in 1 and 2 represents a membrane potential of -70 mv. Experiment was performed at 22°C.

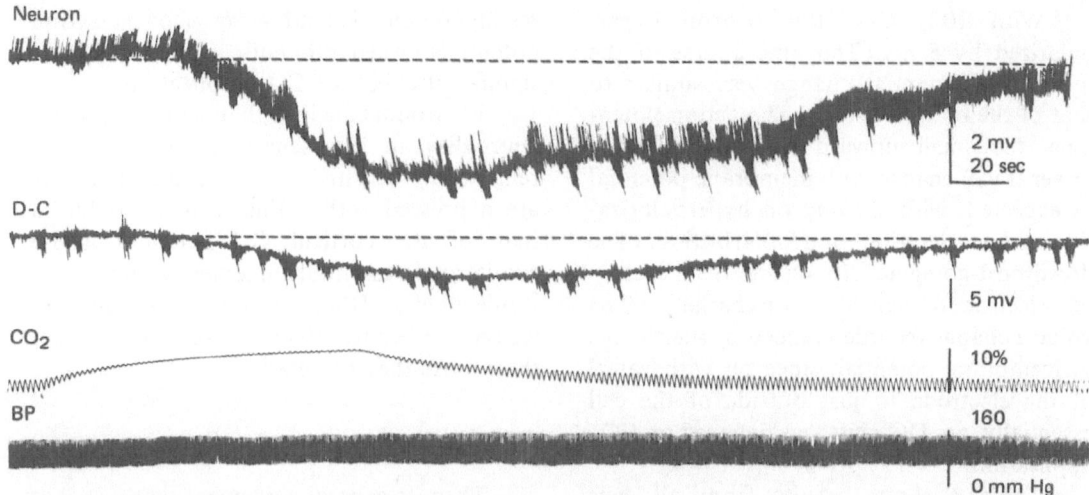

Fig. 2. The effect of 10% CO_2 on membrane potential of a neuron from sensori-motor cortex. The trace marked "neuron" is an intracellular recording through a 15 MΩ microelectrode, while the trace marked "DC" is the surface brain potential recorded through a pore electrode. In both traces negative is indicated by the direction down. The small upward deflections in the intracellular recording are action potentials but are not accurately reproduced by the penwriter. Action potential amplitude was 60 mv. The CO_2 trace monitors expiratory CO_2, while the lowest trace monitors blood pressure.

and variable response with a predominance of pH effects, we turned to mammalian systems to study the effects of CO_2 on single nerve cells.

Carbon Dioxide on Neurons in Sensori-motor Cortex

A series of experiments were done on 15 cats in an attempt to record intracellularly from neurons in sensori-motor cortex. In addition to wanting to add to the number of cortical cells studied by Krnjević et al. [1965], we attempted to relate the time course of the membrane potential changes of single neurons to that of the DC potential shift resulting from the CO_2 application.

Cats were anesthetized with either chlorolose or Nembutal. Results did not differ in experiments with the two different anesthetic agents. Stabilization of the cortex was achieved through wide openings of the bone and by the use of a lucite pressure foot. Microelectrode recordings were made through 15 to 20 mΩK$^+$ citrate electrodes. Signals were recorded through use of a Bak unity gain, high impedance amplifier, and records were photographed from the oscilloscope screen and also were displayed on an Offner penwriter. Cats were given a bilateral pneumothorax, paralyzed with gallamine, and artificially ventilated with room air or 10% CO_2. Expiratory CO_2 was continuously monitored on an infrared Godard capnograph. Other recording procedures were as described by Woody et al. [1970].

Eight neurons were recorded during at least one complete exposure to CO_2 with recovery. An example of the result is shown in Figure 2. The intracellular recording from the neuron is shown in the upper trace. This is a high gain penwriter recording which does not faithfully reproduce the spikes, but does give a small deflection with each action potential. It also accurately records DC changes in resting membrane potential. In this cell the initial resting potential was 40 mv and the action potential spike was 60 mv at the beginning of the trace. The second trace is the brain DC potential recorded through a pore electrode located 1 cm behind the microelectrode tract. The third trace is respiratory CO_2 and the fourth blood pressure.

With 10% CO_2 this neuron hyperpolarized by 5 mv. The time course of the membrane potential change was similar to that of the brain DC shift. The action potentials (the small upward deflections in the upper trace) change with membrane potential as expected, with slowing on hyperpolarization and acceleration on depolarization. (The downward-going activity results from pickup of electrocorticographic discharges). The voltage change recorded reflects a true change in membrane potential, since on withdrawal of the electrode to just outside of the cell essentially no DC shift was detected on CO_2 application.

Table 1 shows results from all cells studied that were held through at least one complete run of exposure to CO_2 and return to room air. Eight neurons were studied for a total of 18 CO_2 trials. These cells showed an average hyperpolarization of 5 mv with 10% CO_2. With good penetration and in preparations with a minimal amount of blood pressure change the results were very reproducible on repeated runs of CO_2. One cell was held through 9 such runs, with essentially identical membrane potential shifts each time. In all cases the time course of the hyperpolarization followed the negative DC shift of the brain potential. This is not to imply that the intracellular potential is the origin of the brain DC shift, for this potential is probably generated primarily across the walls of the cerebral vasculature (HUBBARD, CORRIE, THOMPSON, and MARSHALL [1971]).

Five cells were studied in cortex which have the properties described by Krnjević and Schwartz [1967] and are probably neuroglia. These cells had unusually high resting potentials and never showed action potentials or synaptic noise. They showed no significant effects of CO_2 application.

We would conclude that neurons (but not neuroglia) in the sensorimotor cortex are remarkably sensitive to CO_2, and that they are depressed with a time course similar to that of the cortical DC potential. These results are in essential agreement with those of Krnjević et al. [1965], although the responses we see are less transient and somewhat larger than those they reported.

Carbon Dioxide on Spinal Reflexes

There is general agreement that CO_2 has a depressing effect on the monosynaptic reflex (BROOKS and ECCLES [1947]), although polysynaptic reflexes are affected relatively little (KIRSTEIN [1951]; ESPLIN and ROSENSTEIN [1963]). However, Esplin and Rosenstein showed that monosynaptic transmission through the superior cervical ganglion is not affected by CO_2, and thus suggest that there is something specific about the CO_2 inhibition of the spinal monosynaptic reflex. These observations suggest that CO_2 acts on very specific parts of this neuronal pathway. Because the spinal monosynaptic reflex contains very few elements, experiments were begun to try to determine the site of the CO_2 effect.

Sixteen cats were studied, seven under Nembutal anesthesia and the remainder decerebrated under ether and spinalized just before recording. The leg nerves studied included gastrocnemius-soleus (G-S), sural (S), posterior biceps-semitendinosus (PBST), and semimembranosus-anterior biceps

Table 1. Effects of 10% CO_2 on Cortical cells

	Number studied	Number of tests	Average Δ rmp	Range
Neurons	8	18	+5 mv	+0 to 15 mv
Unresponsive cells	5	7	0	−3 to +4mv

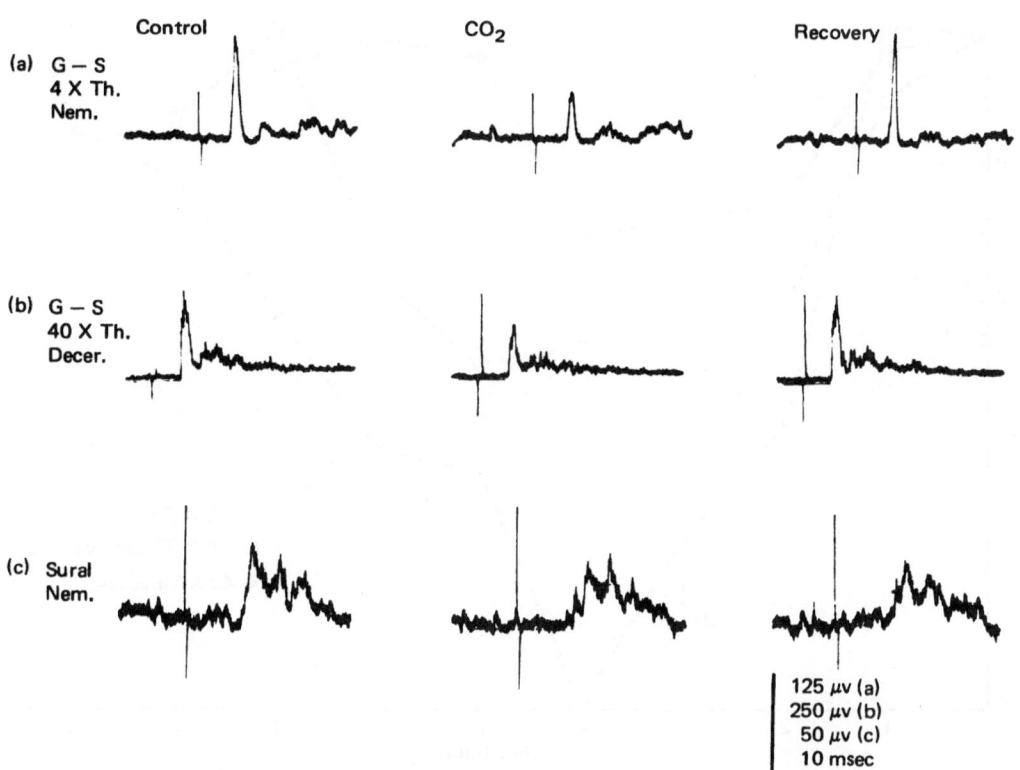

Fig. 3. The effects of CO_2 on mono- and polysynaptic reflexes. Records are selected to show average responses. (A) and (B) show monosynaptic reflexes from G-S in a cat anesthetized with Nembutal [(A)] and in an unanesthetized, decerebrate cat [(B)]. In (C) the response is the polysynaptic reflex resulting from stimulation of the sural nerve, from an experiment on a cat anesthetized with Nembutal. All reflexes were elicited by a single shock to the peripheral nerve and were recorded from the S_1 vertical root.

(SMAB). Except in those experiments on the effects of CO_2 on the afferent discharge these nerves were cut and mounted on silver wire electrodes for stimulation or recording. Ventral roots (L_4–S_2) were cut and S_1 was mounted for recording. All responses were recorded through an Electronics for Life Sciences differential a-c amplifier (ELSDA–1) and photographed from an oscilloscope screen. Cats were paralyzed by gallamine and artificially respired with either room air or 10% CO_2 in air.

Figure 3 shows representative records of the effects of CO_2 on mono- and polysynaptic reflexes from three different experiments. The upper records are monosynaptic reflexes from G-S in a Nembutal cat. These records were

selected to show reasonably average responses in the stated condition. The monosynaptic reflex is normally quite variable because of membrane potential fluctuations of the afferent fiber terminals that result from activity in pathways that give rise to presynaptic inhibition (RUDOMIN and DUTTON [1969]). In CO_2 the monosynaptic reflex is markedly reduced, but recovers on return to air. As shown in the second trace this effect is not a result of the anesthesia, for the same effect of CO_2 is observed in an unanesthetized, decerebrated cat.

There is a polysynaptic as well as a monosynaptic reflex upon stimulating muscle nerves at high intensity. Although as yet these polysynaptic reflexes from muscle have not

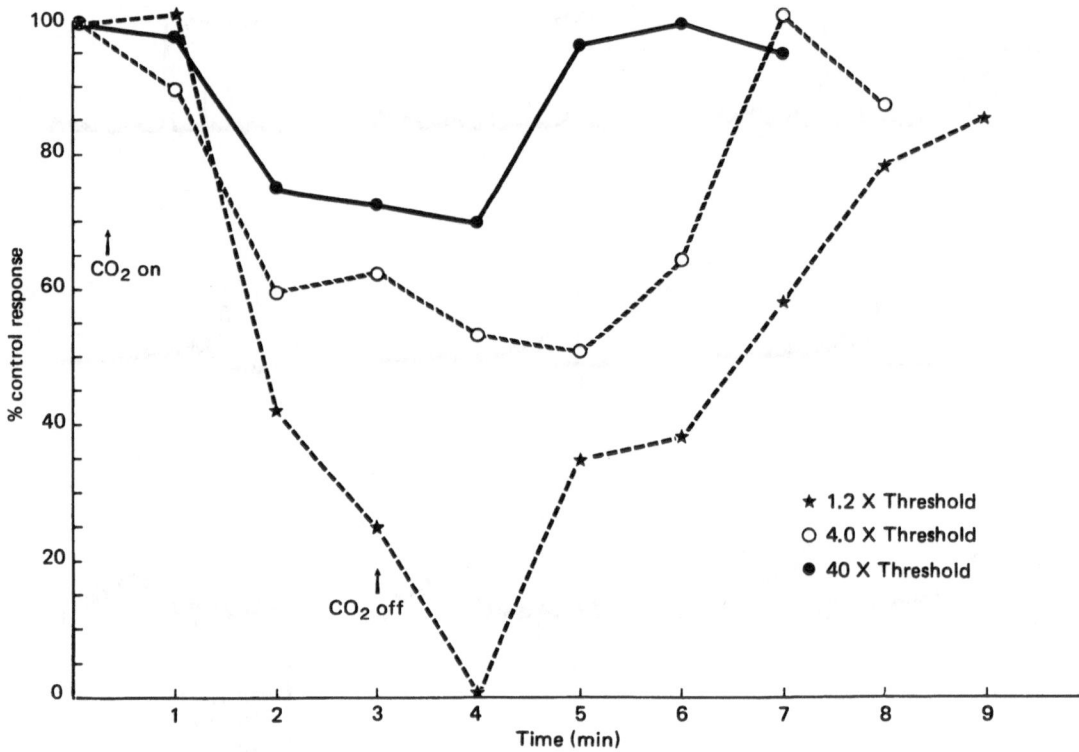

Fig. 4. The effects of 10% CO_2 on the G-S monosynaptic reflex in a decerebrate cat. Reflexes were evoked by stimulation of the G-S nerve, and recordings were made from the S_1 ventral root. The heights of the monosynaptic responses were measured and averaged over 1 min intervals. Response amplitude is expressed as percent of the control response at each stimulus intensity. CO_2 was applied for 3 min between times 0 and 3.

been carefully analyzed, they appear to be somewhat depressed by CO_2, albeit not so dramatically as the monosynaptic reflex. In contrast, the polysynaptic reflex from cutaneous nerves shows little or no effect of CO_2 in either the Nembutal or decerebrate cat (lower traces).

Figure 4 shows a plot of the average depression of the G-S monosynaptic reflex from a decerebrate and spinalized cat. In this plot the average height of the monosynaptic reflex, expressed as the percentage of the control response, is plotted against time. CO_2 was applied at time = 0 and was left on for 3 min. The monosynaptic reflex was completely abolished by 10% CO_2 when the muscle nerve was stimulated at $1.2 \times$ threshold. The latency for this effect was about 1

min, while the time for recovery was somewhat longer and was complete only after 6 or 7 min. At higher intensities of stimulation, the percentage inhibition was less, although the inhibitory effect is clear.

The dramatic inhibition of the monosynaptic reflex by CO_2 without obvious effect on polysynaptic cutaneous reflexes rules out the motor neuron as the site of action of CO_2. Since the only remaining element in the monosynaptic reflex is the annulo-spiral (*1a*) afferent fiber from the muscle spindle, CO_2 must act either on this afferent fiber directly or specifically upon the process of transmitter release from this fiber.

To test general sensitivity of the *1a* afferents to CO_2, experiments were done in which the G-S nerve was left intact to the

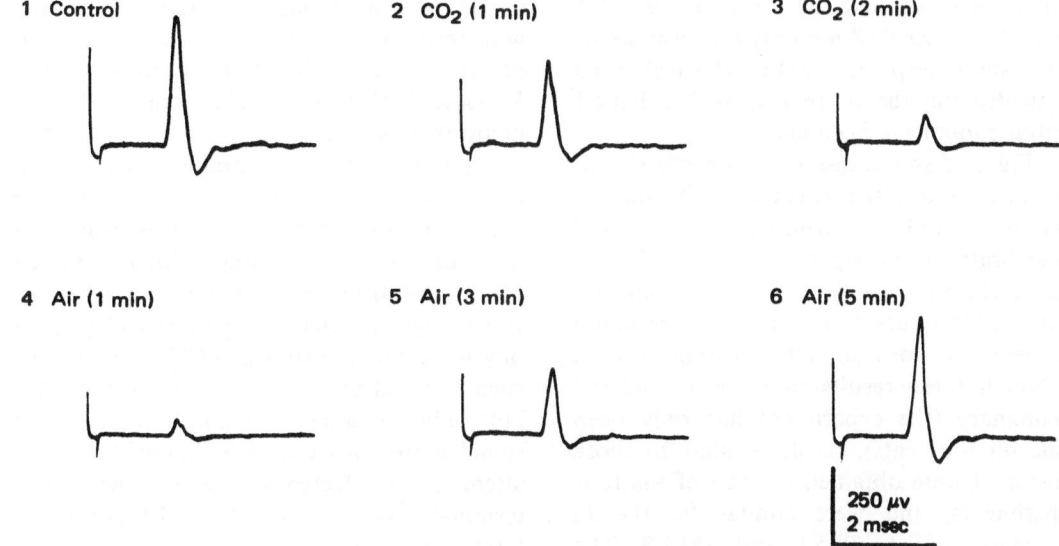

Fig. 5. The effect of 10% CO_2 on the excitability of G-S 1*a* afferent terminals. Records are typical since these responses did not show much variability. Recordings were made from the G-S nerve in a decerebrate-spinalized preparation in which all ventral roots (L_4 to S_2) were sectioned. The stimulation electrode was a 1 MΩ glass mocripipette filled with 2 moles NaCl placed 3 mm deep in the cord in or near to the G-S motor nucleus. Current was passed through the microelectrode from a pulse generator, using a switch at the amplifier head to disconnect the recording. CO_2 was applied for 2 min. The times noted refer to the time after beginning respiration with that gas.

muscle. The muscle with its bony attachment was freed and stretched with tension monitored with a pressure transducer. The S_1 and L_7 dorsal roots were sectioned close to the cord and filaments containing single afferents were separated and mounted for recording as described by Carpenter and Henneman [1966]. *1a* afferent fibers were identified by conduction velocity (greater than 70 mv/sec) and by the fact that they pause discharge during a twitch contraction. None of 10 afferent fibers studied showed changes in discharge frequency to steady applied stretch of the muscle upon exposure to 10% CO_2. This would indicate that the terminals at the muscle end of the fiber are probably not affected by CO_2.

Another site where CO_2 might act to depress monosynaptic transmission from muscle afferents would be at the fiber terminals in the cord. It is known that during presynaptic inhibition, afferent terminals in

the cord are depolarized (ECCLES, MAGNI, and WILLIS [1962]). As a result, the threshold is lowered for antidromic excitation from current passed through a gross microelectrode placed near these terminals (WALL [1962]). In contrast, if the terminals are hyperpolarized the threshold for antidromic excitation is increased (MENDELL and WALL [1964]). Thus, there will be changes in the size of the antidromic afferent volley recorded from the peripheral nerve if CO_2 affects the polarization of the terminals

Four preliminary experiments were done in decerebrate cats using this Wall technique to test for excitability changes in the *1a* terminals The microelectrode was inserted just lateral to the dorsal root entry zone and was used (through a Bak high impedance, unity gain d-c amplifier) to record the field potential of the afferent nerve being stimulated. The electrode was then lowered into the cord until the field potential was large and the tip was near the motor nucleus (at least 2.5 mm deep). Since only the *Ia* afferents terminate so deeply in the cord, this technique stimulates only the *Ia* fibers, provided that all ventral roots have been cut.

Figure 5 shows results of one experiment designed to test the effect of CO_2 on the excitability of G-S *Ia* terminals in a spinalized decerebrate cat. On application of 10% CO_2, the antidromic volley was dramatically reduced. On return to room air, the response recovered to control values within 5 min. Although these results must be considered preliminary (the experiment has only been done on four cats), results similar to those illustrated were obtained in each of the four experiments, and were similar for the *Ia* terminals of G-S, PBST and SMAB. The depression is not a result of blood pressure changes, since it was not seen during hypertension caused by administration of epinephrine. A decreased excitability indicates that the afferent terminals are hyperpolarized by CO_2. This observation is consistent with a general tendency for CO_2 to hyperpolarize neurons, if in fact it has any effect; it is, however, rather surprising in light of the inhibitory effect of CO_2 on the monosynaptic reflex. With moderate increases in terminal membrane potential, synaptic transmission is facilitated rather than inhibited, presumably as a result of a larger action potential in the afferent terminal, resulting in turn in an increase in the transmitter output (TAKEUCHI and TAKEUCHI [1962]). The magnitude of the decreased excitability of the terminals which we observe with CO_2 must reflect a hyperpolarization so large that the impulse is actually blocked from invasion of the afferent terminal. This would then block transmission in that terminal and would explain the reduction of the monosynaptic reflex.

Discussion

The results of these experiments on three entirely different neuronal systems suggest that if a neuron is affected by CO_2 at all, it is hyperpolarized and its discharge is decreased. The exceptions to this generalization are specialized neuronal structures concerned with respiration, such as the chemoreceptors of the carotid body (EYZAGUIRRE and KOYANO [1965]) and brain stem respiratory neurons (COHEN [1968]).

Perhaps the most dramatic conclusion from these experiments is that each type of neuron appears to have its own sensitivity to CO_2, presumably reflecting a difference in its membrane structure or permeability patterns. It is remarkable that an agent of such general physiological importance as CO_2 should show such a variation in its effect on nerve cells. Not only are some cells unaffected (such as spinal motor neurons) but others like the *Ia* afferents are affected at one site (the central terminals) but not another (the peripheral terminals).

However, it probably shouldn't be so surprising that an agent like CO_2 would affect different cells so differently. We are becoming more aware that there may be different responses to and different ionic mechanisms of action by the same agent on different neurons. For instance, in the invertebrate nervous system a number of possible neurotransmitters are excitatory in some cells but inhibitory in others (GERSCHENFELD [1966]). In *Aplysia* it is known that a single interneuron releasing acetylcholine excites one postsynaptic cell but inhibits another (KANDEL, FRAZIER, and COGGESHALL [1967]). At an even more complicated level a single synapse where only one transmitter is liberated may exert two distinct postsynaptic effects (KEHOE [1969]; WACHTEL and KANDEL [1971]). These differing effects of the same transmitter, whether on the same or different neurons, result from the opening of different conductance channels (BLANKENSHIP, WACHTEL, and KANDEL [1971]), presumably secondary to different membrane receptor sites for the neurotransmitter.

It is difficult to see any physiological significance in the pattern of neurons affected or not affected by CO_2. In fact, it would seem more likely that except for specific CO_2 receptor neurons the responses to CO_2 are not specific and are not conveying information useful to the nervous system. These responses may result simply from a chemical interaction with a membrane component present in some cells but not in others. The responses to CO_2 may well be similar to those recently described for neuronal sensitivity to temperature. As a result of the temperature dependence of ionic and metabolic processes, *Aplysia* neurons are all extraordinarily sensitive to changes in temperature (CARPENTER [1967, 1970]). In the mammalian central nervous system there has been a general belief that thermosensitivity of a neuron implied a role for that neuron in transmission of thermal information or in thermoregulation (EISENMAN and EDINGER [1971]). However, the neurons of sensori-motor cortex, which are not known to have a role in thermoregulation, show a very much greater thermosensitivity (BARKER and CARPENTER [1970]) than do those in the region of the hypothalamus concerned with thermoregulation (EISENMAN and JACKSON [1967]). This effect of temperature on sensori-motor neurons and *Aplysia* neurons is probably not a mechanism for detection of temperature but a nonspecific effect of temperature on the membrane processes of the cell. The mechanism of thermosensitivity in those neurons concerned with temperature information may be identical to that in the nonspecific thermosensitive neurons. However, in one case this information is used as a result of the synaptic interactions of the cell, whereas in the other case it apparently is not used. This may be exactly the case with the varying sensitivity of neurons to CO_2, with most of the responses studied in these experiments being unimportant to the functional activity of the animal. This would not, of course, make the response to CO_2 any less interesting for study, since it may supply clues to understanding basic membrane structure and mechanism.

Direct and Indirect Effects of Carbon Dioxide

The effects of CO_2 and H^+ are many times very difficult to separate by virtue of the fact that even in a buffered system some change in pH occurs upon administration of CO_2. However, it is unlikely that the CO_2 effects on cortical cells and the monosynaptic reflex are due to changes in pH. The change in blood pH in the cat resulting from exposure to 10% CO_2 is relatively small. In another series of experiments on 12 cats respired for 3 min with 10% CO_2, we have measured an average fall in pH of 0.41 units. Although the controls of acid injection were not done in these experiments, Bradley, Schlapp, and Spaccarella [1950] found that IV lactic acid given in quantities which changed blood pH by an amount equal to that caused by CO_2 did not depress the monosynaptic reflex. Thus, we conclude that the effect of CO_2 administration on *Ia* afferent terminals and probably also on neurons of sensori-motor cortex is a result of a specific change brought about by CO_2, and not secondary to a change in H^+ concentration.

It is somewhat surprising to find that *Ia* afferent terminals hyperpolarize to an agent which clearly depresses synaptic transmission, since usually the efficacy of transmission increases with membrane potential in the presynaptic terminals (TAKEUCHI and TAKEUCHI [1962]). The simplest explanation for this dilemma is that the hyperpolarization of the afferent terminal is so great that the incoming spike is partially blocked from invasion, thus counteracting any increased synaptic efficacy in terminals not blocked. This explanation would also account for the observation of Esplin and Rosenstein [1963] who observed on CO_2 administration a transient hyperexcitability before the depression of the spinal reflexes, sometimes leading to spontaneous activity of motor neurons. They also sometimes observed a transient hyperexcitability on withdrawal of CO_2. This could result from a situation where most of the terminals are hyperpolarized but not yet blocked by CO_2. It is likely that the transient hyperpolarization seen in some *Aplysia* neurons also represents a specific response to CO_2 although the response was transient and present in relatively few cells. We did not see at any time a biphasic response to pH changes alone in the cells which showed a biphasic response to CO_2. Clearly, the more obvious effect of CO_2 administration to *Aplysia* neurons results from the change in pH.

Possible Mechanisms of Action of Carbon Dioxide

These experiments provide no information as to the mechanisms of action of the direct effect of CO_2 on nerve cells. Those effects mediated by changes in pH in *Aplysia* neurons are always accompanied by a change in conductance of the membrane, probably to Cl^- and K^+, as suggested by Brown and Berman [1970].

The mechanism of the CO_2 effect must either be on some metabolic process or on membrane conductance. Lorente de Nó [1947] suggests but does not prove that CO_2 acts on the metabolic processes controlling membrane potential. Keynes [1965] has shown changes in Na^+ efflux from muscle resulting from CO_2 administration and suggests that these result from changes in internal pH.

There are some observations, primarily on muscle, which suggest that CO_2 may have a direct effect on membrane conductances. Meves and Völkner [1958] report that in frog muscle, CO_2 hyperpolarizes if membrane potential is low but depolarizes if membrane potential is large. This effect is different from that of H^+ and is presumably a direct effect of CO_2. This would suggest that there is an equilibrium potential for the CO_2 effect as would be expected if the mechanism of action were a change in conductance.

The recent study of Williams, Withrow and Woodbury [1971] on effects of CO_2 on membrane potential of rat muscle and liver cells shows that CO_2 does not markedly affect muscle, but rapidly causes a fall in liver cell potentials. They suggest that the action of CO_2 is on membrane permeability, but do not rule out the possibility that it is mediated by a change in intracellular pH.

We may conclude that at least on some neurons CO_2 does have effects caused by some mechanisms other than change in extracellular pH. Whether the mechanism involves changes in intracellular pH, bicarbonate ion, or CO_2 per se is not at all clear.

Bibliography

Arvanitaki, A. and Chalazonitis, N., "Slow waves and associated spiking in nerve cells of *Aplysia*." *Bull. Inst. Oceanogr. (Monaco)*, 1224:1–15 (1961).

Barker, J. L. and Carpenter, D. O., "Thermosensitivity of neurons in the sensorimotor cortex of the cat." *Science*, 169:597–98 (1970).

Blankenship, J. E., Wachtel, H., and Kandel, E. R., "Ionic mechanisms of excitatory, inhibitory, and dual synaptic actions mediated by an identified interneuron in abdominal ganglion of *Aplysia*." *J. Neurophysiol.*, 34: 76–92 (1971).

Bradley, K., Schlapp, W., and Spaccarelli, G., "Effect of carbon dioxide on the spinal reflexes in decapitated cats." *J. Physiol. (London)*, 111:62P (1956).

Brooks, C. McC. and Eccles, J. C., "A study of the effects of anaesthesia and asphyxia on the monosynaptic pathway through the spinal cord." *J. Neurophysiol.*, 10:349–60 (1947).

Brown, A. M. and Berman, P. R., "Mechanism of excitation of *Aplysia* neurons by carbon dioxide." *J. Gen. Physiol.*, 56:543–58 (1970).

Brown, A. M., Walker, J. L. Jr., and Sutton, R. B., "Increased chloride conductance as the proximate cause of hydrogen ion concentration effects in *Aplysia* neurons." *J. Gen. Physiol.*, 56:559–82 (1970).

Carpenter, D. O., "Temperature effects on pacemaker generation, membrane potential, and critical firing threshold in *Aplysia* neurons." *J. Gen. Physiol.*, 50:1469–84 (1967).

Carpenter, D. O., "Membrane potential produced directly by the Na^+ pump in *Aplysia* neurons." *Comp. Biochem. Physiol.*, 35:371–85 (1970).

Carpenter, D. O. and Alving, B. O., "A contribution of an electrogenic Na^+ pump to membrane potential in *Aplysia* neurons." *J. Gen. Physiol.*, 52:1–21 (1968).

Carpenter, D. O. and Henneman, E., "A relation between the threshold of stretch receptors in skeletal muscle and the diameter of their axons." *J. Neurophysiol.*, 29:353–68 (1966).

Chalazonitis, N., "Chémopotentiels des neurones géants fonctionnellement différénciés." *Arch. Sci. Physiol.*, 13:41–78 (1959).

———, "Effects of changes in P_{CO_2} and P_{O_2} on rhythmic potentials from giant neurons." *Ann. N.Y. Acad. Sci.*, 109:451–79 (1963).

————, "Chemopotentials in giant nerve cells (*Aplysia fasciata*)." In Florey, E., ed., *Nervous Inhibition* (Oxford, 1961), pp. 179–93.

Cohen, M. I., "Discharge patterns of brain-stem respiratory neurons in relation to carbon dioxide tension." *J. Neurophysiol.*, 31:142–65 (1968).

Dundee, J. W., Black, G. W., and Nicholl, R. M., "Alterations in response to somatic pain associated with anesthesia." *Brit. J. Anesth.*, 34:24–30 (1962).

Eccles, J. C., Magni, F., and Willis, W. D., "Depolarization of central terminals of group 1 afferent fibers from muscle." *J. Physiol. (London)*, 160:62–93 (1962).

Eisenman, J. S. and Edinger, H. M., "Neuronal thermosensitivity." *Science*, 172:1360–61 (1971).

Eisenman, J. S. and Jackson, D. C., "Thermal response patterns of septal and preoptic neurons in cats." *Exptl. Neurol.*, 19:33–45 (1967).

Esplin, D. W. and Rosenstein, R., "Analysis of spinal depressant actions of carbon dioxide and acetazolamine." *Arch. Int. Pharmacodyn.*, 143:498–513 (1963).

Eyzaguirre, C. and Koyano, H., "Effects of hypoxia, hypercapnia and pH on the chemoreceptor activity of the carotid body in vitro." *J. Physiol. (London)*, 178:385–409 (1965).

Gellhorn, E., "On the physiological action of carbon dioxide on cortex and hypothalamus." *E. E. G. Clin. Neurophysiol.*, 5:401–13 (1953).

Gerschenfeld, H. M., "Chemical transmitters in invertebrate nervous systems." *Soc. Exper. Biol. Sympos.*, 20:299–323 (1966).

Gill, P. K. and Kuno, M., "Properties of phrenic motoneurones." *J. Physiol. (London)*, 168:258–73 (1963).

Hubbard, J. H., Corrie, W. S., Thompson, H. K., and Marshall, W. H., "Beta adrenergic mechanisms influencing brain steady potential in cats and rhesus monkeys." *Internat. J. Neurosci.*, 2:57–67 (1971).

Ivanov, Y. N., "Changes in electrical activity of different brain regions in cats and dogs exposed to carbon dioxide." *Fed. Proc.*, 22:T13–18 (1963).

Jurna, I. and Söderberg, U., "The effect of carbon dioxide, anesthetics and strychnine on jaw reflexes." *Arch. Int. Pharmacodyn.*, 142:323–38 (1963).

Kandel, E. R., Frazier, W. T., and Coggeshall, R. E., "Opposite synaptic actions mediated by different branches of an identifiable interneuron in *Aplysia*." *Science*, 155:346–49 (1967).

Kehoe, J., "Single presynaptic neurone mediates a two component post-synaptic inhibition." *Nature*, 221:866–68 (1969).

Keynes, R. D., "Some further observations on the sodium efflux in frog muscle." *J. Physiol. (London)*, 178:305–25 (1965).

Kirstein, L., "Early effects of oxygen lack and carbon dioxide excess on spinal reflexes." *Acta Physiol. Scand.*, 23:Suppl. 80 (1951).

Krnjević, K., Randić, M., and Siesjö, B. K., "Cortical CO_2 tension and neuronal excitability." *J. Physiol. (London)*, 176:105–22 (1965).

Krnjević, K. and Schwartz, S., "Some properties of unresponsive cells in the cerebral cortex." *Exptl. Brain Res.*, 3:306–19 (1967).

Lorente de Nó, R., "Carbon dioxide and nerve function." *Studies of the Rockefeller Institute for Medical Research*, 131:148–93 (1947).

Mendell, L. M. and Wall, P. D., "Presynaptic hyperpolarization: A role for fine afferent fibres." *J. Physiol. (London)*, 172:274–94 (1964).

Meves, H. and Völkner, K. G., "Die Wirkung von CO_2 auf das Ruhemembranpotential und die elektrischen Konstanten der quergestrieften Muskelfaser." *Pflügers Arch.*, 265:457–76 (1958).

Poulsen, T. "Investigation into the anaesthetic properties of carbon dioxide." *Acta Pharmacol. et toxicol.*, 8:30–46 (1952).

Rapoport, S. I. and Marshall, W. H., "Measurement of cortical pH in spreading cortical depression." *Am. J. Physiol.*, 206:1177–80 (1964).

Rudomin, P. and Dutton, H., "Effects of muscle and cutaneous afferent nerve volleys on excitability fluctuations of 1A terminals." *J. Neurophysiol.*, 32:158–69 (1969).

Takeuchi, A. and Takeuchi, N., "Electrical changes in pre- and postsynaptic axons of the giant synapse of *Loligo*." *J. Gen. Physiol.*, 45:1181–93 (1962).

Wachtal, H. and Kandel, E. R., "Conversion of synaptic excitation to inhibition at a dual chemical synapse." *J. Neurophysiol.*, 34:56–68 (1971).

Wall, P. D., "Excitability changes in afferent fiber terminations and their relation to slow potentials." *J. Physiol.* (*London*), 142:1–21 (1958).

Williams, J. A., Withrow, C. D., and Woodbury, D. M., "Effects of CO_2 on transmembrane potentials of rat liver and muscle *in vivo*." *J. Physiol.* (*London*), 215:539–55 (1971).

Woody, C. D., Marshall, W. H., Besson, J. M., Thompson, H. K., Aleonard, P., and Albe-Fessard, D., "Brain potential shift with respiratory acidosis in the cat and monkey." *Am. J. Physiol.*, 218:275–83 (1970).

Woody, C. D., Thompson, H. K., and Marshall, W. H., "Changes in the steady potential of the brain related to respiratory acidosis and cerebral blood flow." *Trans. Am. Neurol. Assoc.*, 91:32–37 (1966).

Washizu, Y., "Effect of CO_2 and pH on the responses of spinal motoneurons." *Brain and Nerve*, 12:757–66 (1960) (in Japanese).

Carpenter Discussion

LOESCHKE: I should like to contribute a quotation. Drs. Caspers and Speckmann [1969a,b] have investigated postsynaptic potentials in spinal and cortical neurons of the rat. They found that a majority of cells were hyperpolarized during CO_2 inhalation, but that there were a minority of cells which were depolarized.

CARPENTER: Thank you. I was unaware of their studies.

SEVERINGHAUS: I have asked Dr. Matchell's permission, since he couldn't be here, to describe his results with the respiratory center neurons and CO_2. He has now been able to stay inside perhaps half a dozen neurons during changing P_{CO_2} in the cat. Even though the rate of firing of these cells did increase with CO_2, the resting potentials increased. So in spite of the fact that these cells are in the vagal nucleus gigantus cellularus, they are not the chemoreceptor cells. They are being hyperpolarized as a direct effect of CO_2 at the same time they are being synaptically stimulated by the CO_2 chemosensitive neurons.

CARPENTER: These observations are consistent with the generalization that only specific CO_2-sensitive chemoreceptors are depolarized by CO_2, while there is a widespread nonspecific effect of CO_2 tending to increase the membrane potential of neurons.

BROWN: I guess you know that the cerebral blood vessels are probably the most exquisitely sensitive blood vessels anywhere to CO_2. I wonder whether, when you add CO_2, the cerebral blood flow might not be increasing enough to wash out K^+ in the extracellular spaces. This might account for the hyperpolarization you see. For example, the kind of responses you see in the spinal cord could be the difference between the ending itself and the ending that is out in the periphery. There might be a differential effect on flow distribution which changes with external potassium. I have a second question, too.

CARPENTER: May I answer this one first. We cannot absolutely rule out effects on extracellular K^+ resulting from increased blood flow, although it seems to be an unlikely explanation for our results. Glial cells are known to be very sensitive indicators of changes of external potassium (3), and we did not find changes in membrane potential there on changing CO_2.

BROWN: The second question has to do with the fact that CO_2, or the hydrogen ion certainly, inhibits anticholinesterase activity. I wonder whether some of the inhibition of the monosynaptic reflex you see may not, in fact, be related to this.

CARPENTER: That would appear to be highly unlikely since acetylcholine is almost certainly not the transmitter between the annulo-spinal (1a) afferents and the motoneurons.

BROWN: If I may, just one more question for Dr. Severinghaus. In these respiratory center neurons you mentioned which showed a hyperpolarization and increased discharge on CO_2, was the discharge synaptically mediated?

SEVERINGHAUS: Yes, it was. Quite clearly.

Bibliography

Orkand, R. K., Nicholls, J. G., and Kuffler, S. W., "Effect of nerve impulses on the membrane potential of glial cells in the central nervous system of amphibia." *J. Neurophysiol.*, 29:788–806 (1966).

Speckmann, E. J. and Caspers, H., "Verschiebungen des corticalen bestandpotentials bei Veränderungen der ventilationsgrösse." *Pflügers Arch.*, 310:235–50 (1969a).

———, "Inhibitorische CO_2-wirkungen auf spinale zwischen-und motoneurone bei der ratte." *Pflügers Arch.*, 307:R119–20 (1969b).

2. Simultaneous Recordings of pH, P$_{CO_2}$, and Neuronal Activity during Hypercapnic Transients (identifiable Neurons of *Aplysia*)

Nicolas Chalazonitis

Départment de Neurophysiologie Cellulaire
Institut de Neurophysiologie et Psychophysiologie, Marseille, France

Introduction

The aim of investigating ΔpH and ΔP$_{CO_2}$ actions on the giant, identifiable, easily explored neurons of *Aplysia* and *Helix*, endowed with characteristic electrical activity, is, of course, to find out elementary (cellular) mechanisms explaining the well-known reactivities of the central and peripheral chemoreceptive neurons in mammals, which are as yet inaccessible to direct electrophysiological exploration.

Whereas chemoreception is a specific function of some ganglionic and medullary centers in mammals, chemosensitivity (or the ability to respond to small changes of respiratory gas tension) seems to be a general property of a variety of neurons (ARVANITAKI and CHALAZONITIS [1954]; BOISTEL and CORABOEUF [1954]; CHALAZONITIS and SUGAYA [1958]; CHALAZONITIS [1959]).

The biophysical aspect of chemosensitivity lies in the conversion of chemical input to electrical responses, i.e. the excitatory action (CHALAZONITIS [1959, 1961]).

Where and how does this conversion occur? Are there differential chemosensitivities among neurons of a same center? Are chemosensitivities membrane potential dependent, or are they also dependent on membrane structural factors?

Finally, to what extent would the direct chemosensitivity of the nonsynaptic, i.e. nonjunctional somatic membrane, be involved in the chemoreception mechanism? It must be recalled that the somatic membrane of molluscan neurons is devoid of synaptic junctions and thus must be considered as a model of nonjunctional neuromembrane.

On the other hand, the physiological aspect of the excitatory action must be examined according to the different functional types of neurons, such as pacemakers (regularly firing and/or waving-bursting neurons) and the normally silent neurons endowed with stable membrane potential that are only functional during the excitatory actions.

In particular, analysis of the excitatory action on very simple nets of neurons composed of 3 or 4 cells—pacemaker inhibitory and silent-type neurons—has been considered on suitable elementary models performing reciprocal or alternate activities. On such nets any analysis of excitatory action by ΔP$_{CO_2}$ change would lead to simple mechanisms explaining acceleration or deceleration of any reciprocal activity.

The alternative physiological aspect of chemosensitivity is the well-known depressive action of P$_{CO_2}$ on the higher nerve centers (on the cortical centers, for instance) that are normally devoid of any specific chemosensitivity. It also requires interpretation on a cellular basis (GELLHORN [1953]; BRODIE and WOODBURY [1958]; WOODBURY et al. [1958]).

What is the mechanism of these depressive actions? Are they direct CO_2 narcoses, arising either from small CO_2 hyperpolarization or from higher CO_2 excessive depolarization, both leading to inactivation?

Should they also be considered as indirect phenomena resulting in massive inhibitory input on the cortical neurons after CO_2 activation of inhibitory interneurons?

Analysis of these elementary mechanisms leading to depressions on the cortex also requires work on elementary neuronal preparations, which will provide a quantitative estimation of any one chemical or synaptic process leading to depressions.

The remarkable and reversible CO_2 actions on different excitable cells, and the importance of CO_2 as a specific regulator of the nervous activity, gave rise to numerous important investigations. Many of them are quoted in Monnier's excellent review [1962]. In this connection, see also Chalazonitis [1959] and Ducreux [1970].

Material and Methods

Simultaneous recording of the hydrogen ion concentration $[H^+]$ changes, and those of the cell's electrical activity parameters were carried out as described below.

First, some morphologically and functionally identifiable neurons with characteristic electrical parameters were explored intracellularly (Figure 1). Changes in membrane potential were recorded through one intracellular microelectrode, where as a second microelectrode was inserted with a view to injecting direct currents (d-c) and evaluating membrane resistance (MR).

Second, the methods of recording $[H^+]$ (generated by the CO_2 hydrolysis) were based on photometric measurement of the Clark indicator spectral changes (CHALAZONITIS et al. [1969]).

Two indicators were used: in the majority of cases, bromocresol purple (indicating pH 7.0 to pH 5.4) and, to a lesser extent, bromothymol (indicating pH 7.6 to 6.6).

These indicators were diluted either in sea water or in the coelomic fluid of the animal at 100 mg/l.; both may be considered good physiological solutions. They were then incorporated in the ganglion by perfusing the dorsal artery of the animal, which irrigates the visceral ganglion by a collateral. After perfusion, the indicator lies in the glial space, close to the giant neurons.

The cinespectrophotometer described elsewhere (CHALAZONITIS [1968]) is a two-beam instrument. Each wavelength corresponds to the two main absorption bands of the indicator, conversely changing as a function of the pH, the former increasing and the latter decreasing. Thus, the cinespectrophotometer records the difference in transmittancy of both wavelengths during P_{CO_2} transients through a width of ganglionic tissue of approximately 1 mm.

A preliminary study, with a scanning spectrophotometer, of solution containing the same amount of bromocresol purple (corresponding to 10 mg/l., a concentration 10 times less than that shed in the ganglion after perfusion but through a width 10 times larger than the ganglionic thickness, i.e. through a cuvette of 1 cm path) shows that the difference in transmittancy is linearly related to the pH from 5.4 to 6.8 (CHALAZONITIS et al. [1969]), (Figure 2). Therefore, admitting that the same linear relation would hold when the indicator lies in the vascular bed of the ganglion, it turns out that the recorded difference in transmittancy gives the instantaneous value in pH directly.

By electrometric measurement with appropriate electrodes, it was possible to evaluate directly the different pH and P_{CO_2} obtained in seawater (physiological solutions for the *Aplysia* ganglion) when saturated with CO_2 at different levels. A linear relationship was found between the log P_{CO_2} and pH: at 25°C, log $P_{CO_2} = 7.6—0.955$ pH. This relation allows the conversion of any instantaneous pH value into P_{CO_2} values. (Figure 3).

The electrical activity during hypercapnic transitions was recorded for any given identified neuron, simultaneously with the

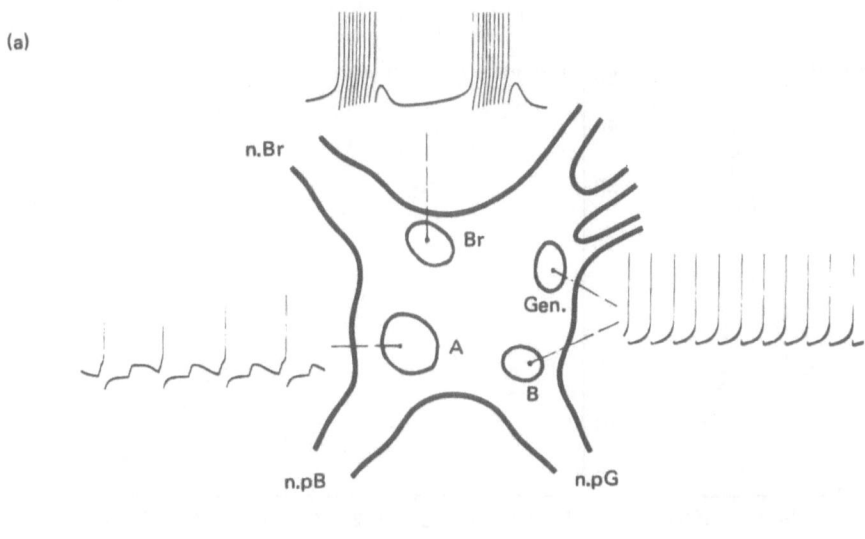

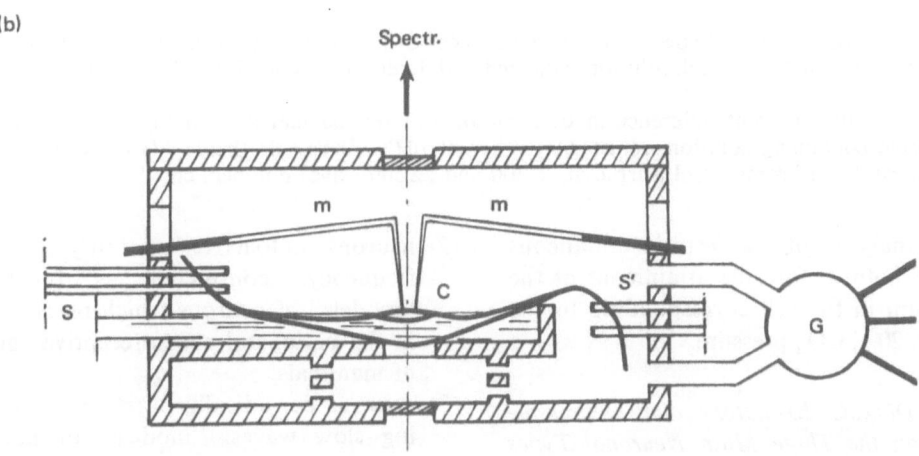

Fig. 1(A). Identifiable giant neurons on the dorsal face of the *Aplysia* visceral ganglion. *A*: Neuron lying near the origin of the pleurobranchial nerve, n. pB, normally silent, responding synaptically only (left pattern). *Gen*: Neuron, near the origin of the genital nerve, spontaneously active with regular spiking frequency (right pattern), or sometimes arhythmic when submitted to a random inhibitory input. *B*: Neuron, near the origin of the pleurogenital nerve, n. pG, with the same behavior as *gen.* neuron. *Br*: Neuron near the origin of the branchial nerve (n. Br), spontaneously active on slow waves (upper pattern).

(B). The preparation in the gas chamber. The isolated ganglion in physiological saline. Two micro-electrodes, *m*, inserted in a cell, *C*. *S*: stimulating electrodes on the pleurobranchial nerve. *S′*: stimulating electrodes on the pleurogenital nerve, and gas admission, *G*. *Arrow* (Spectr.): monochromatic beams transmitted through the ganglion, entering the spectrometer.

pH photometric trace after the insertion of one or two intracellular microelectrodes in the usual way.

The hypercapnic transients were effected with 20% CO_2 + 20% O_2 + 60% N_2. This was adopted as a convenient hypercapnic mixture allowing continuous observation of early, i.e. small, Pco_2 effects, and also of delayed narcotic effects, when the highest Pco_2 value is established in the cells.

It must be pointed out that bioelectric and pH–Pco_2 recordings mainly concern a

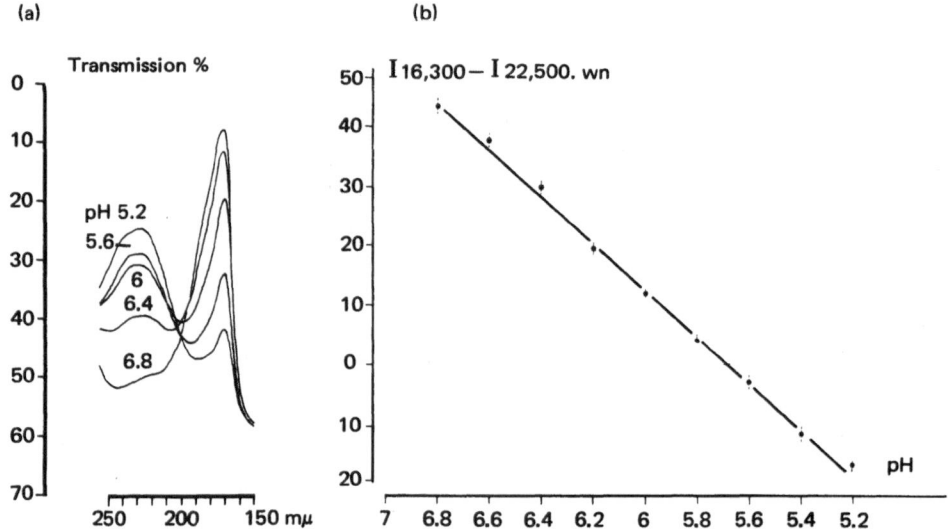

Fig. 2 (A). Superimposed spectrophotometric traces of transmittancy (ordinates) as a function of the wave numbers cm^{-1}, through solutions adjusted at different pH's, containing 9 mg/l. of bromocresol purple.

(B). Ordinates: percent difference in transmittancies (ΔI), calculated from Fig. 2(A), of bromocresol purple containing solution adjusted at different pH's (abcissae); these (ΔI) corresponding to absorption peaks of bromocresol purple at 16,300 and 22,500 waves numbers cm^{-1}.

kinetic analysis of earliest instantaneous values of both, before the attainment of the equilibrium in the cell corresponding to the very high 20% CO_2 pressure.

Carbon Dioxide Excitatory and Depressive Actions on the Three Main Neuronal Types

Direct determinations in the blood (or indirect determinations after *in vivo* measurement of pH values) show *Aplysia* normocapnia as fluctuating between 2.5 mm Hg and 4.3 mm Hg (CHALAZONITIS and NAHAS [1965]). Thus, 20% CO_2 allows a gradual increase of P_{CO_2} in the milieu from 4 mm Hg (normocapnic) to a maximum of 150 mm Hg, corresponding to a pH of 5.65 in the physiological saline injected in the vascular spaces of the ganglion.

As reported previously, three main functional types of neurons exist in *Aplysia* (CHALAZONITIS [1959]) (Figure 1). They are

(1) neurons which are silent, unless under synaptic driving,

(2) neurons autoactive at fairly constant frequency, considered as functional "models" of neurons which predominate in the peripheral chemoreceptive ganglia of mammals,

(3) neurons periodically bursting on repeating slow waves, "models" of neurons which probably predominate in the respiratory centers.

The aim here is to report—using at least the two spontaneously active models—the action of hypercapnia, which for mammalian chemoreceptors is one of the usual respiratory stimuli.

Hypercapnic Activation on Firing Neurons at Regular Frequency

As shown in Figure 4, an initial decrease in pH from 7.1 to 6.7 (corresponding to a P_{CO_2} shift from 6 to 16 mm Hg:10 mm Hg) elicits an increase in instantaneous frequency of about 30%. In the same neuron, the maximum increase was 50% for a final pH of 5.8. The hypercapnic activation on regu-

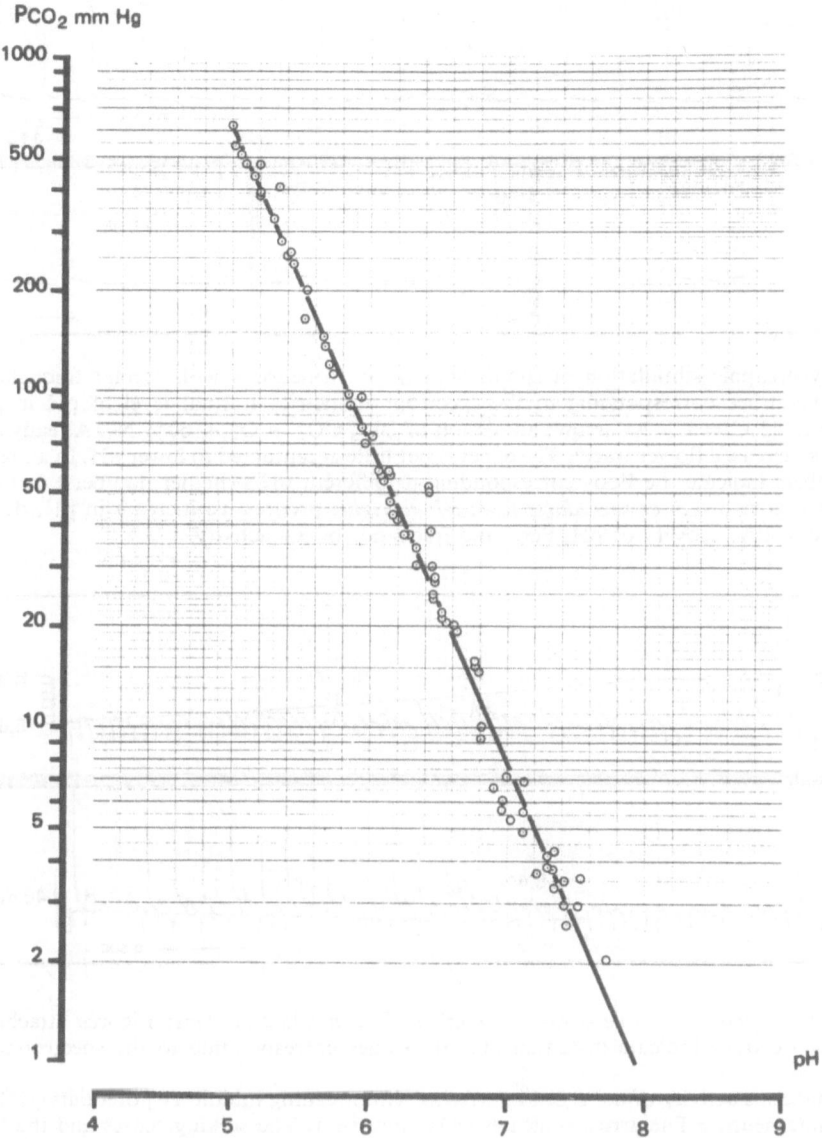

Fig. 3. Log Pco₂ as a function of pH in seawater at 25°C, determined by direct electrometric measurements of pH and Pco₂ in seawater samples equilibrated with different Pco₂'s.

larly firing neurons is not a general phenomenon. In some cases the frequency of firing neurons does not change appreciably with CO_2.

Hypercapnia excitatory effects can also be imitated by extra-neuronal application of hydrogen ions. The extra-neuronal decrease in pH may be carried out in either of two ways: on desheathed neurons by applying physiological saline of pH decreased by HCl; or by lowering the pH very locally—on a small area of the apical neuromembrane —by electrophoretic ejection of H^+ ions through a small pipette filled with acidic saline (CHALAZONITIS and TAKEUCHI [1966]).

Whatever the means of extracellular

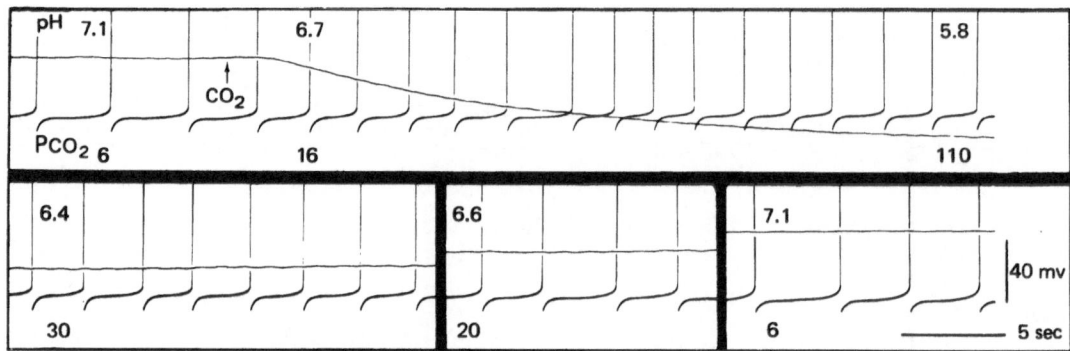

Fig. 4. Hypercapnic stimulation of spontaneously active neurons with regular frequency. *Upper recording*: Upper trace corresponding to the spectrophotometric: normal level of pH in glia, with presence of air at 22°C = 7.7' At arrow: admission of 20% CO_2 + O_2 + 60% N_2. Already at pH 6.7 the frequency is increased (lower trace). The effect is but little accentuated in lower pH. In all recordings, the lower numbers indicate the P_{CO_2} corresponding to different pH's (higher numbers) deduced from the plotting of Figure 3. *Lower recordings from left to right*: progressive increase in pH, during CO_2 elimination and finally recovery of pH, P_{CO_2} and frequency of cell activity.

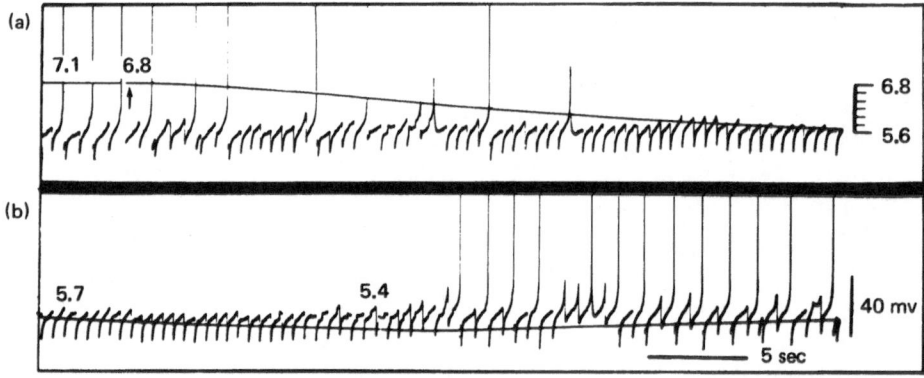

Fig. 5. *Hypercapnic depressive action on inhibitorily controlled neurons*: Figures attached to the spectrophotometric trace indicate instantaneous pH values corresponding to the spectrophotometric trace.

(A). Spontaneous activity of the *B* cell interfering with invading inhibitory potentials (IPSP's) from an associated interneuron. The arrow indicates CO_2 admission: The spiking ceases and the frequency of IPSP's increases.

(B). Reversibility with partial removal of CO_2.

acidification, the general effect is a transient depolarization. This is reversible, either through compensation by the cell buffer systems or by washing out the acidic saline with physiological saline containing buffers such as bicarbonate or THAM.

By using HCl to lower the extracellular glial pH from its normal value (from 7.1 to 5.0), it has been demonstrated that the intracellular pH does not change significantly (ARVANITAKI and CHALAZONITIS [1954]). However, the neuronal membrane is always activated, i.e. depolarized, and extra-activity occurs in neurons firing at regular frequency.

Whereas the external application of low pH (no lower than 5.0, induced by HCl) does not change the intracellular pH but only leads to some consumption of bicarbonate

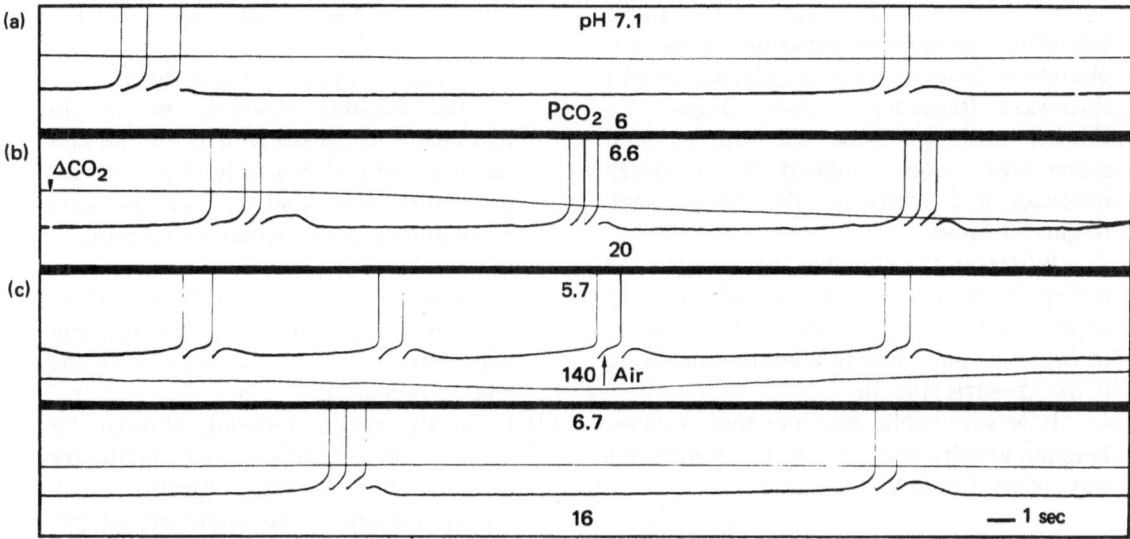

Fig. 6. Hypercapnic activation of waving neurons. In all recordings, upper traces are spectrophotometric and lower traces indicate electrical activity. In this figure, the CO_2 mixture was $40\% \ CO_2 + 20\% \ O_2 + 40\% \ N_2$.

(A). Frequency of bursting in normal conditions (air 22°C).

(B). At arrow, admission of $20\% \ CO_2 \ (+ \ 20\% \ O_2 + 60\% \ N_2)$. Already at pH 6.6 (pCO₂, 20 mm Hg), there is an increase in frequency of bursts.

(C). Highest frequency of bursts at pH 5.7; P_{CO_2} is 140. In all recordings, the lower number indicates glial P_{CO_2} deduced from the plotting of Figure 3.

with CO_2 production, the intracellular change in pH would be performed easily by extracellular increase in P_{CO_2}.

Thus, only CO_2 acts as a real H^+ ion generator inside the cell (ARVANITAKI and CHALAZONITIS [1954]).

Synaptic Inhibitory Control under Small P_{CO_2}, pH Changes

Some *Aplysia* giant neurons [visible on the dorsal face of the ganglion near the origin of the genital nerve trunk (*Gen* cell) or near the pleurogenital nerve cell (*B* cell)], normally of regular frequency, very often undergo a spontaneous inhibitory bombardment from the inhibitory interneurons, which are highly regular in frequency. Consequently, the pattern of their activity will be arythmic.

A pH decrease of about 0.6 units, corresponding to a P_{CO_2} increase of about 19 mm Hg, may cause a measurable decrease in the spontaneous activity of these cells without any measurable influence on the frequency of the inhibitory cell. Later on, and with higher P_{CO_2} and pH displacement, inhibitory cell frequency increases (Figure 5).

Such behavior of the inhibitory interneuron, and of the inhibitorily controlled cell, is suggestive of a possible cellular mechanism of some nerve centers highly depressed by CO_2-H^+ action. The depression is not due solely to a direct hyperpolarizing action, but also to simultaneous indirect action, arising from enhancement of the normal inhibitory bombardment.

Hypercapnic and Low pH Excitatory Effects on Waving Neurons (Bursting on Slow Waves)

The so-called *Br* cells of *Aplysia*, bursting on slow waves of endogenous origin, are also excited by hypercapnic transients. By increasing P_{CO_2} above 6 mm Hg (or decreasing pH below 7.1), a transient depolarization is engendered that augments the slow-wave frequency (Figure 6).

Application of H^+ ions on the apical side of the *Br* cell membrane by the electrophoretic technique elicited depolarization and slow-wave frequency increase (Figure 7). Further washing of the cell with suitable saline (sea water) initiated the recovery processes and return to the initial wave frequency value.

Whatever the stimulus (hypercapnia or low pH), if it is strong enough, it may depolarize the cell to an extent which leads to fusion of the waves in a continuous firing (CHALAZONITIS [1961]).

It is worthwhile recalling that wavingbursting activity may arise in many different ways, described below.

(1) Directly, as in the case of the wavingbursting neuron of *Aplysia*; oscillations and superimposed bursts are of endogenous origin, i.e. they are due to the membrane properties, and not to synaptic

influences (ARVANITAKI and CHALAZONITIS [1964]).

(2) Indirectly, or synaptically, as in the case of the bursting thalamic neuron in mammals (ANDERSEN [1965]); in this case the bursting is due mainly to an afferent excitatory drive and to the alternate auto-inhibition or "recurrent inhibition" of the neuron. The auto-inhibition is performed by a collateral branch of its own axon firing an inhibitory interneuron which in turn stops the activity of the neuron periodically.

(3) Indirectly, arising generally through "a conflict of excitation and inhibitory action"; this bursting function may include the above "recurrent inhibition" and/or the "afferent collateral inhibition", both considered by Eccles [1969].

Conversely, when the bursting activity is indirect, the timing of a multiple action of

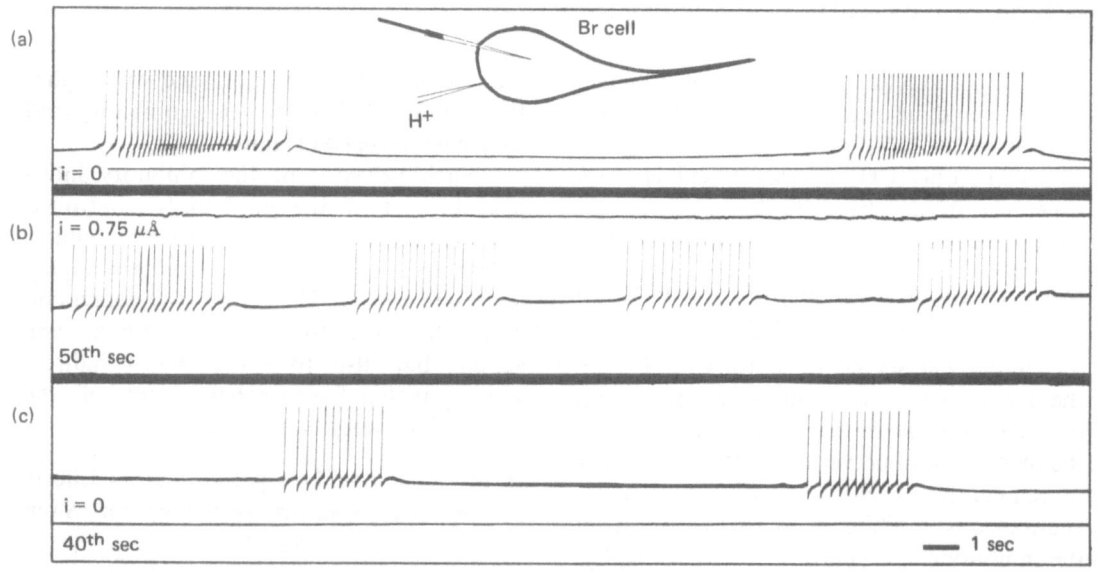

Fig. 7. Microelectrophoretic ejection of H^+ on the surface of the Br (waving or bursting) cell. As in Figure 6, the CO_2 mixture was $40\% \, CO_2 + 20\% \, O_2 + 40\% \, N_2$.

(A). Normal frequency of slow waves.

(B). Just after the electrophoretic ejection of H^+ by a 0.75 μÅ current, during 50 sec (the intensity of the current is deduced from the position of the straight trace in all recordings). After the H^+ ejection the frequency of the waves is increased.

(C). 40 sec after cessation of the H^+ ejection, the frequency of the waving is almost recovered.

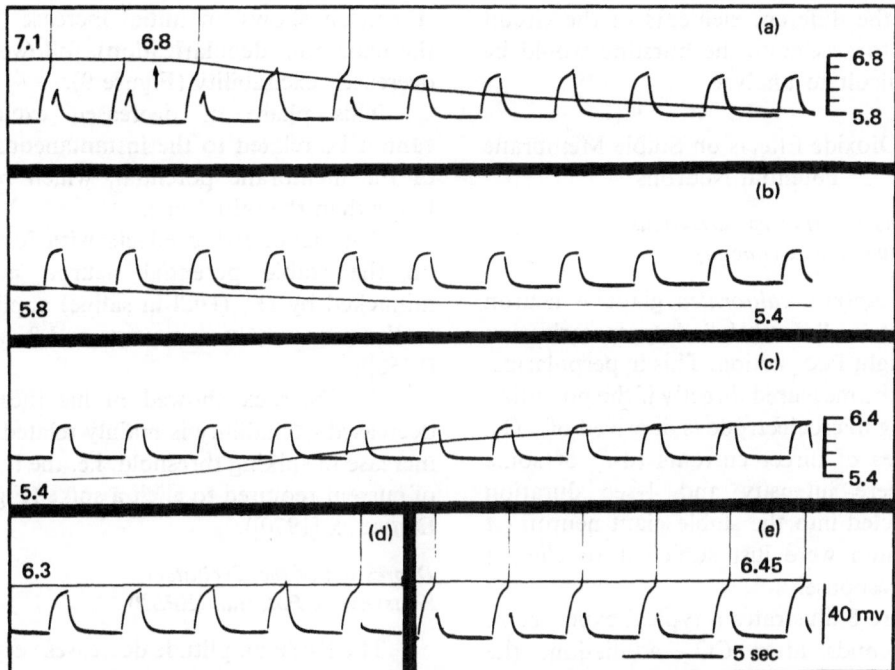

Fig. 8. *Hypercapnic depressive action on the direct excitability of stable neurons.* Bioelectric events were recorded simultaneously with spectrophotometric trace. Figures affixed to the spectrophotometric trace indicate instantaneous pH values. Scales on the right concern the pH values corresponding to the spectrophotometric traces. Neuronal responses to DC of 1 nanocoulomb (1 sec × 1 nanoampere). Arrow indicates admission of CO_2; excitability depression starting at pH 6.5 and reaches a maximum at pH 5.4 [in (B)].In (C), (D), and (E) there is continuous recovery of excitability from pH 5.4 to 6.45.

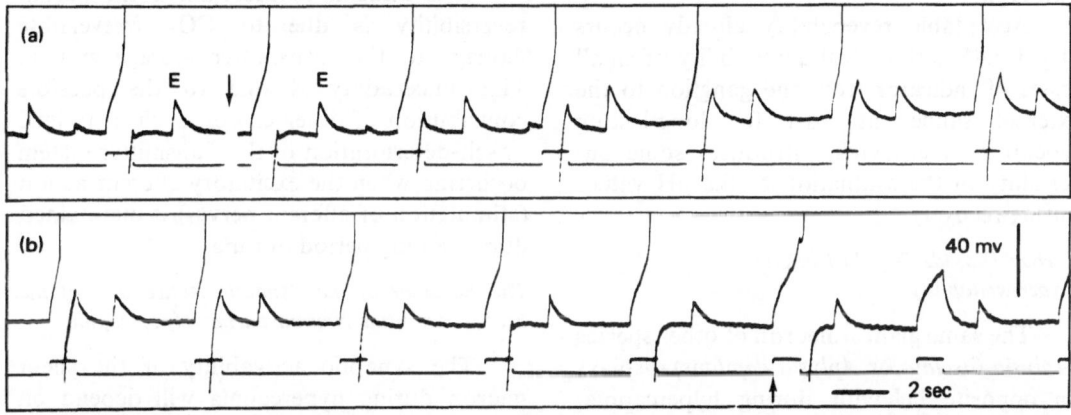

Fig. 9. Simultaneous recording of the somatic excitability and excitory post-snyaptic potential amplitude (EPSP).

(A). Indicated responsiveness of a stable membrane potential neurone to depolarizing DC injection (lower trace) and to synaptic activation (stimulation of the pleurogenital nerve), giving rise to an EPSP [(E)]. The arrow signifies 20% CO_2 admittance. In this case, CO_2 depolarizes the soma and increases excitability. The latency of the spike occurence is shortened, whereas the EPSP amplitude does not change significantly [end of the (A) recording]. Later on, in (B), when the soma displays a decreased excitability to DC, (see arrow), a decrease in EPSP amplitude occurs simultaneously. The photometric trace is omitted, but at the end of the (B) recording, the pH would be approximately 5.6.

CO_2 on the different elements of the circuit in order to accelerate the bursting would be more difficult to analyze.

Carbon Dioxide Effects on Stable Membrane Potential Neurons

Carbon Dioxide Hyperpolarizations: Hypercapnic Hypoexcitability

The *Aplysia californica* giant *A* neuron undergoes a "d'emblée" hyperpolarization during slight P_{CO_2} action. This hyperpolarization may be measured directly if the potential-measuring microelectrode is deprived of CO_2.

Pulses of direct currents (d-c) of some nanoampere intensity and 1-sec duration were injected into the stable giant neuron (*A* neuron) and were just sufficient to elicit a somatic response.

Figure 8 illustrates a typical experiment. Some seconds after CO_2 admission, the injected current elicits a local response only superimposed on the membrane potential displacement at pH 6.2. The earliest sign of excitability decrease is already the equivalent of pH 6.4—in other words, after a P_{CO_2} increase from 16 mm to 30 mm ($\Delta P_{CO_2} = 24$ mm Hg).

Acceptable reversibility already occurs at pH 6.45, although the possibility of small losses of indicator from the ganglion to the external saline, at least for long-lasting repetitive experiments, introduces some uncertainty in the estimation of the pH values during recovery.

Carbon Dioxide Depolarization: Hyperexcitability

The same giant *A* neuron of other species (*Aplysia fasciata* or *Aplysia depilans*) displays an opposite behavior during hypercapnia, i.e. depolarization leading to an increase in excitability. Such an effect has already been described (CHALAZONITIS and NAHAS [1965]) and may occur with a low increase in P_{CO_2}, i.e. with 5%. If P_{CO_2} reaches 20%, the initial depolarizing effect is depressed and the membrane potential starts increasing again. Measurement of the direct excitability of the

A neuron shows an initial increase (during the maximum depolarization), followed by a decreased excitability (Figure 9).

This phase of decreased excitability cannot be related to the instantaneous value of the membrane potential, which remains lower than the initial one.

The depolarizing effects with low P_{CO_2} on the stable potential neuron may be mimicked by H^+ (HCl in saline) application to the neuron (CHALAZONITIS and TAKEUCHI [1966]).

As Ducreux showed in his thesis, the decreased excitability is mainly related to the increase in spiking threshold, i.e. the intensity of current required to elicit a spike (Figure 9; DUCREUX [1970]).

Depression of the Excitatory Postsynaptic Potential (EPSP)

The EPSP amplitude decreases very often when pH is lowered below 6.4 (or P_{CO_2} raised higher than 30 mm Hg) (Figure 10).

Such a decrease is sometimes reversible (Figure 10), but very often only partially so, even when the admission of air exceeds 30 min.

It is difficult to ascertain if the partial reversibility is due to CO_2 irreversible damage to the transmitter storage system. This uncertainty is due to the possible contribution of other causes, such as fatigue or self-deterioration of the transmitter system occurring when the excitatory afferent action (stimulation of afferent nerves) is maintained during a long period of time.

The Behavior of the Synaptic Activability of the Stable Potential Neuron during Hypercapnia

The synaptic activability of the silent neuron during hypercapnia will depend on the kinetics of three different parameters: the MP hypercapnic time course; the EPSP amplitude time course and the threshold potential change during hypercapnia.

If the silent neuron depolarizes with low P_{CO_2} (i.e. 5%) whereas the EPSP's amplitude and the threshold of the spiking do not change, the overall hypercapnic effect will be

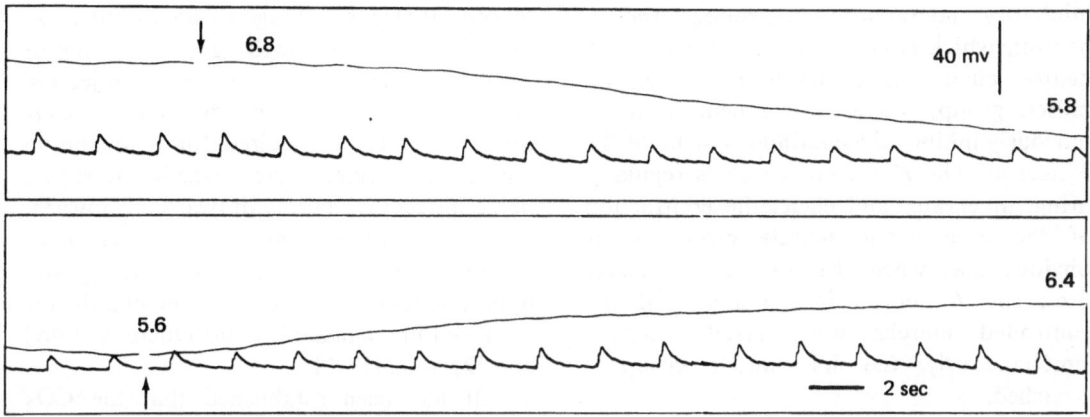

Fig. 10. Hypercapnic depression of the excitory postsynaptic potential (EPSP) elicited on the stable membrane potential neuron [(A soma)]. (A) is the photometric recordings. Numbers indicate the instantaneous pH values. (B) is the EPSP recordings. Both (A) and (B) recordings are continuous.
↓ : admission of 20 % CO_2 gas
↑ : admission of air
Membrane potential increases slightly with CO_2. Already at pH 6.4, the previously depressed EPSP amplitude is restored.

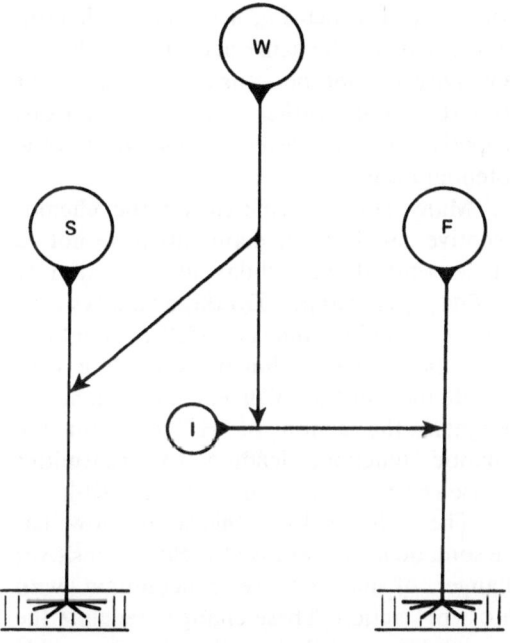

Fig. 11. Alternate activation of two muscle groups by a four-neuron system. *W* is a "waving" neuron, i.e. a pacemaker bursting neuron. This *W* neuron simultaneously activates *S*, the silent neuron (i.e. the neuron of stable membrane potential fired by EPSP's) and the inhibitory interneuron *I*, which stops the continuously firing neuron *F*.

excitatory (CHALAZONITIS and NAHAS [1966]). Conversely, if the CO_2 effect is hyperpolarizing, the synaptic activability of the neuron will be depressed whatever the Pco_2 value.

But a very interesting case is one which concerns differential kinetics of the instantaneous threshold and MP values and EPSP amplitude during hypercapnia. Sometimes the hyperexcitability due to some depolarization may be compensated for by the EPSP's decreased amplitude. In that case the synaptically elicited spiking will not change in frequency.

How Pco_2 Could Accelerate an Elementary Net of Four Neurons Normally Performing Reciprocal Activities to Effectors

A functional elementary net of four neurons was proposed in order to explain, as simply as possible, a reciprocal periodical command of two groups of antagonistic muscles. This net is formed by a waving-bursting neuron, the activity of which is of endogenous origin.

This neuron alternately and excitorily drives two subordinate neurons (Figure 11). The *S* neuron is normally silent, i.e. of stable membrane potential. The *I* neuron is an inhibitory interneuron controlling the *F* neuron, which is continuously firing. The *S* neuron elicits the contraction of the first muscle group, whereas the *I* neuron simultaneously inhibits the continuous firing of the *F* neuron. The *F* neuron, which is regularly firing, innervates and elicits the contraction of the antagonistic muscle group. It is obvious that when the waving pacemaker fires, the *F* neuron is inhibited and the controlled muscles are relaxed, whereas simultaneously, the first muscle group is stretched.

The accelerating action of a transient increase of P_{CO_2} may be exerted on the pacemaker waving-bursting neuron either directly or indirectly: directly as explained above; indirectly by some synaptic excitatory drive coming from the periphery and accelerating the waving-bursting frequency of the pacemaker.

Membrane Potential: Dependence on P_{CO_2}–pH Chemoresponse

It may be concluded from the previous discussion that whereas a large number of neurons show hypercapnic depolarization (excitatory action), the reverse effect (hyperpolarization and inhibition), although less frequent, is observed on other neurons. It also frequently happens that a third category of neurons do not give chemoresponse at all.

On the other hand, should one compare the membrane potential levels in relation to the opposite behavior of neurons to P_{CO_2}–pH action, one finds that the spontaneously active neurons are generally characterized by lower membrane potential levels than the quiescent neurons.

It thus follows that a complementary investigation is indispensable to clarify the extent to which the chemoresponse is governed by the initial membrane potential level. Experiments were therefore carried out as follows (Ducreux and Chalazonitis [1969]).

First, the hypercapnic response was recorded in normal membrane potential. The level of the membrane potential was then dis-placed by means of long-lasting d-c injection into the neuron through the second micro-electrode. The duration of the d-c injection lasted during the 2 min admission of CO_2 mixture, which is required for a maximum effect. The injected current was in the region of some nanoamperes, outward or inward, eliciting a shift in membrane potential of 10 mv to 20 mv, respectively, depolarizing and hyperpolarizing. Further experimental details are given in Chalazonitis and Ducreux [1969] and Ducreux [1970].

It has been established that the CO_2 chemoresponse depends on the membrane potential level. When the membrane is slightly depolarized (MP = 40 mv), the CO_2 depolarization is increased. If MP reaches about 70 mv, there is no more CO_2 response. Conversely, CO_2 exerts a hyperpolarizing action when the MP level exceeds 70 mv. This dependence, although extremely variable from neuron to neuron, nevertheless demonstrates that for the same neuron, the chemosensitivity cannot be considered a constant property, but rather an instantaneous property like the level of the membrane potential itself.

Many studies centered on the chemoreceptive ganglions in mammals have not as yet determined the cellular site of action of the P_{CO_2}, pH changes. Do these changes take place in the epithelioid cells of these ganglions or in their synaptic junctions binding with the efferent fibers? Current ideas tend to designate the action of H^+ ions on the synaptic junction, leading to transmitter release (Eyzaguirre and Zapata [1968]).

The main results of this study show that the somatic membrane is also chemosensitive: changes of its MP are concomitant with P_{CO_2}, pH action. These changes regulate the normal firing of these cells in a forseeable manner and, consequently, its transmission to other cells synaptically. There is no difficulty in transposing this mechanism to the respiratory center neurons; but transposition to the epithelioid cells of the peripheral ganglia of mammals is at present conjectural. However, if the epithelioid cells

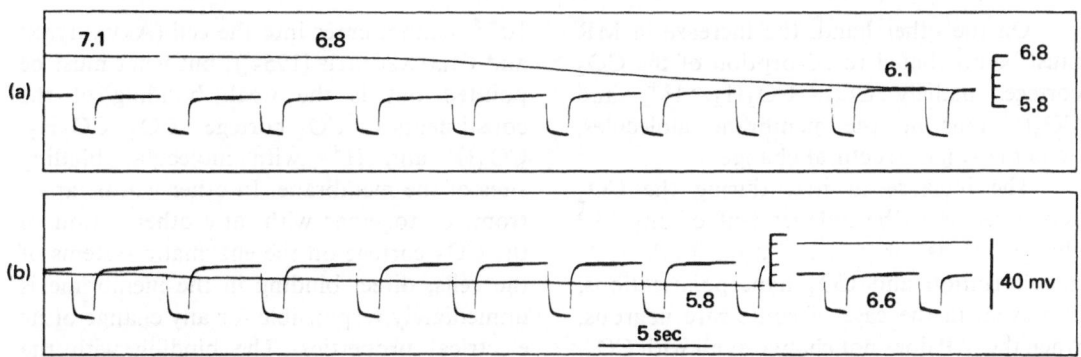

Fig. 12. Increase in membrane resistance during hypercapnia. (A) is photometric traces; (B) shows displacement of the MP by square hyperpolarizing pulses. Recordings from pH 7.1 to 5.8 are continuous. Membrane resistance (MR) of the stable MP neuron increases continuously. At pH 5.8 (P_{CO_2} = 100 mm Hg) MR is 50% increased. The last recording (pH 6.6) is obtained after 20 min recovery in air, when MR reaches its initial value.

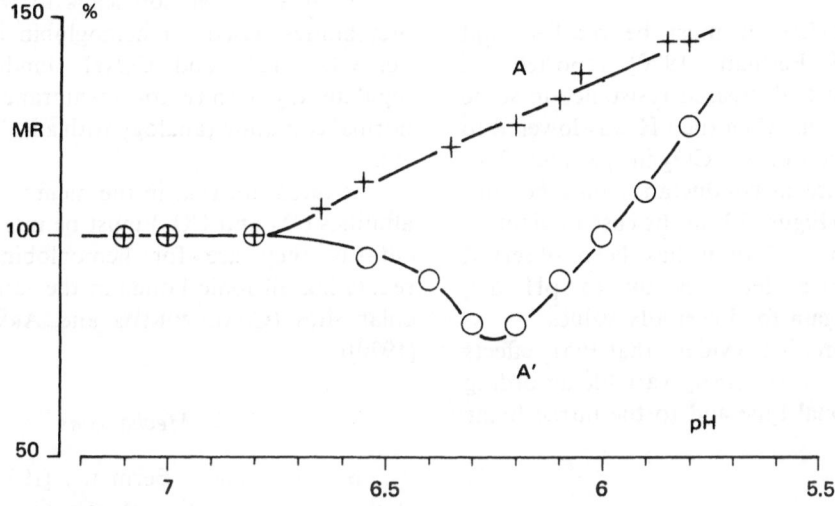

Fig. 13. Membrane resistance as a function of instantaneous pH values during CO_2 transients. *A* and *A'* are identifiable giant cells both of the stable membrane potential type (see CHALAZONITIS [1959]). Whereas the NR of the *A* cells increases continuously during the CO_2 transient, the MR of the *A'* cell reaches a minimum at pH 6.3 (P_{CO_2} = 35 mm Hg) and subsequently increases continuously until pH 5.75 (P_{CO_2} = 110 mm Hg).

are excitable cells, giving a spiking by hypercapnic depolarization, the mechanism of the synaptic transfer of the information remains the same as in the case of *Aplysia* neurons.

Carbon Dioxide Dependence of the Membrance Resistance (MR)

An increase in membrane resistance has already been observed in the case of the *Aplysia*

neuron (CHALAZONITIS and ROMEY [1964]).

A systematic study confirmed these earlier results and, at least for hyperpolarizing pulses, the increase of MP displacement ($+\Delta$MP) during CO_2 action signified a continuous increase in MR. This MR behavior is at least valid for the stable membrane potential neurons, such as the *Aplysia A* neuron (Figures 12 and 13).

On the other hand, the increase in MR must be attributed to adsorption of the CO_2 cortege, namely CO_2, CO_3H_2, H^+, and CO_3H' ions on the membrane molecules, denoting some structural change.

The increase in MR during the CO_2 action seems to be independent of any MP change. It is observed during both CO_2 depolarization and CO_2 hyperpolarizations, and even, in the case of some rare neurons, when the MP does not change at all with CO_2.

But the MR increase with CO_2 apart from any MP change has been demonstrated (DUCREUX [1970]); compensation for any hypercapnic change of the MP by d-c injection restores the MP to its initial level but the membrane resistance still remains increased.

Nevertheless, it must be recalled that Brown and Berman [1970] reported an opposite effect: decreased resistance in some *Aplysia* neurons when the pH was lowered to 6.5 by addition of 5% CO_2 in seawater. This initial increase in conductance may be confirmed here (Figure 13) in the case of giant A' type neurons, where it has been observed that resistance decreases up to pH 6.3, increasing again for lower pH values.

Therefore, it is evident that P_{CO_2} effects on MR may be extremely variable according to the neuronal type and to the intracellular P_{CO_2} level.

Discussion and Conclusions

Two aspects of CO_2 actions will be discussed here: first those at the molecular scale, then those at the cellular scale.

Molecular Scale

For apparent reasons, it is not yet possible to separate the CO_2 and H^+ ion actions within the neuromembrane. On the other hand, unequal diffusibility between CO_2 and H^+ applied extracellularly must be recalled. The inward diffusibility of the CO_2 has been demonstrated, whereas H^+, extracellularly applied at concentration lower than

10^{-5}, cannot enter into the cell (ARVANITAKI and CHALAZONITIS [1954]); but what must be pointed out is the weak bonding of the constituents of CO_2 cortege—CO_2, CO_3H_2, CO_3H' and H^+—with molecular binding sites of the membrane. In other words, apart from, or together with, any other action of the CO_2 cortege on the enzymatic systems of the cells, direct binding in the membrane is immediately responsible for any change of its electrical properties. The binding with the molecular sites of the membranes is by weak bonding, as is the case with the hemoglobin molecule, which is considered a model of the neuromembrane molecular affinities with weak bonding (CHALAZONITIS and ARVANITAKI [1970]).

Such a comparison leads to some predictabilities based on hemoglobin affinities, i.e. CO_2, H^+, and CO_3H' binding may regulate O_2 affinity for membrane sites in normal condition (analogy with a Bohr effect), etc.

It turns out that in the membrane, both affinities (O_2 and CO_2) must be interdependent—as they are for hemoglobin—finally regulating all ionic bonds in the same molecular sites (CHALAZONITIS and ARVANITAKI [1970]).

Ionic Mechanisms

Brown, and Berman [1970] concluded, after a series of experiments with variable P_{CO_2}'s at constant pH in the surrounding saline, that H^+ is the main agent of the CO_2 action. In our opinion such a conclusion may be valid for a number of neurons because of the similarity of H^+ and CO_2 effects on the membrane resistance, but not for all neurons. As a matter of fact, as long as the measurements of CO_2, H^+ and CO_3H' linked to the membrane molecules after the establishment of a given extracellular P_{CO_2} remain unknown, it seems rather difficult to ascribe all P_{CO_2} effects on the main electrical parameters to H^+ only. For many cells, CO_2 cannot duplicate extracellular H^+ actions. For instance, very often

P_{CO_2} increases the resistance of many membranes but H^+ has a reverse action.

On the other hand, recent valuable work done by Brown, Walker, and Sutton [1970] demonstrated that for some neurons the H^+ responsiveness (de- or repolarization) is linked to the transmembrane gradient and conductances of chloride ions.

If the chloride ion is mainly concerned for any direct H^+ effect on the membrane, it must again be recalled that P_{CO_2} and H^+ generally decrease the respiratory rate of nerve tissue (BERGMAN and BERGMAN [1964]) and therefore they could decelerate ionic pumps—the sodium pump, for instance.

But a complete spatiotemporal analysis of P_{CO_2}, pH effects on the sodium pump of *Aplysia* neuromembranes is still lacking and therefore no further attempt would be possible in order to evaluate such indirect effects of P_{CO_2}, pH on the membrane potential.

Cellular Scale

Taking into account the binding of CO_2, H^+, and HCO_3^- molecules on the so-called "receptor molecules" of the membrane, it would seem highly probable that the type and "concentration" of these molecules may be extremely variable from one area to another of a same neuromembrane.

It is well known, for example, how different the bioelectrical properties are from a somatic (nonjunctional) area to an axonal area.

For reasons described in detail in previous work, the heterogeneity of the different areas of the membrane provide an introduction to the concept of a permanent unequal control of the different areas by metabolic endogenous factors giving rise to unequal distribution of the main "forces" that establish the instantaneous value of the membrane potential. To clarify this idea, suppose, for instance, that for a given neuron pumps are permanently more developed near the somatic areas of the membrane and conductances more operative near the axon

hillock. With such a hypothesis, some sodium could be permanently absorbed through the axonal membrane and permanently expelled through the somatic membrane of the same cell. Such a mechanism may depict the presence of permanent ionic currents energizing a spontaneous firing, at least, (for instance, through areas of high oscillatory potentialities) (CHALAZONITIS and ARVANITAKI [1970]).

If such an asymmetrical distribution of "conductances" and "pumps" could be visualized for some neurons, it turns out that the spatiotemporal analysis of CO_2, H^+, and HCO_3^- action would be complicated by the progressive accumulation of these molecules successively in the first area (dominated by pumps) and later in the second area (dominated by the conductances). As a corollary of such a picture any analysis of ionic conductances and/or pumps would concern microtopographic analysis as well as kinetic determinations.

Any P_{CO_2} or pH action would finally lead to change in permanent generator current intensity and/or even direction, thus determining local and overall values of the membrane potential and firing outputs.

In conclusion, development, at least on giant neurons, of a new methodology of precise topographic and kinetic analysis for local electrical properties (for example, local current clamping and extracellular local potential) would be indispensable before any attempt at analyzing ionic movements as contributors to generator current instantaneous value.

Finally, from the overall data of cellular neurophysiology the following conclusions may be suggested.

(1) Because of the absence of synaptic junctions on the perikarya of these giant neurons—their synapses lying deep in the neuropile—any change in MP, if devoid of spontaneous synaptic potentials, must be considered a genuine response of the somatic membrane apart from any possible action of released transmitters.

(2) CO_2 sensitivity is a general property of the somatic neuromembrane measurable by the ratio $\Delta MP/\Delta P\ CO_2$, change in membrane potential (MP) for a given change in P_{CO_2} in mm Hg. A functionally better representation would be $\Delta N/\Delta P_{CO_2}$ consisting of all extra spikes produced for a given ΔP_{CO_2}.

(3) CO_2 sensitivity cannot be a neuromembrane standard property, but is an instantaneous property depending on the initial level of the membrane potential (MP), which is determined by summation of any synaptic influence.

(4) CO_2 sensitivity cannot be the same for two different neurons adjusted at the same MP. Therefore, molecular structural factors inherent in its neuromembrane predetermines its CO_2 sensitivity, apart from its initial MP level.

(5) Direct depolarization by CO_2 of waving-bursting pacemakers performing reciprocal (i.e. alternate) activation of neuron and effectors can directly change the frequency of rythmicities. Indirect influences (i.e. CO_2 acceleration of centripetal excitatory synaptic input) may also indirectly modulate the frequency of the waving-bursting pacemaker.

Summary

The purpose of the work described has been to search for possible excitatory and depressive actions of the CO_2–H^+ system on given neuronal models of *Aplysia* through (a) spectrophotometric recording of absorption changes induced by CO_2 and of suitable pH indicators injected into the ganglion; (b) simultaneous recording of concomitant changes in the bioelectric parameters; (c) establishing the relationship between pH and transmittancy changes giving the instantaneous pH of the glial space (perineuronal) during the P_{CO_2} action; (d) establishing the relationship between pH and P_{CO_2} in seawater (taken as a physiological solution for the isolated ganglion), allowing conversion of the instantaneous pH values into P_{CO_2} values.

Following this approach, effects of the CO_2–H^+ system were demonstrated on giant and identifiable neurons of *Aplysia*.

First, effects were excitatory on the spontaneously active neurons of two types: those firing neurons with regular frequency and those bursting on slow waves.

Secondly, depressive effects of the CO_2–H^+ system were demonstrated on two types of neurons: the stable membrane potential neuron (*A* neuron) and some autoactive but arhythmic neurons, inhibitorily controlled.

In the first case, the depressive effects are due to hyperpolarizing action, decrease in excitatory postsynaptic potential (EPSP) amplitude, and/or increase in the spiking threshold.

In the latter case, the depressive effects were found to be partly due to a decrease in the direct excitability of the examined neuron, and partly to an increase of inhibitory input from associated interneurons.

It was also found that chemosensitivity, defined either as $\Delta MP/\Delta P_{CO_2}$ (change in the membrane potential for a given change in P_{CO_2} or $\Delta F/\Delta P_{CO_2}$ (change in the number of elicited spikes for a given change P_{CO_2}) depends, among other things, on the level of the MP during the CO_2 action. In some cases, this dependence explains why neuronal chemosensitivity is a variable and instantaneous property.

Finally, membrane potential dependence of the CO_2 action and membrane resistance changes during CO_2 action denote a structural change of the molecular conformation of the membrane, substantiating the direct action of CO_2 on the latter.

Acknowledgment   This work was supported in part by the Centre National de la Recherche Scientifique, France, a research grant from the United States Public Health Service under grant Number EY 00440, and a research grant from the United States Army under contract no. DAJA 37–67–C–0971.

Bibliography

Andersen, P., "Rhythmic thalamic activity." In

Studies in Physiology, Springer Verlag (Heidelberg, 1965), pp. 1–6.

Arvanitaki, A. and Chalazonitis, N., "Diffusibilité de l'anhydride carbonique dans l'axone géant, ses effets sur les vitesses de l'activité bioélectrique." *C. R. Soc. Biol.*, 148:952–54 (1954).

———, "Configurations modales de l'activité à différents neurones d'un même centre." *J. Physiol.*, 50:122–25 (1958).

———, "Processus d'excitation d'un neurone autoactif sur ondes lentes." *C. R. Soc. Biol.*, 158:1119–23 (1964).

Bergman, C. and Bergman, J., "Action de l'anhydride carbonique sur la consommation d'oxygène du nerf insolé de grenouille." *C. R. Soc. Biol.*, 158:2000 (1964).

Boistel, J. and Coraboeuf, E., "Action de l'anhydride carbonique sur l'activité électrique du nerf isolé d'insecte." *J. Physiol.*, 46:258–61 (1954).

Brodie, D. A. and Woodbury, D. M., "Acid-base changes in brain and blood of rats exposed to high concentrations of carbon dioxide." *Am. J. Physiol.*, 192:91–100 (1958).

Brown, A. M. and Berman, P. R., "Mechanism of excitation of *Aplysia* neurons by carbon dioxide." *J. Gen. Physiol.*, 56:543–58 (1970).

———, Walker, J. L. Jr., and Sutton, R. B., "Increased chloride conductance as the proximate cause of hydrogen ion concentration effects in *Aplysia* neurons. *J. Gen. Physiol.*, 56:559–82 (1970).

Chalazonitis, N., "Chémopotentiels des neurones géants fonctionnellement différenciés." *Arch. Sci. Physiol.*, 13:41–78 (1959).

———, "Chémopotentials in giant nerve cells (*Aplysia fasciata*)." In *Nervous Inhibition*. Pergamon Press (Oxford, 1961), pp. 179–93.

———, "Intracellular pO$_2$ control on excitability and synaptic activability in *Aplysia* and *Helix* identifiable giant neurons." *Ann. N.Y. Acad. Sci.*, 147:419–59 (1968).

———, and Arvanitaki, A., "Neuromembrane electrogenesis during changes in pO$_2$, pCO$_2$ and pH. *Advances in Biochemical Psychopharmacology*, 2: 245–84 (1970).

———, Chagneux, R., Takeuchi, H., and Ducreux, C., Enregistrement simultané des pH, pCO$_2$ et activité électrique des neurones géants en hypercapnie (neurones indentifiables d'*Aplysia*). *C. R. Soc. Biol.*, 163: 1187–92 (1969).

———, and Nahas, G. G., "Small pCO$_2$ change on neuronal synaptic activation." *Nature (London)*, 205:1016–17 (1965).

———, and Nahas, G. G., "Effets antagonistes, ions-hydrogène-THAM, sur l'activité électrique des neurones géants (*Aplysia et Helix*)." *Ann. Anesthesiol. Franç.*, 7:605–16 (1966).

———, and Romey, G. "Excitabilité directe et conductance de la membrane somatique en fonction de la pression partielle de l'anhydride carbonique (neurone d'*Aplysia*)." *C. R. Soc. Biol.*, 158:2367–72 (1964).

———, and Sugaya, E., "Stimulation-inhibition des neurones géants identifiables d'*Aplysia*, par l'anhydride carbonique." *C. R. Acad. Sci.*, 247:1657–59 (1958).

———, and Takeuchi, H., "Application micro-électrophorétique locale d'ions H$^+$ et variations des paramètres bioélectriques de la membrane neuronique. (Neurones géants d'*Helix pomatia*)." *C. R. Soc. Biol.*, 160:610–15 (1966).

Cohen, M. I., "Discharge patterns of brain-stem, respiratory neurons in relation to carbon dioxide tension." *J. Neurophysiol.*, 31:142–65 (1968).

Ducreux, C., "Propriétés électriques des neuro-membranes en hypercapnie (Neurones d'*Aplysia* et d'*Helix*). Thèse IIIe cycle. Neurophysiologie, Université Aix-Marseille (1970).

———, and Chalazonitis, N., "Réponses hypercapniques du neurone, fonction de son potentiel de membrane (Neurones géants d'*Helix* et d'*Aplysia*)." *C. R. Soc. Biol.*, 163:1183–87 (1969).

Eccles, J. C., "Excitatory and inhibitory mechanisms in brain." In *Basic mechanisms of the epilepsies*. (Boston, 1969), pp. 229–52.

Eyzaguirre, C. and Zapata, P., "Pharmacology of pH effects on carotid body chemoreceptors in vitro." *J. Physiol. (London)*, 195:557–88 (1968).

Gellhorn, E., "On the physiological action of carbon dioxide on cortex and hypothalamus." *E.E.G. J.*, 5:401–13 (1953).

Monnier, A. M., "L'anhydride carbonique régulateur spécifique de l'activité nerveuse." *Arch. Internat. Pharmacod. et Thér.*, 140:189–98 (1962).

Woodbury, D. M., Rollins, L. T., Gardner, M. D., Hirsh, W. L., Hogan, J. R., Rallison,

M. L., Tanner, G. S., and Brodie, D. A., "Effects of carbon dioxide on brain excitability and electrolytes." *Am. J. Physiol.*, 192: 79–90 (1958).

Chalazonitis Discussion

HOLLAND: Perhaps the question is a little aside from your subject, but in the nervous tissue of molluscs, there is always carbonic anhydrase present. What would be the function of carbonic anhydrase in connection with your schema you present?

CHALAZONITIS: What is the real function of carbonic anhydrase schema in the present? I don't know. In order to answer your question to some extent it would be essential to have more precise information on the enzyme localization in relation to the cell species—glial or nervous. Secondly, if carbonic anhydrase exists in nerve cells, one would have to know if it is more concentrated in the soma, axon, or terminals of the molluscan neurons.

SIESJÖ: I've been very impressed by the differences in the action of carbon dioxide on various types of cells and its various concentrations, and I remember when working with Krenovitch and Randig on the cortical cells which Dr. Carpenter was referring to and then we could get excitation with very low concentrations and inhibitions with high concentrations. I wonder if a similar thing is seen with the *Aplysia* neurons?

CHALAZONITIS: Yes. With small concentrations you very often get depolarization and excitation of the cell. With higher concentrations the nerve cell is inactivated, either by excessive depolarization, increased threshold, or sometimes by inhibitory bombardment arising from activated inhibitory interneurons with higher P_{CO_2}'s.

SIESJÖ: I would like to be in agreement with what Dr. Carpenter said about the effects of CO_2 on metabolism, because there are effects on metabolism at substrate levels and also on the transmitter metabolism, and I was just wondering what sort of transmitters you have in *Aplysia*?

CHALAZONITIS: The transmitters found in *Aplysia* nerve cells are acetylcholine dopamine and to a lesser extent 5-hydroxydyptamine. CO_2 action on the *Aplysia* soma—devoid of any synaptic junctions—is exerted directly on the membrane. I also agree that CO_2 effects are exerted on the exergonic metabolism and do control the transmitter release, but these aspects of the CO_2 actions are beyond the limits of my present contribution.

LOESCHKE: I think our idea about the respiratory centers and the chemosensitivity is changing now insofar as it seems that the centers are just a modulating apparatus which must have a supply of constant afferent impulses. I refer to the experiment wherein by using procaine on the surface of the medulla, respiration will stop completely and the procaine will only enter the small layer of the surface, and certainly not reach the center. On the other hand, in the superficial structure of the medulla, Shimata in our laboratory picked up regular trains of action potentials which were dependent upon the superficial pH which was changed in the experiment. These trains of potentials look very similar to what von Euler showed many years ago from the medulla, except that the exact location was not so clear. And so I think the model would now show that there is a place, a chemosensitive structure which sends potentials to the centers, and the centers which modulate them into inspiratory and expiratory activity.

CHALAZONITIS: I agree with your statement that there is, generally speaking, a chemosensitive structure which sends potentials to the centers which then modulate them into inspiratory and expiratory activity. But the modulatory function of the centers is not only inherent in an appropriate circuitry giving rise to periodical bursts—inspiratory and expiratory effectors. This modulatory function is mainly exerted by the endogenous or intrinsic oscillatory properties of some neurone, at least of pacemakers (Fig. 1). A periodical and alternate bursting requires an appropriate circuitry assuring alternatively excitatory and inhibitory influences on neurons already endowed with endogenous oscillatory (or waving) potentialities.

3. Carbon Dioxide Action on Neuronal Membranes

Arthur M. Brown

*Departments of Physiology and Medicine
University of Utah College of Medicine
Salt Lake City, Utah 84112**

Medullary respiratory neurones of mammals are exquisitely sensitive to CO_2, the excitation by this agent providing the main stimulus for respiration (VON EULER and SODERBERG [1952]). On the other hand, cortical and phrenic neurones are inhibited by CO_2 (KINJEVIĆ, RANDIĆ, and SIESJÖ [1965]; GILL and KUNO [1963]). The mechanism whereby CO_2 produced these diverse effects was unknown (LAMBERTSON [1961]), so my colleagues and I undertook a study of this problem. The results of this study have been recently published (BROWN, WALKER and SUTTON [1970]; BROWN and BERMAN [1970]) and are reported briefly here.

The main problems which we anticipated in working with mammalian neurones were technical. The cells are small and cannot be visualized individually. Therefore, we elected to use the largest possible identifiable neurones which hopefully would also have low energy requirements. Fortunately Chalazonitis [1963] had shown clearly that large neurones in the abdominal ganglion of the marine mollusc *Aplysia* were excited by CO_2, and we took this as our lead. We found that CO_2 excited some neurones more than others, that the CO_2 effect is mediated by the increased H^+ outside the neurone, that increased H^+ in turn increased chloride conductance through the neuronal membrane, and finally, that the relationship between the chloride equilibrium potential, E_{Cl}, and

membrane potential, E_M, determined the nature of the response of the neuronal cell to CO_2. When E_{Cl} was less negative than E_M, the neurone was depolarized and excited. When E_{Cl} was more negative, the neurone was hyperpolarized and inhibited.

The methods have been fully described elsewhere (BROWN, WALKER, and SUTTON [1970]; BROWN and BERMAN [1970]). The perfusate which was similar in composition to the extracellular fluid of *Aplysia* had a pH of 8.0. When it was equilibrated with 5% CO_2, the pH fell to 6.5. It should be emphasized that the neurones were exposed to CO_2 for brief periods of 2 to 3 min and that the effects we studied in greatest detail were the initial responses. More prolonged exposure led to complicated changes. In these simpler experiments, we found that some neurones were markedly excited [Figure 1(A)], whereas others were not (Figure 1(B)). The effect of CO_2 was mimicked almost exactly by an equivalent fall in pH produced by a non-volatile acid [Figures 1(C) and (D)]. Such brief changes in external pH are probably not accompanied by alterations in internal pH (CALDWELL [1958]). However, if the perfusate pH was held constantly at 8.0 by continual buffering with $NaHCO_3$, CO_2 was no longer effective [Figure 1(E)]. In this case, intracellular H^+ and HCO_3^- are almost certainly increased (CHALAZONITIS and ROMEY [1964]). The conclusion from these experiments was

*Present address: Dept. of Physiology, University of Texas Medical Branch, Galveston, Texas 77550

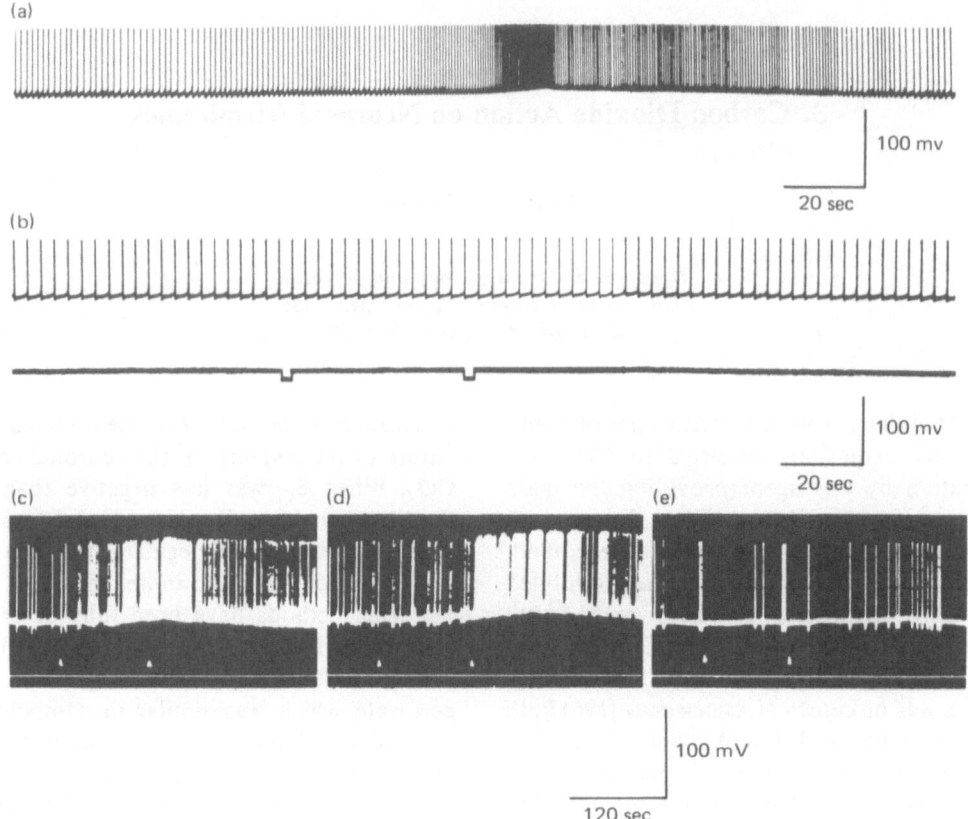

Fig. 1. Action of artificial seawater (ASW) equilibrated with 5% CO_2, pH 6.5 on A, a non-pigmented pacemaker cell, and B, a pigmented pacemaker neurone. Test solution was introduced between signal marks on trace below B. The response of another nonpigmented pacemaker cell to ASW with 5% CO_2, pH 6.5 (C), to ASW with no added Co_2, pH 6.5 (D), and to ASW with 5% CO_2, pH 8.0 (E), are shown here. Test solutions were added between the signal marks on the bottom trace of each panel. Responses in C and D are very similar; test solution in E had no effect.
Figure reprinted by permission from Science, 167:1502 (1970). *Copyright 1970 by the American Association for the Advancement of Science.*

that the CO_2 action was mediated solely by the increased external H^+ (H_o^+).

It is known that increased H_o^+ alters the conductance of muscle membranes (HAGIWARA, GRUENES, SABATA, and GRINNELL [1968]; DEMELLO and HUTTER [1966]; REUBEN, GIRARDIER, and GRUNDFEST [1962]). Therefore, we tested this effect on *Aplysia* neurones. We used solutions having pH 5.0 because they gave the most consistent results. Nevertheless, similar results occurred at higher pH's, up to pH 7.5. Upon exposure

to low pH, the membrane resistance was initially halved at the lower pH (Figure 2). With more prolonged exposure (greater than 5 min.) the membrane resistance changes were more complicated. Therefore, we analyzed only the initial, more reproducible effects. We found that hyperpolarization was converted to depolarization by halving external Cl^- or increasing internal Cl^- electrophoretically. On the other hand, depolarization could be converted to hyperpolarization by prior soaking in zero Cl^- solutions, which

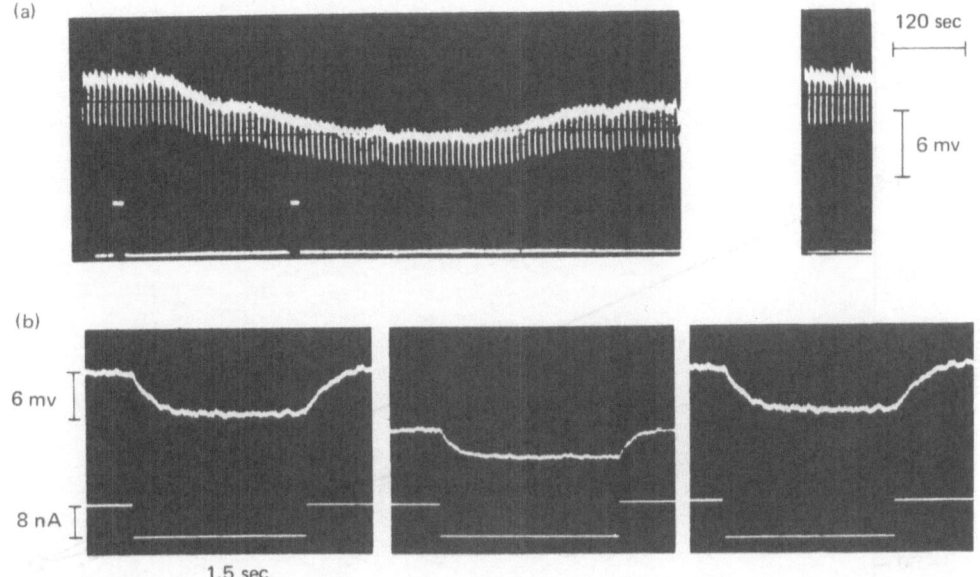

Fig. 2(A). Action of decreasing pH from 8.0 to 5.0 (between signals bottom trace) on membrane potential and resistance of R_2, the giant cell. The cell was hyperpolarized 6 mπ and resistance fell to 58% of control. Far right trace was taken 30 min after return to control. **(B).** Individual voltage responses to constant current pulses during control, peak effect, and recovery, using a fast time base. *Figure reprinted by permission from* J. Gen. Physiol., 56:559 (1970). *Copyright 1970 by the Rockefeller University Press.*

reduced internal Cl^-. This led us to the interpretation that increased H_o^+ increased membrane Cl^- conductance. In order to test this more directly, we studied the effects of alterations in Cl_o^- on E_M at pH 8.0 and 5.0. The slope of the line in Figure 3 gives

$$-\left(\frac{\partial E_M}{\partial \log Cl_o^-}\right)_{J_o} = 58\, T_K$$

where T_{Cl} is the transport number for Cl^- and J_o is external Na^+ and K^+ concentrations. Taking

$$g_{Cl} = T_{Cl} \cdot g_M$$

where g_{Cl} is Cl^- conductance and g_M is $1/R_M$, the total membrane conductance, we found that g_{Cl} at pH 5.0 was three times g_{Cl} at pH 8.0.

The explanation for the variable responses to CO_2 was further clarified when we found that different neurones have different internal Cl^- activities (a^i_{Cl}). We used liquid ion-exchanger microelectrodes to measure a^i_{Cl} in neurones that were hyperpolarized or depolarized by increases in pH. We found that some neurones had an E_{Cl} less negative than E_M and were excited by CO_2, and others had E_{Cl} more negative than E_M and were inhibited (Table 1). Similar differences in a^i_{Cl} amongst molluscan neurones have been noted by others (KERKUT [1966]; AUSTIN [1968]).

In summary, the CO_2 effects are mediated by H^+. Increased H^+ increases Cl^- membrane conductance. Inhibition or excitation ensues, depending upon whether E_{Cl} is more or less negative than E_M.

Acknowledgments This work was supported by USPHS grants HE–10977, HE–13480, and NS 09545.

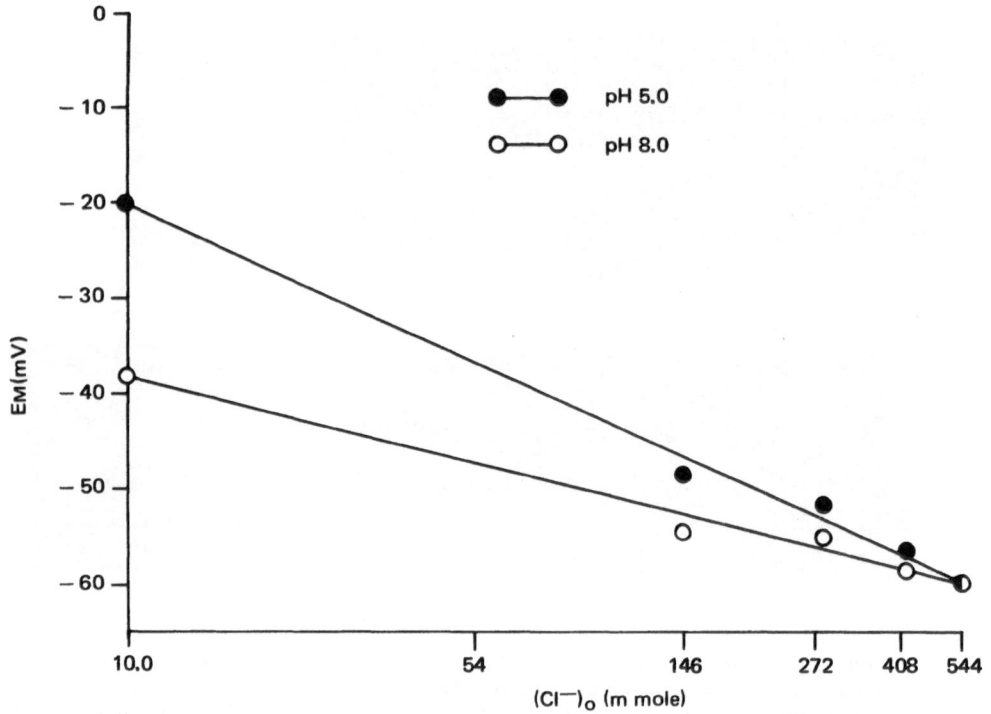

Fig. 3. Effect of decreasing pH from 8.0 to 5.0 on the relation between E_m and $(Cl)_o$. *Figure reprinted by permission from* J. Gen. Physiol., 56:559 (1970). *Copyright 1970 by the Rockefeller University Press.*

Bibliography

Austin, G., Sato, M., Yai, H., and Maruhashi, J. J. Gen. Physiol., 51:321 (1968).

Brown, A. M. and Berman, P. R. J. Gen. Physiol., 56:543 (1970).

———, Walker, J. L. Jr., and Sutton, R. B. J. Gen. Physiol., 56:559 (1970).

Caldwell, P. C. J. Physiol., 142:22 (1958).

Chalazonitis, N. Ann. N.Y. Acad. Sci., 109:451 (1963).

———, and Romey, G. C. R. Hebd. Seances Acad. Sci. Paris, 158:2367 (1964).

DeMello, W. C. and Hutter, O. F. J. Physiol., 183: 11P (1966).

Gill, P. K. and Kuno, M. J. Physiol., 168:258 (1963).

Hagiwara, S., Gruener, R., Hayashi, H., Sabata, H., and Grinnell, A. D. J. Gen. Physiol., 52:773 (1968).

Kerkut, G. A. and Meech, R. W. Life Sci., 5:453 (1966).

Krnjević, K., Randić, M., and Siesjö, B. K. J. Physiol., 176:105 (1965).

Lambertson, D. J., Medical Physiology. St. Louis: C. V. Mosby Co., 1961, p. 613.

Reuben, J. P., Girardier, L., and Grundfest, H. Biol. Bull. (Woods Hole), 123:509 (1962).

Von Euler, C. and Söderberg, U. J. Physiol., 118:545 (1952).

Brown Discussion

SEVERINGHAUS: Could I ask Dr. Brown if he has tried using Ouabain to determine whether the hydrogen ion effect appeared to be only extracellular and whether it has anything to do with sodium transport or hydrogen transport?

BROWN: No.

SIESJÖ: I was fascinated by your results on the chloride conductance. Would you venture to speculate about the bicarbonate ion conductance in the membrane?

Table 1. Intracellular Chloride Activities in 14 *Aplysia* Giant Cells

Cell No.	$a^o{}_{Cl}$*	$a^i{}_{Cl}$	Calculated E_{Cl}†	E_M, pH 8.0	E_M, pH 5.0
	mmoles	mmoles	mv	mv	mv
1	350	26	−65	−58	
2	350	31	−61	−53	−60
3	340	31	−60	−56	
4	340	25	−66	−59	−63
5	340	21	−70	−60	
6	340	25	−66	−57	
7	330	35	−57	−52	−56
Mean ± SEM	341.1 ± 3.6	27.7 ± 1.8	−63.6 ± 1.7	−56.4 ± 1.1	−59.7 ± 2.0
8	330	37	−55	−60	
9	330	40	−53	−55	
10	330	47	−49	−60	−50
11	340	45	−51	−58	−52
12	340	40	−54	−56	
13	340	39	−55	−57	
14	340	37	−56	−60	−57
Mean ± SEM	335.7 ± 3.0	40.7 ± 1.5	−53.3 ± 0.9	−58.0 ± 0.8	−53.0 ± 2.1
	$p > 0.1$	$p < 0.005$	$p < 0.005$	$p > 0.1$	

p values in each column are between cells 1 through 7 as one group and cells 8 through 14 as the other.

* Chloride activity of ASW.

† Chloride equilibrium potential calculated as, $E_{Cl} = \dfrac{RT}{F} \ln \dfrac{a^i{}_{Cl}}{a^o{}_{Cl}}$ where R, T, and F have their usual meaning.

BROWN: We do not know how or whether active transport of chloride is linked to bicarbonate.

SIESJÖ: No, but if chloride permeability is increased, would you generally expect the bicarbonate ion permeability to be changed in the same direction?

BROWN: Well, yes, possibly.

SIESJÖ: What is the equilibrium potential for hydrogen ion, as in your system?

BROWN: We haven't measured internal hydrogen ion activity and I can't answer that. The evidence in squid axion is that hydrogen is pumped out of the cell.

SIESJÖ: Yes.

BROWN: I have no idea whether hydrogen is pumped out of these *Aplysia* neurons.

SIESJÖ: You could have a hydrogen ion pump, but I was just wondering if that could compete with the sodium ions due to a hypercapnia situation where you decrease hydrogen ion concentration itself.

BROWN: Yes, I think there could be. I don't see any reason that hydrogen can't also be exchanging for potassium. Ouabain does not affect the active transport of chloride.

SEVERINGHAUS: Yes, but it's only necessary to say that its active transport is something which results in a movement of chloride; this is not to say that we're dealing with the active transport of chloride.

BROWN: If the chloride equilibrium potential does not equal the membrane potential in the steady state, it equals it when the cell is cooled and becomes unequal upon rewarming. I define this as active transport of chloride.

CHALAZONITIS: May I add a last comment: I was most impressed by your fine work relating the H^+ ion responsiveness (de- or re-polarization) for some neurons to the transmembrane gradient and conductances of chloride ions. On the other hand, I believe that some of the different neurons, being much more controlled by the Na^+ pump, P_{CO_2} and H^+ ions generally decreasing the respiratory rate, could decelerate ionic pumps, thus exerting a supplementary effect on their membrane potential. In this case, space-time analysis of each of these processes (P_{CO_2}, pH linked chloride conductances, and pumps) would clarify fast or delayed changes on the membrane potential.

BROWN: After using a wide variety of exposures and concentrations, we settled upon the method I have described. I don't mean to imply that this is the only response. We have situations where prolonged exposure, for example, will often produce changes that we could never get to reverse, and this was in response to doses of 1% or 2% CO_2, as well as 5% CO_2. Prolonged exposure also had variable effects on membrane resistance.

I think that for the short exposure experiments (less than two minutes), the results were more predictable.

RAHN: I would just like to urge that you try CO_2 concentrations of less than 5%. If we translate this, the normal P_{CO_2} bathing the cells is probably not more than 2 mm or 3 mm, and what you're doing is giving a CO_2 concentration which, translated to man, would be the equivalent of going from 5% to 50% CO_2. That's why you get these fantastic pH changes, and I'd like to urge you to try some concentrations in a more physiological range.

BROWN: Well, as I indicated, we have used 1% CO_2, let's see, 1% gives us 6 mm, is that all right?

RAHN: That's all right. That gives you around 7 mm to 8 mm.

BROWN: This is Salt Lake City, around 6 mm, you know. In general, the results are similar for all doses of CO_2, but the response was more stereotyped at 5% CO_2.

4. Carbon Dioxide in Developmental Processes

John D. Biggers* and Anthony R. Bellvé*

School of Hygiene and Public Health
The Johns Hopkins University
Department of Population Dynamics
615 North Wolfe Street
Baltimore, Maryland 21205

Introduction

Although several scattered reports indicate that CO_2 plays a role in developmental processes, its modes of action are poorly understood. Of these, only the most extensively studied will be discussed—sexual differentiation in coelenterates, CO_2 fixation in cleaving embryos, and uterine implantation of embryos in mammals. Loomis [1957] reviewed the earlier literature, and additional reports are listed in Table 1.

Before reviewing these three topics in detail, it is helpful to make some general comments on the distribution and function of CO_2 in nature. The ultimate source of carbon atoms in most forms of life is CO_2. The importance of this gaseous molecule to life was recognized explicitly by Lawrence J. Henderson during the early part of this century, and discussed in 1913 in his famous monograph: "The Fitness of the environment: An inquiry into the biological significance of the properties of matter." The properties of CO_2 which make it so important are:

(1) It is readily soluble in water. At a pressure of 1 atm and 15°C, CO_2 will dissolve in an equal volume of water.

(2) The dissolved CO_2 reacts with water to yield either H_2CO_3 or a hydrogen ion and a bicarbonate ion, according to the following scheme (EDSALL [1970]):

$$CO_2 + H_2O$$

$$k_{13} \qquad\qquad k_{32}$$
$$k_{31} \qquad k_{23}$$

$$k_{21}$$
$$H^+ + HCO_3^- \qquad\qquad H_2CO_3$$
$$k_{12}$$

where k_{ij} are the rate constants. The values for k_{12} and k_{21} are much greater than the other rate constants.

(3) The solubility of CO_2 in water changes with pH, in that an increase in pH alters the ionization equilibrium in favor of bicarbonate, thereby increasing solubility.

These physico-chemical properties of CO_2 ensure that aquatic and terrestrial organisms contain considerable amounts of CO_2 and bicarbonate ions in their bodies.

Carbon dioxide and bicarbonate ions may be involved in various physiological functions, such as the maintenance of internal pH, and as building blocks in the

* Present address: Dept. of Physiology, Laboratory of Human Reproduction and Reproductive Biology, Harvard Medical School, 45 Shattuck Street, Boston, Massachusetts 02115

Table 1. Examples in Which Carbon Dioxide May Influence Development

Process	Species	Reference
Initiating the development of seeds	*Trifolium subterranean*	BALLARD [1958]
	Trifolium subterranean	BALLARD [1967]
Asexual sporulation of fungi	*Choanephora cucurbitarum*	BARNETT and LILLY [1955]
Development of nematodes	*Ascaris lumbricoides*	FAIRBAIRN [1961]
	Haemonchus contortus	SOMMERVILLE [1964]
	Haemonchus contortus	SOMMERVILLE [1966]
		ROGERS and SOMMERVILLE [1968]
Terminating diapause and initiation of development in insects	*Daphnia pulex*	STROSS [1971]
Sexual differentiation of coelenterates	*Hydra littoralis*	LOOMIS [1957]
	Podocoryne carnea	BRAVERMAN [1962]
Biosynthesis in cleaving embryos	*Psammechinus miliaris* (sea urchin)	HULTIN [1952]
	Psammechinus miliaris	HULTIN and WESSEL [1952]
	Rana temporaria (frog)	FLICKINGER [1954]
	Rana pipiens (frog)	COHEN [1954]
	Rana pipiens ♀ × *Rana sylvatica* ♂ hybrid	COHEN [1963]
	Triton (newt)	TIEDEMANN and TIEDEMANN [1954]
	Salmo salar (salmon)	MOUNIB and EISAN [1969]
	Mus musculus (mouse)	WALES, QUINN, and MURDOCK [1969]
		GRAVES and BIGGERS [1970]
Implantation of embryos in mammals	*Oryctolagus cuniculus* (domestic rabbit)	LUTWAK-MANN and LASER [1954]
		LUTWAK-MANN [1955]
		BÖVING [1959]
	Mus musculus (mouse)	HETHERINGTON [1968]

synthesis of macromolecules. Traditionally, the use of CO_2 for biosynthetic purposes is associated exclusively with photosynthetic processes in plants. It is equally common to think that in the animal kingdom CO_2 is merely an end product of metabolism, and that its primary role is in the regulation of pH. This dichotomy of function between the animal and plant kingdoms, however, is an oversimplification since the utilization of CO_2, for biosynthetic purposes occurs in both autotrophic and heterotrophic organ-isms (WOOD and UTTER [1965]; MARGULIS [1970]). Thus, CO_2 may be involved in the development of animals either by influencing pH or by participating in synthetic processes.

The physiological process in which CO_2 is incorporated into larger molecules is *CO_2 fixation*. This term, however, is imprecise and needs clarification. We now recognize two classes of enzymes, those using CO_2, and those using bicarbonate, in the synthesis of larger molecules. Thus, when an organism is exposed to $Na^{14}CO_3$ the carbon may be incorporated either after ionization of the sodium bicarbonate, or only after conversion of the bicarbonate to CO_2 (see page 87). This subject will be discussed later in this review, and for the moment the term CO_2 fixation will also include the fixation of bicarbonate.

Sexual Differentiation in Coelenterates

The common method of reproduction in coelenterates is asexually by budding. However, under certain conditions, sexual reproduction can be induced. This phenomenon has been studied extensively in the dioecious *Hydra littoralis* (LOOMIS [1957]; PARK, MECCA, and ORTMEYER [1964]; LENHOFF [1968]), and in the marine hydroid *Podocoryne carnea* (BRAVERMAN [1962]).

Lenhoff and Loomis [1957] first suggested that the differentiation of male and female gametes in *H. littoralis* was stimulated by a rise in unhydrated CO_2 in the medium. This suggestion was later confirmed by Loomis [1957] when sexual differentiation was induced in *H. littoralis* by raising the P_{CO_2} for 10 consecutive days. Subsequently, Park, Mecca, and Ortmeyer [1964] questioned the role of CO_2 in inducing sexual differentiation of hydra under natural conditions. Despite this controversy, the earlier work of Loomis and Lenhoff is of interest since it led Lenhoff [1968] to postulate that CO_2 fixation into oxaloacetate is important for the biosynthesis of macromolecules in a developing system. He based his argument on the following evidence:

(1) Substitution of the bicarbonate buffer with Tris(hydroxymethylaminomethane) did not result in sexual differentiation (LOOMIS [1957]).
(2) Carbon is incorporated from $^{14}CO_2$ into the testes, ovaries and cnidoblasts of *H. littoralis* as revealed by autoradiography (LENHOFF [1959]).
(3) The need for CO_2 for sexual differentiation in hydra can be alleviated by the addition of citric acid cycle inter-

mediates, but not by glucose, pyruvate or acetate (LOOMIS [1964]).

Carbon Dioxide Fixation in Embryos

Incorporation of Carbon Dioxide

The first demonstration of CO_2 fixation in embryos was made by Hultin [1952] and Hultin and Wessel [1952] in the sea urchin (*Psammechinus milliaris*). Embryos at different cleavage stages were incubated in $NaH^{14}CO_3$. Subsequent analyses showed the isotope to be present in hypoxanthine, an undefined carbohydrate fraction, the carboxyl carbon of amino acid and proteins, and both adenine and guanine of ribonucleic acid (RNA). Several studies on CO_2 fixation from $NaH^{14}CO_3$ have been made on amphibian embryos (*Rana pipiens*—COHEN [1954]; *Rana temporaria*—FLICKINGER [1954]; *Triton*—TIEDEMANN and TIEDEMANN [1954]; *Rana pipiens* ♀ × *Rana sylvatica* ♂ hybrid—COHEN [1963]). In each case there was general labeling of nucleic acids, proteins and several other compounds (Figure 1).

Bicarbonate ions form a major component of media generally used for the culture of early embryos of the mouse (*Mus muscularis*), rabbit (*Oryctolagus cuniculus*), and deermouse (*Peromyscus maniculatus bairdii*). In the absence of bicarbonate in the medium and 5% CO_2 in the gas phase, embryos fail to develop (WHITTEN [1970]). Replacement of bicarbonate as the buffer system with phosphate, Tris, or HEPES (*N*-2-hydroxyethyl-piperazine-*N'*-2-ethanesulfonic acid) did not allow embryonic development (WALES, QUINN, and MURDOCK [1969]; WHITTEN [1970]). Since bicarbonate appeared to be an essential component of the culture medium, and not acting as a simple buffer system, Biggers, Whittingham, and Donahue [1967] suggested that CO_2 fixation may also occur during the early development of mammalian embryos by the same mechanism that Lenhoff [1968] had coincidentally postulated for the sexually differentiating hydra. The fixation of CO_2 was independently demonstrated to occur in the preimplantation mouse embryo

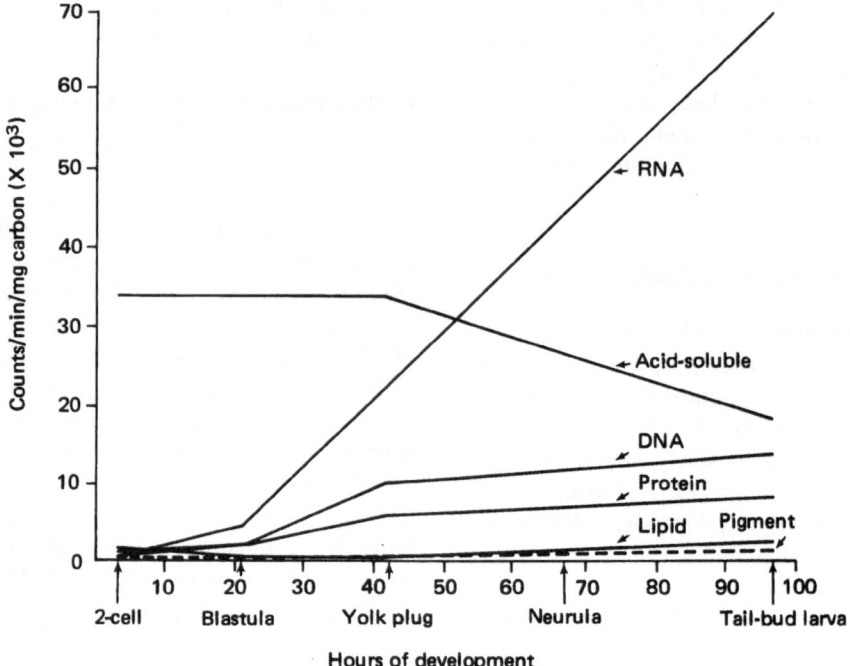

Fig. 1. The incorporation of ^{14}C from $NaHCO_3$ by embryos of *Rana temporaria* (FLICKINGER [1954]).

by Wales, Quinn, and Murdock [1969] and Graves and Biggers [1970].

Graves and Biggers [1970] incubated several stages of the preimplantation mouse embryo for 4 hours in a chemically defined medium containing $NaH^{14}CO_3$ (Table 2). After the incubation period had elapsed the embryos were analyzed for the acid-soluble, lipid, RNA, DNA and protein fractions (Table 3). The ^{14}C atoms were found in the acid-soluble, nucleic acid and protein fractions of each developmental stage. No detectable isotopic incorporation had occurred in the lipid fraction. The results demonstrated a marked increase in CO_2 fixation into protein at the 8-cell stage. Carbon dioxide fixation into RNA and DNA was detected at very low levels in fertilized eggs, and the amount incorporated increased considerably between the 2- and 8-cell stages. Similar results were obtained by Wales, Quinn, and Murdock [1969] following the culture of 8-cell mouse embryos for 24 hours in the presence of $NaH^{14}CO_3$. In

addition to incorporation into the acid-soluble and protein fractions, there was some labeling of the lipid fraction following the longer period of culture. This report seems to be the first demonstration of lipid synthesis in early mammalian embryos. More recently, Murdock and Wales [1971] have shown incorporation of label into soluble RNA, but other classes of RNA were not investigated.

Mechanisms of Carbon Dioxide Fixation

The utilization of CO_2 by heterotrophic organisms was first implied by Wood and Werkman [1935, 1936] in studies on four species of propioniobacterium, and later in the pigeon liver by Evans, Vennesland, and Slotin [1943]. Since that time, a number of biosynthetic pathways have been discovered in which CO_2 or bicarbonate ions are actively involved (WOOD and UTTER [1965]). A general system of classification for the enzymes involved in carboxylation reactions has been derived (LANE [1970]). For this

Table 2. Composition of a Chemically Defined Medium Used to Demonstrate Carbon Dioxide Fixation in Pre-implantation Mouse Embryos (GRAVES and BIGGERS [1970])

Component	Concentration (mmoles/l.)	g/l.
NaCl	94.59	5.54
KCl	4.78	0.356
Ca lactate. $5H_2O$	1.71	0.527
KH_2PO_4	1.19	0.162
$MgSO_4 \cdot 7H_2O$	1.19	0.294
$NaH^{14}CO_3$	25.07	2.106
Na pyruvate	0.25	0.028
Na lactate	21.58	2.416
Glucose	5.56	1.0
Crystalline bovine albumin	—	4.0
Penicillin	—	100,000 I.U.
Streptomycin	—	50 mg

Table 3. Incorporation of Radioactive Carbon from $NaH^{14}CO_3$ into Several Fractions of Pre-implantation Mouse Embryos (counts/min/100 embryos) (GRAVES and BIGGERS [1970])

Stage	Acid-soluble	Lipid	Nucleic acid	RNA	DNA	Protein
Replicate 1						
1-cell, unfertilized	35.4	0	0	—	—	6.3
1-cell, fertilized	40.7	0	0	—	—	7.1
2-cell	26.6	0	1.5	—	—	1.5
Morula	44.3	0	14.2	—	—	13.3
Early blastocyst	37.8	0	15.9	—	—	13.2
Late blastocyst	21.8	0	17.4	—	—	8.8
Replicate 2						
Control*	5.2	0	—	0	0	3.1
1-cell, unfertilized	141.5	0	—	0	4.2	26.9
1-cell, fertilized	77.7	0	—	1.7	0.8	24.1
2-cell	273.5	0	—	5.8	3.2	14.2
8-cell	652.9	0	—	105.2	142.0	138.0
Morula	787.4	0	—	163.9	351.8	423.8
Early blastocyst	1067.4	0	—	234.0	585.4	479.4
Late blastocyst	516.2	0	—	132.4	244.2	372.1

* Treated, then incubated in 1% formalin.

discussion the pathways which are likely to be involved in CO_2 metabolism in developing systems have been listed in Table 4. Those enzymes which utilize bicarbonate ion as substrate have been shown to be biotin-dependent. Reductive carboxylases are characteristic in their requirement of a nicotinamide nucleotide, while the oxidative decarboxylation of pyruvate and 2-oxoglutarate also requires thiamine pyrophosphate in the enzyme complex. The relationship of each individual reaction in the system of metabolic pathways is presented in Figure 2.

Although at the present time little is known about these enzymes in developing systems, there are some indications as to which are functional. Cohen [1954, 1963], using amphibian eggs, has shown that ^{14}C from $NaHCO_3$ appears in citrate, succinate, fumarate, and malate; moreover, the transamination of oxaloacetate and 2-oxoglutarate also occurs, since recovered aspartate and glutamate were highly labeled. This evidence suggests that the citric acid cycle is operative in these embryos. The labeled carbon probably enters the cycle via oxaloacetate and malate. Three possible reactions may be involved:

$$\text{phosphoenolpyruvate} + GDP + CO_2 \underset{\text{(E.C. 4.1.1.32)}}{\overset{\text{phosphoenolpyruvate carboxykinase}}{\rightleftharpoons}} \text{oxaloacetate} + GTP \quad (1)$$

$$\text{pyruvate} + ATP + HCO_3^- \underset{\text{(E.C. 6.4.1.1)}}{\overset{\text{pyruvate carboxylase}}{\rightleftharpoons}} \text{oxaloacetate} + ADP + P_i \quad (2)$$

$$\text{pyruvate} + NADPH + CO_2 \underset{\text{(E.C. 1.1.1.40)}}{\overset{\text{NADP—malate dehydrogenase}}{\rightleftharpoons}} \text{L-malate} + NADP^+ \quad (3)$$

There is no doubt that at least one of these reactions is operating (WALES and WHITTINGHAM [1967]), but direct evidence has yet to be reported. Studies on the nutritional requirements of early mouse embryos (BIGGERS

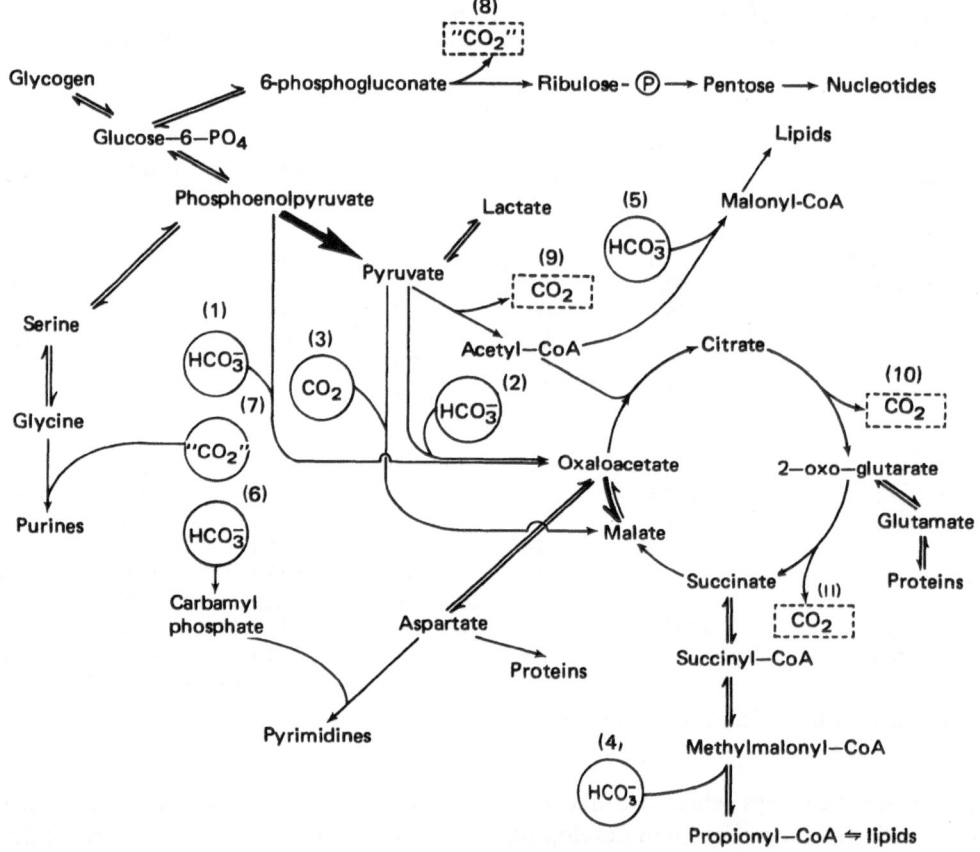

Fig. 2. Possible metabolic pathways involved in CO_2 fixation by developing systems, indication (a) the molecular species involved, (b) the probable carboxylation (circles) and decarboxylation reactions (squares). Reaction numbers coincide with those in Table 4 and the text.

Table 4. Possible Enzymes Involved in Carbon Dioxide Metabolism in Developing Systems

Reaction number	Enzyme	Molecular species	Reference
Acyl-CoA carboxylases			
1	Phosphoenolpyruvate carboxykinase	CO_2	COOPER, TCHEN, WOOD, BENNETT, and FILMER [1970]
2	Pyruvate carboxylase	HCO_3^-	COOPER, TCHEN, WOOD, and BENEDICT [1968]
4	Propionyl-CoA carboxylase	HCO_3^-	KAZIRO, HASS, BOYER, and OCHOA [1962]
5	Acetyl-CoA carboxylase	HCO_3^-	LANE [1970]
6	Carbamyl phosphate synthetase	HCO_3^-	JONES and SPECTOR [1960]
Reductive carboxylases			
3	NADP-malate dehydrogenase	CO_2	DALZIEL and LONDESBOROUGH [1968]
7	Amidazole ribonucleotide carboxylase	"CO_2"*	
8	6-Phosphogluconate dehydrogenase	"CO_2"*	
9	Pyruvate decarboxylase†	"CO_2"*	
10	Isocitrate dehydrogenase	CO_2	DALZIEL and LONDESBOROUGH [1968]
11	2-Oxoglutarate decarboxylase†	"CO_2"*	

* Since biotin is not involved in these reactions, it is likely that CO_2 will prove to be the reactive species.

† Enzymes catalyzing the decarboxylation in reactions 9 and 11 are an integral part of enzyme complexes pyruvate dehydrogenase and 2-oxoglutarate dehydrogenase, respectively.

[1971]) provide some indirect evidence of mechanisms of CO_2 fixation in this species. The 1-cell stage is only supported by either pyruvate or oxaloacetate (BIGGERS, WHITTINGHAM, and DONAHUE [1967]), yet the trichloracetic acid-soluble fraction is labeled with ^{14}C when the embryos are incubated with $NaH^{14}CO_3$ (WALES, QUINN, and MURDOCK [1969]; GRAVES and BIGGERS [1970]). These observations imply, but do not prove, that CO_2 reacts with pyruvate to form oxaloacetate. The inability of oxaloacetate to support development of 8-cell embryos in a system buffered with HEPES (WALES, QUINN, and MURDOCK [1969]) may be due to insufficient CO_2 being generated to supply other essential carboxylation reactions.

An alternative route for CO_2 fixation is via the carboxylation of methylmalonyl-CoA, a residue of lipid degradation.

$$\text{methylmalonyl-CoA} \xrightarrow[\substack{\text{propionyl-CoA} \\ \text{carboxylase} \\ \text{(E.C. 6.5.1.3)}}]{} \text{succinyl-CoA}$$
$$+ ATP + HCO_3^- \qquad\qquad + ADP + P_i$$
$$(4)$$

Ostensibly, this would lead directly into the citric acid cycle by the intermediate succinate, thereby serving a role in providing catalytic quantities of dicarboxylic acids. It is plausible that this series of reactions could be functioning in early mammalian embryos, although neither this nor the presence of a store of degradable lipid has been verified.

Aside from incorporation into citric acid cycle intermediates, fixation may also occur more directly during the synthesis of both lipids and nucleic acids. CO_2 fixation into lipids has been shown to occur in low amounts in embryos of frogs (FLICKINGER [1954]) and mice (WALES, QUINN, and MURDOCK [1969]). The following reaction could be involved:

$$\text{acetyl-CoA} \xrightarrow[\substack{\text{acetyl-CoA} \\ \text{carboxylase} \\ \text{(E.C. 6.4.1.2)}}]{} \text{malonyl-CoA}$$
$$+ ATP + HCO_3^- \qquad\qquad + ADP + P_i$$
$$(5)$$

This reaction is further indicated by the accumulation of labeled malonate in F_1 *Rana pipiens* ♀ × *Rana sylvatica* ♂ hybrids (COHEN [1963]).

Hultin [1952] and Hultin and Wessel [1952], using sea urchin embryos, observed that ^{14}C from $NaHCO_3$ appears in adenine and guanine of RNA. These observations were later extended by Cohen [1954, 1963] when label was found in adenine, guanine, cytosine, uracil, and thymidine isolated from frog embryos. Degradation of the recovered pyrimidines, demonstrated that greater than 78% of the ^{14}C was present in the 2 position of uracil (COHEN [1954]). The fact that carbon 2 or uracil was labeled gives precedence for the following general reaction:

$$\text{L-glutamine} + 2\,\text{ATP} + \text{HCO}_3^- \underset{\substack{\text{carbamyl} \\ \text{phosphate} \\ \text{synthetase} \\ \text{(E.C. 2.7.2.5)}}}{\rightleftharpoons} \text{glutamate} + 2\,\text{ADP} + \text{carbamyl phosphate} \quad (6)$$

Unfortunately, there is no evidence for the direct incorporation of CO_2 into purines in embryos. It could occur via the incorporation of previously labeled glycine by phosphoribosyl-glycineamide synthetase (E.C. 6.3.1.3.), or in the reaction:

$$\text{aminoimidazole ribonucleotide} + \text{CO}_2 \underset{\substack{\text{aminoimidazole} \\ \text{ribonucleotide} \\ \text{carboxylase}}}{\rightleftharpoons} \text{5-aminoimidazole-4-carboxylic acid ribonucleotide} \quad (7)$$

Although CO_2 fixation is possible by reductive carboxylation, as catalyzed by the remaining enzymes listed in Table 4, it would appear unlikely that these would be a major source for incorporation in developing embryos. The acute demand of anabolic processes leading to the synthesis of proteins and nucleic acids would drain the citric acid cycle of intermediates. Reactions involving reductive carboxylation would, therefore, tend to function principally in the direction of oxidative decarboxylation. This tendency does not imply that incorporated CO_2 will be lost in these reactions. The randomization of carbons in citric acid cycle intermediates while passing through the symmetrical di-carboxylic acids succinate and fumarate will ensure that some portion of the labeled carbon will become involved in biosynthetic processes.

Environmental Carbon Dioxide of Mammalian Embryos

Isotopic incorporation of CO_2 by pre-implantation embryos cultured *in vitro* cannot be directly extrapolated to metabolism *in vivo* without experimental verification. Unfortunately, the demonstration of CO_2 fixation *in vivo* using labeled isotopes is difficult and it is necessary to rely on more indirect techniques. Measurements of total CO_2 in the immediate environment of the embryo, the oviducal and uterine secretions, have been reported (Table 5). Values obtained are variable and appear comparable to, or to exceed, that of plasma for a given species (VISHWAKARMA [1962]; RESTALL and WALES [1966]). Vishwakarma compared CO_2 levels of the genital secretions with that of plasma obtained from the same animals, the only realistic approach if differences are to be assessed. The level of CO_2 in genital secretions was considerably greater than that of plasma (24 mM/l.), indicating active transport of bicarbonate into the lumen of the genital tract. Active transport of bicarbonate by the oviduct has also been postulated more recently by Brunton [1969].

The wide variation in reported values (Table 5) may be related to the limitations of the various techniques that have been employed. A major overriding factor has been the small quantity of fluid available for the analyses. Earlier problems associated with collection from slaughtered animals (HALL [1936]) and flushing (HEAP [1962]) have been circumvented by using techniques involving ligation or cannulation (Figure 3). To allow the accumulation of sufficient fluid, ligation of the genital tract into compartments is usually maintained over a period of two to three days (VISHWAKARMA [1962]; DAVID, et al. [1969]). During this period the genital tract becomes abnormally distended and in consequence the epithelial folds grossly

Table 5. Total Carbon Dioxide Content of Mammalian Genital Tract Secretions

Species	Source	Method of collection	HCO₃⁻ concentration (mmoles/l.)	Reference
Rabbit	Oviduct	Ligation	52.19	VISHWAKARMA [1962]
	Oviduct	Cannulation	27.9	HAMNER and WILLIAMS [1965]
	Ampulla	Ligation	27.52	DAVID, BRACKETT, GARCIA, and MASTROIANNI [1969]
	Amp-isth.	Ligation	33.20	DAVID, BRACKETT, GARCIA, and MASTROIANNI [1969]
	Isthmusc	Ligation	41.34	DAVID, BRACKETT, GARCIA, and MASTROIANNI [1969]
Sheep				
(estrus)	Oviduct	Cannulation	22.6	RESTALL and WALES [1966]
(diestrus)	Oviduct	Cannulation	17.0	RESTALL and WALES [1966]
(metestrus)	Oviduct	Cannulation	17.6	RESTALL and WALES [1966]
Rabbit	Uterus	Ligation	53.6	SHIH, KENNEDY, and HUGGINS [1940]
	Uterus	Ligation	50.10	VISHWAKARMA [1962]
Rat	Uterus	Ligation	61.8	SHIH, KENNEDY, and HUGGINS [1940]
Dog	Uterus	Ligation	3.0	SHIH, KENNEDY, and HUGGINS [1940]
Hen	Uterus "plumping"	Aspiration	82.47	EL JACK and LAKE [1967]
	"oviposition"		91.26	EL JACK and LAKE [1967]

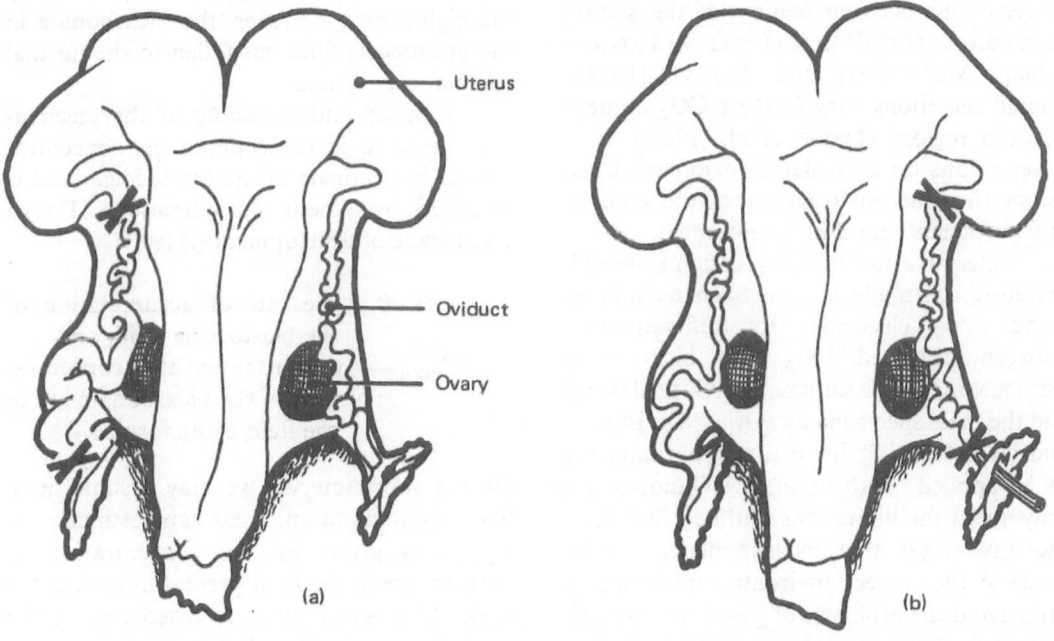

Fig. 3. Methods of collection of oviducal fluids in the ewe (a) by ligation and (b) by cannulation.

distorted. Whether this distended condition, or the period of time involved, has any effect on the CO_2 content of the secretions has not been adequately investigated. In contrast, prolonged cannulation of the genital tract (CLEWE and MASTROIANNI [1960]; RESTALL [1966]; BELLVÉ and MCDONALD [1968]) does not cause distension, but as with ligation, it involves a delay between the time of secretion and its subsequent collection in the chamber outside the body. This delay arises from the dead space in the cannulae, since secretions reach the external collection chamber solely by displacement. The rate of displacement will, therefore, depend on the volume of the cannula and subsequent rates of secretion. In sheep, displacement time may range from 12 hours to 2 days, depending on the stage of the estrous cycle. Catabolism of macromolecules, such as carbohydrates, in the cellular detritus during this period, even in the absence of bacterial contamination, could lead to a spurious production of CO_2.

Both ligation and cannulation involve ligatures placed at appropriate sites on the genital tract to isolate the regions under study. This practice prevents the free exchange of secretions between regions of the genital tract (BJORK [1959]; BELLVÉ and MCDONALD [1968]; MCDONALD and BELLVÉ [1969]). Should secretions vary in their CO_2 content between regions (DAVID et al. [1969]), then observations on an isolated region need not reflect the true environment of the embryo at a particular period in development.

Determination of CO_2 content should, therefore, be made *in situ*. Such techniques using P_{CO_2} electrodes for differentiating between dissolved CO_2 and bicarbonate (SEVERINGHAUS, HAMILTON, and COTEV [1969]) and the mass spectrometer (GURTNER, BURNS, and DAVIES [1972]) are available but have yet to be applied. Both of these techniques not only avoid the limitations outlined, but have the advantages that measurements can be made at the correct environmental temperature, avoid the problems of gaseous exchange, and also allow greater magnitudes of sensitivity.

Implantation

Four to five days after fertilization the mammalian embryo reaches the uterus after migration down the oviduct. The embryo then adheres to the endometrial lining of the uterus, and an intimate, fixed relationship develops between the mother and embryo. This process is called implantation.

The possibility that CO_2 is involved in implantation was first raised by the discovery of high concentrations of bicarbonate in the young blastocyst, and of high concentrations of carbonic anhydrase at the time of implantation in the rabbit uterus (LUTWAK-MANN and LASER [1954]). Since then, a specific role of CO_2 in implantation has been postulated by Böving [1959] in the rabbit and by McLaren [1969] in the mouse.

Bicarbonate Content of the Blastocoele Fluid

The bicarbonate content of the blastocoele fluid of the rabbit changes with development (LUTWAK-MANN and LASER [1954]; LUTWAK-MANN [1962]). Initially, the concentration of bicarbonate is about four times higher than that in the maternal plasma; by the eighth day, however, the bicarbonate in the blastocoele fluid has fallen to the normal plasma level (Table 6).

A better understanding of the mechanisms involved in determining the concentration of bicarbonate in the blastocoele fluid is obtained by kinetic considerations. For a given stage of development (t) let:

$$dV/dt = \text{the rate of accumulation of the blastocoele fluid, and}$$
$$C_{HCO_3^-} = \text{the instantaneous concentration of the bicarbonate ion in the fluid being formed.}$$

Over a short interval we may assume, as a first approximation, that an estimate of $C_{HCO_3^-}$ is given by the concentration of bicarbonate in the fluid present in the blastocoele. This assumption is reasonable if the concentration in the blastocoele fluid is not changing rapidly. It follows that the net rate

Table 6. The Rate of Accumulation of Blastocoele Fluid (dV/dt), Concentration of HCO_3^-, and the Net Rate of Accumulation of HCO_3^- ($dA/dt_{HCO_3}^-$) in the Blastocoele Fluid of the Rabbit

Age (days)	dV/dt* (μl./hr)	Concentration HCO_3^-† (nmoles/l.)	$dA/dt_{HCO_3}^-$ (nmoles/hr)
5	0.068	84.4	5.74
$5\frac{1}{2}$	—	—	—
6	0.8	62.5	50
$6\frac{1}{2}$	2.29	53.6	123
7	5.6	—	—
$7\frac{1}{2}$	10.5	33.5	352
Maternal plasma	—	22.3	—

* DANIEL [1964]. Estimates for $6\frac{1}{2}$ and $7\frac{1}{2}$ days have been made by interpolation.

† LUTWAK-MANN [1962]. These estimates are approximations obtained from Figure 1, and they are assuming that the results were expressed at N.T.P.

of bicarbonate accumulation at time t is given by

$$dA/dt_{HCO_3}- = C_{HCO_3}- dV/dt.$$

Sufficient data are present in the literature for approximate estimates of $dA/dt_{HCO_3}-$ to be made at different stages of development (Table 6). The calculations indicate that an increasing net accumulation of bicarbonate occurs in the blastocoele fluid with development, and that the observed fall in concentration is due to the more rapid accumulation of water.

The source of bicarbonate which accumulates in the blastocoele fluid is presumably the cells of the blastocyst. These cells are capable of producing considerable quantities

Table 7. The Rate of Carbon Dioxide Production by 5- and 6-day-old Rabbit Blastocysts from Glucose, Pyruvate, and Lactate

Substrate	CO_2 production (nmoles/embryo/hr)	
	Five days	six days
Glucose*	1.34	4.90
Pyruvate†	2.03	9.88
Lactate†	0.66	3.84

* BRINSTER [1968].

† BRINSTER [1971].

of CO_2 *in vitro* from glucose, pyruvate, and lactate in the rabbit (BRINSTER [1968]) and mouse (BRINSTER [1967a,b; 1971]; MENKE and McLAREN [1970a,b]). The results obtained on the rabbit are shown in Table 7. Under these conditions the rate of CO_2 production from all three substrates fall far short of the equivalent amount of bicarbonate accumulated by the blastocyst. However, the measurements have been made under very limited conditions, and much greater outputs of CO_2 may be observed with other media and concentrations of substrate. Thus, it is impossible to determine the extent of the contribution of bicarbonate to the blastocoele fluid by the embryonal cells, and whether there is a surplus or deficit.

Carbonic Anhydrase (E.C. 4.2.1.1) in the Uterus

The hydration of CO_2 either to H_2CO_3 or the bicarbonate ion, are reversible reactions, but they are inherently slow because of the extensive electronic rearrangements involved (EDSALL [1970]). The isoenzymes of carbonic anhydrase catalyze these reactions, and thus can rapidly alter the pools of CO_2, H_2CO_3, and bicarbonate within cells.

LUTWAK-MANN and LASER [1954] reported that high concentrations of the enzyme occur in the uterine mucosa of rabbits on the

Table 8. Species Variations in Uterine Carbonic Anhydrase Concentrations (Modified from OGAWA and PINCUS [1962])

Conditions	Mouse	Rat	Rabbit
Estrous cycle—maximum at	Early estrus	Diestrus	Luteal phase
Ovariectomy	Decrease	Increase	Decrease
Estrogen	Increase	Decrease	Decrease
Progesterone	Decrease	Little effect	Increase
Estrogen/progesterone jointly	Antagonism	Antagonism	Antagonism

sixth to seventh days of pregnancy, and that the residual blood in the tissues could only account for 5 % to 10 % of the total enzymatic activity. LUTWAK-MANN [1955] then found that the enzyme is completely absent in the nonpregant uterus, and the interplacental areas of the endometrium of the rat, hamster, and guinea pig. However, it was present in the maternal portion of the placenta. In contrast, Miyake and Pincus [1959] demonstrated carbonic anhydrase in the uterus of nonpregant rats. The differences between the results obtained by the two laboratories are probably due to differences in the sensitivity of the methods of assay (OGAWA and PINCUS [1960]; BIALY and PINCUS [1960]). Many studies have now been made on the carbonic anhydrase content of the uterus. The results have shown that carbonic anhydrase is present in the uterus of the rabbit, rat, mouse, hamster, guinea pig, sheep, and human. Although the enzyme has not been found in the nonpregnant uterus of the mare, sow, cat, and dog (LUTWAK-MANN [1955]), this again may be due to the lack of sensitivity in the assay procedure.

The results have also demonstrated that in some species the content of carbonic anhydrase in the uterus changes with the reproductive cycles and is under hormonal control. However, the effects of the hormones vary between species (Table 8). The literature on the endocrinological control of uterine carbonic anhydrase can be gained through the papers of Miyake [1962]; Pincus and Bialy [1962]; Korhonen, et al. [1966]; Maren [1967]; Nicholls and Board [1967]; and Board [1970]. Only those papers concerned

with implantation and decidua formation will be discussed further.

Since the original observations of Lutwak-Mann and Laser [1954], many observations have been made on the uterine carbonic anhydrase of the rabbit. The results show that carbonic anhydrase increases in the endometrium of both pregnant and pseudopregnant rabbits, and reaches high levels by the sixth day after mating or the injection of gonadotropin, respectively (Figure 4) (LUTWAK-MANN [1955]; PINCUS and BIALY [1962]; LUTWAK-MANN and MCINTOSH [1969]; MAKLER and MORRIS [1971]). Recently, evidence has been obtained which suggests that this increase in uterine carbonic anhydrase is due to a specific uterine isoenzyme (MCINTOSH [1970]). McIntosh purified two isoenzymes of carbonic anhydrase obtained from the rabbit endometrium (Figure 5). One isoenzyme (C2) was indistinguishable from rabbit erythrocyte isoenzyme and it was presumed that it came from residual blood in the uterus. The second endometrial isoenzyme (C1) is absent from blood and appears to be the form which increases during early pregnancy.

It is clear that carbonic anhydrase increases in the uterus in early pregnancy, but it is not concentrated in the implantation site. Pincus and Bialy [1962] compared the concentration of enzyme in the endometrium at the implantation and interimplantation sites of the rabbit. On the sixth day the concentrations were equal, whereas on the seventh and eighth days the concentration was less in the implantation site. The interpretation of these results is difficult since

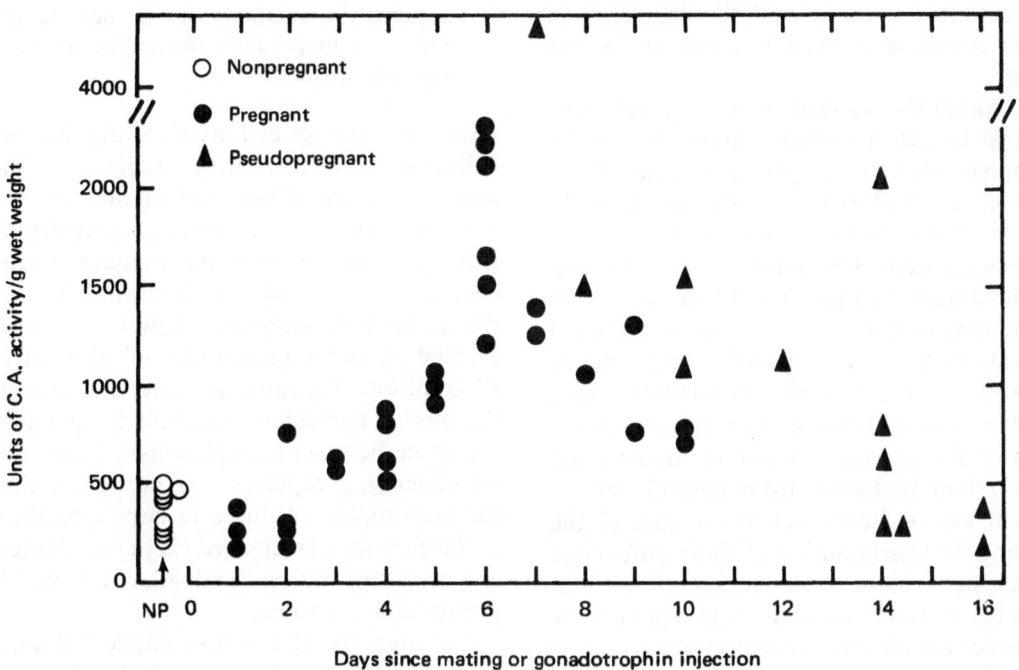

Fig. 4. Assay of carbonic anhydrase in the rabbit. ○—nonpregnant; ●—pregnant; ▲—pseudo-pregnant (after LUTWAK-MANN and MCINTOSH [1969]).

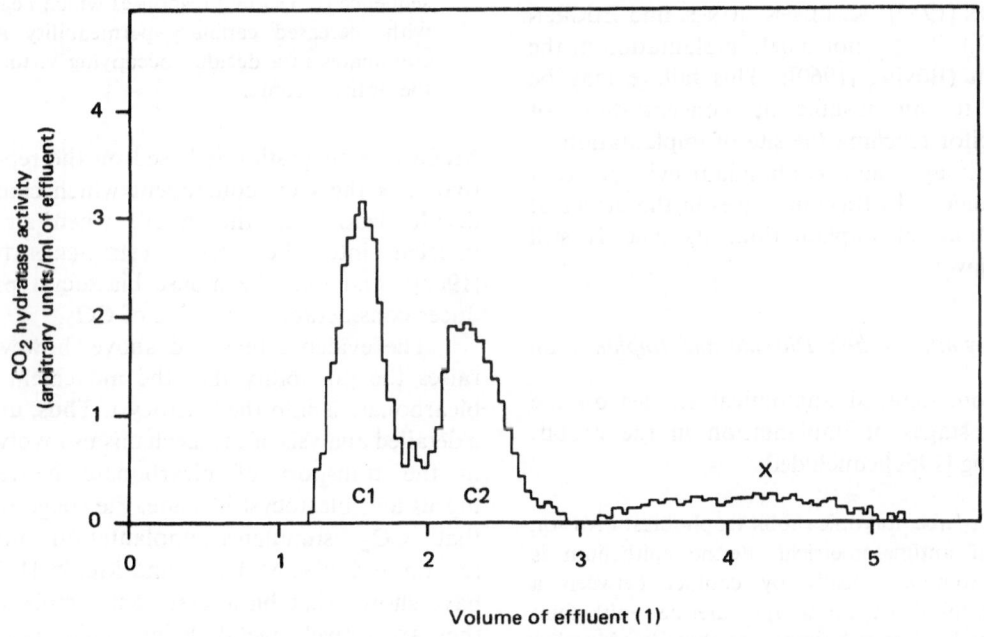

Fig. 5. The carbonic acid isozymes from the uterus of the rabbit. C1 is specific to the uterus and C2 coincides with one of the rabbit erythrocyte isozymes (after MCINTOSH [1970]).

concentrations are related to differences in other components, such as water, at the two sites.

Although Lutwak-Mann [1955] was unable to detect carbonic anhydrase in the nonpregnant and interplacental areas of the endometrium of the rat, Johnson, Lutwak-Mann, and Shelesnyak [1959], using the same technique, were able to measure it in induced deciduomata. The presence of the enzyme in deciduomata has also been shown in the rat (BIALY and PINCUS [1960]) and mouse (MADJEREK and VAN DER VIES [1961]). Both studies showed, however, that the concentration of the enzyme is lower in the decidual tissue than in tissues from control contralateral uterine horns. As in the case of the rabbit, the interpretation of these differences is difficult, since concomitant differential changes in water content could significantly influence the observed concentrations.

While *in vivo* administration of acetylaminothiadiazole sulphonamide (Diamox), a potent inhibitor of carbonic anhydrase, depresses the activity of enzyme extracted from the uterus of rats and rabbits (LUTWAK-MANN [1955]; KNUDSEN, JONES, and EDGREN [1969]), it does not block implantation in the rabbit (Böving [1960]). This failure may be due to an insufficient concentration of inhibitor reaching the site of implantation.

Although there is abundant evidence that carbonic anhydrase increases in the uterus at the time of implantation, its role is still unknown.

Embryonic Carbon Dioxide and Implantation

From detailed anatomical studies on the early stages of implantation in the rabbit, Böving [1959] concluded:

> . . . abembryonic rabbit trophoblast invasion of antimesometrical uterine epithelium is promoted locally by contact between a trophoblast knob and uterine epithelium with a vessel beneath. At that site, invasion is promoted by a chemical that is produced in the blastocyst and transferred to the maternal circulation; it is not locally promoted by products secreted or stored in the endometrium.

Using the findings of Lutwak-Mann and her colleagues, together with studies on the localization of silver precipitates in the neighborhood of implanting blastocysts, Böving proposed that bicarbonate is the chemical promoting implantation in the rabbit. Böving's suggestion, however, is based on finding heavy precipitates of silver after silver nitrate injection, between the cells of the uterine epithelium, particularly spanning the space between a trophoblastic knob and an underlying capillary. He postulates that the bicarbonate produced in large quantities in the blastocyst is removed via the capillaries, and that this causes local alkalinity which precipitates the silver.

McLaren [1969] has also implicated CO_2 from the blastocyst as a stimulus for implantation. She writes:

> . . . it [the blastocyst] "puffs" CO_2 at the uterine epithelium, and this sets off a sequence of decidual responses which begins with increased capillary permeability and culminates in a decidua occupying virtually the entire stroma.

McLaren's suggestion is based on the report that it is the CO_2 component which causes decidualization in the mouse when air is injected into the uterus (HETHERINGTON [1968]), and that the mouse blastocyst produces considerable quantities of CO_2.

The evidence reviewed above, however, raises the possibility that the movement of bicarbonate is into the blastocyst. Thus, until a detailed analysis of the mechanisms involved in the transport of bicarbonate between uterus and blastocyst is made, the suggestion that CO_2 stimulates implantation must remain in doubt. McLaren and Menke [1971] have shown that blastocysts only implant if they are actively metabolizing. This may be a necessary condition, but not the only requirement, for implantation to occur.

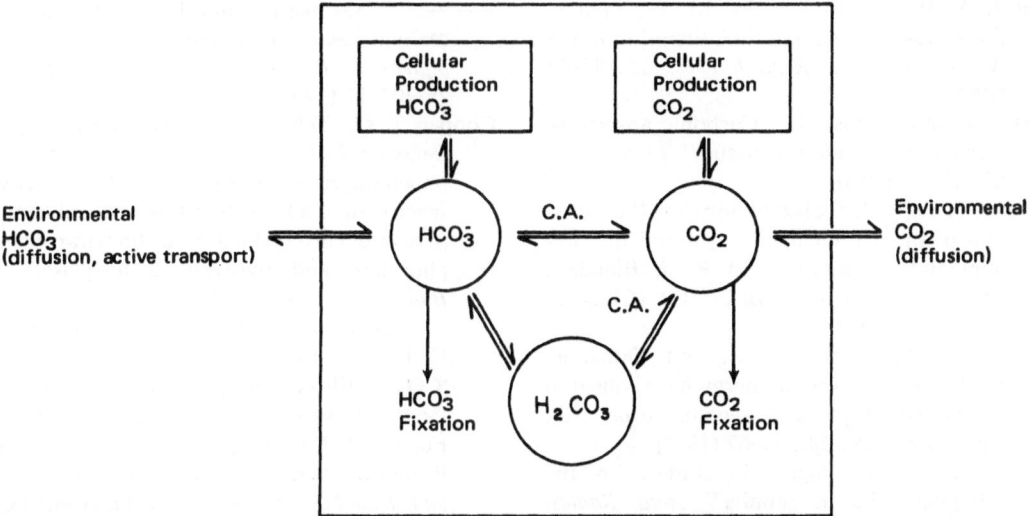

Fig. 6. A hypothetical system showing the factors influencing the CO_2, H_2CO_3, and bicarbonate pools in a developing system. C.A. represents the site of action of carbonic anhydrase.

Conclusion

From the reactions involved in the reversible hydration of CO_2, it is possible to postulate a model in which organisms (uni- and multicellular) have three pools—CO_2, H_2CO_3, and bicarbonate. The equilibrium between the three pools is disturbed by addition to the system of CO_2 or bicarbonate, either from environmental and/or the cellular production of CO_2 or bicarbonate. It is this system of reactions between the three pools that provides the well-known buffering function of bicarbonate. The equilibrium is also disturbed by the removal of CO_2 irreversibly from the system as would occur by CO_2 fixation for biosynthetic purposes, as in developing embryos, and the transport of bicarbonate to extracellular regions, as in the formation of the blastocoele fluid. A summary of the relationships involved is shown in Figure 6. In order to apply this model in the analysis of the specific systems, such as early mammalian development, it is necessary to determine which enzyme systems are functional and the direction of the reactions they catalyze, the extent and mechanism of fixation of CO_2 and bicarbonate, and the extent and mechanism of movement of CO_2 and bicarbonate into extra- and intra-embryonic spaces. In order to understand the role of CO_2 in implantation, the extent and mechanism of movement of CO_2 and bicarbonate between mother and embryo must be determined. The development of new techniques is now making these studies possible.

Acknowledgments The preparation of this paper has been made possible by grants from the Ford Foundation, the National Institute of Child Health and Human Development, and the Population Council.

Bibliography

Ballard, L. A. T., "Studies of dormancy in the seeds of subterranean clover (*trifoliam subterraneum L.*) I. Breaking of dormancy by carbon dioxide and by activated carbon." *Aust. J. Biol. Sci.*, 11:246–60 (1958).

———, "Effect of carbon dioxide on the germination of leguminous seeds." In N. Borliss, ed., *Physiology, Ecology and Biochemistry of Germination.* (Greifswald, 1967), pp. 209–19.

Barnett, H. L. and Lilly, V. G., "The effects of humidity, temperature and carbon dioxide on the sporulation of *Choanephora cucurbitarum.*" *Mycologia*, 47:26–29 (1955).

Bellvé, A. R. and McDonald, M. F., "Directional flow of fallopian tube secretion in the Romney ewe." *J. Reprod. Fert.*, 15:357–64 (1968).

Bialy, G. and Pincus, G., "Carbonic anhydrase activity of rat uterine tissue." *Endocrinol.*, 67:728–29 (1960).

Biggers, J. D., "New observations on the nutrition of the mammalian oocyte and the pre-implantation embryo." In R. J. Blandau, ed., *The Biology of the Blastocyst.* (Chicago, 1971), pp. 319–27.

————, Whittingham, D. G., and Donahue, R. P., "The pattern of energy metabolism in the mouse oocyte and zygote." *Proc. Nat. Acad. Sci., U.S.*, 58:560–67 (1967).

Bjork, L., "Cineradiographic studies on the fallopian tube in rabbits." *Acta Radiol. Suppl.*, 176 (1959).

Board, J. A., "Endometrial carbonic anhydrase after diethylstibestrol as a postcoital anti-fertility agent." *Obstet. Gynec.*, 36:347–49 (1970).

Böving, B. G., "The biology of trophoblast." *Ann. N.Y. Acad. Sci.*, 80:21–43 (1959).

————, "Endocrine influences on implantation." In *Endocrinology of Reproduction.* (New York, 1960).

Braverman, M. H., "Studies in hydroid differentiation: I. *Podocoryne carnea*, culture methods and carbon dioxide induced sexuality." *Exp. Cell Res.*, 27:301–06 (1962).

Brinster, R. L., "Carbon dioxide production from glucose by the preimplantation mouse embryo." *Exp. Cell Res.*, 47:271 (1967*a*).

————, "Carbon dioxide production from lactate and pyruvate by the preimplantation mouse embryo." *Exp. Cell Res.*, 47:634–37 (1967*b*).

————, "Carbon dioxide production from glucose by the preimplantation rabbit embryo." *Exp. Cell Res.*, 51:330–34 (1968).

————, "Mammalian embryo metabolism." In R. J. Blaundau, ed., *The Biology of the Blastocyst.* (Chicago, 1971), pp. 303–18.

Brunton, W. J., *Active transport of chloride by the isolated rabbit oviduct.* Ph.D. Thesis, University of Pennsylvania, 1969.

Clewe, T. H. and Mastroianni, L., "A method for continuous volumetric collection of oviduct secretions." *J. Reprod. Fert.*, 1:146–50 (1960).

Cohen, S., "The metabolism of $^{14}CO_2$ during amphibian development." *J. Biol. Chem.*, 211:337–54 (1954).

————, "$^{14}CO_2$ fixation and the accumulation of malonic acid in amphibian hybrids (*R. pipiens* ♀ × *R. sylvatica* ♂)." *Exp. Cell Res.*, 29:207–11 (1963).

Cooper, T. G., Tchen, T. T., Wood, H. G., and Benedict, C. R., "The carboxylation of phosphoenolpyruvate and pyruvate. I. The active species of 'CO_2' utilized by phosphoenolpyruvate carboxykinase, tarboxytransphosphorylase and pyruvate carboxylase." *J. Biol. Chem.*, 243:3857–63 (1968).

————, Tchen, T. T., Wood, H. G., Benedict, C. R., and Filmer, D. L., "The species of 'CO_2' utilized in the carboxylation of P-enolpyruvate and pyruvate." In R. E. Forster, J. Edsall, A. B. Otis, and F. J. W. Roughton, eds., *CO₂: Chemical, biochemical, and physiological aspects.* (Washington, D.C., 1970).

Dalziel, K. and Londesborough, J. C., "The mechanisms of reductive carboxylation reactions." *Biochem. J.*, 110:223–30 (1968).

Daniel, J. C., "Early growth of rabbit trophoblast." *Amer. Nat.*, 98:85–98 (1964).

David, A., Brackett, B. G., Garcia, C-R., and Mastroianni, L., "Composition of rabbit oviduct fluid in ligated segments of the fallopian tube." *J. Reprod. Fert.*, 19:285–89 (1969).

Edsall, J. T., "Carbon dioxide, carbonic acid, and bicarbonate ion: Physical properties and kinetics of interconversion." In R. E. Forster, J. Edsall, A. B. Otis, and F. J. W. Roughton, eds., *CO₂: Chemical, biochemical, and physiological aspects.* (Washington, D.C., 1970), pp. 15–27.

El Jack, M. H. and Lake, P. E., "The content of the principal inorganic ions and carbon dioxide in uterine fluids of the domestic hen." *J. Reprod. Fert.*, 13:127–32 (1967).

Evans, E. A. Jr., Vennesland, B., and Slotin, L., "The mechanism of carbon dioxide fixation in cell-free extracts of pigeon liver." *J. Biol. Chem.*, 147:771–84 (1943).

Fairbairn, D., "The *in vitro* hatching of *Ascaris lumbricoides* eggs." *Can. J. Zool.*, 39:153–62 (1961).

Flickinger, R. A., "Utilization of $^{14}CO_2$ by developing amphibian embryos, with special reference to regional incorporation into individual embryos." *Exp. Cell Res.*, 6:172–80 (1954).

Graves, C. N. and Biggers, J. D., "Carbon dioxide fixation by mouse embryos prior to implantation." *Science*, 167:1506–08 (1970).

Gurtner, G. H., Burns, B., and Davies, D. G., "Relationship between blood and extra-vascular pCO_2, H^+ and HCO_3^-, lung, cerebrospinal fluid and brain." In *Carbon dioxide in metabolic regulations* (New York, 1974).

Hall, B. V., "Variations in acidity and oxidation reduction potential of rodent uterine fluids." *Physiol. Zool.*, 9:471–97 (1936).

Hamner, C. E. and Williams, W. L., "Composition of rabbit oviduct secretions." *Fert. Ster.*, 16:170–76 (1965).

Heap, R. B., "Some chemical constituents of uterine washings: A method of analysis with results from various species." *J. Endocrinol.*, 24:367–78 (1962).

Hetherington, C. M., "Induction of deciduomata in the mouse by carbon dioxide." *Nature*, 219:863–64 (1968).

Hultin, T., "Incorporation of C^{-14}-labelled carbonate and acetate into sea urchin embryos." *Arkiv Kemi*, 6:195–200 (1952).

——, and Wessel, G., "Incorporation of C^{14}-labelled carbon dioxide into the proteins of developing sea urchin eggs." *Exp. Cell Res.*, 3:613–16 (1952).

Johnson, T. H., Lutwak-Mann, C., and Shelesnyak, M. C., "Carbonic anhydrase in the deciduoma of the rat." *Nature*, 184:961–62 (1959).

Jones, M. E. and Spector, L., "The pathway of carbonate in the biosynthesis of carbamyl phosphate." *J. Biol. Chem.*, 235:2897–2901 (1960).

Kaziro, Y., Hass, L. F., Boyer, P. D., and Ochoa, S., "Mechanism of the propionyl carboxylase reaction. II. Isotopic exchange and tracer experiments." *J. Biol. Chem.*, 237: 1460–68 (1962).

Knudsen, K. A., Jones, R. C., and Edgren, R. A., "Effect of a carbonic anhydrase inhibitor (Diamox) on the progesterone-stimulated rabbit uterus." *Endocrinol.*, 85:1204–05 (1969).

Korhonen, L. K., Korhonen, E., Hyyppa, M., and Punnonen, R., "Histochemical demonstration of carbonic anhydrase activity in the uterus." *Histochemie*, 6:164–67 (1966).

Lane, M. D., "Comparison of enzymatic carboxylation mechanisms." In R. E. Forster, J. Edsall, A. B. Otis, and F. J. W. Roughton, eds., *CO₂: Chemical, biochemical, and physiological aspects.* (Washington, D.C., 1970).

Lenhoff, H. M., "Migration of C^{14}-labelled cnidoblasts." *Exp. Cell Res.*, 17:570–73 (1959).

——, "Some prospects for investigating hydra cells *in vitro*." *In Vitro*, 3:33–48 (1968).

——, and Loomis, W. F., "Environmental factors controlling respiration in hydra." *J. Exp. Zool.*, 134:171–82 (1957).

Loomis, W. F., "Sexual differentiation in hydra: Control by carbon dioxide tension." *Science*, 126:735–39 (1957).

——, "Microenvironmental control of sexual differentiation in hydra." *J. Exp. Zool.*, 156: 289–306 (1964).

Lutwak-Mann, C., "Carbonic anhydrase in the female reproductive tract: Occurrence, distribution and hormonal dependence." *J. Endocrinol.*, 13:26–38 (1955).

——, "Glucose, lactic acid and bicarbonate in rabbit blastocyst fluid." *Nature*, 193:653 (1962).

——, and Laser, H., "Bicarbonate content of the blastocyst fluid and carbonic anhydrase in the pregnant rabbit uterus." *Nature*, 173: 268–70 (1954).

——, and McIntosh, J. E. A., "Zinc and carbonic anhydrase in the rabbit uterus." *Nature*, 221:1111–14 (1969).

McDonald, M. F. and Bellvé, A. R., "Influence of oestrogen and progesterone on flow of fluid from the fallopian in the tube ovariectomized ewe." *J. Reprod. Fert.*, 20:51–61 (1969).

McIntosh, J. E. A., "Carbonic anhydrase isoenzymes in the erythrocytes and uterus of the rabbit." *Biochem. J.*, 120:299–310 (1970).

McLaren, A., "Stimulus and response during early pregnancy in the mouse." *Nature*, 221:739–41 (1969).

——, and Menke, T. M., "CO_2 output of mouse blastocysts *in vitro*, in normal pregnancy and in delay." *J. Reprod. Fert.*, *Suppl.*, 14:23–29 (1971).

Madjerek, Z. and Van der Vies, J., "Carbonic anhydrase activity in the uteri of mice under various experimental conditions." *Acta Endocrinol.*, 38:315–20 (1961).

Makler, A. and Morris, J. M., "Effect of postcoital estrogen on uterine carbonic anhydrase." *Fert. Steril.*, 22:204–08 (1971).

Maren, T. H., "Carbonic anhydrase: Chemistry, physiology and inhibition." *Physiol. Rev.*, 47:595–781 (1967).

Margulis, L., *Origin of Eukaryotic Cells.* New Haven: Yale University Press, 1970.

Menke, T. M. and McLaren, A., "Mouse blastocysts grown *in vivo* and *in vitro*: Carbon dioxide production and trophoblast outgrowth." *J. Reprod. Fert.*, 23:117–27 (1970*a*).

————, and McLaren, A. "Carbon dioxide production by mouse blastocysts during lactational delay of implantation or after ovariectomy." *J. Reprod. Fert.*, 23:287–94 (1970*b*).

Miyake, T., "Progestational substances." In R. I. Dorfman, ed., *Methods in Hormone Research*, Vol. 2. New York: Academic Press, pp. 127–78 (1962).

————, and Pincus, G., "Hormonal influences on the carbonic anhydrase concentration in the accessory reproductive tracts of the rat." *Endocrinol.*, 65:64–72 (1959).

Mounib, M. S. and Eisan, J. S., "Metabolism of pyruvate and glyoxylate by eggs of salmon (*Salmo salar*)." *Comp. Biochem. Physiol.*, 29:259–64 (1969).

Murdoch, R. N. and Wales, R. G., "The synthesis of soluble-RNA in developing preimplantation mouse embryos cultured *in vitro* in the presence of ^{14}C-labelled pyruvate, glucose and carbon dioxide." *J. Reprod. Fert.*, 24:287–90 (1971).

Nicholls, R. A. and Board, J. A., "Carbonic anhydrase concentration in endometrium after oral progestins." *Amer. J. Obstet. Gynec.*, 99:829–32 (1967).

Ogawa, Y. and Pincus, G., "Micro-determination of carbonic anhydrase activity in animal tissue." *Endocrinol.*, 67:551–58 (1960).

————, and Pincus, G. "Estrogen effects on the carbonic anhydrase content of mouse uteri." *Endocrinology*, 70:359–64 (1962).

Park, H. D., Mecca, C. E., and Ortmeyer, A. B., "Carbon dioxide tension and sexual differentiation in hydra." *Biol. Bull.*, 126:121–32 (1964).

Pincus, G. and Bialy, G., "Carbonic anhydrase in steroid-responsive tissues." *Recent Progr. Horm. Res.*, 19:201–42 (1962).

Restall, B. J., "The influence of progesterone and oestrogen on the secretory activities of the fallopian tube." *Aust. J. Biol. Sci.*, 19:187 (1966).

————, and Wales, R. J., "The fallopian tube of the sheep. III. The chemical composition of the fluid from the fallopian tube." *Aust. J. Biol. Sci.*, 19:687–98 (1966).

Rogers, W. P. and Sommerville, R. I., "The infectious process and its reaction to the development of early parasitic stages of nematodes." In B. Dawes, ed., *Advanced Parasitology*. York: Academic New Press, 1968, pp. 327–48.

Severinghaus, J. W., Hamilton, F. N., and Cotev, S., "Carbonic acid production and the role of carbonic anhydrase in decarboxylation in brain." *Biochem. J.*, 114:703–05 (1969).

Shih, H. E., Kennedy, J., and Huggins, C., "Chemical composition of uterine secretions." *Amer. J. Physiol.*, 130:287–91 (1940).

Sommerville, R. I., "The effect of carbon dioxide on the development of third stage larvae of *Haemonchus contortus in vitro*." *Nature*, 202:316–17 (1964).

————, "The development of *Haemonchus contortus* to the fourth stage *in vitro*." *J. Parasitol.*, 52:127–36 (1966).

Stross, R. G., "Photoperiod control of diapause in Daphnia. IV. Light and CO_2-sensitive phases within the cycle of activation." *Biol. Bull.*, 140:137–55 (1971).

Tiedemann, H. and Tiedemann, H., "Einbau von $^{14}CO_2$ in gefurchte und ungefurchte eihalften und in verchiedene entwicklungstadien von tritron." *Naturwissenchaften*, 41:535 (1954).

Vishwakarma, P., "The pH and bicarbonate-ion content of the oviduct and uterine fluids. *Fert. Steril.*, 13:481–85 (1962).

Wales, R. G., Quinn, P., and Murdoch, R. N., "The fixation of carbon dioxide by the eight-cell mouse embryo." *J. Reprod. Fert.*, 20:541–43 (1969).

————, and Whittingham, D. G., "A comparison of the uptake and utilization of lactate and pyruvate by one- and two-cell mouse embryos." *Biochim. Biophys. Acta*, 148:703–12 (1967).

Whitten, W. K., "Nutrient requirements for the culture of preimplantation embryos *in vitro*." *Adv. Biosciences*, 6:129–41 (1970).

Wood, H. G. and Werkman, C. H., "The utilization of CO_2 by the propionic acid bacteria in the dissimilation of glycerol." *J. Bacteriology*, 30:332 (1935).

————, and Werkman, C. H. "The utilization of CO_2 in the dissimilation of glycerol by the propionic acid bacteria." *Biochem. J.*, 30:48–53 (1936).

————, and Utter, M. F., "The role of CO_2 fixation in metabolism." In P. N. Campbell and G. D. Greville, eds., *Essays in Biochemistry*, Vol. 1. (London, 1965), pp. 1–27.

Biggers Discussion

SEVERINGHAUS: I find this extremely interesting. I'm thinking about the pH of the fallopian tube environment since you, I suppose, would assume that the P_{CO_2} is controlled by the mother. The fact that you find a high bicarbonate in the blastocyst along toward the time of implantation would imply a rather alkaline pH. Has it been possible to put micro-pH electrodes into the fallopian tube and see whether the environment is also alkaline or whether it's just the inside of the blastocyst?

BIGGERS: I have, a grant to measure this right now, but I haven't gotten around to doing it.

SEVERINGHAUS: It's also interesting that early lactate metabolism appears to be the primary source of metabolism and that at about the time of implantation glucose metabolism begins to take place, and that this change occurs at the time when it must be most alkaline. We also know that alkalinity directly stimulates glycolysis to lactate. I'm not sure what the relationship is.

BIGGERS: When you start with the egg entering the uterus, it's a ball of cells in one particular place, located excentrically; a cavity starts to form and this swells to give rise to this cyst-like structure which is the blastocoele cavity. This region is accumulating water and potassium, sodium and bicarbonate in very large quantities, so it is presumably being produced from the cells of the trophoplast. So we have the input of these ions and bicarbonate into the blastocoele cavity, and then we're talking about a gradient from inside maternal back to the capillary.

NAHAS: Do carbonic anhydrase inhibitors inhibit implantation, and has it been studied as a possible contraceptive method?

BIGGERS: Yes, people have been interested in this in the development of contraceptive methods. They just don't seem to work, at least in rodents, I talked to someone about this some years ago and he seemed to believe that it was probably difficult to get the inhibitors in sufficient concentrations into the uterine lumen.

RAHN: Can you give me the approximate concentration of bicarbonate in relation to the blood of the mother? Is it two times or three times higher?

BIGGERS: Well, that depends on whose paper you look at.

RAHN: Well, approximately?

BIGGERS: There are such big discrepancies in the literature, bicarbonate concentrations vary between 27.5 and 50 mmoles/l.

RAHN: I have another question. You spoke about breaking the diapause in some of the early eggs. Have you speculated at all upon breaking the diapause in the development of certain mammals where the implantation, I believe, is stopped for long periods of time?

BIGGERS: First of all, some animals naturally have the blastocysts rest for several months before development. For example, a bear will mate in July and the blastocysts form in about a week and then they won't do anything until October when it implants and continues on from the blastocyst stage. You can produce this experimentally in mice and rats by ovariectomizing them two days after mating and giving them progesterone; they will remain arrested until such time as you give them some estrogen, and it can be three or four months that they will stay in this state. I don't know of anybody who has tried to put these animals in an atmosphere of high CO_2. I don't know of any work that is relevant to your question.

RECTOR: With respect to the question of Dr. Severinghaus, Dr. Pierre Mongine, who is now working in our laboratory, has been studying bicarbonate secretion in the uterus of the chicken. I don't know whether this is applicable to the mammalian system or not, but when the egg enters the uterus in a chicken, bicarbonate secretion is initiated and this proceeds for about 5 hours until calcium secretion begins, and then you get the formation of the shell. This can be blocked by acetazolomide. Whether there's a similar system in the mammalian uterus I don't know, but it certainly could be answered by *in vivo* pH measurements.

TRUH: Are there any effects of CO_2 on the sperm that you know of?

BIGGERS: CO_2 fixation is described in sperm; there's an extensive literature on this. I'm really not very familiar with it.

TURINO: Is there any data on the relationship between the appearance of this high concentration of bicarbonate and the O_2 utilization by the eggs at this particular point? In other words, is this high HCO_3^- timed to a point when oxygen utilization may increase and metabolic CO_2 be produced in larger amounts?

BIGGERS: The O_2 consumption is being measured pretty well in mice embryos by the Cartesian diver technique. There is a significant uptake of O_2 right from the time of fertilization, but it really goes up exponentially after the eight-cell stage. The eight-cell stage is a very critical stage in the mice, where metabolism changes and also rapidly increases. This is not correlated with the bicarbonate levels that I know of.

5. Mechanisms of Carbon Dioxide and pH Effects on Metabolism

Gabriel G. Nahas

College of Physicians and Surgeons
Columbia University
630 West 168th Street
New York, New York 10632

Introduction

The physiological effects of acidemia are well established. It depresses the functional activity of all vital organs. The cardiovascular system is primarily affected (CLOWES et al. [1961]). Both cardiac conduction and the contractile force of the myocardium are depressed and there is vasodilatation in the peripheral circulation and cerebral vessels. By contrast, vasoconstriction develops in the lung vasculature. In the liver enzymatic activity is generally depressed. Acidemia has a thromboplastic effect and increases coagulation, contributing to intravascular clotting, as described by Hardaway [1966].

It is also known that acidosis decreases catecholamine activity (BURGET and VISSCHER [1927]). Adrenaline and noradrenaline, at acid pH, influence heart rate and blood pressure less than at normal pH. It should, however, be remembered that acidosis is also a profound stimulus to catecholamine production (NAHAS et al. [1967]). These two antagonistic effects of acidosis result in a new, unstable condition which will vary from one individual to the next and will depend upon the degree of sympatho-adrenal stimulation and the degree of inhibition of catecholamine activity produced by a given level of acidosis. In the present paper I will describe primarily the effects of acidosis on catecholamine activity and some steps of intermediary metabolism and will finally mention recent experiments describing pH effects on leukocyte motility.

Effects of Acidemia on Adrenal Function

Fenn and Asano reported in 1956 that hypercapnia was accompanied by an increase in sympatho-adrenal activity in the cat. Subsequently Tenney [1956] showed that CO_2 serves as a potent stimulus to increase the titre of circulating sympatho-adrenal catecholamines in the cat. In 1960 we attempted to quantitate these changes. Hypercapnic acidosis was produced in dogs by the process of "apneic oxygenation," and arterial blood pH was decreased to 7.0 while Pa_{CO_2} was increased to about 100 mm Hg (NAHAS, LIGOU, and MEHLMAN [1960]). Under these conditions, plasma concentrations of adrenaline and noradrenaline increased, while O_2 uptake did not, although an increase in catecholamine is usually accompanied by increased O_2 uptake (STEINBERG et al. [1964]). Furthermore, mean blood pressure did not change much in these animals. However, when the acidosis was corrected there was a sudden increase in O_2 uptake and blood pressure. These observations were interpreted as indicating that correction of acidosis restored a normal hydrogen-ion concentration and catecholamines exerted their optimal metabolic activity.

Similar observations were made on animals ventilated with 10% CO_2 and 30% O_2 so that arterial pH fell to 7.0. There was no increase in O_2 uptake and no increase in non-esterified fatty acids (FFA) or glycerol concentrations in plasma. When pH was restored to normal, there were marked increases in FFA and glycerol concentrations and in O_2 uptake (POYART and NAHAS [1966]). These experiments indicate further that catecholamines endogenously released by hypercapnic acidosis will resume their metabolic activity when pH is restored to normal.

It was shown that the rise in circulating plasma catecholamines during acidosis could be attributed to an increased release from peripheral nerve endings (EULER and LISHAJKO [1963]) and also from the adrenal gland (NAHAS et al. [1967]). The isolated adrenal gland of the dog was perfused at constant flow at ·37°C with diluted homologous blood at normal and acid pH. It was shown that this medium preserved the integrity of the fine structure of the adrenal gland. The perfusion medium was made acid by equilibration with hypercapnic mixtures or addition of lactic acid. Noradrenaline and adrenaline concentrations were measured in the diluted blood after perfusion and adrenal catecholamine output was calculated. At normal pH, it averaged 70 ng/gland/min. Adrenal catecholamine output was increased by 100% following perfusion with hypercapnic mixtures at a pH of 6.96 to 7.10 (Pa_{CO_2} 70, 118 mm Hg) and 660% with a mixture at a pH of 6.79 to 6.92 (Pa_{CO_2} 125, 210 mm Hg). This increase was primarily due to a rise in adrenaline concentration. Similar results were obtained following perfusion with media made acid by the addition of lactic acid. These results indicate that increases in $[H^-]$ directly stimulate adrenal medullary secretion.

It was also observed (MITTELMAN et al. [1962]) that hypercapnic acidosis in the dog significantly increased cortisol output. The physiological importance of catecholamine release during hypercapnia was demonstrated by observations (NAHAS and CAVERT

[1957]) which showed that giving adrenaline or noradrenaline reversed or prevented the acute myocardial failure produced by respiratory acidosis which was first observed by Jerusalem and Starling [1910] in the heart-lung preparation.

The increased catecholamine output of acidemia related to an augmentation of catecholamine synthesis in rats (NAHAS and STEINSLAND [1968]). It was first observed that exposure to hypercapnia was not accompanied by significant depletion of catecholamine stores: In a group of rats exposed to 20% CO_2, 25% O_2, balance N_2, for periods of up to 5 hours, there were no significant changes in the noradrenaline content of the heart, salivary glands, and brain, or in the catecholamine content of the adrenal gland compared with a control group breathing air. Another group of rats was given intraperitoneally 300 mg/kg of L-α-methyl-*p*-tyrosine in three divided doses before a similar period of hypercapnia. They presented a 37.7% decrease in the noradrenaline content of the heart and a 34.3% decrease in the catecholamine content of the adrenals. Rats treated with L-α-methyl-*p*-tyrosine and breathing room air did not present significant changes in the catecholamine content of heart or adrenal gland. Forty hours after the administration of dopa-^{3}H, exposure to hypercapnia significantly decreased specific activity of catecholamines in the adrenal gland. Conversion of tyrosine-^{3}H to labeled catecholamines was also increased in rats during hypercapnia. These results indicate that the rate of catecholamine synthesis is increased during hypercapnia and enables the animal to sustain the elevated catecholamine release required to maintain vital physiological functions.

Lotspeich [1967] has reported that metabolic acidosis produces in the rat an increase in glutaminase enzymes and in the hexose monophosphate shunt enzymes. Kidney hypertrophy is also present and can be explained by an incorporation of the glutamine carbon skeleton into renal tissue components. When protein synthesis was blocked by actinomycin D, the hypertrophy of metabolic adicosis did not occur. This led Lotspeich to postulate that the increased [H⁺] of NH_4Cl acidosis might derepress a gene site in kidney cells responsible for protein and enzyme synthesis. In our experiments, the adrenals of hypercapnic rats were not weighed; however, it was previously reported (SCHAEFER et al. [1955]) that, after one hour of exposure to 30% CO_2, the weight of the adrenal gland in guinea pigs was significantly increased, indicating that hypercapnia might also produce a hypertrophy of the adrenals. However, further investigations are required to ascertain if the increased rate of synthesis of adrenal catecholamine is also accompanied by an increased synthesis of the enzymes that convert tyrosine into dopa and dopamine. Acidosis profoundly alters sympatho-adrenal regulation, producing an increase in catecholamine synthesis and release, and at the same time decreasing the metabolic activity of these amines.

Effects of Acidemia on the Metabolic Activity of the Catecholamines

During hypercapnia, the increase in enzyme activity that controls catecholamine synthesis contrasts with the inhibitory effect of [H⁺] on enzymes which regulate intermediary metabolism and which are activated by these catecholamines. This inhibition was observed *in vivo* as well as *in vitro*.

Experiments *in vivo*

For the experiments *in vivo*, pedigree beagles were used because they have constant and reliable substrate and acid-base levels (POYART and NAHAS [1966]). They were given a standard dose of noradrenaline or adrenaline (1.5 μg/kg/min for 30 min) while being mechanically ventilated with room air. (Arterial pH was 7.42 and Pco_2 30 mm Hg). A week later, the animals received the same dose of catecholamine, but this time were ventilated with a mixture of 10% CO_2 and 25% O_2 in N_2 so their average pHa was 7.0

and average Pa_{CO_2} was 100 mm Hg. Noradrenaline infusion, when ventilation was with room air, produced 25% to 30% increments in O_2 uptake that persisted for at least an hour after the end of the 30-min infusion. By contrast, when the same animals were made hypercapnic a week later, O_2 uptake was not significantly different from the control uptake. Changes in free fatty acid levels with noradrenaline infusion also occurred. There was a marked increase in free fatty acids when pH was maintained at normal. At pH 7.0 the lipolytic activity of noradrenaline was depressed by 70%. Similar alterations in free fatty acids, glucose, and lactic acid blood concentrations also occurred with adrenaline infusion. At normal pH, there was a marked increase in free fatty acid and glycerol concentrations; during acidosis, these substances did not increase significantly. Under conditions of normal pH, glucose concentrations rose from 100 mg% to 300 mg% and lactic acid levels also rose. During hypercapnic acidosis, there was still a significant increase in glucose, but no change in lactic acid. This would indicate that while glycogenolysis does proceed during acidosis, glucose utilization might be impaired.

In an additional group of dogs metabolic acidosis was induced by the intravenous administration of ammonium chloride (0.15M) for 48 to 60 hours until pHa was decreased to between 7.05 and 7.15 (NAHAS and POYART [1967]). During the experiment, ventilation was adjusted to maintain pHa and Pa_{CO_2} at this level and noradrenaline was then infused for 30 min. Before the noradrenaline infusion, blood concentrations of free fatty acids, glycerol, glucose, and lactic acid were the same as at normal pH, while VO_2 was slightly higher. No significant increases in VO_2 and free fatty acids occurred following noradrenaline infusion, and the increase in glycerol, although significant, was small and comparable to the change in free fatty acids. As compared with controls, the increase of VO_2 induced by noradrenaline during acidosis was inhibited by 60%, free fatty acids by 68%, and glycerol by 80%. There were no significant changes in blood glucose or lactic acid concentrations.

Similar experiments were performed to study the effect of respiratory and metabolic alkalosis on noradrenaline-induced calorigenesis and lipolysis (NAHAS and POYART [1967]). Three groups of dogs were either hyperventilated mechanically or alkalosis was induced by the infusion of THAM (0.3 M) or sodium bicarbonate (0.3 M). Neither metabolic nor respiratory alkalosis significantly altered control values. When noradrenaline was simultaneously infused with alkali, there was a slight but not significant enhancement of lipolysis. There were no significant differences in changes in blood glucose and lactic acid except for a marked hypoglycemia while THAM was being infused. When noradrenaline was infused during hyperventilation, the increase in VO_2 was significantly higher than the increase produced by noradrenaline at normal pHa. At the end of noradrenaline infusion during hyperventilation, plasma free acid concentrations were also significantly higher than at

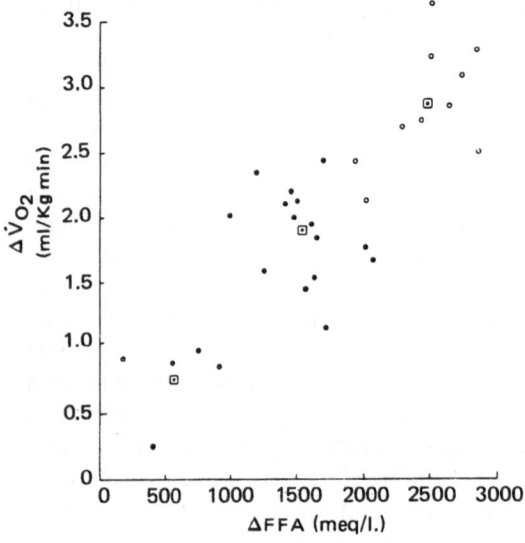

Fig. 1. Relationship between changes in O_2 consumption (VO_2) and FFA during noradrenaline infusion (1.5 μg/kg/min for 30 min) in 30 beagles which had normal, acid, or alkaline pHa. (From NAHAS and POYART [1967]).

normal pHa, but there was only a slight change in glycerol.

Alterations of the metabolic effects of noradrenaline are, therefore, related to changes in [H^+] rather than to changes in Pa_{CO_2} or [HCO_3^-]. Acid pH, produced either by hypercapnia or by infusion of NH_4Cl, inhibits to the same extent noradrenaline-induced lipolysis and calorigenesis. On the other hand, a decrease in [H^+], either by means of hyperventilation or by administration of base, results in higher VO_2 and slightly higher release of free fatty acids. Figure 1 shows the correlation between the increase in VO_2 and the plasma concentration of free fatty acids, the latter being determined by the [H^+] of the blood at the end of the noradrenaline infusion.

Experiments *in vitro*

This inhibition of activated lipolysis by acid pH was also observed *in vitro*. Rat epididymal adipose tissue was incubated in Krebs–Ringer phosphate medium with 5% albumin, without glucose but with glucagon, ACTH, and noradrenaline or cyclic 3′, 5′-AMP dibutyrate. The pH of the medium was varied from 7.4 to 6.6. Glycerol release was measured and taken as the index of lipolytic activity. In a first series of experiments at pH 7.4, noradrenaline, ACTH, and glucagon-activated lipolysis was potentiated by increasing doses of theophylline. In a second series, with the pH of the medium at 6.6, the lipolytic effects of these three hormones were significantly inhibited. When theophylline (10^{-2} M) was added in combination with optimal doses of the hormones, the rate of glycerol release was similar at normal and acid pH. These results were interpreted as indicating that H^+ might exert its inhibitory effect on a common mechanism which results in cyclic 3′, 5′-AMP formation (TRINER and NAHAS [1965]). This hypothesis was confirmed: When cyclic 3′, 5′-AMP dibutyrate (10^{-3} M) was added to the medium, the same glycerol release was found at pH 7.4 and 6.6 (POYART and NAHAS [1968]).

When combined with noradrenaline, cyclic 3', 5'-AMP dibutyrate also reversed the inhibitory effects of acidosis. These results, when analyzed according to the drug-receptor theory, would indicate that acidosis might inhibit, at least in part, the different lipolytic drugs used in this study by hindering the formation of the drug-receptor complexes which activate lipolysis.

Effects of Acidosis on Glucose Metabolism

The effects of variations in extracellular pH on glucose metabolism have been studied in different tissues. In rat liver slices, epididymal fat pad, and diaphragm muscle, a direct relationship was found between the rate of lactate production and the pH of the incubation medium (GEVERS and DOWDLE [1963]). During acidosis, glucose uptake in human red blood cells was inhibited and lactate production decreased. It was suggested that this inhibiting effect of acidosis was exerted between the hexose phosphate and the triose phosphate stages (MURPHY [1960]). Conversely, during alkalosis, accelerated glycolysis and a higher glucose uptake and production of lactate were observed in erythrocytes (TRINER et al. [1964]). In the perfused rat heart, Delcher and Shipp [1966] observed increased glucose uptake, lactate production, and glycogen breakdown. The activities of several enzymes are sensitive to changes of pH; Reynolds and Haugaard [1967] observed decreased phosphorylase activity in diaphragm muscle and Trivedi and Danforth [1966] demonstrated a significant fall in the activity of phosphofructokinase from frog skeletal muscle at low pH. The purpose of the study performed on the rat diaphragm was to investigate further the effect of acid pH on the concentration of some intermediates in the glycolytic pathway in skeletal muscle. At pH 6.8 glucose uptake was significantly decreased (-23%), while glycogen content was significantly increased over control ($+22\%$) at pH 7.4 (Table 1). Both lactate and pyruvate production were significantly decreased (-38% and -20%,

respectively). In the muscle there was a significant increase in glucose-6-phosphate (G-6-P, $+22\%$) but not in glucose-1-phosphate (G-1-P, $+12\%$) or fructose-6-phosphate (F-6-P, $+11\%$) concentrations, while fructose-1,6-diphosphate (F-1,6-P) concentration was significantly lower (-29%) (Table 2). These changes indicate that acid pH inhibits phosphofructokinase activity in mammalian skeletal muscle, the rate-limiting step in the glycolytic pathway. There were no significant changes in O_2 consumption or citrate concentration in the muscle with acid pH (Table 3), indicating that the Krebs cycle and electron transfer through the respiratory chain are not inhibited by this degree of acidosis. Similarly, there was no change in O_2 uptake *in vivo* during hypercapnic or metabolic acidosis.

Metabolic changes occurring in K^+-free medium are similar to those at acid pH. When K^+ is not present in the medium, there is a shift of K^+ and other ions from the intra- to the extracellular compartment and it's known that similar shifts of K^+ occur at low pH (FENN and COBB [1934]). The importance of ions, such as K^+, in the activation of certain enzymes of the glycolytic pathway has often been demonstrated and recently reviewed by Bygrave [1967]. An elevated K^+ concentration in the incubation medium increases glucose metabolism in liver slices (ASHMORE et al. [1957]) and glycogen breakdown in heart muscle (STADIE, HAUGAARD, and PERLMUTTER [1947]).

Changes in intermediates of the glycolytic pathway at low pH suggest that the activity of the enzymes, phosphorylase and phosphofructokinase, which require phosphate ions for their actions, are inhibited. These enzymes are also very sensitive to changes in concentration of cyclic 3',5'-AMP. The results of this study do not show whether or not metabolic changes due to acid pH and ouabain are caused by an inhibition of the adenyl cyclase system. However, since the effect of cyclic 3',5'-AMP on phosphorylase activity of skeletal muscle is not pH-dependent (REYNOLDS and HAUGAARD [1967]),

Table 1. The effect of acid pH on glycogen content in muscle and on lactate and pyruvate concentrations in medium*

| | Krebs-Ringer phosphate | |
Medium	pH7.4	pH6.8
Glycogen	7.15 ± 0.56	8.76 ± 0.62†
(μmol glucose/g wet tissue)	(11)	(11)
Glucose uptake	15.36 ± 1.39	10.24 ± 1.62†
(μmol glucose/g wet tissue)	(14)	(13)
Lactate	31.58 ± 1.26	19.74 ± 1.06
(μmol lactate/g wet tissue)	(16)	(15)
Pyruvate	1.41 ± 0.00	1.13 ± 0.00†
(μmol pyruvate/g wet tissue)	(15)	(15)

* Values are means ± SE. Figures in parentheses represent number of experiments.
† Significantly different ($p < 0.05$) from control values (pH 7.4).

Table 2. The effect of acid pH on the concentration of hexose phosphates in muscle (μmol/100 g wet tissue)*

| | Krebs-Ringer phosphate | |
Medium	pH7.4	pH6.8
Glucose-1-phosphate	4.0 ± 0.7	4.5 ± 1.3
	(14)	(13)
Glucose-6-phosphate	16.1 ± 0.8	19.6 ± 1.1†
	(17)	(15)
Fructose-6-phosphate	4.3 ± 0.3	4.8 ± 0.5
	(13)	(13)
Fructose-1,6-diphosphate	7.5 ± 0.5	5.3 ± 0.5†
	(13)	(10)

* Values are means ± SE. Figures in parentheses represent number of experiments.
† Significantly different ($p < 0.05$) from control values (pH 7.4).

Table 3. The lack of effect of acid pH on oxygen consumption and citrate concentration of rat diaphragm*

| | Krebs-Ringer phosphate | |
Medium	pH7.4	pH6.8
Oxygen consumption	3.35 ± 0.14	3.14 ± 0.15
(μl O_2/mg dry tissue/hour)	(15)	(16)
Citrate concentration	220 ± 22	204 ± 31
(μg/g wet tissue)	(13)	(13)

* Values are means ± SE. Figures in parentheses represent number of experiments.

at low pH there might be a decreased formation of cyclic 3′,5′-AMP.

Effects of pH on Leukocyte Motility

The last series of experiments to be presented illustrate the complexity of pH effects (NAHAS, TANNIERES, and LENNON [1971]). Most of the data that we have discussed indicate that acidosis exerts an inhibitory effect on function and enzymatic activity. However, we already noted the experiments of Lotspeich [1967] which indicate that increased $[H^+]$ increases the activity of the glutaminase enzymes and, with Steinsland (NAHAS and STEINSLAND [1968]), we have shown that acidmia increases tyrosine hydroxylase activity and catecholamine synthesis in the adrenal gland.

The present experiments on leukocyte motility indicate that marked increases in $[H^+]$ do not alter leukocyte motility while alkalosis inhibits this basic function.

A special system (Figure 2) was designed to study polymorphonuclear neutrophils (PMN) under conditions of a constant microenvironment. This system was comprised of two parts: a series of equilibrating tonometers (Eschweiler) and a micro-observation chamber in communication with the latter. The equilibrating tonometers (volume, 15 ml) were immersed in a constant temperature bath. They were connected through humidifiers to gas mixtures of known concentrations of O_2, N_2, and CO_2. The observation chamber was made of a glass slide and a cover slip sealed with resin and connected with two polyethylene tubes (0.5 mm i.d.). One of the tubes was connected to the equilibrating tonometer, the other to a syringe. The system allowed for an anaerobic filling of the observation chamber after the blood cells had been equilibrated in the tonometer. The observation chamber was placed under a phase contrast microscope. The objective of the microscope was fitted with a device (LENNON [1970]) which maintained constant the temperature of the

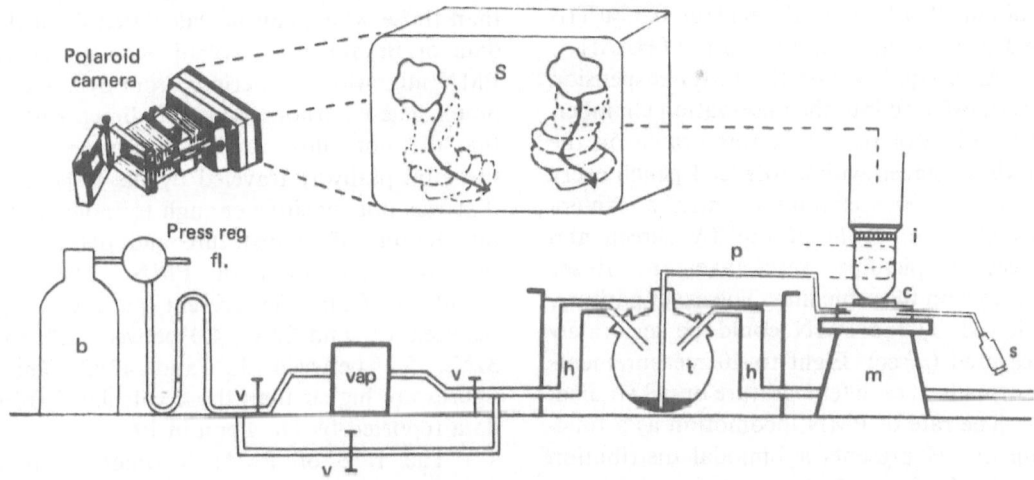

Fig. 2. System for the direct study of blood cells under controlled microenvironment. This system comprises: a tank (b) containing known concentration of equilibrating gases with pressure reducer (*Press Reg*) and flowmeter (*fl*); a calibrated vaporizer for each of the anaesthetic vapors utilized; a series of valves (v) for bypassing or using the vaporizer; a thermostated bath with tonometer (*t*) and humidifiers (h); a microscopic air-sealed observation chamber connected to the tonometer by means of a polyethylene tube (p) and to a syringe (s) for filling; a phase contrast microscope (m) and an objective that is thermally controlled and isolated from the microscope by means of an insulating ring; a television screen (s) for observing the blood cells; a Polaroid camera which can be triggered at regular intervals. (From NAHAS, TANNIERES, and LENNON [1971]).

preparation under microscopic observation. This device consisted of a metal coil placed around the objective of the microscope. Temperature could be rapidly modified from 0° to 50°C by circulating through the coil warm water or supercooled alcohol. The objective was isolated from the microscope by an insulating ring; changes in temperature were only transmitted to the center of the glass observation chamber. Temperatures could be continuously recorded by means of a thermocouple placed next to the cover slip. The image of the preparation under the microscope was transmitted to a television screen, according to the technique described by Bessis [1964].

PMN from healthy human donors were sampled according to conventional techniques and equilibrated in the tonometers. The Po_2 of the equilibrating gases was maintained at 150 mm Hg. The Pco_2 was changed from 15 mm Hg to 150 mm Hg. The pH of the plasma in which the PMN were suspended was varied over the range of 5.0 to 8.1, either by changing Pco_2 or by addition of 0.15 M lactic acid or 0.3 M Tris (hydroxymethyl) aminomethane (THAM).

After equilibration the PMN suspension was transferred into the observation chamber. The outline of the PMN was drawn on the television screen with a soft lead pencil every 10 sec for 90 sec. Subsequently, a camera was placed in front of the TV screen and successive pictures were taken at 10-sec intervals on the same film. The exact pathway followed by the PMN could be accurately measured (μ/sec). Eight to 20 measurements were made at each temperature or pH studied.

The rate of PMN locomotion as a function of pH presents a bimodal distribution that is observed when temperature increases above 23°C. The inhibitory effect of alkaline pH beyond 7.6 contrasts with the lack of effect of acid pH until 6.5 (Figure 3).

Rate of locomotion of PMN is markedly affected by temperature, especially between 23° and 42°C. This rise in temperature is associated with a ninefold increase in velocity. The maximum velocity observed for human PMN (0.94 μ/sec ± 0.006) was at pH 7.43

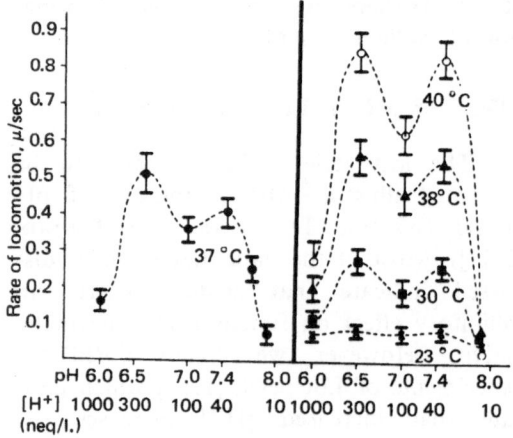

Fig. 3. Rate of locomotion of human polymorphonuclear neutrophils in function of pH and temperature. (From NAHAS, TANNIERES, and LENNON [1971]).

and 42°C. This value is at variance with that reported by McCutcheon [1923], who observed a maximum velocity of 0.65 μ/sec ± 0.002 at 40°C, with a sharp drop thereafter. But McCutcheon did not control pH. These velocities are also three times greater than those which can be calculated from the data of Bryant et al. [1966], who measured PMN migration for periods from over 1 to 4 hours. These authors used an indirect method that did not allow for the measurement of the total pathway traveled by the PMN and that was not sensitive enough to indicate the interactions of temperature and pH on the rate of locomotion of PMN. The Q_{10} calculated from the present data was 3.1 between 12° and 22°C, 4.0 between 22° and 32°C, 5.2 between 32° and 42°C. These figures are higher than those calculated from data reported by Dr. Fenn in 1922.

The rate of PMN locomotion as a function of pH (Figure 3) presents a bimodal distribution similar to that reported for amoeba Proteus (PITTS and MAST [1933]), with peak velocities at pH 6.5 and 7.4. Such a bimodal distribution was observed at four different temperatures. Changes of pH toward acidity over a significant range from pH 7.4 to 6.5 does not alter or even increase rate of locomotion. By contrast, alkaline pH beyond 7.6 produces a significant decrease in rate of locomotion that is completely and irreversibly inhibited at pH 7.9 for all temperatures. This contrast is more apparent when $[H^+]$ concentration is used in neq/l., instead of pH. Rate of PMN locomotion is not greatly affected when $[H^+]$ changes from 40 neq/l. (pH 7.4) to 320 neq/l. (pH 6.5). However, it is totally inhibited when $[H^+]$ decreases from 32 neq/l. (pH 7.5) to 10 neq/l. (pH 8.0). When blood is collected in open tubes with heparin, CO_2 escapes and pH of the plasma tends to become alkaline (pH 7.5–7.7), a factor which will decrease rate of PMN motility.

Conclusion

All of the experiments that we have described illustrate the very complex and often antagonistic effects of pH on cellular function. When all of these effects are considered, it is remarkable to see how a constant optimal pH can be maintained at all of these different cellular levels. It is also remarkable that basal metabolic functions are still able to proceed in the total organism when plasma pH is changed from 7.5 to 7.0 (30 to 100 neq/l.).

The present experiments in leukocyte motility indicate that marked increases in $[H^+]$ do not alter leukocyte motility while alkalosis inhibits this basic function.

Acknowledgments   The author gratefully acknowledges the advice and support of Professor Marcel Bessis, Director of the Institute of Cellular Pathology, Hospital Bicêtre, Le Kremlin-Bicêtre, France.

This work was supported, in part, by a National Institutes of Health grant, GM–09069–06 and –07; Army contract DADA–17–67–C–7126; the Robert Sterling Clark Foundation Inc., and the Dolores and Bob Hope gift for the study of shock.

Bibliography

Ashmore, J., Cahill, G. F. Jr., Hastings, A. B., and Zottu, S., "Studies on carbohydrate metabolism in rat liver slices. VIII. Effect of ions and hormones on pathway of glucose-6-phosphate metabolism." *J. Biol. Chem.*, 224:225–35 (1957).

Bessis, M., In *Cellular Injury*. Ciba Foundation Symposium. (Boston: Little Brown, 1963), p. 287.

Bryant, R. E., Desprez, R. M., Vanway, M. H., and Rogers, D. E., "Studies on human leukocyte motility." *J. Exp. Med.*, 124:483–99 (1966).

Burget, G. E. and Visscher, M. B., "Variations of pH of blood and the response of the vascular system to adrenalin." *Amer. J. Physiol.*, 81: 113–23 (1927).

Bygrave, F. L., "The ionic environment and metabolic control." *Nature*, (*London*), 214: 667–71 (1967).

Clowes, G. H. A. Jr., Sabga, G. A., Konitaxis, A., Tomin, R., Hughes, M., and Simeone, F. A., "Effects of acidosis on cardiovascular function in surgical patients." *Ann. Surg.*, 154:524–55 (1961).

Comandon, J., "Influence de la temperature sur la reptation leukocytaire." *C. R. Soc. Biol.*, 82: 1305 (1914).

Delcher, H. K. and Shipp, J. C., "Effect of pH, pCO_2 and bicarbonate on metabolism of glucose by perfused rat heart." *Biochim. biophys. Acta* (*Amsterdam*), 121:250–60 (1966).

Euler, U. S. V. and Lishajko, F., "Influence of pH on uptake and release of noradrenaline in adrenergic nerve granules." *J. Neurochem.*, 10:145–49 (1963).

Fenn, W. O., "Leukocyte motility and Q_{10}." *J. Gen. Physiol.*, 4:331 (1922).

———, and Asano, T., "Effects of carbon dioxide inhalation on potassium liberation from the liver." *Amer. J. Physiol.*, 185: 567–76 (1956).

———, and Cobb, D. M., "The potassium equilibrium in muscle." *J. Gen. Physiol.*, 17:629–56 (1934).

Geevers, W. and Dowdle, E., "The effect of pH on glycolysis in vitro." *Clin. Sci.*, 25:343–49 (1963).

Hardaway, R. M. III, *Syndromes of disseminated intravascular coagulation*. Springfield, Ill.: Thomas, 1966.

Jerusalem, E. and Starling, E. H., "On the significance of carbon dioxide for the heartbeat." *J. Physiol.*, 40:279–94 (1910).

Lennon, J. F., "Mesure et contrôle de la température des préparations sous microscope."

C. R. Soc. Biol., 164:1433–1937 (1933–37).

Lotspeich, W. D., "Metabolic aspects of acid-base change. Interrelated biochemical responses, in the kidney and other organs, are associated with metabolic acidosis." *Science*, 155:1066–75 (1967).

McCutcheon, M., "The effects of temperature on the rate of locomotion of human neutrophilic leukocytes in vitro." *Am. J. Physiol.*, 66:185 (1923).

Mittelman, A., Dos, S. J., Barker, H. G., and Nahas, G. G., "Adrenal-cortical response during corrected and uncorrected hypercapnic acidosis." *Amer. J. Physiol.*, 202:334–36 (1962).

Murphy, J. R., "Erythrocyte metabolism. II. Glucose metabolism and pathways." *J. Lab. Clin. Med.*, 55:286–302 (1960).

Nahas, G. G. and Cavert, H. M., "Cardiac depressant effect of CO_2 and its reversal." *Amer. J. Physiol.*, 190:483–91.

———, Ligou, J. C., and Mehlman, B., "Effects of pH changes on O_2 uptake and plasma catecholamine levels in the dog." *Amer. J. Physiol.*, 198:60–66 (1960).

———, and Poyart, C., "Effect of arterial pH alterations on metabolic activity of norepinephrine." *Amer. J. Physiol.*, 212:765–72 (1967).

———, and Steinsland, O. S. "Increased rate of catecholamine synthesis during respiratory acidosis." *Resp. Physiol.*, 5:108–17 (1968).

———, Tannieres, M. L., and Lennon, J. F., "Direct measurement of leukocyte motility: Effects of pH and temperature." *Proc. Soc. Exp. Biol. Med.*, 138:350–52 (1971).

———, Zagury, D., Milhaud, A., Manger, W. M., and Pappas, G. D., "Acidemia and catecholamine output of the isolated canine adrenal gland." *Amer. J. Physiol.*, 213:1186–92 (1967).

Pitts, R. F. and Mast, S. O., "Relation between inorganic salt concentration [H+] and physiological process in amoeba Proteus." *J. Cell Comp. Physiol.*, 3:449–62 (1933).

Poyart, C. and Nahas, G. G., "Inhibition of catecholamine-induced calorigenesis and lipolysis by hypercapnic acidosis." *Amer. J. Physiol.*, 211:161–68 (1966).

———, and Nahas, G. G., "Inhibition of activated lipolysis by acidosis." *Molec. Pharmacol.*, 4:389–401 (1968).

Reynolds, R. C. and Haugaard, N., "The effect of variations of pH upon the activation of phosphorylase by epinephrine in perfused contracting heart, liver slices and skeletal muscle." *J. Pharmacol. Exp. Ther.*, 156:417–25 (1967).

Schaefer, K. E., King, C. T. G., Mego, J. L., and Williams, E. E., "Effect of a narcotic level of CO_2 on adrenal cortical activity and carbohydrate metabolism." *Amer. J. Physiol.*, 183:53–62 (1955).

Stadie, W. C., Haugaard, N., and Perlmutter, M., "The synthesis of glycogen by rat heart slices." *J. Biol. Chem.*, 171:419–29 (1947).

Steinberg, D., Nestel, P. J., Buskirk, E. R., and Thompson, R. H., "Calorigenic effect of norepinephrine correlated with plasma free fatty acid turnover and oxidation." *J. Clin. Invest.*, 43:167–76 (1964).

Tenney, S. M., "Sympatho-adrenal stimulation by carbon dioxide and the inhibitory effect of carbonic acid on epinephrine response." *Amer. J. Physiol.*, 187:341–46 (1956).

Triner, L., Kypson, J., Mróz, M., and Zicha, B., "The influence of acidosis on the utilization of glucose by the red blood cells in shock." *Med. Exp. (Basel)*, 10:103–10 (1964).

———, and Nahas, G. G., "Acidosis: effect on lipolytic activity of norepinephrine in isolated fat cells." *Science*, 150:1725–27 (1965).

Trivedi, B. and Danforth, W. H., "Effect of pH on the kinetics of frog muscle phosphofructokinase." *J. Biol. Chem.*, 241:4110–12 (1966).

Nahas Discussion

SIESJÖ: I was very glad to see your results because there have been very few reports of the actual site where acidosis acts on glycolysis, except for Triverdi and Danforth [*J. Biol. Chem.*, 241:4110 (1966)] who showed that phosphofructokinase was inhibited at low pH. I don't think they had any measurements to show that the phosphorylase also was affected. I wonder if you have the equivalent experiment where you have shown an increased flux through the glycolytic pathway during alkalosis; and the second question is, Do you also measure lactate and pyruvate in the tissue during an acidotic state?

NAHAS: To answer your first question, we have some data which indicate that the opposite pattern occurs during alkalosis. This is also true for the flow of substrates.

SIESJÖ: I meant the fructose-1, 1-6-diphosphate concentration. That goes up, then?

NAHAS: Yes, that's right. And, as to your second question, we haven't measured lactate in the tissue.

SCHAEFER: We have found similar results in chronic hypercapnia, confirming your beautiful studies. The activity of phosphofructokinase decreased 55% after a 1-hour exposure of guinea pigs to 15% CO_2 and remains at a lower level (-33%) during prolonged exposure for 7 days. On the other hand, glycolytic inhibition indicated in a decrease in lactate and increase in glucose is limited to a 3-day period until a physiological compensation of the respiratory acidosis is reached. These pH-dependent changes in glycolysis correlate well with the pH-dependent changes in 2-3-diphosphoglycerate.

CHERNIAK: Have you also measured O_2 consumption in alkalosis? Does that go up?

NAHAS: Oh, yes. Oxygen consumption goes up during simple hyperventilation because there is probably an increase in sympaticomimetic activity. It's not a great increase, but it's measurable on the order of 15%. [Nahas and Poyart, *Am. J. Physiol.*, 212:765 (1967)].

FITZGERALD: Would you account for the increases in serum inorganic phosphorus by the interruption of these metabolic pathways?

NAHAS: Well, yes, I would.

FITZGERALD: Well, in that case, did you make or notice any differentiation or do any experiments whereby you differentiated between metabolic and respiratory acidosis? The reason I ask this is because we only monitor serum inorganic phosphorus. I'm very new at this game and I'm not quite sure what to look at. We found a big difference between whether you make the animal acidotic with CO_2 or with equivalent drops due to the infusion of hydrochloric acid and, in fact, there's a 60% increase in serum inorganic phosphates with respiratory acidosis and about 10% with metabolic acidosis. Then in answer to the previous question that was asked, the reverse of that—making the animal metabolically or respiratorily alkalotic—did not reduce the serum inorganic phosphorus very much (only by about 30%), whereas the respiratory acidosis increased the serum inorganic phosphorus by 60%. Have you any information on this, on the difference between the two?

NAHAS: No, we do not measure those factors systematically in animal preparation and certainly not in the *in vitro* studies.

SIESJÖ: I think I may have a good explanation for the increase in the inorganic phosphate concentration. In the brain, and that may also be valid for muscle tissue, if you increase the tissue CO_2 tension you get an intracellular acidosis that shifts the creatinine phosphokinase reaction to the right. This will lead to a decreased phosphocreatine concentration with a stoichiometrical increase in the inorganic phosphate concentration and that may leak out into the plasma and give an increased plasma inorganic phosphate concentration.

NAHAS: But as far as the isolated enzyme itself is concerned, it doesn't matter whether the pH is changed by increasing P_{CO_2} or by increasing an organic acid.

ALBERS: As far as Dr. Fitzgerald's question was concerned, with the metabolic acidosis or respiratory acidosis we did not find any difference in oxygen consumption whether we changed the pH by increasing the P_{CO_2} or by adding ammonium chloride, or with decreasing P_{CO_2} and adding bicarbonate. It had the same effect on the O_2 consumption when the pH of the arterial blood was changed by the same amount.

6. Carbon Dioxide, Respiratory Regulation, and Chronobiology

Michael Smolensky, Franz Halberg,
Alain Reinberg, Maurice Stupfel

*Chronobiology Laboratories, Dept. of Pathology, Medical School,
Minneapolis, Minn. 55455
and
Air Pollution Center, INSERM, 3 Rue Leon,
Bonnat, Paris, XVIe, France*

Chronobiology

Today a section of biology, which may be called chronobiology, is achieving the objective description of biologic time structure—the sum total of nonrandom, and thus predictable, temporal aspects of organismic behavior, including rhythms as well as changes related to growth, development and aging.

It is now recognized that biologic time structure characterizes individuals as well as groups or populations of organisms or their subdivisions: organ-systems, organs, tissues, cells and intracellular elements (including electron-microscopic ultrastructure). While evidence continuing to accumulate reveals that several aspects of biologic rhythms are innate, these rhythms nevertheless are eminently adaptive: They are readily amenable to synchronization, modulation or at least "influencing" by a broad range of environmental frequencies characterizing several social as well as geophysical factors.

Chronobiology has now gathered many facts which have been the subject of annual review articles in *Physiology* (HALBERG [1969]) and *Pharmacology* (REINBERG and HALBERG [1971]). These same reviews present special electronic computer methods developed particularly to analyze rhythms. By these techniques, evidence has been obtained to document the view of regulation for periodicity of most, if not at all, body functions. Such regulation for rhythmicity includes, with respiration in health and in disease rather generally, a variety of CO_2 measures in experimental animals as well as in man.

Studies have been carried out in several laboratories that demonstrated how two kinds of computer-prepared displays of rhythm characteristics on microfilm—serial sections and the cosinor—are capable of quantifying a circadian rhythm in CO_2 emission of grouped rats. Moreover, a gradual rather than abrupt phase-shifting of this rhythm was observed following a sudden inversion of a regimen of 12 hours light alternating with 12 hours darkness, findings that are of interest to students of CO_2 and regulation. (Stupfel *et al.* [1973]).

Why Rhythmometry?

The rhythm characteristics such as acrophase, amplitude and rhythm-adjusted mean represent sensitive endpoints for those concerned with circadian- or about-yearly (circannual) rhythms. In the case of unequidistant time series the fitted mesor i.e., the rhythm-adjusted value is more descriptive of the location of all data than the mean of a sampling period. It is this mesor that may be gauged for monitoring pollution along the 24-hour scale, as previously suggested by us for the city at large (REINBERG et al. [1970]), as well as for closed environments (STUPFEL, HALBERG, and HALBERG [1971]) such as space capsules (STUPFEL et al. [1970]). Under these circumstances and many others, rhythms represent the interaction of environmental factors with intrinsic periodic regulatory mechanisms exhibiting a multitude of frequencies, including the circadian and circannual ones.

Rhythms in Health and Disease

Among rhythms in respiratory function, variations in concentrations of either CO_2 or O_2 in the blood or pulmonary air have been examined for about-24-hour (or circadian), as well as for about-yearly (or circannual) rhythms. Rhythms with both frequencies, as well as about-weekly and other bioperiodicities, have been reported by investigators who often presented their findings in theses or little known journals. In certain cases, experiments originally designed to study aspects of respiratory function other than rhythms resulted in findings useful for documenting the latter. Herein, data from such investigations as well as from others aimed specifically at rhythmometry are summarized to construct circadian maps by the use of specially designed electronic computer procedures—cosine fitting by least squares and cosinor analyses. Findings presented herein can be discussed as they may relate to similar-frequency rhythms in

asthmatic and bronchitic complaints and to the optimal phasing of therapy in such illness. The same data also are pertinent for the monitoring of physiologic responses to air pollutants through the longitudinal self-assessment of biologic changes with time—autorhythmometry (REINBERG et al. [1970]).

Table 1 reveals analyses of a pioneering series collected on himself by A. Baird Hastings (HASTINGS [1940]), now at the University of California at San Diego. Actually, the data relate to the second of two experiments only—i.e. the one that yielded the (statistically significant) results shown. These results are in keeping with those from a first experiment for which a sinusoidal circadian rhythm was not demonstrated; in the first experiment, a 24-hour cosine curve accounted for only 20% of the variability on hand, while in the second (tabulated) experiment on the same subject, the fit of a 24-hour cosine curve accounted for 77% of the overall variability. In any event, the first experiment yielded an acrophase differing by only 24° from that in the second experiment, and an amplitude of 2.9 mm Hg. These results agree well also with those on patients with chronic respiratory insufficiency published 28 years later by Atlan et al. [1968], also shown in Table 1—as far as both the amplitude and the acrophase of CO_2 pressure are concerned and in spite of drastic differences in the overall mesor of CO_2 pressure.

Table 2 shows a more complete analysis

Table 1. CO_2 Pressure (mm Hg) of Arterial Blood in a Healthy Subject and in Subjects with Chronic Respiratory Insufficiency

Source of data (subjects)[†]	Probability value	Mesor M ± SE (mm/Hg)	Amplitude, A ± SE (mm/Hg)	Acrophase, ∅* (0.95 confidence arc)
Hastings (1H)[‡]	<0.01	44.3 ± .5	3.5 ± .8	−360° (−332 to −18)
Atlan et al. (10 CRI)	<0.001	58.0 ± 1.0	3.8 ± .8	−352° (−312 to −29)

* Acrophase given in degrees with $360° \equiv 24$ hours, $15° = 1$ hour. Reference = middle of habitual daily sleep span.

† H = healthy; CRI = chronic respiratory insufficiency.

‡ Second experiment. See text.

of the original data by Atlan et al. [1968]. Rhythms are quantified for a number of variables of interest to respiratory regulations —in human arterial blood from patients with chronic respiratory insufficiency. It indeed should be noted that a marked and statistically highly significant rhythm characterizes these variables; also that there are rather drastic differences in the rhythm's timing, apparent from the last column of acrophases.

Table 3 shows the circadian rhythm in peak expiratory flow in health and in asthmatics. The timing of this rhythm reveals chronopathology in patients with byssinosis, who have an altered acrophase of $-97°$, as compared to acrophases ranging from $-195°$ to $-225°$ in other subjects. There is no overlap between the confidence arc for the circadian peak expiratory flow acrophase of 12 patients with byssinosis, on the one hand, and for 50 patients with asthma or for 27 healthy subjects, on the other hand. Another

Table 2. Circadian Variations in Gases of Arterial Human Blood in Patients with Chronic Respiratory Insufficiency

Variable investigated (unit)	Probability value of rhythm description	Mesor $M \pm SE$ (liters/min)	Amplitude, A (liters/min)	Acrophase, $ø*$ (0.95 confidence arc)
$SaCO_2$ (%)	0.006	84.5 ± 0.8	2.5 (0.8 to 4.1)	$-222°$ (-172 to -257)
CO_2T (vol. %)	<0.001	76.7 ± 0.8	2.0 (1.4 to 2.6)	$-40°$ (-359 to -70)
Pa_{CO_2} (mm Hg)	<0.001	58.0 ± 1.0	3.8 (2.2 to 5.5)	$-37°$ (-357 to -74)
R.A. (meq/l.)	<0.001	32.7 ± 0.4	0.8 (0.5 to 1.1)	$-39°$ (-356 to -70)
pH	0.006	7.4 ± 0.1	0.02 (.01 to 0.03)	$-218°$ (-170 to -267)
Pa_{O_2} (mm Hg)	0.05	53.4 ± 1.2	2.6 (0.01 to 5.1)	$-203°$ (-125 to -298)

Data from: G. Atlan, R. Bydlowski, C. Hatzfeld, and D. Brille, "Étude des variations des gaz du sang arteriel au cours du nyothemère chez les insuffisants respiratoires chroniques. Path.-Biol., 16: 1666 (1968). From Table 2 on page 63.

* ø referred to local midnight. $15° = 1$ hour.

Table 3. Circadian Rhythm in Expiratory Peak Flow

Source of data (subjects)†	Probability value	Mesor $M \pm SE$ (liters/min)	Amplitude, $A \pm SE$ (liters/min)	Acrophase, $ø*$ (0.95 confidence arc)
Günther et al. (9H)	<0.01	528 ± 36	15 ± 3	$-217°$ (-187 to -228)
Smolensky (18H)	<0.01	583 ± 4	10 ± 3	$-202°$ (-180 to -225)
Reindl et al. (11AR)	<0.05	230 ± 67	45 ± 8	$-208°$ (-191 to -227)
(15MA)	<0.05	204 ± 72	42 ± 15	$-195°$ (-172 to -216)
(14SA)	<0.05	144 ± 47	33 ± 11	$-225°$ (-209 to -241)
Zuidema (10A)	<0.05	294 ± 4	25 ± 5	$-217°$ (-188 to -246)
McKerrow (12BY)	<0.01	349 ± 8	23 ± 7	$-97°$ (-359 to -136)

* referred to local midnight. $15° = 1$ hour.

† H = healthy; A = asthmatic; MA = mild asthma; AR = asthma in remission (controlled with bronchodilators without steroids); SA = severe steroid-dependent asthmatic; BY = byssinotic subjects.

aspect of chronopathology is an increase in amplitude of rhythm which is larger in asthmatics than in healthy subjects.

Table 4 suggests again a different acrophase for circadian changes in airway resistance of patients with byssinosis as compared to others.

Table 5 shows that for forced expiratory volume a rhythm cannot be detected in groups of healthy subjects by the cosinor method, yet the acrophases are so similar

that they can hardly be random.

Table 6 shows that in many cases a rhythm indeed is statistically significant for the forced expiratory volume of patients with asthma and respiratory disease. In this table and in others, the lack of a confidence arc next to the acrophase indicates a lack of rhythm description by the method used. For vital capacity, Table 7 (healthy subjects) and Table 8 (hospitalized patients) show that a rhythm is more readily detected in patients

Table 4. Circadian Rhythm in Airway Resistance*

Source of data (subjects)‡	Probability value	Mesor M ± SE (liters/min)	Amplitude, A ± SE* (liters/min)	Acrophase, ø† (.95 confidence arc)
McDermott (H)	< 0.01	0.99 ± .04	0.13 ± 0.02	−29° (−360 to −58)
Sherrer (H)	> 0.05	3.53 ± .03	0.10 ± 0.08	− 40°
[A(1)]§	< 0.05	7.63 ± .45	2.24 + 0.62	−21° (−355 to −47)
[A(2)]§	< 0.01	11.67 ± .54	2.99 ± 0.16	−20° (− 3 to −37)
[A(3)]§	< 0.05	16.31 ± .75	4.08 ± 0.73	−14° (−360 to −27)
[A(4)]§	< 0.05	20.73 ± .94	3.96 ± 1.18	−352° (−338 to − 6)
[A(5)]§	< 0.05	8.26 ± .16	1.35 ± 0.50	−4° (−351 to −16)
[A(6)]§	< 0.05	9.55 ± .87	3.84 + 0.94	−31° (−3 to −59)
Zuidema (A)	< 0.01	8.65 ± .28	1.78 ± 0.19	−13° (−359 to −38)
(A)	< 0.01	9.38 ± .28	1.71 ± 0.26	−16° (−354 to −38)
McKerrow (BY)	> 0.05	6.60 ± .03	.90 ± 0.16	−261°

* Assesment of airway resistance by "esophageal interruption", except for McDermott who utilized whole body plethysmography Units in $cmH_2O/L./Sec.$
† referred to local midnight. 15° = 1 hour.
‡ H = healthy; A = asthmatic; BY = byssinotic subjects.
§ Asthmatics characterized by: (1) no, (2) slight, (3) moderate, and (4) severe dyspnoea at rest; (5) moderate, and (6) chronic airway obstruction.

Table 5. Circadian Rhythm in Forced Expiratory Volume (0.75- or 1.0-second forced volume assessed by spirometry) in Healthy Subjects

Source of data (number of subjects)	Mesor M ± SE (liters/min)	Amplitude, A ± SE (liters/min)	Acrophase, ø* (0.95 confidence arc)
Israels (12)	3836 ± 21	92 ± 48	−246°
Lewinsohn (5)	3224 ± 16	26 ± 13	−220°
Straeten (11)	3434 ± 28	7 ± 5	−219°
Tammeling (10)	3221 ± 65	59 ± 30	−224°
Smolensky (18)	2777 ± 43	46 ± 26	−251°

* ø referred to local midnight. 15° = 1 hour. Point estimate only is given since the fits of a 24-h cosine curve summarized by mean cosinor do not yield statistically significance for any one of the series.

Table 6. Circadian Rhythm in Forced Expiratory Volume (0.75-or 1.0-second forced volume assessed by spirometry) in Patients with Asthma and Other Respiratory Diseases

Source of data (subjects)†	Probability value	Mesor M ± SE (liters/min)	Amplitude, A ± SE (liters/min)	Acrophase, ø* (.95 confidence arc)
DeVries (5B & E)	> 0.05	811 ± 21	27 ± 22	− 240°
DeVries (11A)	< 0.01	1985 ± 88	187 ± 67	− 199° (− 120 to − 216)
Israels (12A)	< 0.01	2052 ± 22	396 ± 76	− 210° (− 180 to − 230)
Lewinsohn (4MA)	> 0.05	1942 ± 70	272 ± 150	− 226° (− 204 to − 248)**
Lewinsohn (12SA)	< 0.01	749 ± 15	66 ± 20	− 236° (− 200 to − 272)
Straeton (12A)	< 0.01	2139 ± 53	33 ± 9	− 221° (− 203 to − 236)
Straeten (11A)	< 0.01	1347 ± 62	19 ± 4	− 211° (− 179 to − 236)
Tammeling (15A&B)	< 0.05	2628 ± 97	242 ± 60	− 220° (− 190 to − 260)
Tammeling (13A*)	> 0.05	1660 ± 48	79 ± 40	− 199°
Zuidema (10A)	< 0.01	2222 ± 11	7 ± 2	− 242° (− 184 to − 300)

* ø referred to local midnight. 15° = 1 hour.
† A = asthmatic; MA = mild asthmatic; SA = severe asthmatic; B = bronchitic; E = emphysemic subjects.
**Confidence arc from single cosinor rather than mean cosinor.

Table 7. Circadian Rhythm in Vital Capacity of Healthy Subjects (assessed by spirometry)

Source of data (number of subjects)	Probability value	Mesor M ± SE (liters/min)	Amplitude, A ± SE (liters/min)	Acrophase, ø* (0.95 confidence arc)
Kroetz (2)	< 0.05	3975 ± 90	224 ± 65	− 187° (− 155 to − 217)
Lewinsohn (5)	> 0.05	4228 ± 15	59 ± 30	− 123°
Hildebrandt (1)	< 0.01	3631 ± 29	206 ± 22	− 207° (− 185 to − 228)
Israels (12)	> 0.05	5032 ± 21	65 ± 33	− 245°
Straeten (11)	> 0.05	4580 ± 10	3 ± 4	− 176°
Tammeling (10)	> 0.05	4521 ± 65	29 ± 15	− 226°
Smolensky (18)	> 0.05	4898 ± 31	9 ± 2	− 242°

* ø referred to local midnight. 15° = 1 hour.

and, as a rule, increases in amplitude with the occurrence of respiratory disease.

Importance of Chronobiology

Even if the many rhythms in health and disease are ignored and only the most extreme situation, "death," is considered—and one's view is further restricted to a population (of healthy experimental animals or human patients rather than to an individual)—one indeed finds rhythms with different periods, or amplitudes, each rhythm sufficiently important to tip the scale between death or

survival in response to identical external conditions or stimuli. The dramatic importance of circadian and circannual rhythms in human populations, accounting for the difference between life or death on a global scale, represents a persuasive reason prompting us to define health positively by the spectrum of those quantifiable rhythms that underlie our periodic changes in resistance to challenge.

In concluding, we may want to point out that in Minnesota as well as in Florida (in a state with cold winters as well as another with relatively mild ones), and on both

Table 8. Circadian Rhythm in Vital Capacity of Hospitalized Subjects (assessed by spirometry)

Source of data (subjects)†	Probability value	Mesor M ± SE (liters/min)	Amplitude, A ± SE (liters/min)	Acrophase, ø* (.95 confidence arc)
Oechsler (7C)	< 0.05	2519 ± 235	164 ± 63	−206° (−152 to −248)
Kroetz (1C)	< .01	2651 ± 56	273 ± 38	−195° (−161 to −228)
Lewinsohn (4MA)	> .05	3599 ± 89	298 ± 188	−237°
Lewinsohn (12SA)	< .01	1794 ± 42	194 ± 44	−234° (−214 to −256)
Oechsler (6A)	< .05	2476 ± 90	493 ± 230	−218° (−131 to −266)
Israels (12A)	< .01	3850 ± 37	307 ± 97	−216° (−176 to −240)
Straeten (12A)	< .01	3830 ± 95	28 ± 20	−232° (−202 to −260)
Straeten (11A)	< .01	3068 ± 97	28 ± 7	−218° (−165 to −241)
Tammeling(15A & B)	< .05	4135 ± 93	169 ± 42	−212° (−166 to −282)
Tammeling(12A & B)	> .05	3484 ± 86	66 ± 82	−244°
Zuidema (10A)	< .01	3919 ± 15	94 ± 16	−229° (−196 to −262)
DeVries (11A)	> .05	3838 ± 71	57 ± 38	−78°
DeVries (5B & E)	> .05	2164 ± 40	42 ± 80	−168°
Sauer (11P)	< .01	2612 ± 116	384 ± 144	−175° (−126 to −211)
Oechsler (10P)	< .01	3784 ± 331	178 ± 38	−216° (−194 to −236)

* ø referred to local midnight. 15° = 1 hour.

† H = healthy; C = cardiac; A = asthmatic; MA = mild asthma; SA = severe asthma; B = bronchitic; E = emphysemic; P = miscellaneous.

hemispheres, respiratory and cardiac mortality show a similar circannual timing. (Smolensky, Halberg and Sargent [1972]). However, we may indeed conclude by saying that such data serve to underline the importance of rhythms. The task now on hand is to replace a negative as well as narrow definition of health (viewed as the absence of detectable illness and based only upon group studies) by rhythm measurement for a *positive quantitative* and *individualized* assessment of health status. Chronobiology deals with time not only because it resolves temporal characteristics of body functions, respiratory and other, but also because rhythmometry should start in time before the onset of disease, and this can be done by rhythm assessment in schools.

Bibliography

Apfelbaum, M., Reinberg, A., Lacatis, D., Abulker, C., Bostsarron, J., and Riou, F., "Rythme circadien de la consommation d'oxygene et du quotient respiratoire de femmes adultes jeunes en alimentation spontanee et après restriction calorique."

Rev. Europ. Etudes Clin. Biol., 16:135–43 (1971).

Atlan, G., Bydlowski, R., Hatzfeld, C., and Brille, D., "Etude des variations des gaz du sang arteriel au cours du nycthemère chez les insuffisants respiratoires chroniques." *Path.-Biol.*, 16:61–66 (1968).

Halberg, F., "Chronobiology." *Ann. Rev. Physiol.*, 31:675–725 (1969).

———, Tong, Y. L., and Johnson, E. A., "Circadian system phase—an aspect of temporal morphology; procedures and illustrative examples." Proc. Int. Cong. of Anatomists. In *The Cellular Aspects of Biorhythms* (New York, 1967), pp. 20–48.

Hastings, A. B., "Diurnal variations in acid base balance." *Proc. Soc. Exp. Bio. Med.*, 43:308 (1940).

Reinberg, A., Gervais, P., Frambourg, J.-C., Halberg, F., Abulker, C., Vignaud, D., and Dupont, J., "Rythmes circadiens de fonctions respiratoires et de la temperature d'asthmatiques sejournant en milieu hypoallergenique." *Presse Med.*, 78:1817–21 (1970).

———, and Halberg, F., "Circadian chronopharmacology." *Ann. Rev. Pharmacol.*, 2: 455–92 (1971).

Smolensky, M., Halberg, F., and Sargent II, F. "Chronobiology of the Life Sequence in advances in Clinatic Physiology, S.Ttoh, K. Ogata and H. Yoshimura, eds. Igaku Shoin, Ltd, Tokyo, 1972. pp. 281–318.

Stupfel, M., Halberg, Francine, and Halberg, F., "Synchronisation par l'alternance lumière-obscurité de l'emission rythmique circadienne de gaz carbonique par un groupe de rats." *C. R. Acad. Sci., Paris*, 272:2001–04 (1971).

———, Nelson, W., Halberg, J., and Halberg, F., "Multiple-purpose monitoring of carbon dioxide in closed organism-environment systems, including biosatellites." *Space Life Sci.*, 2:33–39.

Stupfel, M., Francine Halberg, F. Halberg, E. Halberg and J. K. Lee: (1973). Computer-prepared displays of feeding-time and lighting effects upon circadian rhythms in CO_2 emission by rats. *Intl. J. Chronobiology*, in press.

Halberg Discussion

SEVERINGHAUS: Do you have data on the P_{CO_2} as a function of day time that would be of interest to those of us who are interested in the regulation of respiration?

REINBERG: No, I've no data of this kind.

SEVERINGHAUS: Perhaps others may have some. I only have some data we collected at high altitude some years ago, on five subjects over four days. There was a variation in P_{CO_2} (that is peak-average variation) 2.5 mm of pCO_2 plus or minus 1.2 mm. The lowest pCO_2 being at noon, the highest at midnight.

KELLOG: I can add a few random observations to this same story. We measured the position of the CO_2 response curve some years ago, both at sea level and at altitude, in a small group of subjects, and found that the position during the day and the position between 10 P.M. and midnight was about the same. However, since then we have looked at two different spot times during the day, between 6 and 7 A.M. and about the same time in the P.M., and there is a difference of about 2mm Hg.

Part III

Carbon Dioxide and pH Effect on Oxygen
and Carbon Dioxide Transport

1. Effect of Acid-base Status on Oxygen Transport by Whole Blood

Claude Lenfant

National Heart and Lung Institute
National Institute of Health
Bethesda, Maryland
20014

Despite the frequent appearance of acid-base disturbances in clinical medicine, there seem to be few studies that assess their effect on oxygen transport. Moreover, by virtue of its relative complexity, oxygen transport seems to be a rather vulnerable process.

Indeed, oxygen transport from the environment to the mitochondria is achieved by four linked transport mechanisms: ventilation, pulmonary gas exchange, circulation, and tissue diffusion. Each of these mechanisms includes several components whose integrity is necessary for a continuous flow of oxygen to the tissues. Table 1 lists the four transport mechanisms and their components. Although acid-base changes affect almost all of them, this discussion is exclusively concerned with those components which are part of the circulatory transport mechanism: blood flow, hemoglobin concentration, and the O_2-Hb dissociation curve.

Effect on Cardiac Output

There are very few data reported in the literature on the effect of acid-base changes on cardiac output. Furthermore, all the available data were obtained following rapidly induced pH changes and not in chronic states. There seems to be species differences, and the response to acidosis and alkalosis appears to depend on the method used to induce pH change.

In unanesthetized dogs experiencing a pH change from 7.40 to 7.26 while breathing 6% carbon dioxide, the cardiac output decreases suddenly by about 11%. If carbon dioxide exposure is continued, this decrease persists as long as 30 min (HORWITZ, BISHOP, and STONE [1968]). In man, inhalation of 7% carbon dioxide (pH change from 7.38 to 7.25) causes an increase in cardiac output (RICHARDSON, WASSERMAN, and PATTERSON [1961]) of nearly 20%. Vigorous hyperventilation has a similar effect; i.e. increase in cardiac output (BURNUM, HICKAM, and MCINTOSH [1954]). This increase is related to the change in Pa_{CO_2}, since it does not occur if Pa_{CO_2} is kept constant by carbon dioxide inhalation during hyperventilation.

When acid-base changes are induced by injection of acid or base, the blood flow response is different: Alkalosis is accompanied by a conspicuous increase in cardiac output, but no change occurs with induced acidosis (RICHARDSON, WASSERMAN, and PATTERSON [1961]).

Effect on Hemoglobin Concentration

Although there are no data suggesting a relationship between acid-base status and whole blood hemoglobin concentration, there is some evidence that the mean corpuscular hemoglobin concentration (MCHC) is affected by plasma pH. This was first observed by

Table 1. Oxygen Transport Mechanisms (After RAHN [1966])

Mechanisms	Components
Ventilation	Alveolar ventilation (role of dead space)
Gas to blood exchange	Diffusion
	Ventilation to perfusion ratios distribution
	Anatomical shunt
Circulation	Blood flow
	Hemoglobin concentration
	O_2-Hb dissociation curve
Tissue diffusion	Solubility and diffusion coefficients
	Distance between capillaries

Granbarth et al. [1953]. More recent observations have confirmed these early observations (BELLINGHAM, DETTER, and LENFANT [1971]). A change in MCHC affects oxygen transport in two ways: First, when MCHC increases, as in alkalosis, a given volume of red cells will carry more oxygen, than if MCHC were lower. With acidosis, the opposite effect is observed. Second, and much more significant, is the interaction between hemoglobin concentration and hemoglobin affinity for oxygen. This interaction, which results in a decrease in affinity with increasing hemoglobin concentration, has been observed in hemoglobin solution (RADFORD et al. [1967]), and also has been found to be enhanced with increasing 2,3-diphosphoglycerate (DPG) concentration (FORSTER [1972]). Similar observations have been made in whole blood and *in vivo* (BELLINGHAM, DETTER, and LENFANT [1970, 1971]). These latter observations demonstrated that this effect is independent of, and in fact additive to, the effects of pH on the O_2-Hb dissociation curve that are described in the next section. However, some very recent work by Wranne et al. [1972] did not confirm Bellingham et al.'s findings; hence, there is still considerable uncertainty as to whether or not acid-base changes modify the transport of O_2 through an effect on the hemoglobin concentration.

Effect on the O_2-Hb Dissociation Curve

The oxygen transport parameter which is most unquestionably affected by acid-base

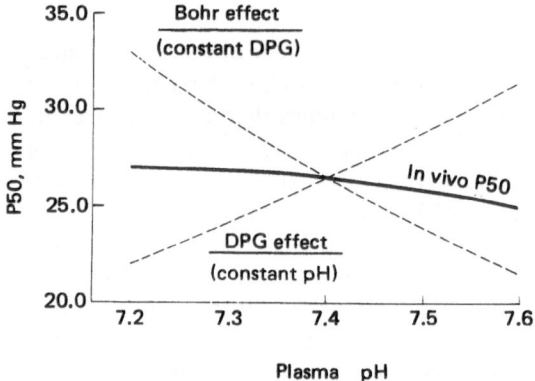

Fig. 1. Effect of chronic pH change on the affinity of hemoglobin for O_2 (as shown by P50) shows (1) the Bohr effect, (2) the DPG effect, and (3) the combined Bohr and DPG effects.

changes is the O_2-Hb dissociation curve. The effect of pH on the curve may be direct or indirect. With acute pH change, only the direct effect plays a role, whereas in chronic acid-base disturbance the overall change results from both direct and indirect effects.

Direct Effect: Bohr Effect

The Bohr effect (Figure 1) (BOHR, HASSELBALCH, and KROGH [1904]) is well known. It has always been considered an important physiological phenomenon at rest as well as during exercise since it facilitates the delivery of oxygen into the tissues. Some recent observations have shown that the magnitude of the Bohr effect (expressed as $\Delta \log P50/\Delta pH$) is related to the DPG concentration (WRANNE, WOODSON, and DETTER [1972]) and also to the hemoglobin oxygen saturation (GARBY and ZAAR [1972]).

Indirect Effect: DPG Effect

The pH plays a major role on the O_2-Hb dissociation curve through its effect on the DPG concentration: increase in pH stimulates DPG production, but when pH decreases, DPG diminishes. The DPG effect was first shown by Benesch and Benesch [1967] and Chanutin and Curnish [1967], who demonstrated that an increase in DPG causes a decrease in hemoglobin affinity for oxygen (or an increase in P50, i.e. partial pressure of oxygen corresponding to 50% saturation of blood with oxygen.) (Figure 2). Since pH effects are acting in opposite directions, two questions arise, as discussed below.

First, what is the time course of the DPG pH-induced changes? Bellingham et al. [1971] showed that the DPG change subsequent to a sudden alteration in pH was delayed by about three hours (upper rows in Figure 3). It is important to note that these observations were made at only one magnitude of pH change; hence, further studies are necessary to establish whether the time course of the DPG change is related to the magnitude of the pH change.

The second question is whether, in chronic acid-base disturbance, the pH effect is fully compensated for by the DPG effect. To answer this question, one must consider the two ways P50 can be expressed. As shown in Figure 2, the DPG effect is usually related to P50 at a standard pH of 7.4. But of course it is more important to determine the position of the curve at the *in vivo* pH. The two lower rows in Figure 3 show the change in P50 at standard pH and at *in vivo* pH. It can be seen that in the latter condition, the compensation of the DPG effect seems to be almost complete. Figure 1 illustrates more precisely the respective and combined effects of pH and DPG, showing that the direct pH effect on P50 at *in vivo* pH is slightly predominant in acidosis as in alkalosis. It must further be

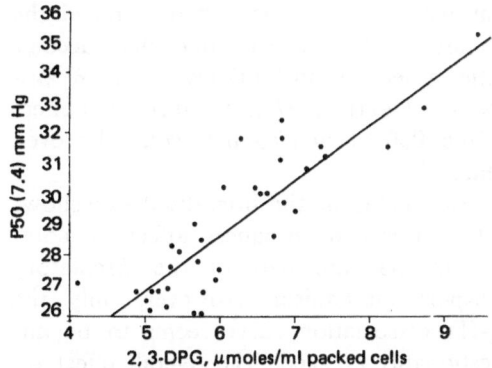

Fig. 2. Effect of DPG change on P50 at standard pH (7.4).

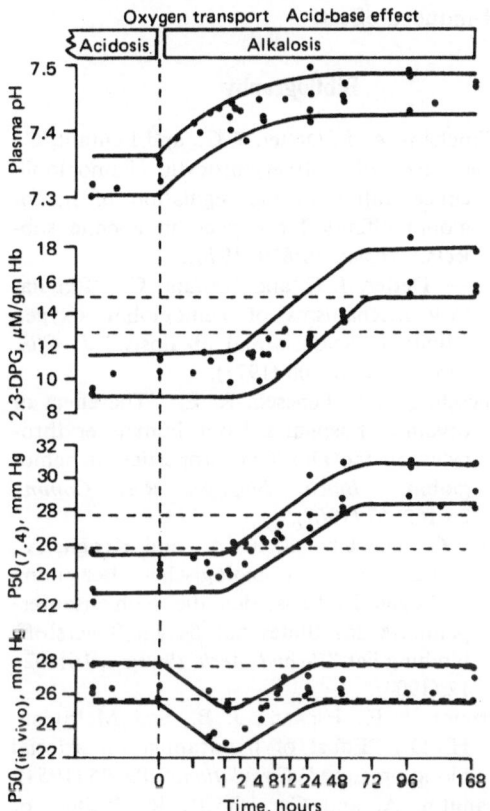

Fig. 3. Effect of induced pH changes on red-cell 2, 3-DPG, P50 at standard pH (7.4) and P50 at *in vivo* pH.

pointed out that the Bohr effect shown in this figure is an underestimate, since a constant value was used irrespective of the pH and, thus, of the DPG concentration. If, on the contrary, the calculations had included the increase in Bohr effect value that accompanies a decrease in DPG (WRANNE, WOODSON, and DETTER [1972]), the direct pH effect on the P50 at *in vivo* pH would be even greater.

In conclusion, this brief discussion shows that acid-base disturbances affect all components that are part of the circulatory transport mechanism. However, only the O_2-Hb dissociation curve seems to be unquestionably affected. The overall effect on the *in vivo* O_2-Hb dissociation curve is such that the direct pH effect by the DPG seems to be nearly completely compensated for by pH-induced effect.

Bibliography

Bellingham, A. J., Detter, J. C., and Lenfant, C., "The role of intraerythrocytic hemoglobin concentration in the regulation of hemoglobin affinity for oxygen in anemic subjects." *Blood*, 36:850 (1970).

———, Detter, J. C. and Lenfant, C., "Regulatory mechanisms of hemoglobin oxygen affinity in acidosis and alkalosis." *J. Clin. Invest.*, 50:700–06 (1971).

Benesch, R. and Benesch, R. E., "The effect of organic phosphates from human erythrocytes on the allostenic properties of hemoglobin." *Bioch. Biophys. Res. Comm.*, 26:162–67 (1967).

Bohr, C., Hasselbalch, K. A., and Krogh, A., "Uber einen in biologischer Beziehung wichtigen Einfleiss, den die Kohlensaurespannung des Blutes auf dessen Sauerstoffbindung hat." *Scand. Arch. Physiol.*, 16:402–12 (1904).

Burnum, J. F., Hickam, J. B., and McIntosh, H. D., "Effect of hypocapnia on arterial blood pressure." *Circulation*, 9:89–95 (1954).

Chanutin, A. and Curnish, R. R., "Effect of organic and inorganic phosphatoses on the oxygen equilibrium of human erythrocyte." *Arch. Biochem. Biophys.*, 121:96–102 (1967).

Forster, R. E., "The effect of dilution of saline on the oxygen affinity of hemoglobin. In P. Astrup and M. Rorth, eds., *Fourth Alfred Benzon Symposium: O_2 affinity of hemoglobin and red cell acid base status* (Copenhagen, 1972), pp. 162–65.

Garby, L., Robert, M., and Zaar, B., "Proton and carbamino-linked oxygen affinity of normal human blood." *Acta. Physiol. Scand.* (in press, 1972).

Granbarth, H., Mackler, B., and Guest, G. M., "Effect of acidosis on utilization of glucose in erythrocytes and leucocytes." *Amer. J. Physiol.*, 172:301–08 (1953).

Horwitz, L. D., Bishop, V. S., and Stone, H. L., "Effect of hypercapnia on the cardiovascular system of conscious dogs." *J. Appl. Physiol.*, 25:346–48 (1968).

Radford, E. P., Torrelli, G., Celentano, F., and d'Angelo, E., "Concentration dependence of O_2-hemoglobin equilibrium." *Fed. Proc.*, 26:333 (1967).

Rahn, H., "Conductance of O_2 from the environment to the tissues at high altitude." In L. E. Farhi and H. Rahn, eds., *Studies in pulmonary physiology: mechanics, chemistry and circulation of the lung.* Vol. II. AMRL–TDR–63–103(2):34–41.

Richardson, D. W., Wasserman, A. J., and Patterson, J. L., "General and regional circulatory responses to change in blood pH and carbon dioxide tension." *J. Clin. Invest.*, 40:31–43 (1961).

Wranne, B., Woodson, R. D., and Detter, J. C., "The Bohr effect: interaction between H^+, CO_2 and 2, 3 DPG in fresh and stored blood." *J. Appl. Physiol.*, 32 (in press, 1972).

Lenfant Discussion

RAHN: Thank you very much, Dr. Lenfant, for this beautiful picture that you have given us. I think that for the first time I'm beginning to understand the various relationships, and I'd like to open this up for discussion.

FENCL: May I ask you a question? Have you any data on the effect of these combined shifts produced by pH and DPG on patients with severe acidosis, such as patients undergoing chronic dialysis in chronic uremia?

LENFANT: Well, we did not study patients undergoing dialysis, but we looked at patients who were in diabetic keto-acidosis. If these patients stay in severe acidosis for a long time they deplete their DPG. In this case you can observe a tremendous shift to the left of their curve corrected to pH = 7.40. But at the same time the Bohr effect comes into play and brings the *in vivo* curve back to normal. The point that I think is very important is that although we are talking of severe acidosis with tremendous DPG depletion, the circulating blood remains normal because these two effects compensate each other in chronic conditions. I believe it could be very dangerous to correct acidosis rapidly because we would have that shift of the *in vivo* curve that you saw in Figure 3.

ENSON: I was intrigued with the observation of an increase in cardiac output with induced metabolic alkalosis. I wonder, what stimulus was used to produce the alkalosis?

LENFANT: Bicarbonate.

ENSON: Well, that is probably an unspecific effect of the hypertonic solution that was used. If isosmotic solutions are used, the effect is quite the opposite, actually, as I'll indicate subsequently. Severe acidosis, at a given blood volume, causes a redistribution of the blood volume to the central circulation and then increases the output that way.

LENFANT: Yes, I would accept that indeed. I think you may have a point there.

BECK: May I return once more to DPG? If you induce acidosis or alkalosis and change the concentration of DPG *in vivo*, and now withdraw a sample to determine pH and so on, will the DPG concentration stay as it was *in vivo* or will it, *in vitro*, return to its normal level? That is, is there enough substrate in the red cell to continue in DPG metabolism?

LENFANT: No. If you store blood, DPG is going to keep on going down.

RYBACK: I would like to know whether you have any explanation of the effect of the organic phosphates at the molecular level?

LENFANT: Well, I am really on thin ice here because this is out of my field. Let me tell you what my biochemist friends have told me, and what I understand from what they said. I understand that there is a dual effect of DPG—one which is due to binding of DPG on the hemoglobin molecule (especially when the hemoglobin molecule is in the deoxy form), but also DPG is an acid and, like all acids, it is ionized; hence, there is an increase in H^+ inside the red cells. Thus, there is a shift of the curve by virtue of the Bohr effect but *inside* the red cells. We don't see a pH change in the plasma. What I am saying is that there is an increase in the hydrogen concentration gradient between plasma and red cells.

RYBACK: Is that not the explanation given by Perutz in a recent paper in *Nature* in '70?

LENFANT: I believe that in this paper he was primarily discussing binding.

RYBACK: He spoke also about the Bohr effect and the organic phosphate, looking at the heme-heme interaction. He gives the explanation you summarized just now.

LENFANT: Maybe, I am not really familiar with that paper.

CRAIG: Is there any evidence, or what *is* the evidence, that this is a pH effect on DPG and not on CO_2?

LENFANT: The evidence is pretty good. You can change pH at constant CO_2 and you will observe what pH does. It plays a role on the glycolytic pathway at the level preceding the appearance of DPG; it acts on some of the enzymes there.

SCHAEFER: One short remark: We have similar results *in vivo* with animals, guinea pigs, exposed to 15% for seven days, and we found the DPG decrease beginning within one hour but reaching the maximum fall at 24 hours. Simultaneously the Bohr effect is increased, compensating for the DPG depletion. But it takes some time to get the full decrease in DPG, although the maximum inhibition of glycolysis is reached within one hour.

2. The Influence of pH and Oxygen on the Erythrocyte Content of 2,3-Diphosphoglycerate

Peter R. B. Caldwell, Ernst R. Jaffé, and Ronald L. Nagel

Departments of Medicine,
College of Physicians and Surgeons,
Columbia University,
630 West 168th Street,
New York, New York 10032,
and
Albert Einstein College of Medicine,
of Yeshiva University,
1300 Morris Park Ave.,
New York, New York

In 1917 Hasselbalch first demonstrated a displacement of the oxygen dissociation curve in the blood of patients with disease (HASSELBALCH [1917]), thus challenging the concept that the oxygen equilibrium of blood was constant for any given conditions of temperature and pH. Ten years later Richards and Strauss showed a rightward shift of the oxygen dissociation curve in patients with anemia (RICHARDS and STRAUSS [1927]), but could not identify the cause for the abnormality. During the next decade, studies at altitude by Dill and coworkers (DILL et al. [1931]) and Keys, Hall, and Guzman [1936] showed the same abnormality in acclimatized normal man, suggesting that the alteration might be an adaptive mechanism related to oxygen transport by the blood. In 1938 Keys and Snell demonstrated the displacement in patients with liver disease and proposed that there might be a reduction in the affinity of hemoglobin for oxygen to account for it (KEYS and SNELL [1938]). In 1943 McCarthy observed that fetal hemoglobin had a lower affinity for oxygen than adult hemoglobin when studied in dilute solution, while fetal blood showed a higher affinity than maternal blood (McCARTHY [1943]). He postulated that some erythrocytic factor might be responsible for the difference in behavior between adult and fetal blood. The observations of Valtis and Kennedy [1954], who showed a shift in the oxygen dissociation curve of stored blood which was corrected *in vivo* after transfusion, strengthened the view that unknown physiologic factors influenced the oxygen equilibrium of blood. Finally, the demonstration, *in vivo*, of a displacement of the oxygen dissociation curve in patients with anemia (RODMAN, CLOSE, and PURCELL [1960]) or liver disease (CALDWELL, FRITTS, and COURNAND [1965]) confirmed the validity of the earlier studies done *in vitro*. Yet the agent or mechanism responsible for the apparent change in oxygen affinity of the blood remained unknown. In this regard, Gomez modified the association coefficients of Adair's formulation for the oxygen equilibrium of hemoglobin and demonstrated that the new equation fit the oxygen dissociation curves for both whole blood and dilute hemoglobin solutions (GOMEZ [1961]). He postulated that some intracellular factor, as yet unidentified, influenced the affinity of hemoglobin for oxygen. Further, since his modification entailed using different values of the association constants for different oxygen tensions, he predicted that the mechanism would be influenced by the level of oxygen saturation.

Following the discovery of the effect of 2,3-diphosphoglycerate (2,3-DPG) (BENESCH and BENESCH [1967]; CHANUTIN and CURNISH [1967]) on the oxygen affinity of hemoglobin, it was shown that the erythrocyte content of this glycolytic intermediate correlated well with the oxygen equilibrium of blood from patients with anemia (TORRANCE et al.) or liver disease (THOMAS, CALDWELL, and FRITTS [in preparation]) and in persons acclimatized at high altitudes (LENFANT, et al. [1968]). In addition, the studies of Tyuma and Shimizu indicated that the aforementioned anomalous behavior of fetal blood might be explained by a difference in the response of fetal hemoglobin to 2,3-DPG, compared to that of adult hemoglobin (TYUMA and SHIMIZU [1969]).

Attention has shifted recently to a consideration of the factors which influence the level of 2,3-DPG in the erythrocyte. Benesch, Benesch and Yu [1968] demonstrated that 2,3-DPG binds to completely deoxygenated but not to fully oxygenated hemoglobin. This differential binding was presumed to be related to the difference in oxygen affinity of these two forms of hemoglobin. It was further suggested that the differential binding might play a role in controlling the erythrocyte content of 2,3-DPG, since its binding would reduce the inhibition of diphosphoglycerate mutase by free 2,3-DPG (ROSE [1970]). Since blood *in vivo* exists at levels of oxygen tension intermediate to those studied previously, we investigated 2,3-DPG binding to hemoglobin at physiologic levels of oxygen saturation. In addition, we measured the change in erythrocyte content of 2,3-DPG during incubation over the full range of oxygen saturation. In both experiments, we used a tonometer system in which gas tension could be controlled precisely.

Dilute hemoglobin solutions (1×10^{-4}M)

were freshly prepared, stripped of 2,3-DPG (CALDWELL, NAGEL, and JAFFE [1971]), and buffered in 0.05 M bis Tris, 0.1 M NaCl at the desired pH. Aliquots were put into dialysis sacs which were then placed in the same buffer solution inside a tonometer flask pre-equilibrated at the desired gas tension. 2,3-DPG-U-^{14}C (0.3 μCi/μmole) was added to the buffer outside the dialysis sac. Incubation at 20°C was then continued until equilibration, as measured by distribution of radioactivity, was complete and measurements were made.

The effect of pH on the binding of 2,3-DPG to both oxy- and deoxyhemoglobin is shown in Figure 1. Binding is linearly related to pH within the physiologic range. There is measurable, though minimal, binding to oxyhemoglobin.

Under fixed conditions of pH (7.2), there is a linear relationship between binding and oxygen saturation as shown in Figure 2.

In the second set of experiments, freshly drawn blood was separated by centrifugation. The denser older erythrocytes were discarded and the lighter younger cells were resuspended in glucose-enriched plasma to a packed cell volume of 20%. An aliquot was analyzed for 2,3-DPG content and incubation was begun at 37°C with the desired oxygen tension and a carbon dioxide tension of 40 mm Hg. After 4 hours of incubation 2,3-DPG was measured again. The change in erythrocyte content during the incubation period is plotted against the mean oxygen saturation for the 4-hour period in Figure 3. Each point represents an average of five or more experiments using blood from five different individuals. The change in erythrocyte content of 2,3-DPG is linearly related to oxygen saturation. While the relation appears to be clear-cut, its interpretation is less certain because of the change in pH which occurs with a change in oxygen saturation (Bohr effect). Figure 4 shows the time course of pH change for one blood sample incubated at three different oxygen tensions. The alkalosis associated with deoxygenation favors glycolysis, thereby increasing the erythrocyte content of 2,3-DPG,

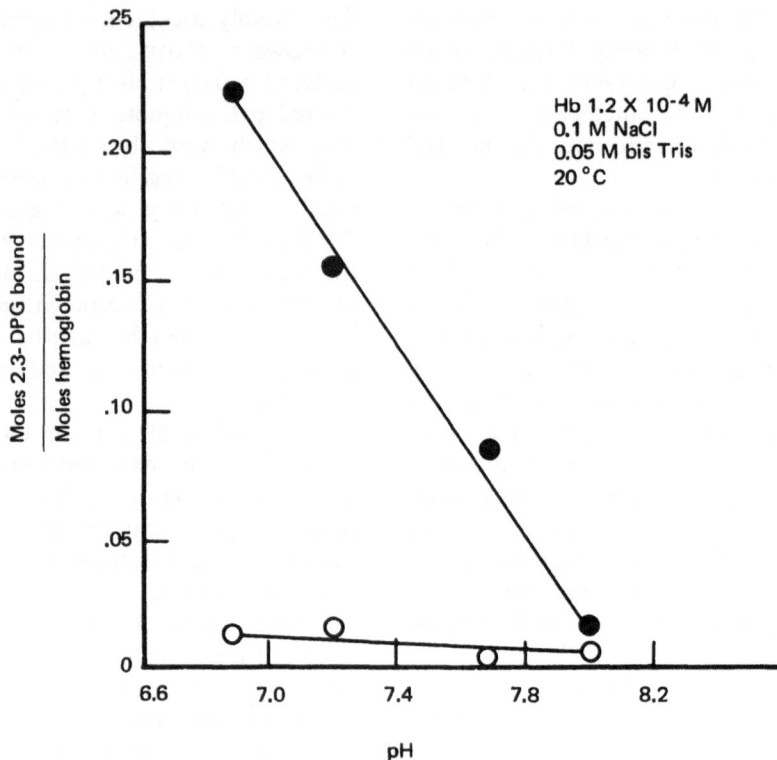

Fig. 1. The effect of pH on 2,3–DPG binding to deoxy—(0) and oxy—(0) hemoglobin. Hb $1.2 \times 10^{-4}M$, 0.1M NaCl, 0.05M bis Tris, 20°C.

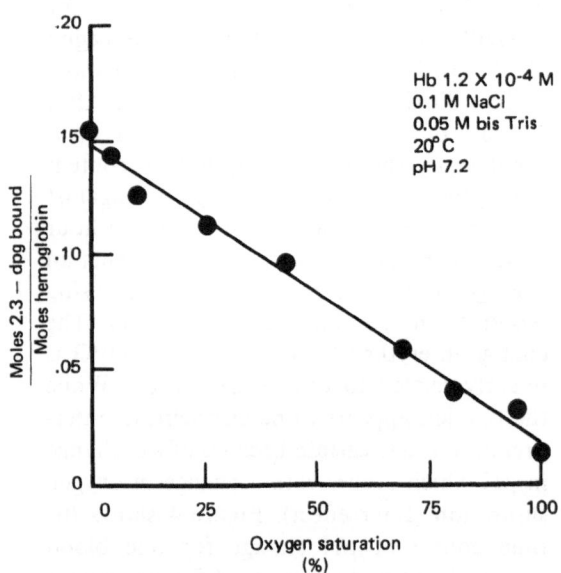

Fig. 2. The binding of 2,3–DPG to hemoglobin versus oxygen saturation. Hb $1.2 \times 10^{-4}M$, 0.1M Na Cl, 0.05M bis Tris, pH 7.2, 20°C.

while acidosis does the opposite (MINAKAMI and YOSHIKAWA [1966]; ASAKURA et al. [1966]). Hence, the relation of 2,3-DPG content and oxygen saturation depicted in Figure 3 must be determined, at least in part, by a change in pH. Efforts to buffer the change in pH attendant to change in oxygen saturation have not been successful, owing to the high erythrocytic content of hemoglobin ($4-5 \times 10^{-3}$ M).

ADDENDUM: Part of this work has appeared in Biochemical, Biophysical Research Communications 44:1504, 1971, where preliminary observations on the binding site of hemoglobin for 2,3-DPG are presented.

Acknowledgment   This work was supported by USPHS Grants HE-02001, HE-05741, HE-05443, AM-13430, AM-13698, AM-5435, AM-15053, and a grant-in-aid

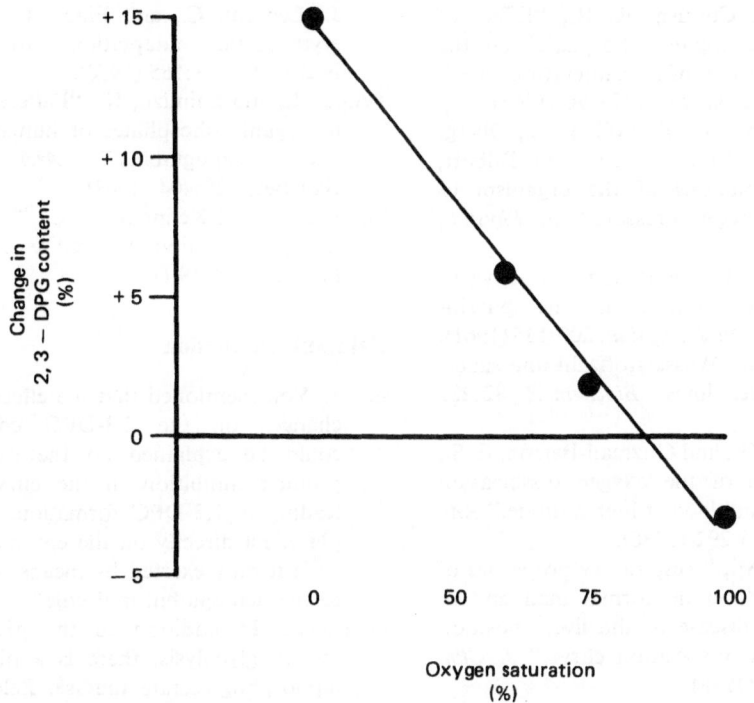

Fig. 3. The change in erythrocyte content of 2,3–DPG versus mean oxygen saturation. Packed cell volume 20%, glucose enriched plasma, P_{CO_2} 40 mm Hg, 37°C.

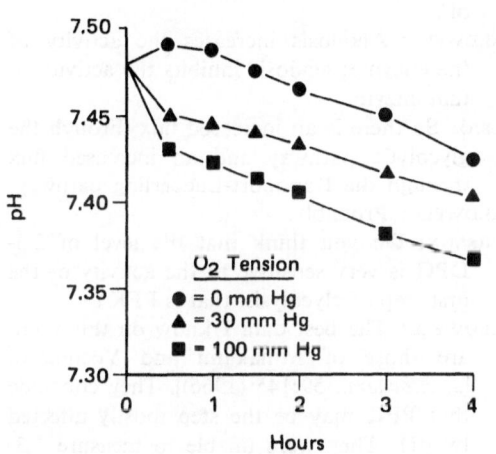

Fig. 4. The time course of pH change in blood during the 4-hour incubation.

from the New York Heart Association. The authors are career scientists of the Health Research Council of the City of New York.

Bibliography

Asakura, T., Sato, Y., Minakami, S., and Yoshikawa, H., "pH dependency of 2,3-diphosphoglycerate content in red blood cells." *Clin. Chim. Acta*, 14:840 (1966).

Benesch, R. and Benesch, R. E., "The effect of organic phosphates from the human erythrocyte on the allosteric properties of hemoglobin." *Biochem. Biophys. Res. Comm.*, 26:162 (1967).

———, and Yu, C. I., "Reciprocal binding of oxygen and diphosphoglycerate by human hemoglobin." *Proc. Nat. Acad. Sci.*, 59:526 (1968).

Caldwell, P. R. B., Fritts, H. W. Jr., and Cournand, A., "Oxyhemoglobin dissociation curve in liver disease." *J. Appl. Physiol.*, 20:316 (1965).

———, Nagel, R. L., and Jaffe, E. R., "The effect of oxygen, carbon dioxide, pH and cyanate on the binding of 2,3-diphosphoglycerate to human hemoglobin." *Biochem. Biophys. Res. Comm.*, 44:1504 (1971).

Chanutin, A. and Curnish, R. R., "Effect of organic and inorganic phosphates on the oxygen equilibrium of human erythrocytes." *Arch. Biochem. Biophys.*, 121:96 (1967).

Dill, D. B., Edwards, H. T., Folling, A., Oberg, S. A., Pappenhiemer, A. M., and Talbott, J. H., "Adaptations of the organism to changes in oxygen pressure." *J. Physiol.*, 71:47 (1931).

Gomez, D. M., "Considerations of oxygen-hemoglobin equilibrium in the physiological state." *Am. J. Physiol.*, 200:135 (1961).

Hasselbalch, K. A., "Wasserstoffzahl und sauerstoffbindung des elutes." *Biochem. Z.*, 82:282 (1917).

Keys, A., Hall, F. G., and Guzman-Barron, E. S., "The position of the oxygen dissociation curve of human blood at high altitude." *Am. J. Physiol.*, 115:292 (1936).

———, Snell, A. M., "Respiratory properties of the arterial blood in normal man and in patients with disease of the liver: position of the oxygen dissociation curve." *J. Clin. Invest.*, 17:59 (1938).

Lenfant, C., Torrance, J., English, E., Finch, C. A., Reynafarje, C., Ramos, J., and Faura, J., "Effect of altitude on oxygen binding by hemoglobin and on organic phosphate levels." *J. Clin. Invest.*, 47:2652 (1968).

McCarthy, E. F., "The oxygen affinity of human maternal and foetal hemoglobin." *J. Physiol.*, 102:55 (1943).

Minakami, S. and Yoshikawa, H., "Studies on erythrocyte glycolysis. III. The effects of active cation transport, pH and inorganic phosphate concentration on erythrocyte glycolysis." *J. Biochem.*, 59:145 (1966).

Richards D. W. Jr. and Strauss, M. L., "Oxyhemoglobin dissociation curves of whole blood in anemia." *J. Clin. Invest.*, 4:105 (1927).

Rodman, T., Close, H. P., and Purcell, M. K., "The oxyhemoglobin dissociation curve in anemia." *Ann. Int. Med.*, 52:295 (1960).

Rose, Z. B., "Enzymes controlling 2,3-diphosphoglycerate in human erythrocytes." *Fed. Proceed.*, 29:1105 (1970).

Thomas, H. M. III, Caldwell, P. R. B., and Fritts, H. W. Jr., "Blood oxygen affinity and acid-base state in patients with liver disease and in normals." (In preparation.)

Torrance, J., Jacobs, P., Restrepo, A., Eschbach, J., Lenfant, C., and Finch, C. A., "Intra-erythrocytic adaptation to anemia." *N.E.J.M.*, 283:165 (1970).

Tyuma, I., and Shimizu, K., "Different response to organic phosphates of human fetal and adult hemoglobins." *Arch. Biochem. Biophys.*, 129:404 (1969).

Valtis, D. J. and Kennedy, A. C., "Defective gas transport function of stored red blood cells." *Lancet*, 266:119 (1954).

Caldwell Discussion

SIESJÖ: You mentioned that the effect of the pH changes on the 2,3-DPG concentration could be explained on the basis of end product inhibition in the enzymatic step leading to 2,3-DPG formation. Is there no pH effect directly on the enzymatic activity or is it only exerted by means of a binding to the hemoglobin molecule?

CALDWELL: In addition to the pH effect on overall glycolysis, there is a pH effect on diphosphoglycerate mutase. Zelda Rose of the Cancer Research Institute in Philadelphia has unpublished data showing that the enzyme is sensitive to pH change in the physiologic range between 7.0 and 8.0.

SIESJÖ: In what direction is the change you speak of?

CALDWELL: Alkalosis increases the activity of the enzyme; acidosis inhibits the activity of that enzyme.

SIESJÖ: So there is an increased flux through the glycolytic pathway and an increased flux through the Rapoport-Lueberling pathway.

CALDWELL: Probably.

BURSAUX: Do you think that the level of 2,3-DPG is very sensitive to the activity of the first step of glycolysis, that is PFK?

CALDWELL: The best data I know on this point are those of Minakami and Yoshikawa [*J. Biochem.*, 59:145 (1966)]. They conclude that PFK may be the step mostly affected by pH. They were unable to measure 1,3-DPG, so they do not comment on the separate effect of pH on 2,3-DPG mutase.

LUFT: Now I'm not quite clear; what is the definition of deoxyhemoglobin? Is it synonymous with what we used to call reduced hemoglobin or does it refer to any hemoglobin that is deoxygenated? And the point I am coming to is this: How do other hemoglobin combinations affect this relationship, for instance carboxyhemoglobin, methemoglobin, and possible others?

CALDWELL: In our experience, when the hemes are liganded, whether by oxygen or water, there is very little binding of 2,3-DPG. The mechanism of interference with binding by carbon dioxide is perhaps different, since carbon dioxide binds the N terminal amino groups [*BBRC*, 44:1504 (1971)].

SEVERINGHAUS: You showed that 4 hours of incubation caused an incremental change in erythrocyte 2,3-DPG content, depending on the saturation of the blood during incubation. Could you tell us how much the oxygen dissociation curve (P50) would shift after 4 hours at each of the two ends of that curve?

CALDWELL: We didn't measure the p_{50} in these studies. Perhaps Dr. Lenfant could answer the question.

LENFANT: In whole blood, as I recall, for one micromole increase of 2,3-DPG per gram of hemoglobin, there's a 0.6 mm Hg shift.

———: Have you any information on the effect of hemoglobin concentration on the binding activity?

CALDWELL: Preliminary studies indicate that there is no effect over a range of 0.5 to 12 g% of hemoglobin concentration.

SIESJÖ: The Swedish group has shown a very definite effect of hemoglobin concentration.

CALDWELL: These studies are done with freshly prepared hemolysates. If you let the hemolysate age in the refrigerator for ten days, the binding is reduced by 50%. If you agitate the hemoglobin and produce met-hemoglobin, you can reduce the binding markedly, so I think we would have to be certain about the conditions of those studies.

3. Carbon Dioxide Transport

John W. Severinghaus

University of California Medical Center
551 Parnassus Avenue
San Francisco, California 94122

We learned yesterday of the healthy sexual effect of CO_2 on the hydra, converting the creature from homosexuality, or reproduction by sporting, into heterosexuality. Perhaps the CO_2 effect was put in its true perspective best by Piet Hein in his book called *Hint and Suggestion*: "The human spirit sublimates the impulses it thwarts. A healthy sex life mitigates the lust for other sports." I suppose that's a CO_2 transport of delight.

CO_2 transport is an enormous subject, fortunately come of age—that is, well covered in texts. For the connoisseur, Roughton is the scripture in the *Handbook of Physiology*, Respiration, Volume 1. A brief chapter that is useful for students and almost up-to-date appears in John Nunn's textbook, *Applied Respiratory Physiology* (Butterworth, 1969).

Two aspects of CO_2 physiology which are not adequately covered in texts, and in which I have some personal experience, are to be my subject this morning. They are CO_2 narcosis and cerebral carbonic anhydrase. First to CO_2 narcosis.

While most of the physiologic biochemical effects of CO_2 are now recognized as mediated by hydrogen ions (somewhere, often beyond an ion impermeable cell wall such as the blood brain barrier) CO_2 narcosis has been a reasonably viable candidate for a direct or non-H^+ effect. Drs. Eisele, Eger and Muallem have rather effectively demolished

even this possibility. They showed that during metabolic acidosis and alkalosis, the narcotic potency of CO_2 correlated well with CSF pH but poorly with P_{CO_2} (EISELE, EGER, and MUALLEM [1967]). Before I describe their experiments, their antecedents deserve mention.

In the mid-nineteenth century, Henry Hill Hickman discovered and used the anesthetic effect of CO_2, primarily in animals. In 1927 Ralph Waters, the father of modern anesthesia, anesthetized two women with 30% CO_2 for minor surgery. Since they both convulsed after awakening, he didn't pursue it. About 10 years ago McAleavy and his colleagues, of which I was one, devised a way of titrating CO_2 against N_2O in volunteers in order to determine the anesthetic potency of CO_2. Since this titrating technique led to Eisele's approach, I would like to describe it. McAleavy determined the alveolar N_2O concentration at which consciousness was lost in volunteers (MCALEAVY et al. [1961]). He found he could obtain a reasonably reproducible end point if the subject was forced to perform a coordinated task as N_2O was slowly increased or, if necessary, decreased to the point where the coordination failed to an arbitrary degree. Arbitrariness, it turned out, was unnecessary since the point coincided with loss of consciousness, which was virtually like falling asleep, an all-or-nothing quantum jump.

McAleavy then varied P_{CO_2} in the

subjects, waiting for a steady state at P_{CO_2} of 25, 40 and 55 torr, before adding N_2O. N_2O was then added slowly until the loss of coordination end point. As illustrated in Figure 1, the effective concentration of N_2O was found to be higher at low P_{CO_2} and lower at high P_{CO_2}. When both P_{N_2O} and P_{CO_2} are given in mm Hg, the slope of the regression line of the data was -5. An increase of P_{CO_2} of 10 mm Hg permitted the anesthesia end point to be attained with 50 mm Hg less N_2O pressure.

That would mean CO_2 has five times the anesthetic potency of N_2O. Eger and his associates have shown that any two inhalation anesthetic agents are additive when used together. That is, when the concentration of each is expressed as a fraction of its MAC (the minimum alveolar concentration producing a nonresponsive anesthetic state), the fractions for two agents used together add up to 1.0 when just enough is used to produce this anesthetic state. This additive concept is a critical precursor to Eisele's experiments with CO_2 in dogs. He reasoned that he could differentiate between CO_2 and H^+ as the

anesthetic agent by using a similar method—withdrawing some volatile anesthetic as CO_2 was added and plotting P_{CO_2} against the anesthetic pressure, each point being a steady-state point at which the total effect of the CO_2 and anesthetic just sufficed to keep the dog from moving in response to a standardized pain stimulus. At each point, after 30 min he sampled CSF pH and P_{CO_2} as well as blood pH and P_{CO_2}. In the same dogs on different days he induced metabolic acidosis and alkalosis long enough to raise or lower CSF HCO_3 by 5–10 meq/l. He then could plot halothane requirement either as a function of P_{CO_2} or CSF-pH, as illustrated in Figure 2. The results suggested that the halothane requirement fell to zero, that is CO_2 became sufficiently anesthetic of itself (as H^+) when CSF pH fell to about 6.8. The P_{CO_2} at this end point was lower when brain HCO_3^- was lowered (central acidosis), indicating that H^+ of ECF rather than P_{CO_2} was the effective anesthetic.

I now turn to the cerebral carbonic anhydrase story. The role of the enzyme in brain has recently been clarified. If metabolism yields CO_2 gas as its direct end product, rather than H^+ and HCO_3 (or carbonic acid), then this gas only need to diffuse into the passing blood to be carried away.

Maren and his colleagues had published experiments that suggested to them that metabolism did indeed yield CO_2 rather than H_2CO_3. However, two discordant experiments left room for doubt. Siesjö showed that total brain extractable CO_2 was increased by Diamox even when animals were ventilated enough to keep brain P_{CO_2} constant. My colleagues and I mounted pH and P_{CO_2} electrodes on dog brain cortical surface. Diamox administration greatly increased cerebral blood flow, slightly raised tissue P_{CO_2}, and lowered ECF pH about 0.15 unit, when ventilation was altered to keep tissue P_{CO_2} constant. Putting Siesjö's and our experiments together suggests ECF acidosis and intracellular alkalosis, a puzzling conclusion, or more probably an increase of both

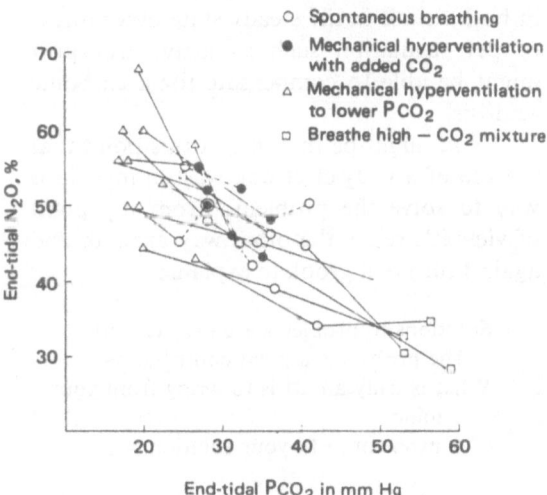

Fig. 1. The anesthetic potency of N_2O is altered by P_{CO_2}, such that less N_2O is required to obtund consciousness at higher P_{CO_2}, suggesting that CO_2 (or H^+) have anesthetic potency five times as great as N_2O.

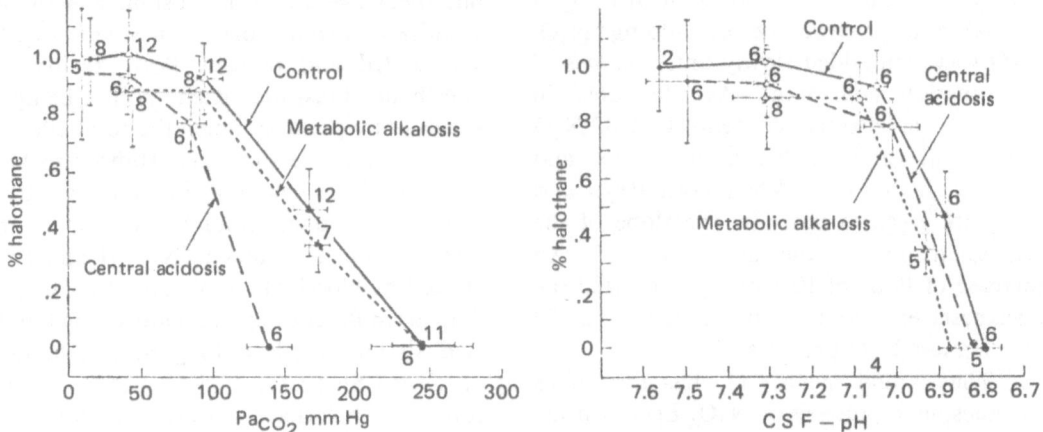

Fig. 2. The effect of CO_2 acidosis on anesthetic potency of halothane. Ordinate is percent halothane required to prevent head movement of anesthetized dogs in response to tail clamping. When cerebral ECF HCO_3^- was altered by several hours of systematic acidosis or alkalosis, the anesthetic effect of CO_2 correlated better with the cerebral ECF pH than with arterial P_{CO_2}, and suggested that anesthesia is produced by cerebral ECF acidosis alone at pH = 6.85 ± .05.

H^+ and HCO_3^- at constant P_{CO_2}. That is carbonic acidosis, due to uncatalyzed dehydration of metabolically newly formed H_2CO_3.

We needed a way to test directly the possibility that brain metabolism generates, separately, H^+ and HCO_3^- (or H_2CO_3), rather than molecular CO_2. We reasoned that if we could suddenly oxygenate brain homogenate and keep its P_{CO_2} constant, we could observe its pH (SEVERINGHAUS et al. [1969]). If the homogenate contained Diamox, the effect of oxygenation on pH would depend on whether CO_2 or H_2CO_3 was produced. We did the experiment as described below.

Homogenate was made with a mock intracellular fluid without buffers except for 10 meq of HCO_3^-. We put a drop of homogenate in place of the usual electrolyte in a CO_2 electrode—that is, between the glass pH electrode and the teflon membrane. We could thus control its gas tensions by flowing gases through the CO_2 electrode cuvette and measure the effect of sudden oxygenation at constant P_{CO_2}. The results confirmed the production of H_2CO_3 by metabolism. That is, oxygenation produced a greater acid shift

when Diamox was added, preventing the rapid dehydration of H_2CO_3 to CO_2 and escape through the teflon membrane.

This suggests that the enzyme in brain plays a pH regulating role. Possibly this is most important where rapid changes are occurring in either metabolism or flow (or in both), since in the steady state other forms of pH regulation such as active transport might be able to compensate for a carbonic acidosis.

You might be thinking at this point that the use of a CO_2 electrode was an ingenious way to solve the problem. From my point of view it's really the other way around, and again I turn to a grook to explain:

Solutions to problems are easy to find
    The problem's a great contribution
What is truly an art is to wring from your mind
    A problem to fit your solution.

Bibliography

Eisele, J. H., Eger, E. I., II, and Muallem, M., "Narcotic properties of carbon dioxide in the dog." *Anesthesiology*, 28:856 (1967).

McAleavy, J. C., Way, W. L., Altstatt, A. H., Guadagni, N. P., and Severinghaus, J. W., "The effect of pCO_2 on the depth of anesthesia." *Anesthesiology*, 22:260 (1961).

Severinghaus, J. W., Hamilton, F. N., and Cotev, S., "Carbonic acid as an intermediate in brain decarboxylation." *Biochem. J.*, 114: 703 (1969).

Severinghaus Discussion

RAHN: I would like to open up the discussion by referring to the first graph you presented, which I think reveals a fascinating approach to the problem of inert gases. I wonder whether you would like to comment on whether you believe that the first graph you've shown us would also be applicable to nitrogen narcosis, for example?

SEVERINGHAUS: Yes, it has been shown to be. Eger and his colleagues have, in fact, tested nitrogen, helium and other inert agents, and in all of them have found additive abilities. The one interesting exception is helium, which has been said to have no anesthetic effect. It has now become apparent that this is because helium has two effects. It does have an anesthetic effect, but in order to get this you must use enormous pressures, and pressure has an anti-anesthetic effect. To be specific, at 200 atm of pressure one has to add an anesthetic to keep an animal at an appropriate degree of normality. So one needs about 50% nitrous oxide, or half an atmosphere of nitrous oxide in a chamber with 200 atm of helium to keep a mouse happily awake and eating and running around. Now if you take away the nitrous oxide he convulses, so the helium effect is an additive of the anesthetic or narcotic effect plus the pressure effect, or the simple hydrostatic effect. And nitrogen fits the same scale. The more carefully the experiments have been done, the better all of these agents fit on a curve of the amount dissolved in the lipid phase of the animal's brain.

RAHN: But you indicated that the solubility coefficients have to be altered somewhat from the standard ones. Is that right, to make this fit or that prediction? I thought you mentioned that the CO_2 solubility, for example, was not according to Hoyle, so to say.

SEVERINGHAUS: No, I just said I didn't have the figure. If you use the CO_2 lipid solubility figure it fits on the curve, but I don't have the exact number which results.

RYBACK: About homogenates, I'd like to draw attention about the fact that one must be very careful about the conclusion because when you homogenate a tissue you put together molecules which are not contiguous in the intact cells and I wonder, in your case, what the initial pH of your homogenate was?

SEVERINGHAUS: Well, the problem of measuring the pH accurately depends on having a good liquid junction. I can tell you that the pH approximated 6.9 in most cases, but I wouldn't give that as an accurate figure since we didn't make an effort to form a good liquid junction. We just put it inside the CO_2 electrode as a drop, then filled the rest of it with CO_2 electrolyte. The whole brain homogenate pH I think has been measured by others. I think perhaps Dr. Siesjö would give us his figure.

SIESJÖ: I think if you add 10 meq equivalents of bicarbonate to it you should have a pH around 6.9.

SEVERINGHAUS: This was at pCO_2 40, I should explain.

SIESJÖ: I wonder, Dr. Rahn, could I add comments to the discussion? The first one is about the pCO_2 narcosis; it's a very important observation you have made that the narcotic effect from CO_2 relates to the extracellular pH. I just should like to add that we have been giving up to 40% CO_2 to rats which have been artificially ventilated with nitrous oxide as the only anesthetic, and we can say that there is definitely no interference with the energy state of the tissue under circumstances, so the narcotic effect has nothing to do with the depletion of energy in the tissue and I think this a very important observation. The second point relates to the results on Diamox you were mentioning. We found that at a constant tissue CO_2 tension we had an increased bicarbonate concentration in intracellular space. We were also very puzzled by this observation and of course had a feeling that the intracellular space should be acidotic. Thus, we tried to find another way of measuring the intracellular pH under these circumstances. And at least we got some indication, by using the lactate and pyruvate concentrations of the tissue and the L/P ratio, that the tissue was really acidotic because both the lactate and pyruvate concentrations went down at constant pCO_2 during Diamox-carbonic anhydrase inhibition, and I don't know of any direct effect of Diamox on glycolysis. It should be a pH effect, and the pH effect on the LDH equilibrium should shift the L/P ratio upwards; it did, so we had to conclude that at constant pCO_2, and at an increased bicarbonate concentration, the tissue was acid and the only solution we could come upon was to say that there is H_2CO_3 acidosis under these circumstances with a disequilibrium between H_2CO_3 and CO_2. So I think we completely agree with your observations.

SCHAEFER: I would like to refer to CO_2 narcosis. I think we have to realize that different areas of the brain, as pointed out previously, have different sensitivities, and I refer to some experiments which show that, for instance, the threshold of the motor cortex with 30% CO_2 is greatly raised. On the other hand, the hypothalamus has the same excitability, and there are some old data of Barcroft who used different, higher concentrations of CO_2 to narcotize different structures in the brain. So I think the CO_2 narcosis has many levels and I wanted to point that out because one could get the impression that there is but one.

SEVERINGHAUS: Yes, that's quite important; thank you. Perhaps it's worth pointing out that the test of anesthetic potency that Cullen used, which is movement in response to a painful stimulus, only tests one kind of overall sensitivity and that it doesn't say anything about other systems in the brain. What we use in patients as a test of anesthetic potency is whether the patient moves when the surgeon slits his skin with a knife.

LOESCHKE: I am somewhat mixed up and I hope you will help me. I understand that the CO_2 anesthesia is following the law of lipid solubility on the one side and on the other it seems to me you have demonstrated that it acts by H^+: If both are correct, I must ask whether that holds for all gaseous anesthetics? In that case I think we should investigate whether all these would cause such a H^+ concentration in the cerebral spinal fluid.

SEVERINGHAUS: I'm sorry, I think I mixed you up. I said that CO_2, if it followed the ordinary lipid theory, would require five times higher pCO_2 to produce anesthesia than it does. It is working by H^+. No one has tested its lipid-like anesthetic activity because of the fact that it produces acidotic anesthesia at far lower levels.

RAHN: I'm glad you straightened me out, too. Thank you very much.

DUBOIS: Could you clarify something for me? It was mentioned that the anesthetic effect was related to extracellular hydrogen ion concentration. Does this rule out the possibility that there was also a change in intracellular hydrogen ion concentration, or were you just using extracellular as a measure of something?

SEVERINGHAUS: We were only using spinal fluid, and it's not even correct to extrapolate from spinal fluid to extracellular fluid. In fact, at least during hypoxia, we know that spinal fluid does not become as acid as extracellular fluid, but at least with hypercapniac acidosis there's a very good agreement between the two. We don't know anything about intracellular pH, and I wouldn't extrapolate from this to say anything about that; and Cullen's experiments can only be interpreted to say that there is a good correlation with extracellular fluid H^+.

DUBOIS: Yes. This, then, is a limitation of experimental method and conceptually we can't differentiate at this point between the anesthetic effect of a change in extracellular versus the anesthetic effect of a change in intracellular H^+.

SEVERINGHAUS: As far as I know, we can't. Dr. Siesjö, can you make any predictions about the effect of chronic metabolic acidosis and alkalosis on intracellular fluid pH versus that on extracellular?

SIESJÖ: I would expect that during the time periods you were starting the animals—that was about a few hours, wasn't it?—there should be very small changes, if any, in the intracellular pH at a constant CO_2 tension; so if you have a decrease in bicarbonate in the extracellular fluid, I wouldn't expect to find any in the intracellular fluid, or very small ones at most. But I should like to add that the effect could also be due to an intracellular acidosis, of course, and we can't rule it out since we have some experiments with pure hypoxemia where, going down to very low O_2 tensions in the arterial blood, the only thing we can see until we get to extremely low values is an acidosis inside the cells, and we know that at these O_2 tensions the animals are unconcscious. So we are just starting to wonder if intracellular acidosis doesn't in some way make the animals lose their consciousness.

FENCL: May I comment on what you have said? I think the tissue pCO_2's at this point, at a pH point of 6.80, are different depending on the acidosis and alkalosis. So if you assume that there is no change in, say, intracellular bicarbonate concentration in the brain, there should probably be a difference in the intracellular pH as well.

4. Carbon Dioxide and the Utilization of Oxygen

Claus Albers

Lehrstuhl Physiologie
Universität Regensburg
Regensburg, Germany

Carbon dioxide and hydrogen ions may act on the utilization of oxygen at different levels of integration. The lowest level of integration is represented by the chemical reactions. From the papers presented earlier it seems likely that many metabolic reactions depend on pH, e.g. all reactions where NAD is involved. A somewhat higher level of integration, though closely related to the level of chemical reactions, is represented by carbon dioxide effects on the oxygen dissociation curve. A still higher level of integration with respect to the effects of carbon dioxide are reactions of organs and organ systems as, for instance, the stimulatory effect of carbon dioxide on the respiration or on the cerebral blood flow. Such reactions affect profoundly the supply of oxygen to the different organs. As a consequence of the aforementioned effects of carbon dioxide, the utilization of oxygen and the oxygen consumption of the whole organism could well be altered by carbon dioxide. In this paper, examples for the effects of carbon dioxide at different levels of integration will be discussed. Furthermore, I shall attempt to reduce these effects to a common denominator by defining a quantitative index of oxygen utilization.

An example for the effect of pH on a chemical reaction involving NAD is shown in Figure 1. It is the dehydrogenation of malic acid by NAD in the presence of malate dehydrogenase at different pH values. The ordinate is the extinction due to NADH. Obviously the equilibrium is shifted to NADH if the pH is increased, as has been described earlier by BERGMEYER and MOELLERING [1966].

Since there is a great number of such reactions, it seems impossible to predict how carbon dioxide acts on the overall oxygen consumption. Experiments in artificially ventilated dogs under nembutal-curare anesthesia were done in our laboratory by USINGER and SPAICH [1970]. The results

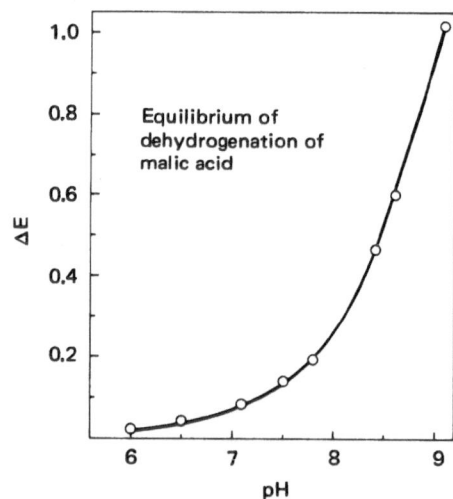

Fig. 1. Effect of pH on the equilibrium of the dehydrogenation of malic acid with NAD. On the ordinate the extinction difference due to the formation of NADH. (ALBERS, unpublished data).

demonstrated an unequivocal, though small, decrease in oxygen consumption when the arterial pH was lowered. The relationship was described by the equation

$$\log \dot{V}O_2 = 0.265 \text{ pH} - 1.165$$

when the oxygen consumption is expressed in ml/min^{-1} kg^{-1}. The positive correlation between pH and oxygen consumption did not depend on how the arterial pH was altered. Increasing the arterial carbon dioxide tension had the same effect as infusion of acids with the arterial carbon dioxide tension kept constant. These findings indicate that the metabolic effects of carbon dioxide are mediated at least to some extent by hydrogen ions.

It is important to note that the effect of carbon dioxide on the ventilation, and hence the increase in the work of breathing, were prevented by paralyzing the animals. The effect of hydrogen ions therefore must be related to the resting metabolism of the tissues.

The well-known effects of carbon dioxide on the oxygen dissociation curve, on the ventilation, and on the perfusion of the brain have the greatest impact on the utilization of oxygen. For a better understanding of these relationships it seems necessary to describe the utilization of oxygen in a more quantitative manner.

Certainly the utilization of oxygen depends on how much oxygen is offered to the tissues by the arterial blood. However, if the tissues would take up the total amount of oxygen in the blood, severe damage due to anoxia would result. To guarantee a sufficient supply of oxygen, a minimum oxygen tension in the tissue has to be maintained, which in turn requires a minimum oxygen tension in the venous blood leaving the tissue. Actually, it is an empirical fact that some organs do not show any sign of hypoxic dysfunction unless the venous Po_2 falls below a critical level. For example, NOELL and SCHNEIDER [1942] showed more than 30 years ago that the first sign of hypoxia in the brain is observed if

the oxygen tension in the cerebral venous blood is less than 19 torr.

The maximal amount of oxygen available for the tissues is limited therefore by the oxygen content in the arterial blood and by the oxygen content in the venous blood at the critical venous tension. We may call the difference between these two values the critical arterio-venous difference.

We may relate the critical a–v difference to the actual a–v difference of an organ and define the ratio of these two as the oxygen utilization index (U).

$$U = \frac{\text{critical a–v } O_2 \text{ difference}}{\text{actual a–v } O_2 \text{ difference}} \quad (1)$$

If the oxygen utilization index is unity, the tissue uses just as much oxygen as is allowed by the critical oxygen a–v difference. If this index is less than unity, the actual extraction of oxygen is too high and hypoxia ensues; if the index is greater than unity, the oxygen supply of the tissues does not offer any difficulties. A closer examination of the oxygen utilization index reveals that it depends on three factors: From the Fick principle it follows that

$$U = \frac{\dot{Q} \times (\text{critical a–v } O_2 \text{ difference})}{\dot{V}O_2} . \quad (2)$$

Therefore U varies linearly with the perfusion $\dot{Q}$ and the critical a–v oxygen difference and varies inversely with the oxygen consumption of the tissue. With the aid of these relationships the effect of carbon dioxide on the utilization of oxygen is now easily depicted.

Let us first consider the oxygen consumption. As shown above, an increase in pH tends to be associated with an increase in oxygen consumption. This in turn will decrease the oxygen utilization index.

We have next to consider the critical a–v difference, which is influenced by the pH due to the Bohr effect. To demonstrate this effect, I should like to present the oxygen dissociation curve in a somewhat unusual manner. Figure 2 shows the percentage oxygen saturation as a function of pH for selected values of the oxygen tension. The curves are derived from the oxygen dissociation curve of dog blood at $T = 37°C$ and pH = 7.4 (BARTELS and HARMS [1959]) with Δ *ln* $Po_2/\Delta pH = 1.088$. The curves were calculated by a computer using the Hill-Equation with $n = 3.091$, $K = 3.125 \times 10^{-5}$ for $Po_2 \geqslant 18.1$ torr and $n = 1.487$, $K = 3.368 \times 10^{-3}$ for $Po_2 \leqslant 18.0$ torr. This graph tells us two important facts: At the top and at the bottom of the oxygen dissociation curve, represented by the lines for an oxygen tension of 100 torr and 10 torr, there is only a small effect of pH on the oxygen saturation. On the other hand, at oxygen tensions between 60 torr and 20 torr the effect of pH on the oxygen saturation increases remarkably, especially in the region of elevated pH values. Obviously neither the uptake of oxygen in the lungs nor the oxygen content of the venous blood at very low oxygen tensions is affected by the pH, whereas at intermediate values of oxygen tensions the oxygen content depends appreciably on the pH.

The consequences for the critical a–v difference are shown in Figure 3. The two organs chosen differ in the critical venous oxygen tension: For the brain a value in the region of 16 torr to 20 torr seems quite well established by many authors, whereas for the heart the work of Bretschneider et al. [1957] indicates a critical Po_2 of about 5 torr. It is at once evident that the critical a–v difference for the heart should be almost independent of the pH, whereas for the brain an increase in pH should decrease the critical a–v difference and hence the availability of oxygen. Again more striking effects can be expected at a more elevated pH.

It is necessary to stress that the critical a–v difference depends, of course, on the value given to the arterial oxygen content. The examples given in this paper are based on an arterial oxygen content corresponding to $Pa_{O_2} = 100$ torr and a hemoglobin content of 15 g %, which we found as the average in our experiments on cerebral blood flow. For other values of the arterial oxygen content, the critical a–v difference has to be recalculated. It is only at very low arterial oxygen tensions, however, that the critical a–v difference will not change with pH, as is obvious from the curves of Figure 2.

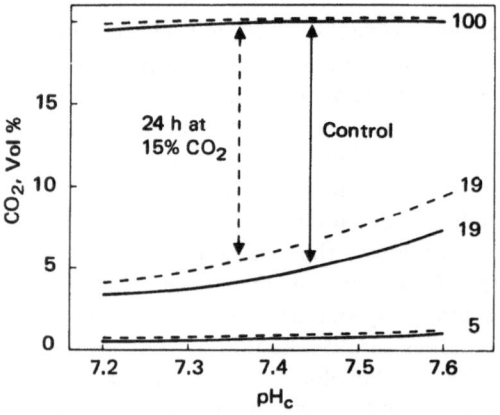

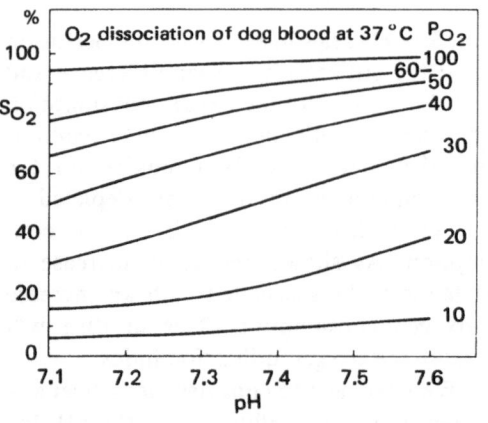

Fig. 2. Oxygen saturation in percent as a function of pH at different levels of oxygen tension (Po_2), based on data of Bartels and Harms [1959].

Fig. 3. Total oxygen content as a function of pH for arterial blood ($Po_2 = 100$ torr) and for venous blood (Po_2 equals 19 torr and 5 torr, corresponding to the critical venous oxygen tension of the brain and of the heart respectively), calculated for a hemoglobin concentration of 15g%. The solid line is the normal oxygen dissociation curve; the dashed line is the oxygen dissociation curve shifted to the left by exposure to 15% carbon dioxide *in vivo*. The arrows indicate the critical a-v difference.

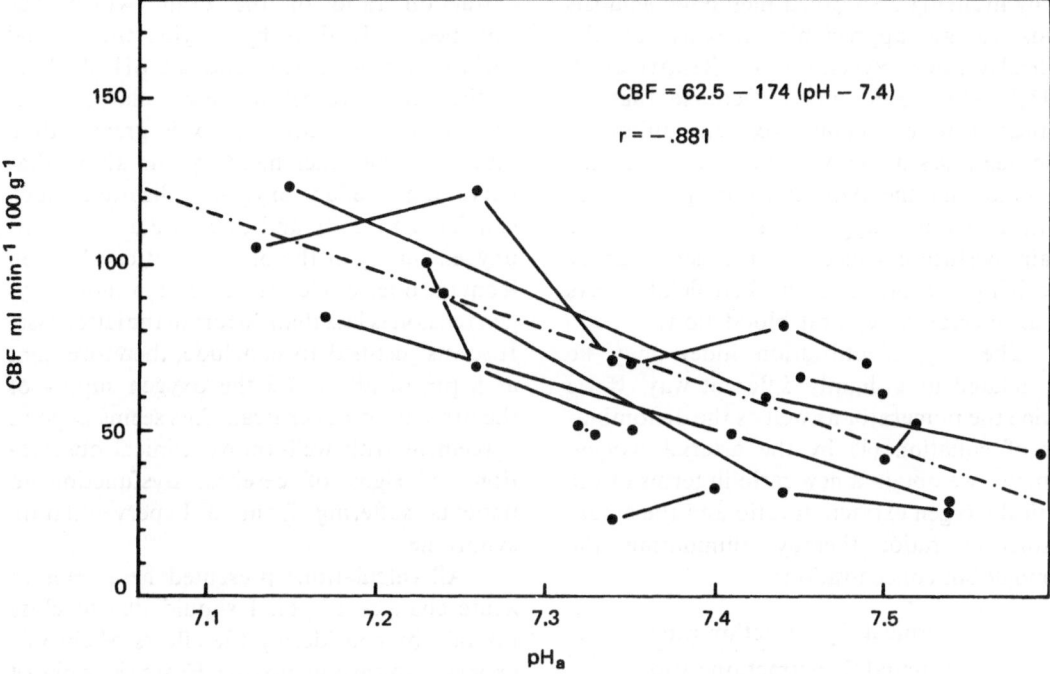

Fig. 4. Cerebral blood flow in anesthetized dogs as a function of the arterial pH.

If we now turn to the last factor in the equation given above we have to consider the effects of carbon dioxide and pH on the perfusion of the different organs. The organ most thoroughly investigated with respect to such effects is certainly the brain. The well-known effect of Pco_2 on the cerebral blood flow may be described in terms of pH rather than Pco_2. From experiments done in our laboratory (DEMERS, SPAICH, and USINGER [1969]), cerebral blood flow has been plotted against arterial pH to derive Figure 4. There is a fairly uniform increase in cerebral blood flow when the pH decreases. Over the observed range of pH, the overall regression coefficient is about 174 ml/min/100g, indicating that a decrease in the arterial pH of 0.1 will lead to an increase in cerebral blood flow by 17 ml/100g/min. With respect to the oxygen utilization index we see again that an elevation of the pH leads to a decrease in cerebral blood flow and must result in a decrease of the oxygen utilization index also. A similar

effect may be expected for the heart, since it is known that the coronary blood flow also increases with carbon dioxide (KAMMERMEIER et al. [1968]), though the quantitative relationship between pH and Pco_2 on one side and the coronary blood flow on the other side are not as well established as the relationship for the brain.

If we now reexamine equation (2), we see at once that the effects of an elevation of the pH on the three variables on the right side of the equation all tend to decrease the oxygen utilization index.

The opposite conclusion—that a decrease in pH should increase the oxygen utilization index and hence the availability of oxygen to the organs—does not seem possible. We have treated hitherto the critical a–v difference as if the critical venous oxygen tension itself did not depend on the pH. Recent work on the critical venous oxygen tension of the brain indicates, however, that lowering the pH either by inducing a respiratory acidosis or by inducing a so-called metabolic acidosis leads to an appreciable increase in the critical venous oxygen tension (GROTE et al. [1971]). This would imply, of course, that the critical arterio venous oxygen difference also decreases if the pH is lowered. It seems possible that the two effects of pH on the critical venous oxygen tension and on the brain perfusion cancel each other, thereby depriving the brain of the beneficial effects of an increased cerebral blood flow.

The oxygen utilization index may be formulated in a slightly different way. If we divide the numerator as well as the denominator of equation (1) by the arterial oxygen content, we obtain a new ratio in terms of the critical oxygen extraction ratio and the actual extraction ratio, thereby eliminating the hemoglobin concentration:

$$U = \frac{\text{critical } O_2 \text{ extraction ratio}}{\text{actual } O_2 \text{ extraction ratio}}. \quad (3)$$

The dimensionless extraction ratios are well suited to demonstrate experimental effects, as is shown in Figure 5 for the critical oxygen extraction ratio of the brain. The curve represents the critical oxygen extraction ratio calculated from the data in Figure 3. The experimental points show the actual oxygen

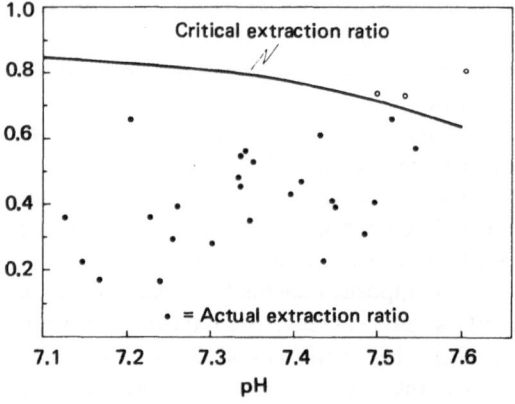

Fig. 5. Critical oxygen extraction ratio of the brain, calculated from Figure 3 (solid line), and experimentally observed oxygen extraction ratios. Po$_2$ in the cerebral venous blood greater than 19 torr is represented by closed circles, and that less than 19 torr by open circles.

extraction ratio of the brain which was obtained in 12 dogs by varying the arterial carbon dioxide tension and the pH. As long as the points are below the calculated curve, the oxygen utilization index is greater than unity. On the other hand, points above that curve indicate an oxygen utilization index smaller than unity and therefore an impaired oxygen supply of the brain. As it can be seen from the open circles, the cerebral venous oxygen tension is less than 20 torr in the latter case. It seems justified to conclude, therefore, that at a pH of about 7.5 the oxygen supply of the brain becomes critical. This seems in good agreement with well-known clinical observations of signs of cerebral dysfunction in patients suffering from a hyperventilation syndrome.

All calculations presented here refer to acute changes of pH. I should like to close my talk by considering the effects of chronic exposure to carbon dioxide. From the work of Schaefer et al. [1970] it is known that during the first days of exposure to 15% carbon dioxide, dissociation curve shows a marked shift to the left. The effect of such shift on the critical a–v difference is indicated in Figure 3 by the dashed lines. The curves for Po$_2$ = 100 and Po$_2$ = 5 torr are not much affected. The curve for the critical venous oxygen tension of the brain, however, is appreciably elevated, which in turn means that the critical a–v difference is diminished. Unfortunately, the guinea pigs of Dr. Schaefer did not tell how they felt. But it would seem to be as a pretty reasonable type of regulation that the animals succeeded in bringing the oxygen dissociation curve back to the right place.

Bibliography

Bergmeyer, H. U. and Moellering, H., "Enzymatische bestimmung von acetat." *Biochem. Z.*, 344:167–89 (1966).

Bretschneider, H. J., Frank, A., Kanzow, E., Bernard, U., "Über den kritischen Wert und die physiologische Abhängigkeit der Sauerstoff-Sättigung des venösen coronarblutes." *Pflügers Arch. Ges. Physiol.*, 264:399 (1957).

Demers, H. G., Spaich, P., Usinger, W., "Der hirnkreislauf bei erhöhter körpertemperatur." *Verh. Dtsch. Ges. Kreislaufforschg.*, 35:340–43 (1969).

Grote, J., Kreuscher, H., Schubert, R., Russ, H. J., "Investigations on the influence of PaO_2 and $PaCO_2$ on the regulation of cerebral blood flow in dogs." In *Brain and Blood Flow* (London, 1971), pp. 200–04.

Kammermeier, H., Rudroff, W., Gerlach, E., "Beeinflussung von kontraktilität, kroonarfluß und intrazellulären metaboliten des isolierten herzens bei variation von pH, PCO_2 und bikarbonat." H. Reindell, J. Keul, and E. Doll, eds. *Herzinsuffizienz*, 242–47 (Stuttgart: Thieme, 1968).

Noell, W., Schneider, M., "Über die durchblutung und die sauerstoffversorgung des gehirns im akuten sauerstoffmangel. III Mitteilung. Die arterio-venöse Sauerstoff- und Kohlensäuredifferenz. *Pflügers Arch. Ges. Physiol.*, 246:207–49 (1942).

Schaefer, K. E., Messier, A. A., Morgan, C. C., "Displacement of oxygen dissociation curves and red cell cation exchange in chronic hypercapnia." *Resp. Physiol.*, 10:299–312 (1970).

Usinger, W., Spaich, P., Sauerstoffverbrauch und kreislauf bei akuten Änderungen des arteriellen pH. *Int. Z. Angew. Physiol.*, 28:181–92 (1970).

Albers Discussion

COURNAND: I think that the notion of a critical a-v difference for oxygen is a rather interesting one, but I am just wondering whether you have some information about another ratio which is critically related to the notion which you introduced—the ratio of oxygen transport to oxygen utilization (oxygen transport is oxygen content times flow). I would like to report to you some observations that we made about 30 years ago in studying shock, where we were able to relate this ratio of oxygen transport—over oxygen utilization—to the formation of lactic acid. It's very interesting and I just wonder whether you have some information on this subject, too? Now this is based on the approximately 120 cases that have been studied in which we related transport of oxygen to lactic acid formation.

RAHN: And what is your definition of oxygen utilization? I want to be sure that we have the right meaning.

COURNAND: Oxygen utilization means the difference between the inspired and expired oxygen.

RAHN: The oxygen uptake.

ALBERS: Thank you very much. I guess this could easily be changed to give an equation similar to that I have just proposed. As far as your data are concerned, they refer to the total organism, is that right? If so, I don't think we can formulate an oxygen utilization index for a whole organism because all things I have said refer to special organs where we know at least what the venous Po_2 has to be. But for the total circulation we cannot define such a critical level of mixed venous Po_2.

SIESJÖ: As Dr. Albers mentioned, it is well known that extreme hyperventilation can reduce the cerebral blood flow to values of about 50% of the normal; it has been speculated for a very long time if this reduction of the cerebral blood flow can give straightforward hypoxia in the tissue, and the symptoms as you mentioned that you get during extreme hyperventilation are consistent with the view that there is hypoxia during hyperventilation. We have studied this for a number of years and these are data which Dr. Graunholm, in my laboratory, has obtained using cats, hyperventilated for 45 min with measurements of intra- and extracellular lactate and pyruvate concentrations; and since we have the pH values too, we can calculate the cytoplasmotic $NAD/NADH^+$ ratio. And you see that if the PCO_2 is reduced from 40, at a PCO_2 of below 20 you get a very sharp increase in the intracellular lactate/pyruvate ratio. And now if you combine these values with the pH values, we can also determine that there is an increase in the $NAD/NADH^+$ ratio. Now, this redox change could be interpreted to show that there is hypoxia in the tissue. However, if you also measure the organic phosphates and calculate what Atkinson has called the energy charge potential (ADP divided by 0.5 times ADP divided by ADP+ADP+AMP), there is no change whatsoever at these low values. So it indicates that even if a slight hypoxia is induced in the tissue during extreme hyperventilation, it is not of such a degree that the energy state of the tissue is affected. We've also combined pure respiratory alkalosis with metabolic respiratory alkalosis. In this way we can get the pH of the blood to increase in the first group from 7.4 to about 7.55 and to about 7.75 in this group. So this alters the dissociation curve so much that any hypoxia in the tissue should be exaggerated. Now you can see that by combining the two, there is an increase in the intracellular lactate concentration and there is a slight increase in the NAD/NADH$^+$ ratio. However, even under these circumstances, there is no indication that the energy state is affected during extreme hyperventilation, and this then also applies to a situation where the blood is extremely alkalotic. It has been shown from Gothenberg that when you reach these very low values of the venous Po$_2$ and try to reduce the Po$_2$ even further by manipulating the pH of the blood, there is an increase in the cerebral blood flow, so the tissue always protects itself by increasing the blood flow under these circumstances. I don't think it's possible to induce a state of severe hypoxia in the tissue by hyperventilation or by manipulating the pH of blood. Thank you.

RAHN: Dr. Albers, would you like to comment?

ALBERS: Which anesthesia did you use on your cats?

SIESJÖ: With the cats it was Nembutal. We had exactly the same results with nitrous oxide anesthesia in rats or very superficial halotherm anesthesia (0.6%).

ALBERS: Well, first I'll answer your last point—that there's a kind of self-protecting increase in cerebral blood flow if the Pco$_2$ gets too low. This has been described many times, but always in circumstances where the arterial Po$_2$ was either normal or lower, due to hypoxic breathing. In our experiments we had artificial ventilation with pure oxygen and on the arterial side we always had a Po$_2$ of about 500 torr. We never observed an increase in cerebral blood flow when we changed the pH to 7.6–7.7 and got a decrease in cerebral blood flow and a tremendous decrease in cerebral venous Po$_2$ down to about 10 mm Hg. So I wonder whether the lack of the self-protecting increase in blood flow in our experiments is due to the high arterial Po$_2$ and hence to the inactivation of the chemoreceptors of the carotid body.

SIESJÖ: I don't think so. These results have been reported both by Alexander and his co-workers in Philadelphia in 1969 and by the Gothenberg group.

CHERNIAK: In answer to Dr. Cournand's question, we have data that relate oxygen delivery flow times oxygen content of the arterial blood to oxygen consumption, in muscle and in brain. As you decrease the oxygen flow or delivery, oxygen consumption falls in both organs after the flow is decreased about 20% below its normal level. And in alkalosis in muscle, despite the shift of the oxyhemoglobin dissociation curve, for any given level of oxygen delivery there's a greater oxygen consumption, not less.

NAHAS: The data that Dr. Siesjö presented is very comforting to the anesthesiologist, who doesn't hesitate to hyperventilate the patient down to Po$_2$ of 20 torr in neurosurgical procedures where the brain is exposed and may be traumatized, and it seems by empirical findings that these procedures have been very well tolerated. In this respect, it's very interesting to see that on the basis of your data, Dr. Siesjö, under conditions of this hyperventilation, the intracellular pH of the brain does not change very much; in fact, it remains constant. So I wonder if the closed loop signal that actually is required in any type of regulation is not determined by the intracellular pH in the brain cell which, in itself, is ultimately regulated by metabolic changes occurring there. These changes may also be triggered by the alteration in extracellular pH and which tend, of course, to maintain this intracellular pH at a constant level.

ALBERS: Well, you are quite happy. My coworkers always resist when I say we start the experiment with a hyperventilation period because if we started with a very drastic hyperventilation, we lost 50% or 60% of our dogs, but I don't know whether this is due to the brain or due to the heart. In our experiments hyperventilation was always more critical than hypoventilation. Again,

I wonder whether the chemical inactivation of the chemoreceptors is involved.

OTIS: In your definition of critical a-v difference you include the condition that the arterial blood, the incoming blood, is fully oxygenated. Now if this were not the case, then you would have a different value for the critical a-v difference, would you not? Do you have to redefine it in each circumstance of oxygenation?

ALBERS: Actually, one has to recalculate for each oxygen saturation if one wants to be very correct, but if you do so for oxygen tensions between 100 torr and 80 torr, this makes not a great difference. If you have a severe cyanosis, then of course things are different.

SEVERINGHAUS: My question has to do with your rather low jugular venous or cerebral sagital venous oxygen tensions with hyperventilation. A number of other investigators have reported that they have not been able to produce sufficient vaso constriction to get the P_{O_2} below about 17 or 18 torr, no matter how much they hyperventilate, provided hypertension doesn't occur. I wondered whether your animals were hypotensive as well, or whether you deliberately reduced the pressure to get the P_{O_2} down?

ALBERS: No, they were not hypotensive. They had a mean arterial blood pressure of 105 mm Hg to 120 mm Hg.

SEVERINGHAUS: In other words, you do not find the kind of cerebral blood flow plateau below a P_{CO_2} of 20 torr that McDowell, Harper, Lassen, and others have reported?

ALBERS: No, we did not find that. But our smallest P_{CO_2} was 12 torr and at that low P_{CO_2} we found a very low cerebral blood flow. Using the Kety-Schmidt method, from the plot of the nitrous oxide values you see immediately that there was a very low brain perfusion even with a very low cerebral venous P_{O_2}.

SEVERINGHAUS: These were directly measured P_{O_2}'s?

ALBERS: Directly measured—electrode measured P_{O_2} and P_{CO_2}.

SEVERINGHAUS: And the animal, and the anesthesia?

ALBERS: Nembutal and curare were used for anesthesia. Dogs served as experimental animals and were artificially ventilated.

SEVERINGHAUS: Then do you agree this is a discrepancy with most of the other data in the literature?

ALBERS: Yes, but I don't know the reason, unfortunately.

BÖNIG: The concentration of inorganic phosphate is decreased during short hyperventilation in man of 30 min to half its beginning value. Perhaps this may be explained as an effect of formation of energy-rich phosphate compounds in the whole body during hyperventilation. Second, the question to Dr. Albers: The critical oxygen tension must depend on the distance of the cells from the capillaries. Is it possible to calculate changes in this distance during hyperventilation, perhaps in changes of blood pressure?

ALBERS: No, we did no such calculations, but we assumed that the geometry of the tissues and the capillaries within the brain, at least, should not change with the pH. But may I have one question for Dr. Siesjö? Do you think that the phosphate ratio you have given is the true indicator of hypoxia? If the $NAD/NADH^+$ ratio changes, what then happens to cytochrome oxidase? This should also be in a more reduced state then. The second point is that it might be that the phosphate is perfectly okay; but our chairman told me some weeks ago that when he let his people hyperventilate, at this pH of about 7.5 he almost inevitably got signs of bad performance on psychological tests, if I understood you right.

RAHN: Oh yes, it's well known, that when the arterial pH goes up in voluntary subjects hyperventilating, your performance decreases with the alveolar P_{CO_2} and the arterial pH.

SIESJÖ: I do agree with you that there may be slight hypoxia in the tissue. My point is that this hypoxia is not of a degree which will, so to speak, jeopardize the viability of the tissue. I think it's quite possible that you get a redox change before you get a sufficient decrease in the rate of oxidative phosphorilization. This does mean that the electrones are being delivered from a higher level than before, but it doesn't say anything about the rate of phosphorilization.

5. P_{CO_2} pH and Body Temperature

Hermann Rahn

*Laboratoire de Physiologie Respiratoire, C.N.R.S.,
67-Strasbourg, France,
and
Department of Physiology,
State University of New York at Buffalo,
Buffalo, New York 14214*

One of the most impressive regulations of the *milieu intérieur* is the constancy of blood pH in homeotherms. This is accomplished by the renal control of the plasma bicarbonate concentration on the one hand and the ventilatory control of the plasma H_2CO_3 concentration on the other. The ratio between this buffer pair is normally 20:1, which at 37°C maintains a pH of 7.4 or a H^+ concentration of 40 nmoles/l. This constancy of blood pH and P_{CO_2} throughout the life of most homeotherms is so remarkable that at first glance one might consider a pH of 7.4 to be the proper reference standard of acid-base balance for other vertebrates, even those that live at body temperatures other than 37°C.

While poikilotherm vertebrates appear to regulate their acid-base balance in a manner similar to homeotherms, it is at first rather discomforting to observe that these animals require for each body temperature a different pH, H^+, and blood P_{CO_2} in order to stay in acid-base balance. As I will try to show, a pH of 7.4 is for most of these forms a state of acidosis.

These alterations of pH with body temperature have a profound effect upon the P_{CO_2} of the blood and, therefore, upon ventilation. As the body temperature falls, so does the P_{CO_2}, and therefore the relative ventilation (i.e. relative to the transport of a unit quantity of CO_2) must increase. I would first like to present some evidence of how P_{CO_2} behaves when blood is cooled *in vitro*, when blood cools *in vivo*, and lastly, how the ventilation in cold-blooded animals responds to these changes.

Neutrality of Water

Long ago the physicist established the degree of ionization of water and how it changes with temperature. The ionization constant for water, Kw, can be translated into pH, and Figure 1 shows how the pH or the pOH of neutral water, pN, changes as a function of temperature. [The abscissa is $1/(K°)^2$ with centigrade values superimposed. This graphical procedure has the advantage that the pN line is straight.]

In this figure I have also indicated the blood pH and tissue pH of man at 37°C. At chemical neutrality, pH = 6.8, the H^+ concentration is about four times greater than in the blood while the tissues are close to neutrality. The question now arises what the blood or tissue pH values are when the temperature is less than or greater than 37°C. Should man's reference point at 37°C, namely a pH of 7.4, be maintained or will it be shifted relative to the chemical neutrality of water? I hope to provide evidence from poikilotherm vertebrates to uphold the latter

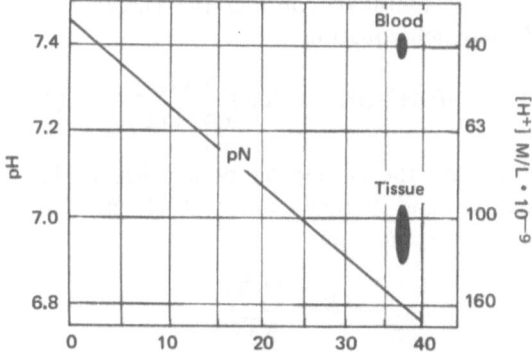

Fig. 1. pN, the neutrality of water where pH = pOH, as a function of temperature. Temperature scale is plotted as $1/(K°)^2$. On the right hand ordinate the H$^+$ concentration is expressed assuming an activity coefficient of 1.0. Shaded areas at 37°C represent typical values of blood and tissues of homeotherms.

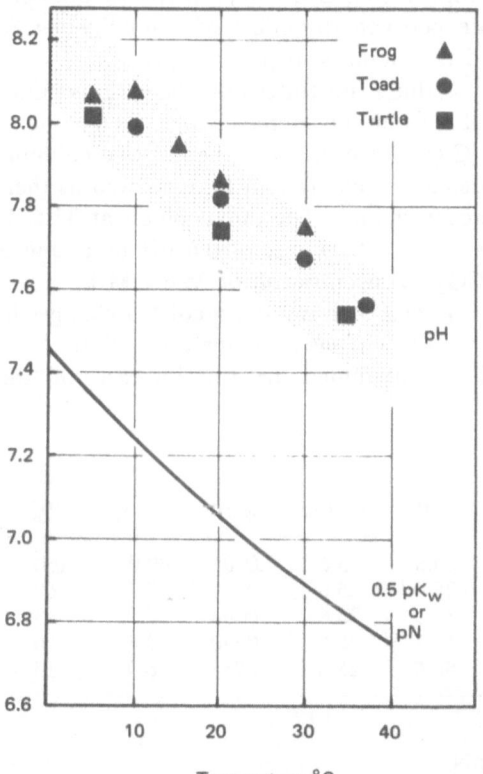

Fig. 2. Normal arterial pH values of poikilotherms as a function of body temperature, illustrating the parallel behavior between pH and pN. This difference represents the constant relative alkalinity—or the constant OH$^-$/H$^+$ ratio in the blood. (From HOWELL et al. [1970]).

alternative. This in turn requires an increasing pH number as the temperature falls so that the difference between blood pH and pN remains constant.

In Figure 2 you will see the normal pH values for three species of poikilotherms and how these values maintain a constant relationship to neutrality of water, pN. It is this constant difference between pH and pN that we have called *constant relative alkalinity*. The antilog of pH − pN expresses the ratio of H$^+$ neutrality to H$^+$ blood and the antilog of 2 (pH − pN) the ratio of OH$^-$ blood to H$^+$ blood. It would appear that these 2 ratios are regulated at all temperatures and kept constant (HOWELL et al. [1970]).

Behavior of Blood pH *in vitro*

One approach to testing these assumptions is to cool blood anaerobically and to measure the pH. Rosenthal [1948] was one of the first to do this systematically and found that the pH of whole blood increased. This has been confirmed on various species of mammals including hibernators. Robin [1962] was the first to establish this in the blood (*in vitro*) of a cold-blooded species, the turtle. More recently Howell et al. [1970] reported similar results in the frog and another species of turtle and pointed out that the changes in pH upon cooling the blood do, indeed, parallel the changes in pH of neutral water and that by this criterion, the blood did not become more "alkaline" upon cooling but maintained a constant relative alkalinity or a constant ratio of OH$^-$ to H$^+$ ions.

Behavior of Blood PCO$_2$ *in vitro*

When blood is cooled anaerobically, the total CO$_2$ concentration cannot change. There is a possible change in the partition of HCO$_3^-$ between the plasma and red cells, but at least in the turtle blood the HCO$_3^-$ concentration of the plasma remained constant (ROBIN [1962]). Thus, as Albers [1962] pointed out, it is possible to predict the change in PCO$_2$ with cooling, if the plasma

HCO_3^- concentration remains constant and the change in pH is known.

Method of Calculation

As pointed out above, the pH of blood cooled anaerobically *in vitro* can, for any temperature, best be described by the simple relationship

$$pH - pN = k$$
or
$$pH = pN + k \quad (1)$$

where k varies between 0.6 and 0.8 pH units, depending upon the particular species, and pN is the pH of neutrality at a given temperature (or 0.5 pKw, the dissociation constant of water).

With these considerations it is possible to predict the behavior of Pco_2 when blood is cooled anaerobically (*in vitro*). The basic assumption is that the plasma HCO_3^- remains constant and that the pH of the blood at any temperature is equal to $pN + k$. In addition, one must consider the changes in pK' of the H_2CO_3, as it is affected by (1) temperature, as well as pH, and (2) the changes in solubility of CO_2 in plasma. These changes can be taken from the data of Severinghaus et al. [1965] and extrapolated to 5°C.

It is useful to consider the Henderson-Hasselbalch equation

$$(pH - pK') = \log\frac{[HCO_3^-]}{\alpha CO_2 \cdot Pco_2} \quad (2)$$

If we take the antilog on both sides of the equation and designate antilog $(pH - pK')$ as B then we can write

$$B = \frac{HCO_3^-}{\alpha \cdot Pco_2}$$
or
$$Pco_2 = \frac{HCO_3^-}{\alpha \cdot B} \quad (3)$$

As the temperature falls both α and B will increase. B will increase because the change in pK' is very small compared to the change in pH. One can furthermore differentiate between the effect of solubility *per se* and the changes in pH and pK'.

Table 1 illustrates how the various values that must be considered change when blood at 37°C is cooled *in vitro*. The last two columns indicate the changes in Pco_2 as well as their percent change. The initial blood at 37°C is assumed to have a k of 0.6 pH units and a HCO_3^- concentration of 25.6 mM/l.

Figure 3 shows the predicted changes in Pco_2 with change in temperature. Part of the fall is attributed to the increase of the

Table 1.

T	0.5 pKw	k	pH	pK'	pH − pK'	B	HCO_3^-	αCO_2	Pco_2	%
37	6.810	0.6	7.410	6.091	1.319	20.8	25.6	.0308	40.0	100
29	6.933	0.6	7.533	6.128	1.405	25.4	25.6	.0371	27.2	68
21	7.066	0.6	7.666	6.161	1.505	32.0	25.6	.0464	17.2	43
13	7.210	0.6	7.810	6.190	1.620	41.7	25.6	.0590	10.4	26
5	7.367	0.6	7.967	6.214	1.753	56.6	25.6	.0755	6.0	15

$$T = °C$$
$$0.5\,pKw = pH \text{ of neutrality} = pN$$
$$pH = 0.5\,pKw + 0.6$$
$$pK' = \text{apparent dissociation constant for } H_2CO_3$$
$$B = \text{antilog } (pH - pK')$$
$$[HCO_3^-] = 25.6 \text{ mmoles/l.}$$
$$\alpha CO_2 = \text{mmoles/l.}$$
$$Pco_2 = 25.6/(\alpha CO_2 \cdot B) \quad \text{equation (3)}$$
$$\% = \text{change in } Pco_2 \text{ when } 40 = 100\%$$

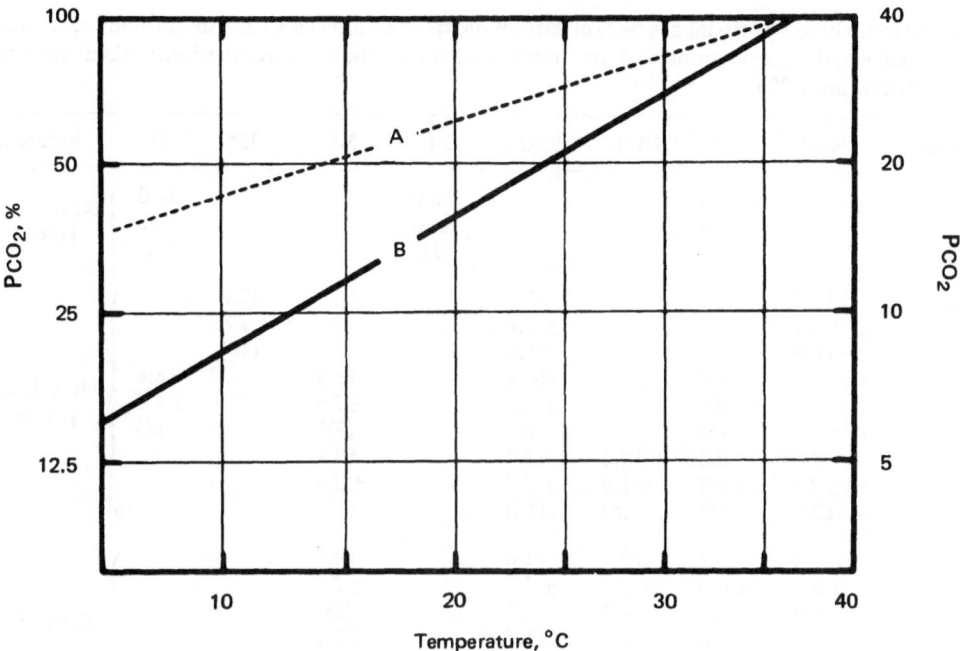

Fig. 3. Calculated values of PCO$_2$ as a function of temperature when a blood sample taken at 37°C is cooled anaerobically *in vitro*. Calculations appear in Table 1. The slope of the PCO$_2$ line is a function of changes in the pH and pK' of H$_2$CO$_3$ (*A*) and, in addition, to the change in solubility of CO$_2$ (*B*).

difference (pH − pK') and is shown by the dotted line *A*. When in addition the changes in solubility of CO$_2$ in plasma are considered, we note the total change, line *B*. A change in the plasma bicarbonate concentration of the initial blood or the assumption of a different *k* value only alter the absolute values of PCO$_2$ in such a graph, but not the slope of the line which, on a semilog plot, is linear if the abscissa has the temperature expressed as 1/(K°)^2, as in Figure 1.

One may therefore predict the relative changes in PCO$_2$ of whole blood *in vitro* with changes in temperature, provided the *k* value and the HCO$_3$$^-$ concentration remain constant. Between 10°C and 40°C the PCO$_2$ increases 85% for every 10°C increase in temperature. Thus, the Q$_{10}$ for PCO$_2$ is 1.85.

In vivo PCO$_2$ **Changes with Temperature**

We must now ask what the *in vivo* changes in PCO$_2$ are, since this value is established and maintained by the ratio between the metabolic CO$_2$ production and the ventilation. Campbell [1926] was probably the first to call our attention to the fact that in cold-blooded vertebrates the PCO$_2$ increased with body temperature. He established gas pockets in the toad, *Bufo*, and after equilibration removed this gas for analysis. More recently Torre [1967] tested systematically the PCO$_2$ in subcutaneous and intraperitoneal gas pocket of *Rana catesbiana* between 4°C and 30°C. That such tissue values reflect the gas tensions changes in blood is attested to by the parallel behavior between these two values (Table 2). Table 2 shows all available values for PCO$_2$ of blood (155 observations) and tissues (70 observations) of poikilotherm animals as a function of body temperature. When these values are plotted on a log scale against temperature (Figure 4), we see that they have a similar slope. The slope value has been calculated between 10°C and 30°C (Table 3) for each species and

Table 2. Arterial blood or tissue gas pocket carbon dioxide tensions as a function of body temperature, their standard deviations and the number of observations (parenthesized). Total number of observations 225.

Species	4–5°	10°	15–16°	20–22°	24°	30°	35°	37°	References
Pseudemys		18.6 ± 6 (11)			28.0 ± 10 (11)			56.0 ± 12 (11)	} Robin [1962]
Chelydra	12.2 ± 1.4 (12)			25.2 ± 1.4 (13)			47.0 ± 12.3 (10)		
Bufo		6.9 ± 0.5 (5)		10.4 ± 0.5 (6)		15.9 ± 1.6 (8)		18.6 ± 1.3 (8)	} Howell et al. [1970]
Rana	5.5 ± 2.0 (20)	6.2 ± 0.8 (5)	10.2 ± 1.6 (8)	12.7 ± 3.8 (16)		17.4 ± 3.4 (11)			
*Rana S.C.**	5.4 ± 0.6 (8)	7.1 ± 0.6 (5)	10.7 ± 0.6 (7)	13.4 ± 1.2 (7)		19.1 ± 1.0 (8)			} Torre [1967]
Rana I.P.†	7.7 ± 0.6 (8)	7.9 ± 0.6 (5)	13.1 ± 1.1 (7)	17.5 ± 1.6 (7)		22.1 ± 1.7 (8)			

* *S.C.*   subcutaneous gas pocket
† *I.P.*   intraperitoneal gas pocket

Table 3. The Q_{10} for P_{CO_2} between 30°C and 10°C calculated from actual or interpolated values at two temperatures (see Table 2). The mean Q_{10} for P_{CO_2} is 1.66.

Species	30°	10°	$\sqrt{30°/10°}$	Tissue
Pseudemys	40.0	18.0	1.49	
Chelydra	40.0	15.0	1.64	} Blood
Bufo	15.9	6.9	1.52	
Rana	17.4	6.2	1.67	
Sub. Cut.	19.1	5.4	1.88	} Gas Pockets
1. Perit.	22.1	7.7	1.70	

yields a mean Q_{10} for P_{CO_2} of 1.64. This value can now be compared with the value of 1.85 for *in vitro* changes of P_{CO_2}.

The difference between these two values is either due to the fact that the *k* value (or constant relative alkalinity) was not maintained or that the plasma HCO_3^- concentration changed. It appears that the lesser slope of the *in vivo* P_{CO_2} changes are due to a slight increase in HCO_3^- concentration as these animals acclimated to lower tempera-

tures. From the data of Howell et al. [1970] the average changes of HCO_3^- with acclimation can be calculated. This has been done for the temperature range between 10°C and 30°C (Table 4) and gives a mean Q_{10} value of -1.18.

These findings can be interpreted as follows. As the body temperature falls, the maintenance of a constant relative alkalinity requires a large fall in blood P_{CO_2}. However, this change is not quite as great as occurs

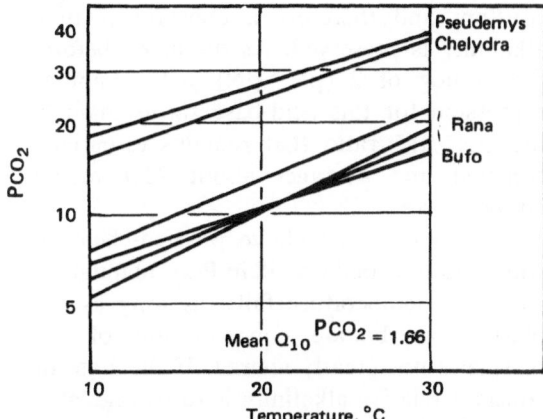

Fig. 4. Average behavior of P_{CO_2} in the blood and tissues of four species of poikilotherms as a function of temperature. While the absolute P_{CO_2} levels differ among these species, the slope on the semilog scale plot is similar. Data were taken from Tables 2 and 3.

Table 4. The Q_{10} for plasma bicarbonate, mmoles/l. between 10°C and 30°C calculated from the values of Howell et al. [1970] at two temperatures. Q_{10} for plasma bicarbonate is −1.18.

Species	10°	30°	$\sqrt{10°/30°}$
Chelydra	57	44	−1.14
Rana	36	26	−1.17
Bufo	30	20	−1.22

when blood is cooled *in vitro*, because *in vivo* a small increase in plasma HCO_3^- occurs during acclimation to cold.

Regulation of Ventilation

We have all been imprinted with the concept that our ventilation is regulated to maintain a constant P_{CO_2} which, in the presence of a given plasma bicarbonate level, provides for the maintenance of a rather precise pH level in the blood. How is the regulation of ventilation steered in the poikilotherm vertebrate where, as we have seen, each temperature requires a different optimal pH or H^+ value, a different P_{CO_2} value, and in addition, is accompanied by a

different metabolic rate or CO_2 production? Dr. E. Robin [1962] was the first to ask precisely this question some 10 years ago: "Since the turtle does not maintain a constant P_{CO_2} when temperature of the body is varied, it seems likely that the regulation of ventilation in the turtle does not depend on the CO_2 tension or the pH of extracellular fluid."

Our interests were originally stimulated by these observations. Today, some 10 years later, I will attempt to provide an explanation of the regulation of ventilation in the turtle. This is based upon more recent contributions from Dr. Robin's laboratory [1969], our own laboratory (HOWELL et al. [1970]), and particularly the recent experiments of Dr. Jackson [1971] at the University of Pennsylvania, who has measured the metabolic rate and ventilation in the awake and relatively unrestrained turtle, *Pseudemys elegans*. I am particularly indebted to Dr. Jackson for the privilege of presenting some of his observations which have just appeared [1971].

Changes in Metabolic Rate and Blood P_{CO_2} with Temperature

However, before presenting the ventilation rates, I would like to predict these values for different temperatures and then compare them with the measured values. As I suggested some years ago (RAHN [1966]), both P_{CO_2}, as well as metabolic CO_2 production, are lowered when the temperature falls. If both of these values fall at the same rate, then one would predict no change in ventilation. This can be appreciated from the alveolar ventilation equation where

$$\dot{V}_A = k(\dot{V}_{CO_2}/P_{A_{CO_2}})$$

Figure 5 shows the $\dot{V}_{O_2}$ values of Jackson [1971] at 10°C, 20°C, and 30°C on a log scale. The mean Q_{10} is approximately 1.72. If we assume that the respiratory exchange ratio is constant, then this slope also applies to the CO_2 production or $\dot{V}_{CO_2}$. Below this curve I have plotted the *in vivo* arterial P_{CO_2} values of Robin [1962] for the same species of turtle and the data of Howell et al. [1970] for the turtle species *Chelydra*. The slope of this curve is based upon the latter species and is estimated to have a Q_{10} for P_{CO_2} of 1.64. One can appreciate that the slopes of these curves are very similar and that on this basis one would predict relatively little change in absolute ventilation between 30°C and 10°C, in spite of the fact that the CO_2 production is reduced nearly four-fold. Above the lines of Figure 5 I have plotted on a linear scale the actual ventilation that Jackson measured. Each value is based on 30 observations. The standard error is of the order of 10% and there was no significant change in tidal volume and frequency at these three temperatures. These observations on the ventilation are particularly interesting from another point of view since they demonstrate a functional activity which appears to be independent over a 20°C change in body temperature.

In Table 5 I have listed the metabolic rates and ventilation flow rates of Jackson, and below I indicated the acid-base values of the *Chelydra* turtle.

On the basis of these data one is able to speculate about the acid-base regulation and the role of ventilation as the body temperature varies. First of all, the observed changes in blood pH do not reflect a change in the acid-base status, but merely reflect the change in degree of ionization of the H^+ as well as the OH^- ions. The difference between pH and pN (the pH state of neutrality) remains

constant and therefore a constant relative alkalinity is preserved. As discussed before, the antilog of 2 (pH − pN) yields another expression for this acid-base status, namely the OH^-/H^+ ratio that remains essentially constant and averages about 23:1 at all temperatures.

As we have seen above, physico-chemical considerations make a fall in P_{CO_2} mandatory when the temperature falls, as long as the plasma bicarbonate concentration of the plasma is not greatly altered. If the state of constant relative alkalinity is to be regulated by the H_2CO_3 buffer system, then the ventilation must adjust itself to the dictated changes in the P_{CO_2} level, and this appears to be the case. In the turtle the relative changes in P_{CO_2} and $\dot{V}_{CO_2}$ with changes in temperature are similar, and in this animal we then have no change in the absolute ventilation rate although the relative ventilation increased several times. To what extent other animals will behave in a similar fashion remains to be seen. However, from these considerations it seems unlikely that the metabolic rate is the only determiner of the ventilation rate and that the maintenance of the relative alkalinity must also be considered.

In light of these observations it is of interest to speculate about the acid-base regulation and ventilation of homeotherms. It would appear that all vertebrates maintain a given degree of alkalinity with reference to the neutrality of water or, as Reeves [1969] and Robin et al. [1969] have suggested, maintain a constant protein buffer ratio. Thus, the absolute pH of the blood at any temperature must vary with the changes in the ionization of water or the ionization constant of particular protein buffers. Since the pK of imidazole changes with temperature in a manner parallel to the changes in neutrality of water, it is difficult to distinguish between their relative importance in the maintenance of a constant relative alkalinity. I would like to argue that the protein buffers were specially selected during the evolution to comply with the ionization changes of water.

Table 5. Oxygen uptake and ventilation of *Pseudemys* (JACKSON [1971]). Below are indicated the acid-base values from the turtle *Chelydra* (HOWELL et al [1970]).

	10°C	20°	30°
$\dot{V}_{O_2}$ ml min⁻¹ kg⁻¹	0.31	0.68	1.15
$\dot{V}_E$ ml min⁻¹ kg⁻¹	23.9	24.8	23.5
Pa_{CO_2}	15	25	40
pH	7.94	7.76	7.60
pH − pN	0.67	0.69	0.68
OH^-/H^+	22:1	24:1	23:1

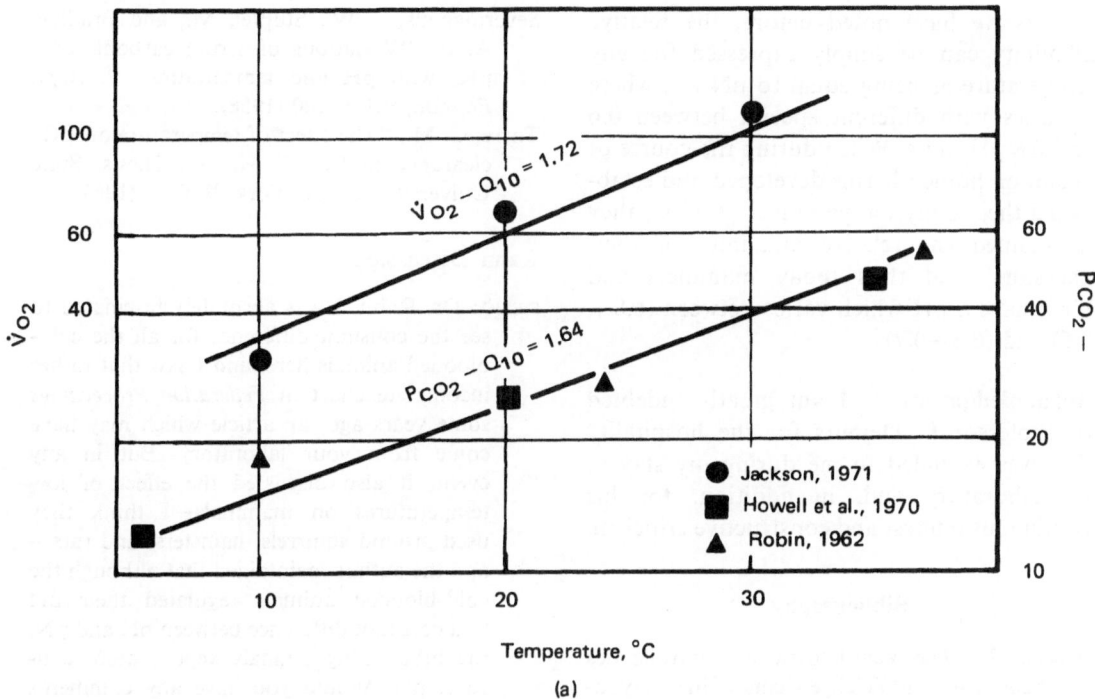

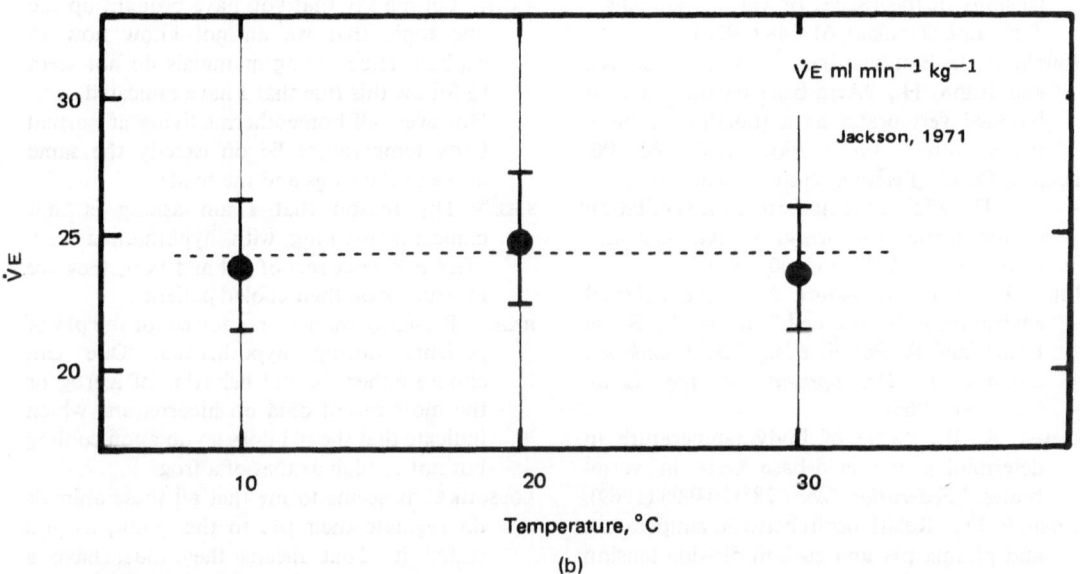

Fig. 5(A). Comparison of the changes in V_{O_2} of the turtle *Pseudemys* (Jackson [1971]) and the arterial blood P_{CO_2} of *Pseudemys* (ROBIN [1962]) and *Chelydra* (HOWELL *et al.* [1970]) as a function of body temperature. From these two slopes only a small change in absolute ventilation would be predicted between 30°C and 10°C.

(B) Ventilation of the turtle *Pseudemys* showing essentially a constant ventilation flow rate between 10°C and 30°C. (JACKSON [1971]).

As we have noted before, the relative alkalinity can be simply expressed for any temperature as being equal to pN + k, where k varies with different species between 0.6 and 0.8 pH units. When during the course of evolution homeotherms developed and established their body temperatures at 37°C, they maintained the relative alkalinity of their ancestors, and thus today mammals and birds have a pH which varies between (6.8 + 0.6) and (6.8 + 0.7).

Acknowledgments   I am greatly indebted to Professor P. Dejours for the hospitality that was extended to me during my stay at his laboratory and, in addition, for his continuous interest and constructive criticism.

Bibliography

Albers, C., "Die Ventilatorische Kontrolle des Saüren-Basen-Gleichgewichts in Hypothermie." *Der Anaesthetist*, 11:43–51 (1962).

Campbell, J. A., "The normal CO_2 and O_2 tensions in the tissues of various animals." *J. Physiol.* (*London*), 61:248 (1926).

Howell, B. J., Baumgardner, F. W., Bondi, K., and Rahn, H., "Acid-base balance in cold blooded vertebrates as a function of body temperature." *Am. J. Physiol.*, 218:600–06.

Jackson, D. C. (Personal communication).

———. "The effect of temperature on ventilation in the turtle, *Pseudemys scripta elegans*." *Respir. Physiol.*, 12:131–40 (1971).

Rahn, H., "Gas transport from the external environment to the cell." In A. V. S. de Reuck and R. Porter, eds., *Ciba Foundation Symposium. Development of the Lung.* (London, 1966).

Reeves, R. B., "Role of body temperature in determining the acid-base state in vertebrates." *Federation Proc.*, 28:1204–08 (1969).

Robin, E. D., "Relationship between temperature and plasma pH and carbon dioxide tension in the turtle." *Nature*, 195:249–51 (1962).

———, Bromberg, P. A., and Cross, C. E., "Some aspects of the evolution of vertebrate acid-base regulation." *Yale J. Biol. Med.*, 41:448–67 (1969).

Rosenthal, T. B., "The effect of temperature on the pH of blood and plasma *in vitro*." *J. Biol. Chem.*, 173:25–30 (1948).

Severinghaus, J. W., Stupfel, M., and Bradley, A. F., "Variations of serum carbonic acid pK′ with pH and temperature." *J. Appl. Physiol.*, 9:179–200 (1956).

Torre, C. M., "The effect of temperature on CO_2 clearance in frogs." Masters Thesis, State University of New York, Buffalo (1967).

Rahn Discussion

SIESJÖ: Dr. Rahn, I was absolutely fascinated to see the constant difference for all the cold-blooded animals here, and I saw that rather incomplete chart in *Federation Proceedings* some years ago, an article which may have come from your laboratory. But in any event, it also discussed the effect of low temperatures on mammals—I think they used ground squirrels, hamsters, and rats—and the author maintained that although the cold-blooded animals regulated their pH to a constant difference between pH and pN, the hibernating animals kept a more constant pH. Would you have any comments on that article and on the kind of experiments it was based on?

RAHN: Let me say that you have brought up the one topic that we do not know how to explain. Hibernating mammals do not seem to follow this rule that I have indicated here. However, all homeotherms living at normal body temperature lie on exactly the same curve as the frogs and the toads.

SIESJÖ: The reason that I am asking is that clinicians working with hypothermia very often ask what sort of pH and P_{CO_2} they are measuring on their cooled patients.

RAHN: Presently we have no advice for the pH of patients during hypothermia. One can choose either the pH behavior of a frog or the most recent data on hibernators, which indicate that the pH does go up upon cooling but not as high as that of a frog.

LOESCHKE: It seems to me that all these animals do regulate their pH to this point, as you stated it. That means they must have a receptor to measure the ratio H^+ to OH^-—of course this is the receptor which we all investigate by ventilation—and my question is whether there is any model to date that could explain such a measurement?

RAHN: A model for the ventilation-regulating receptor that specifically monitors (and defends) an OH^-/H^+ ratio has not been put forward. However, a model has been suggested by R. B. Reeves [*Resp. Physiol.*, (1972)] with the same end result as if a receptor were envisaged with two important properties: (1) the receptor must contain a dissociable group with a pK' in the physiological pH range; and (2) the change in pK' with temperature must be similar to the slope of the pN-temperature curve—i.e. a $\Delta H° = 7000$ cal mole^{-1} (Albery and Lloyd). It is possible to picture a protein component whose charge-state and conformation are sensitive to the animal's acid-base status at any body temperature. It might be thought of in terms of an "ion-gating protein" component in the membrane of a respiratory pacemaker neuron, the dissociation of which is written in terms of the imidazole group of the histidine moieties in protein peptide linkages, unique among biological compounds for satisfying the two important conditions already mentioned. The dissociation can be written HIm$^+$ = H$^+$ + Im, and the fractional dissociation $\alpha =$ (Im)/(HIm$^+$) + (Im). The latter can be related to the buffer ratio. (Im)/(HIm$^+$) = $\alpha/1 - \alpha$. The model proposes that the pacemaker for ventilation is governed by α-imidazole at a specific protein locus, and that a set-point is defended over all physiological temperatures (i.e. the system functions as an alpha-stat for a specific imidazole locus or loci). The difference between expressing ventilation sensitivity classically and as pH versus α can only be detected in systems where comparisons at different body temperatures are made.

STUPFEL: Can the results from fishes be compared to the other data?

RAHN: Yes, I did not present the data. The fish lie on the same line.

BERNDT: Dr. Rahn, whenever I look at the actions of protons, I'm looking for some parameter which depends very distinctly upon the concentration of protons, and one such parameter is the degree of dissociation of calcium compounds which, of course, is quite important for the action of neurons and so on. Now my question is whether anything is known about the pK of calcium compounds and its dependency upon temperature as compared with water. This probably runs parallel also.

RAHN: I do not know.

BERNDT: Well, probably this would be exactly what might happen. But in a case like that, if you have a solution which is alkaline, say of a pH of 8 at 37°C, then you have a very low concentration of ionized calcium; and one unit lower, at a pH of 7, you have about 30 times the ionized calcium. This dependency of ionization upon pH probably changes with temperature.

RAHN: You have brought up an important point which we will have to consider.

ALBERS: Dr. Nahas, some minutes ago, asked for the intracellular pH as a very important regulated variable, and now these lines which you just have drawn refer to the extracellular buffers, especially the buffers of the hemoglobin, the histidines. But if you go to the intracellular buffer, the slope seems to be much greater, and this seems to be different from organ to organ. This makes the question of Dr. Siesjö very difficult to answer. If you have an organ where you can maintain a very fine OH$^-$/H$^+$ ratio as you suggest (and as Dr. Severinghaus has suggested, many years ago when he told an anesthesiologist to ventilate that the carbon dioxide content is constant which is exactly the same as the OH$^-$/H$^+$ ratio) you may have a good ratio, let us say, for the brain and then for the liver it is terrible, or you may make it good for the liver and then it is bad for the heart, and so on, and so on. So I doubt that with hypothermic conditions which are absolutely abnormal for man, you will ever have a normal ventilatory regimen.

RECTOR: My colleague, Dr. Carter, has measured intracellular pH with his microelectrode in a number of different species at different temperatures. In the rat, the barnacle, the frog, and the crab he finds that the intracellular pH is in electrochemical equilibrium with the extracellular fluid. The determinant of intracellular pH is the extracellular pH and the membrane potential. In the poikilothermic animals he finds that the membrane potential is relatively constant over about a 15 to 20 degree temperature change, so that the intracellular pH would parallel your pN line except that it would be below it. Now in contrast, if you cool a homeothermic animal, the membrane potential does not remain constant but begins to drop, so as you cool the animal you now have a dissociation between the intracellular pH and your pN line, which might explain some of the discrepancies in the hibernating animals.

RAHN: I just want to say that these are very important observations. Obviously, we're very much concerned about what the intracellular pH is. Intracellular pH measurements by Reeves in the skeletal muscles of frogs indicate that it runs parallel to our pN line, and it's exactly what you have indicated from your direct approach of intracellular pH measurements.

COURNAND: Would you care to comment on the significance of the shivering that is observed in the human on the mechanism that you described?

RAHN: No, Dr. Cournand, I'm afraid that I have never thought about this problem.

COURNAND: I think that the effect of pH blood is not a primary effect on thermal regulation. The primary regulation of temperature is by the hypothalamus. The hypothalamus controls temperature by hyperpnea against hyperthermia and by vasoconstriction against hypothermia. One can get a great hyperthermia in the animals only by injection of some poison in the brain, or by a chemical change. For example, we can produce a temperature about 43°C in the rabbit only by injection of a little quantity of blood mixed with methylene blue. So in these animals we haven't any change of pH blood, but the temperature is changed from 38°C to 42°C.

6. Carbon Dioxide and Temperature Regulation of Homeothermic Mammals

Maurice Stupfel

Air Pollution Research Center of the
French National Institute of Health and Medical Research (INSERM),
3 rue Léon Bonnat, Paris, 16e, France

Carbon dioxide, which is ubiquitous in the biosphere at the concentration of 0.03 %, can be related in part to volcanic activity, plant metabolism, and secondarily to human air pollution.

Being the product of carbon combustion, CO_2 as well as CO, can be originated in hot environments, as in foundries, blast furnaces, glass works, and other similar industries. In all such manufactories, a sufficient ventilation is ordinarily required by legislation to abate the H_2CO_3 gas concentration below 0.1 %. During great fires such as occurred during the bombings of World War II, CO_2, whether or not associated with hypoxia, carbon monoxide, and very high temperatures, has been reported as the cause of pathological symptoms and even of mortality. Death also occurred among firemen using CO_2 extinguishers to fight fires.

At the opposite gradations of the thermometer, carbon dioxide is encountered in the cold industry, sometimes as dry ice emanations, where it is used for refrigeration of meat and food. When in such cold storage ventilation is insufficient, intoxication due to this gas has been observed.

In closed environments such as submarines, diving, space flights, and bomb shelters, when difficulties occur in air conditioning and gas absorbers circuits, it is possible to observe H_2CO_3 gas accumulation, generally associated with hypoxia, abnormal temperatures, and elevated hygrometries.

As it can be seen, it is possible to find dangerous concentrations of CO_2 in thermal environmental conditions quite far from the normal ones; however, the action of CO_2 on the temperature regulation has been ignored for a long time.

In 1873 Paul Bert presented an observation on the hypothermic death, at rectal temperature between 23°C and 28°C, of a dog rebreathing in a bag filled with O_2, when its CO_2 concentration increases to a level of 35 % to 45 %. Veselkin, in 1913 demonstrated by calorimetric experiment an augmentation of the thermolysis and a decrease of the thermogenesis in dogs and rabbits; the change was due to the action of 10 % CO_2 and also to an increase of the fever in hyperthermic animals. In 1937 Gellhorn published that in rats and mice, 3 % CO_2 enhances the hypothermic effect resulting from hypoxia. Giaja, toward 1953, was the promoter of a method associating hypoxia and hypercapnia (obtained by rebreathing) to external cooling, to cool rats and mice. Using that procedure, Andjus and Smith [1955] refrigerated rats to body temperatures of 0°C to 2°C and succeeded in reanimating some of them by a thoracic local and progressive rewarming. The progressive decrease of the O_2 and increase of the CO_2 content of the confined atmosphere at the end of such a cooling results in about 5 % O_2 and 10 % CO_2.

Concerning the effect of CO_2 alone on temperature regulation, an interesting study was made in 1943 by Barbour and Seevers on rats placed at 5°C in a 10% CO_2 atmosphere. In the subsequent hours, the rectal temperature fell rapidly and according to the degree of the rats' body cooling, the following observations were made: cessation of voluntary movements at 23°C, disappearance of corneal reflexes and pulse at 30 c/min to 100 c/min, respiratory frequency of 1 c/min to 20 c/min at 17°C, and finally death at 14°C. These authors succeeded in maintaining what they called "narcosis" in these rodents for 24 hours, with 10% CO_2 at an external temperature of 18°C to 20°C.

As hypothermia was developed as a mean of anesthesia between 1955 and 1957, attempting to reduce the O_2 consumption and the stress reaction of the body, hypercapnia was tried as an adjunct to anesthesia to prevent shivering during the cooling and, eventually, to increase cerebral flood flow. Such researches, apparently directed toward these purposes, were published by the Americans Niazi and Lewis [1957], who used monkeys, and by Russian biologists such as Repin [1959], who experimented in rabbits. The mechanisms of the dysfunction of temperature regulation by CO_2 has been experimentally studied, mostly by Good and Sellers [1957] and E. B. Brown [1956] on dogs, by Stupfel et al. [1957, 1958, 1959, 1960], Broom [1962], Chapin and Edgar [1963] on rats, and by Chapot [1966, 1970] on cats. Finally, the effect of small concentrations of 3% to 6% carbon dioxide on the human temperature regulatory reactions to a warm or a cold environment have been investigated by Bullard and Crise [1961, 1964].

This report will be limited to homeothermic mammals. The modifications by CO_2 of the metabolism, and consequently of the variations of the internal temperatures of poikilothermic animals, will be discarded. Although hibernating mammals will not be considered, it is impossible to review the effects of carbonic gas on temperature regulation without mentioning the theory of Raphaël Dubois [1895, 1896] on the "carbonic narcosis" and "autonarcosis." According-

ing to him, marmot builds up an excess of CO_2 in its burrow and this causes the animal to hibernate. To prove that, in giving CO_2 to breathe to an awake marmot, he succeeded in lowering its temperature from 37.4°C to 20.4°C. Inversely, by the inhalation of more than 45% CO_2, he obtained, after a considerable increase of its respiratory rate, the arousal of this animal in state of hibernation at a rectal temperature of 12°C. Since that time and with the work of Kayser [1939, 1961] and of Lyman and Hastings [1951], the increase of CO_2 content and the decrease of Pco_2 in hibernating mammals in the hibernating state has mostly been considered the consequence and not the cause of their hypothermia.

For reviewing the action of H_2CO_3 gas on the temperature regulation of homeothermic mammals, the subsequent outline will be followed:

(1) The possibility of the effects of carbon dioxide on temperature regulation will be first experimentally demonstrated in rats, rabbits, dogs, and cats.
(2) Data on men, mostly medical observations and a few experiments, will be presented.
(3) A critical essay to compare these experimental data and observations, obtained from such different mammals and such various experimental conditions, will follow. Finally, an attempt will be made to unite the action of carbon dioxide on the physical, physiological, and biochemical mechanisms of the temperature regulation of the homeothermic mammals and to bring out its chief significances.

Experimental Effects of Carbon Dioxide on the Temperature Regulation of Different Mammals

The effects of a toxic can only be safely estimated on animals and its influence on temperature regulation can only be fully appreciated without any anesthesia; in addition, the test for such effects must be done in an environment that is well controlled thermally and on a sufficient number of individuals. *Rats, rabbits, dogs* and *cats* have been used for experimenting with the effects of carbon dioxide on the temperature regulation of mammals.

Rat

For the previously discussed reasons, also because it is an animal that is easy to handle and to put in sufficient number into small containers where CO_2, as well as O_2, temperature, and hygrometry can be well controlled, Stupfel [1960] chose the rat to experiment with. On a total of 500 albino rats (*Rattus Norvegicus*), he obtained the following results.

The Effect of 10% Carbon Dioxide on the Colic Temperature of Rats Exposed to Ambient Temperatures between +5°C and 42°C

Among a total of 101 male rats, the group of 61 animals used as controls was placed in an airtight container filled with 0.3% CO_2 and 20.9% O_2. A second group of 40 rats, in that same container, breathed 9.7% CO_2 and 26% O_2. In Figure 1, the abcissas are the ambient water-saturated temperatures. In regard to the ordinates, point 0 corresponds to the mean colic temperature (measured at a depth of 7 cm to 10 cm beyond the rectal sphincter) which is $38.1 \pm 1.2°C$ ($\bar{x} \pm \sigma$) before the exposure; + or − means the warming up or the cooling of colic temperature in °C. Hollow circles

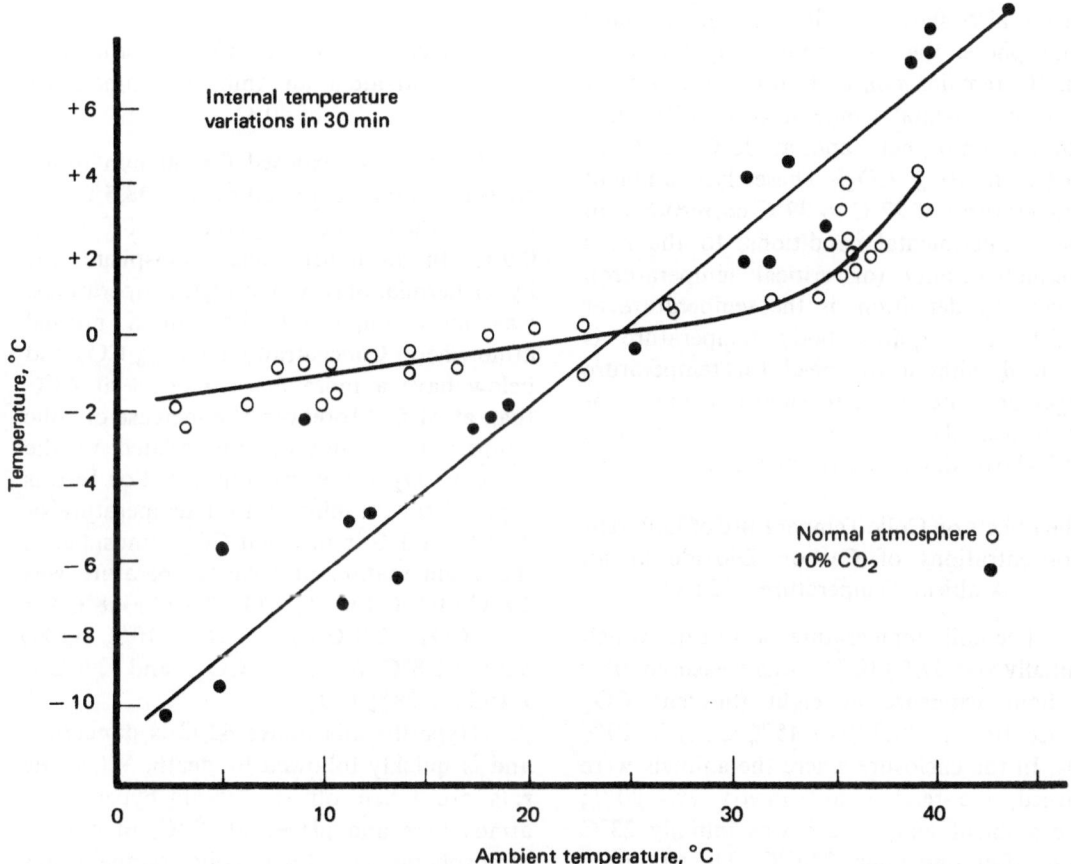

Fig. 1. Variations of rats' colic temperatures after an exposure of 30 min to different ambient temperatures, in a normal atmosphere or in an atmosphere of 10% CO_2.

represent the temperatures of the control rats (20.9 % O_2 and 0.3 % CO_2) and black points the temperatures of the rats in the hypercapnic atmosphere (9.7 % CO_2 and 26 % O_2). In order to avoid adaptive phenomena, one different rat was taken for each experiment. It can be seen that for ambient temperatures between 8°C and 31°C, there is a plateau for the colic temperature of rats in an environment of normal atmospheric gaseous composition. On the contrary, the cold temperature of the animals in the 9.7 % CO_2 atmosphere varies with the ambient temperature. At 30 min of exposure, a straight linear relationship exists between the ambient temperatures (from 5°C to 44°C) and the colic temperature variations (from −10°C to +6°C), which correspond to colic temperatures between 28°C and 44°C. These curves also show that in a water-saturated atmosphere, the rat's colic temperature of 38.1°C remains constant (0°C variation) at an environmental temperature of 26°C in a normal atmosphere and at 28°C (27°C to 29°C) in 10 % CO_2. These last ambient temperatures of 27°C to 29°C correspond, in these experimental conditions, to the rat's thermoneutrality (or critical temperature), which, by definition, is the temperature at which the required body temperature is attained without the need for temperature regulation. Below these environmental temperatures, the rat tends to hypothermia, and above them to hyperthermia.

The Effects on Colic Temperature of Different Concentrations of Carbon Dioxide at an Ambient Temperature of 24°C

The colic temperature of 45 rats, which initially was $37.5 \pm 0.5°C$, was measured after 1 hour exposure at eight different CO_2 concentrations (0.3 % to 45 % CO_2) in 20 % O_2. In the enclosure where the animals were placed, the relative hygrometry was 80 %; the ambient temperature was initially 23°C and, after one hour, 24.6°C. The graph of Figure 2 (each point is a mean and each bar corresponds to 2σ) shows that at an ambient temperature of 24°C there is a fairly linear relationship between the CO_2 concentration, from 0.03 % to 20 %, and the hourly decrease of the rat's colic temperature. Until the concentration of 20 % CO_2, the motility of the animals is apparently normal. Above that concentration, motility is markedly depressed but sensibility to pinching still persists. Above 30 % CO_2, a certain percentage of mortality occurs among the rats, and all the animals die after a one-hour sojourn in a 40 % CO_2 atmosphere, 80 % water saturated. So above 30 %, the high concentration of CO_2 dangerously impeding the circulatory and respiratory functions, the cooling rate tends to follow the physical laws which condition the thermodeperdition of dead corpses (MOLNAR, HURLEY, and FORD [1954]).

The Effect of Different Concentrations of Carbon Dioxide at an Ambient Temperature of 40°C

Sixteen rats exposed for 30 min to an environmental temperature of 38.5°C increased their colic temperature of $0.8°C \pm 0.9°C$. In an hypercapnic atmosphere, the hyperthermia, observed at high temperatures, was more important than in a normal atmosphere. Concentrations of 5 % CO_2 and below have a more marked effect at 43°C than at 24°C. Moreover, the increase of colic temperature is not directly related to the percent CO_2 of the environment. For 16 rats exposed for 30 minutes to a temperature of $39.7°C \pm 1.3°C$ in different CO_2 atmospheres, the augmentation of colic temperature was $2.8°C \pm 0.9°C$ for 3 % CO_2, $3.2°C \pm 0.8°C$ for 5 % CO_2, $2.8°C \pm 1.2°C$ for 10 % CO_2, $5.2°C \pm 0.8°C$ for 22 % CO_2, and $2.6°C \pm 1.4°C$ for 28 % CO_2.

Hyperthermia above 43°C is dangerous and is quickly followed by death. When the rats are taken off the warm hypercapnic atmosphere and placed at 22°C, in normal atmospheric air, their colic temperatures decrease rapidly—for instance from 41.8°C to 39.0°C in 10 min. The recovery of a normal

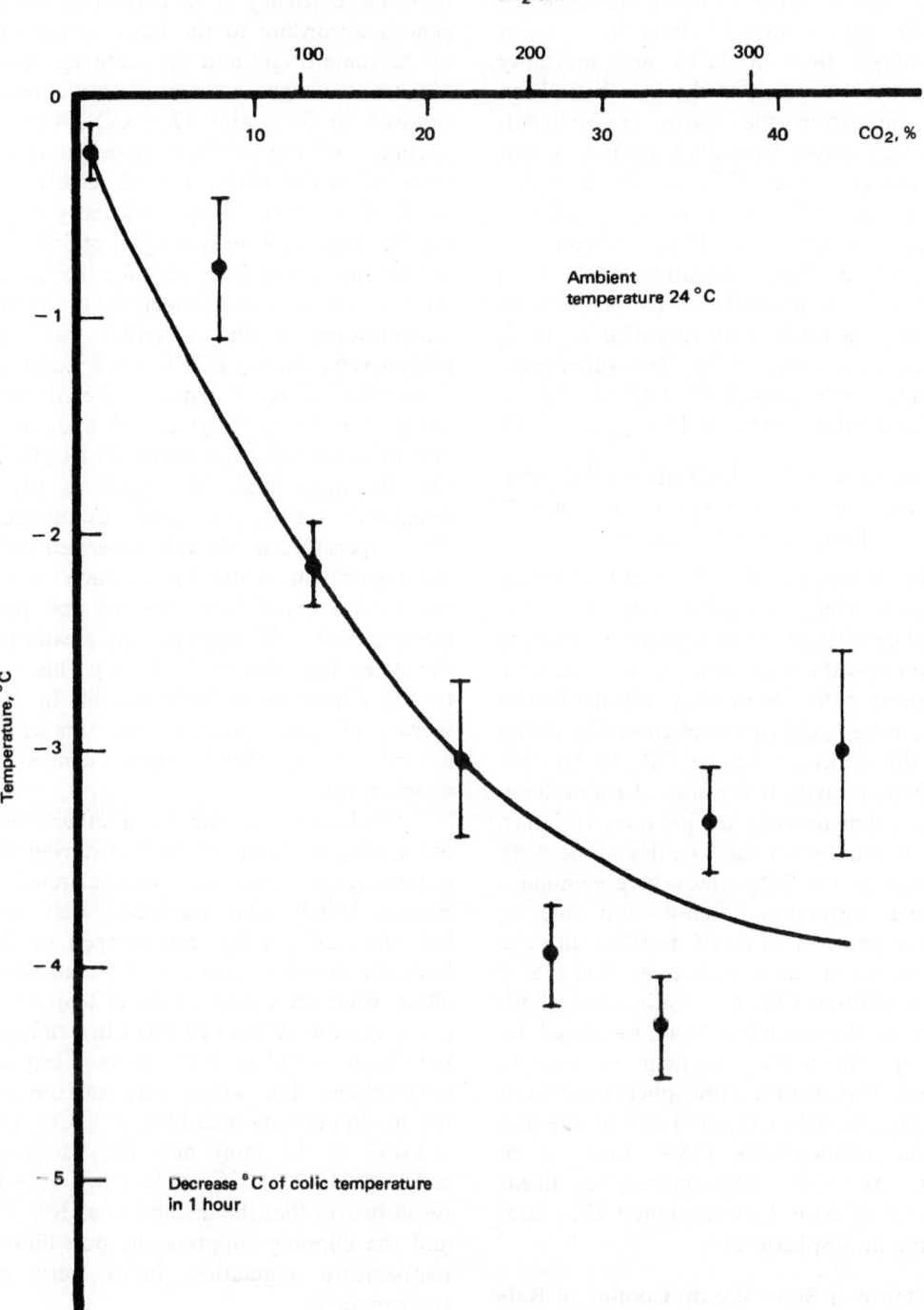

Fig. 2. Hourly decrease of colic temperature of various groups of rats, at different concentrations of CO_2, at an ambient temperature of 24°C.

motility and behavior is much slower when the CO_2 intoxication is done in a warm environment than at 24°C, and mortality has been observed after the rats have been taken out from the warm environment, respiratory arrest preceding cardiac arrest. As a matter of fact, CO_2 toxicity is higher in a warm environment than at ordinary laboratory temperature. If the mortality is cumulated for CO_2 concentrations between 0 and 40% at an ambient temperature of 25°C, 6 of a total of 68 rats died at 40°C, 27 died of a total of 78. The subsequent mortality percentages (8.8% and 34.6%) are significantly different ($\chi^2 = 13.81$; $p < 0.001$).

The Necessity of the Penetration of Carbon Dioxide in the Organism to influence Temperature Regulation

To investigate if CO_2 could influence the temperature regulation only by local contact or whether it could penetrate through the skin into the organism, experiments were performed, either by putting only the bodies of rats in a 8% CO_2 atmospheres or by giving them this concentration of CO_2 to breathe, their bodies staying in the normal atmosphere. The fact that no colic temperature variation was observed when rats' bodies alone were immersed in the CO_2 atmosphere eliminates a direct vasomotor phenomenon due to carbonic gas as a cause of its effect on colic temperature, at least at a concentration of 8%.

In addition CO_2 penetration and elimination in the organism were measured by checking blood CO_2 content of rats in different hypercapnic atmospheres (between 0% CO_2 and 40% CO_2) and at two different ambient temperatures (25°C and 38 to 42°C). At both temperatures, a linear relationship exists between blood CO_2 content and atmospheric CO_2.

Importance of Body Size on Cooling of Rats by 34% to 37% Carbon Dioxide at an Ambient Temperature of 24°C

To investigate the importance of the physical thermodeperdition (radiation, convection, and conduction) and also to deter-

mine the efficiency of its correlated thermogenesis according to the body surface, rats of the same origin and the same age, but of different weights, were simultaneously exposed to 34% and 37% CO_2. For that purpose, 107 rats of the same origin and age were taken (55 males and 52 females), the sexual dimorphism being particularly marked for the sizes, with body weights of 352 ± 55 g for the males and 219 ± 52 g for the females. At the end of a first experiment, the colic temperatures of the surviving rats were, respectively, 34.76 ± 1.20°C for 8 males and 33.98 ± 1.47°C for 8 females (the difference being statistically insignificant) and, at the end of a second experiment, 35.88 ± 0.71°C for 19 males and 34.14 ± 0.91°C for 12 females ($t = 5.80$; $p < 0.001$). Compared to the temperature of the rats measured before the experiment, it can be concluded that in the second experiment, the females' hypothermia (-4.2°C) is significantly greater than the males' hypothermia (-2.1°C). This is due to the difference of body weight, in other words, of body surface; the smaller the animal is, the quicker its internal temperature drops down.

Insulation by fur is another factor influencing the rate of cooling during CO_2 hypothermia. This was demonstrated by Broom [1962] who published that when breathing 20% CO_2, rats clipped of their body fur cooled quicker than those unclipped, either when they were at room temperature (varying from 19°C to 23°C) or in a refrigerator (from -4°C to 0°C). In that last cold environment, the cooling rate was the same for 10 clipped rats breathing 20% CO_2 (11.2 ± 1.0°C in 30 min) and for 10 clipped cadavers (10.2 ± 1.2°C in 30 min). This last result proves that the inhalation of 20% CO_2 and the clipping suppress the possibility of temperature regulation in a very cold environment.

Vasomotor Effects of 10% to 30% Carbon Dioxide at 20°C

As the body surface thermal exchanges are very important, peripheral vasometricity and water shifts intervene on living animals. To judge the vasomotor effects of CO_2 on rats, Stupfel [1960], using thermocouples measured peripheral temperatures (skin, paws, tail) and central temperatures (nose, colon) in unanesthetized rats. From a few measurements he concluded that at an ambient temperature of 20°C, concentrations of CO_2 of 10% and 33% provoke a diminution of the circulation of the peripheral shell of the body and an increase of the caloric deperdition by the respiratory upper ways. At this level, it will be observed that hypercapnia produces a higher increase of the respiratory frequency at an ambient temperature of 39°C than at 25°C.

Water Losses

It can be supposed that CO_2, by its increase of the respiratory rate and its peripheral vasoconstrictive effect, can modify the rat's water losses, either through its respiratory airways or through its body surface. A procedure was imagined to separate the water losses of the respiratory upper ways from those issued through the skin body surface. A group of 14 male rats, deprived of water and food for 18 hours before the measurement, was used for that determination, which lasted one hour. A 10% CO_2 atmosphere increases water elimination between 26°C and 33°C and decreases water elimination above 33.5°C; the partition of the water losses between skin and airways is not modified by this concentration of H_2CO_3 gas.

Oxygen Consumption

Oxygen consumption was measured on 49 rats at 8 different environmental temperatures and in 7 different hypercapnic atmospheres: 8.7%, 13.4%, 18.5%, 19.5%, 28.2%, 32.5% and 36.2% CO_2, in mixtures containing between 19.9% and 35.8% O_2. Simultaneously the same measurements were made with the same apparatus in control rats, in atmosphere containing no CO_2 and between 20.9% and 32.7% O_2. During a 8.7% CO_2 exposure in a cold environment, contrary to what happens in controls, there is no increase of O_2 consumption, but a decrease of colic temperature. For temperatures over 30°C, no significant differences of O_2 consumption appear between hypercapnia and normoxia. As concerns the effects of high doses of CO_2 on O_2 consumption, at 24°C concentrations of 19.5% and 32.5% CO_2 decrease the O_2 consumption even below the basal metabolic rate; for high environmental temperatures (38.5°C to 39.5°C), in comparison to controls, 13.4% CO_2 increases the O_2 consumption, 18.5% and 28.2% CO_2 does not change it, and 36.2% CO_2 decreases it at a level even lower than the basal metabolic rate.

Summary of the Investigations Made on Rats of the Effects of Carbon Dioxide on the Different Physiological Factors of Temperature Regulation

To sum up, the O_2 consumption and evaporative losses, expressed in hourly calories per unit of body surface, and the hourly variations of colic temperature at different environmental temperatures in a normal or in a 10% CO_2 atmosphere, are presented in Figure 3. Two vertical lines at the ambient temperatures of 29°C (thermoneutrality) and 35°C, cutting the three curves (O_2 consumption, evaporative losses, and colic temperature variations) corresponding to measurements made either in normal or hypercapnic atmosphere (10% CO_2 and 21% O_2), delimit on the graph three zones numerated 1, 2, and 3.

In zone 1, corresponding to environmental temperatures below 29°C, hypothermia results from hypercapnia. The caloric losses, due to the cold environment, are normally compensated by the increase of the O_2 consumption observed in the upper curve. But as hypercapnia prevents that compensating increase in metabolism, a lowering of colic temperature (the more important the cooler the environment) has been measured in the hypercapnic rats. As concerns the evaporative water losses, the 10% CO_2 atmosphere does not much interfere with them for ambient temperatures between 7°C

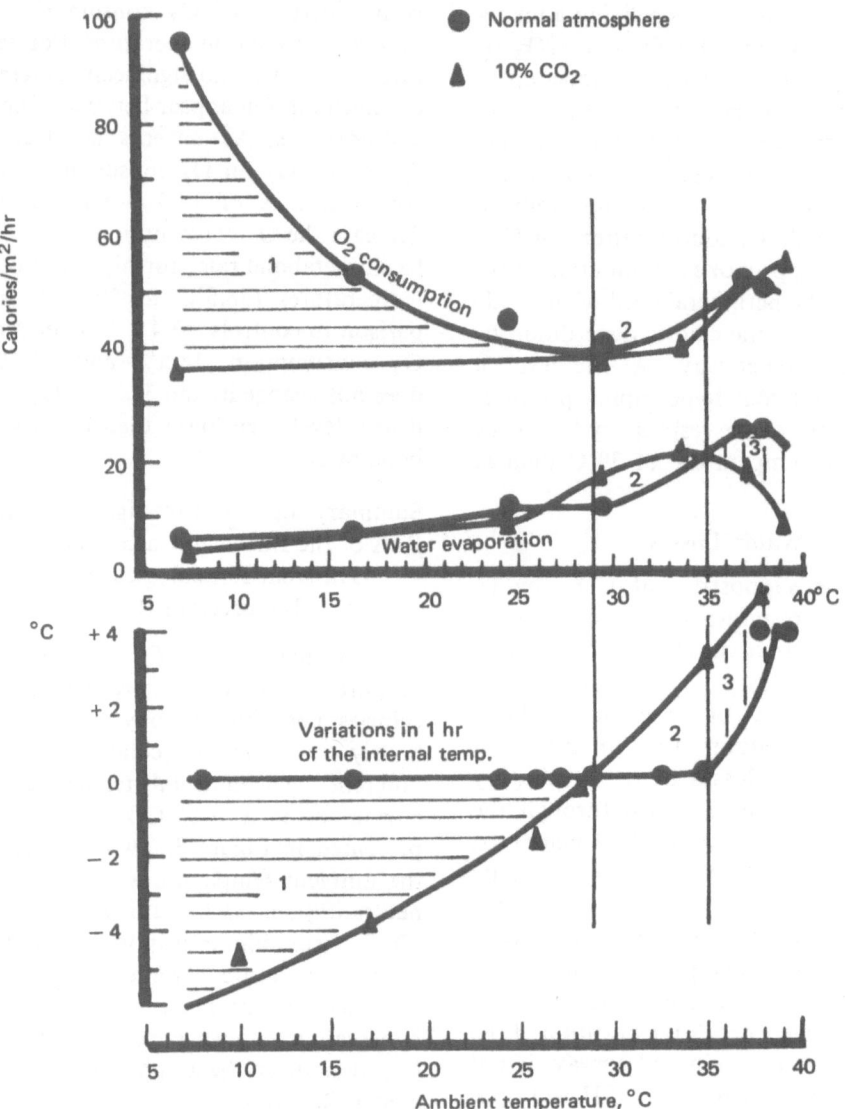

Fig. 3. Summary of the action of a 10% CO_2 atmosphere on O_2 consumption, total water evaporation and hourly variations of colic temperature, at different ambient temperatures.

and 26°C, but increases them above 26°C, which is a factor of hypothermia.

In zone 2, there is a neat increase of the evaporative water losses, while O_2 consumption is but little decreased by 10% CO_2. Therefore the caloric deperdition is less than in a normal atmosphere, which results in the increase in colic temperature depicted in the lower curve.

In zone 3, the 10% CO_2 atmosphere diminishes the evaporation of water and increases metabolism, which provokes hyperthermia and quickly brings the cardiovascular collapse of the animal. Death is preceded by a diminution of the O_2 consumption and of the evaporative water losses. The ambient temperatures of 34°C to 35°C which delimit the lower part of zone 3 appear to be the frontier of the maintenance of homeothermia.

Rabbit

In 1878 Friedlander and Herter, studying the toxicity of CO_2, noted that rabbits could breathe 20% CO_2 during one hour with apparently no toxic effects, otherwise that an increase of the cardiac and respiratory activities occurred. At 30% CO_2 in air, toxicity appears, unconsciousness, a progressive fall of the rectal temperature, and death. A mixture of 80% CO_2 and 20% O_2 rapidly induces narcosis and a rapid decrease of rectal temperature. If the animal is put back in normal air after 15 minutes of such an inhalation, recovery is obtained. Russian pathologists, interested since Veselkin [1913] in the effects of high doses of CO_2 (20% to 30%) on temperature regulation, have used the rabbit as experimental animal (Golodof [1946]). Particularly in 1959, Repin, at Leningrad, published the results of his work on 72 unanesthetized rabbits, breathing through a mask without artificial respiration, mixtures of 5% to 20% CO_2 in air. Skin, muscular, rectal (12 cm beyond the anal sphincter) temperatures, and electromyograms were recorded, and in 6 animals the total thermoproduction was measured by means of a calorimeter. At an ambient temperature of 18°C to 22°C, the hourly decrease in the temperature was 2.3°C for 20% CO_2, of 1.3°C for 10% CO_2, and of 0.8°C for 5% CO_2 concentration, which appeared to be the threshold of the hypothermic action. In most of these experiments, the rabbits breathed 20% CO_2 for a period of 6 to 8 hours. Figure 4 shows the cooling effects, by two separate inhalations, on the rectum, muscle, and thorax temperatures; but meanwhile, the ears' temperature behaves differently. To see whether the apparent ear vasodilation observed could influence the internal temperature cooling by CO_2, the ears of a few rabbits were cut off, which did not influence their central temperature evolution. Figure 5 presents the records of the myogram of the thigh at different times of

the cooling. For lines 1 to 3: from 30 to 75 min after fixation on a table, temperature lowers from 38.9°C to 38.1°C; lines 4 and 5: a hot water bag is placed under the back, rectal temperature is 38.4°C; lines 6 and 7: ice bags, rectal temperature is 38.2°C; lines 8, 9 and 10: inhalation of 5% CO_2 to 20% CO_2 as the rabbit put into ice water is lowering its temperature to 26.3°C (line 10); lines 11 and 12: 40 sec and 2 min after cessation of inhalation of CO_2; line 13: intercostal recording during the cooling under CO_2, with respiratory movements and ECG tracings. As well as these myograms illustrated the cessation of shivering by inhalation of these high concentrations of CO_2, calorimetric

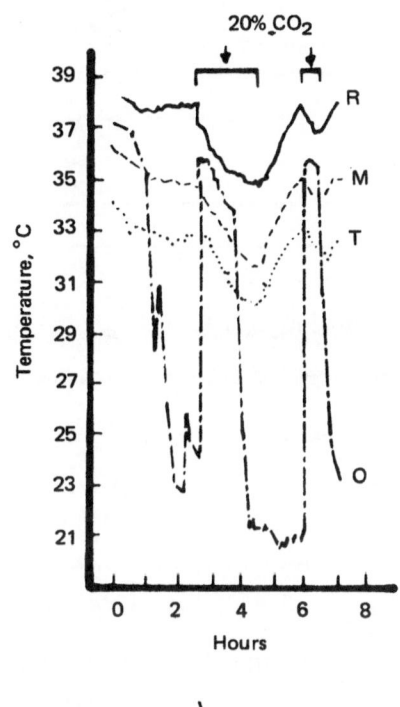

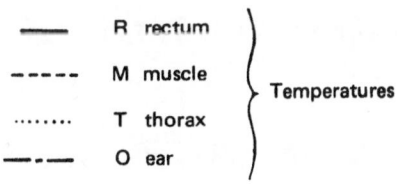

Fig. 4. Temperatures of the rectum, of the muscles, of the skin (thorax) and of the ears in a rabbit, inhaling, during two different intervals of time, a concentration of 20% CO_2. (From REPIN [1954].)

measurements showed that 20% CO_2 diminished the temperature production nearly 50% while the rectal temperatures decreased. Always, according to Repin, the blocking of the shivering by that high dose of CO_2 does not depend on its hypoxic Bohr effect, for it is still observed when 50% O_2 is added to the 20% CO_2 inhaled.

Dog

Good and Sellers [1957] exposed 6 unanesthetized dogs to $-35°C$ for 30 min. The dogs were equipped with thermistors in

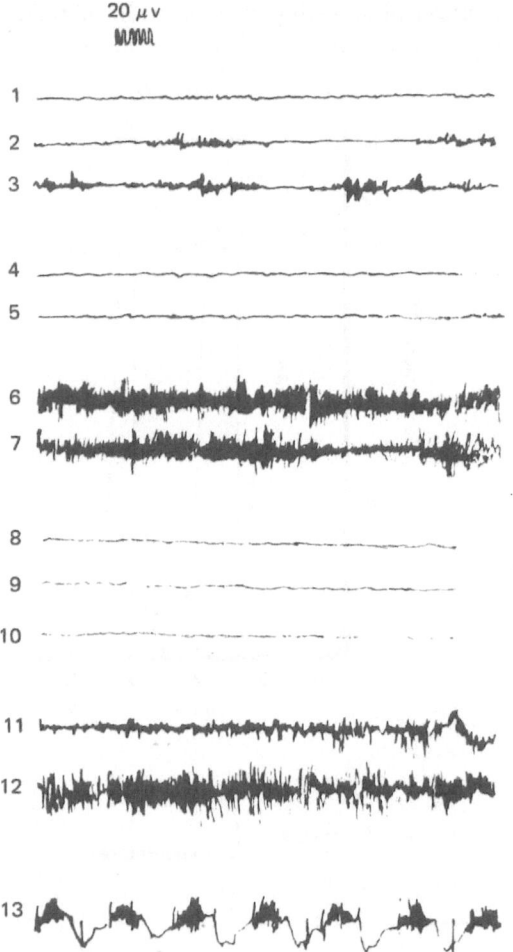

Fig. 5. Electromyograms of a rabbit being cooled and inhaling 5 to 20% CO_2 (lines 8, 9, and 10). The explanation of the different tracings is in the text. (From Repin [1959].)

the pulmonary artery, hepatic vein, rectum, and at different locations of the skin (thorax, forearm, and paw). In practically all experiments, immediately upon exposure to cold the animals shivered, the blood and rectal temperatures increased, and the skin temperatures declined. An inhalation of 4% CO_2 in all cases decreased the visible shivering and, in a few instances, stopped it completely, diminishing the blood and rectal temperatures without changing the skin temperature. Ten minutes after the gas was turned off, the intensity of shivering increased and concurrently blood and rectal temperatures rose. The authors interpret the action of the H_2CO_3 gas as its effect on the cutaneous vasoconstriction due to intense cold, which augments blood and rectal temperatures, while it diminishes cutaneous temperatures. They also noted, "The emotional stress that may have been induced in the animals because of the (CO_2) hyperpnia and feeling of air hunger."

The action of CO_2 on the behavior of dogs to heat stress has been studied by Garrelon and Langlois [1907]: they observed that a concentration of CO_2 above 3.5% prevented the onset of the thermal polypnea. Anrep and Hammouda [1932] observed that 4% to 7.6% of CO_2 increased the total ventilation of a dog in the state of "thermal polypnea," while it decreased its respiratory rate. That phenomenon, not modified by vagotomy, has, according to these authors, a central nervous origin. More recently, Brown [1956] elevated of $2°C$ to $3°C$, the body temperature of 10 pentothal anesthetized dogs, by inhalation of warm moist oxygen, and by infrared lamps and heating pad application. This hyperthermia decreased the tolerance (as judged by blood pressure, arterial pH, and ECG) of the animals to the inhalation of 30% CO_2 plus 70% O_2 in accelerating the cardio-vascular collapse.

Cat

The effects of CO_2 on a cat's temperature regulation has been studied by Chapot [1966, 1967, 1970]. On 5 of these curarized and artificially ventilated animals at room temperatures between 23°C and 25°C, the inhalation during 3 hours of 4.8% CO_2 diminished the O_2 consumption and also the rectal temperature. As soon as normal air was given back, the O_2 consumption increased and the cooling was simultaneously reduced. In other experiments, made with the same technique and on cats as well, metabolism decreased when FA_{CO_2} of 4% to 7% was obtained. In 16 cats, anesthetized and artificially ventilated (and with section of the medulla and of the vagosympathetic trunks to isolate the motoneurones from the encephale), shivering, obtained by immersion in cold water baths, was diminished when FA_{CO_2} was raised from 2% to 6%.

Reports of the Effects of Carbon Dioxide on Man's Temperature Regulation

There are old and numerous reports about the action of CO_2 on man's temperature, either locally (mainly in the carbogaseous baths) and more rarely by inhalation. However, as soon as 1862, in France, Ozanam, using a mixture of 75% CO_2 in air for general anesthesia to incise an abscess of the thigh, noted a profuse sweating of the face of his patient. In spite of their number, most of the observations, on the effects of CO_2 on man's temperature regulation, are difficult to interpret for lack of measurements and lack of precision about the associated conditions. Just in recent years, a few experiments (BULLARD and CRISE [1961]; BULLARD [1964]) are of a real scientific interest, but the medical ones could not just be ignored.

Local Thermic Effects

The carbogaseous baths attracted attention to the action of CO_2 on peripheral temperature sensibility. Liljestrand and Magnus [1922], in the course of a study at Saint-Moritz, noted that the peripheral vasoconstriction normally observed in a cold bath is replaced, in a carbogaseous one, by a marked cutaneous vasodilation with a sub-jective sensation of warmth. The increase of the caloric deperdition can diminish by 1°C the rectal temperature of the subject. These observations were subsequently confirmed by Gollwitzer-Meier [1937], who described a cutaneous redness accompanying the sensation of warmth. Burton and Bazett [1936], measuring the exchanges of heat and vasomotor responses by means of a bath calorimeter, bubbled CO_2 into the tube where a man was immersed until they got a P_{CO_2} of 180 torr of the water; they added then an excess of baryta water to remove the H_2CO_3 gas. During these procedures, they obtained barely measurable changes in conductivity (less than 8%) and only fleeting sensations of temperature.

The observations of the local effects of CO_2 as a gas are not so numerous. However, in 1855, Boussingault, visiting a mine of sulphur in New Granada, noted that the natural gas released near a volcano "provokes a sensation of unpleasant warmth and pricklings like a sinapism, when the ambient air temperature is only 19.5°C." Goldscheider [1887], DuBois-Reymond [1893], Goldscheider and Ehrmann [1924], plunging the hand in a CO_2 dry or humid atmosphere, felt a sensation of warmth without local erythema. According to these last authors, on man's hand H_2CO_3 gas should lower, by 5°C to 7°C, the threshold of the sensation of warmth; in other terms, a hand immersed at 18°C in a pure CO_2 atmosphere would have the same sensation of warmth as if it were immersed in air at 25°C. It was stated by Schindewolf and Weigmann [1952], who explored with tiny thermoelectrodes the points of the back of the hand sensitive to the warmth and the cold, that CO_2, in gas or in solution, suppresses the excitability of the cold thermoreceptors and increases that of the warm receptors. Moreover, it must be remembered, as it will be seen later, that in pure H_2CO_3 gas, thermoconductivity is greater than in air. According to Weigmann and Schindewolf [1954], CO_2 would also suppress the cutaneous sensitivity to pain. The suppression of these peripheral excitations is even more difficult to prove during a sojourn in a hypercapnic atmosphere where, in addition to objective symptoms such as hyperventilation resulting from inhalation of the H_2CO_3 gas, many other subjective and psychological factors can interfere and affect sensitivity, shivering, or sudation.

In 6 experiments, made on 2 subjects, Stupfel did not observe any local action of pure CO_2 on the sweating of hands for ambient temperatures between 32°C and 42°C and interdigital temperatures between 36°C and 37°C.

Concerning the vasodilating or anesthetic local effect of high concentrations of CO_2 in water solution or as a gas, the possibility of a diffusion through the skin into the organism must be considered (SHAW and MESSER [1931]; KRAMER and SARRE [1935]; GENAUD and GROS [1954]). It is the opinion of certain physicians that during carbogaseous water baths, the diffusion of CO_2 through the skin would explain the erythematous reaction of the immersed part of the body and even a lowering of the blood pressure by a direct action of the gas on the skin vessels and on their innervation.

Effects of Inhalation

The main thermal effects that CO_2 has on man, when it is inhaled in small concentrations, are modifications of temperature sensations, sweating, and shivering. It will be stressed again that many times, it is difficult to distinguish them from the other physiological effects of CO_2. The most important of these actions and the most easily observed is the progressive augmentation of the respiratory volume for CO_2 concentration increasing from 3% to 10% (COMROE [1965]), with some interindividual variations (SCHAEFER [1958]), mixtures containing more than 10% decreasing the ventilation. These conditions of discomfort can influence thermoreactions such as sweating and shivering that are physiological phenomena on which psychological and stress factors can be of a determining importance.

Thermal Sensitivity

During 2% to 5% CO_2 inhalation, subjects generally feel warmer. It has been proposed that the breathing of the gas, like its direct contact with the skin, inhibits the activity of the cold thermoreceptors. However, Bullard and Crise [1961], in two subjects breathing 6% CO_2, did not find any effect of the gas on the thermal impressions due to the cooling by a thermode, and the reports of Schaefer [1958] pointed out their individual variations.

Sweating

Sweating, provoked in man by inhalation of CO_2 has been known a long time ago (Ozanam [1862]). Later, Haldane and Smith [1893] noted transpiration appearing in a man rebreathing in a balloon, and sweating is given as a sign of CO_2 retention in manuals of anesthesia. Adachi [1936] reported, unfortunately at unknown environmental temperatures, that sweating appears on the forehead, the chest, the axillas, the palms of the hands, and the soles of the feet, in subjects breathing 4% to 10% CO_2. If the inhalations of H_2CO_3 gas are repeated, sweating is not obtained any more. E. W. Brown [1930] noted that 6% CO_2 breathed with a mask provoked a respiratory uneasiness, dyspnea, throat irritation, a sensation of fainting, and also sweating of the face. Schaefer [1958] has observed that, at room temperature, sweating during CO_2 inhalation was greater in subjects who showed the highest ventilatory responses. Estimating sweating by measurement of resistance hygrometry, Bullard [1964] studied 9 male subjects exposed in a controlled environmental chamber at either 27°C, 38°C, or 49°C with low relative humidity. At these three temperatures, the inhalation of 6% CO_2 provoked, on the arm, a significant increase of the sweating rate and was much more pronounced at 49°C than at 27°C (Figure 6). The skin temperature decreased during the CO_2 inhalation and the sweating. Using the weighing method, Houdas [1971] observed that subjects placed

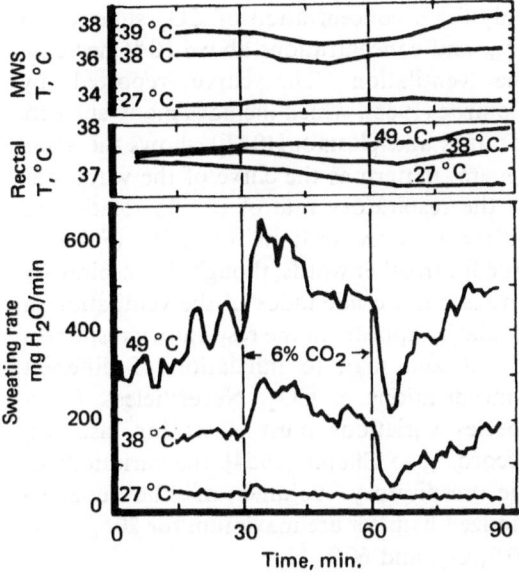

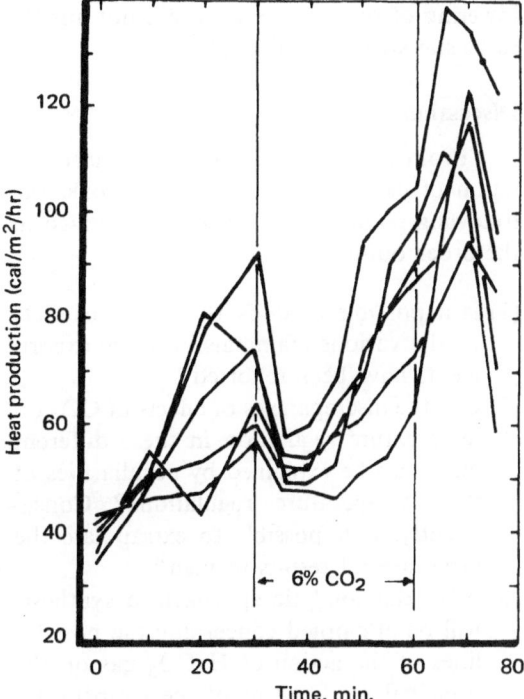

Fig. 6. Effects of 6% CO_2 on sweating rates recorded from the arm in a plastic chamber, rectal temperature, and mean weighted skin temperature. These different ambient temperatures were used. Each curve represents the mean of six experiments. (From BULLARD [1964/ 1961].)

Fig. 7. Heat production of six subjects exposed to 5°C; 6% CO_2 breathed from 30th to 60th[i] minute of exposure time. (From BULLARD and CRISE [1961].)

at 40°C and inhaling 4% CO_2 increase their sweating rate while their cutaneous, rectal, and tympanic temperatures are decreased. After 15 mins whether inhalation is continued or not, the sweating rate comes back to its initial level.

Shivering

In 1949 Hensel reported that an inhalation of 3% CO_2 produces shivering in a naked subject entering into a cold room at a temperature of 10°C, without modifying his rectal and cutaneous temperatures. But Bullard and Crise [1961] did not confirm that observation. On the contrary, in 6 men exposed to an ambient temperature of 5°C for 75-min periods, they reported that the breathing of 6% CO_2 inhibited shivering. However, when the inhalation lasted 30 min, the shivering was overcome. Concurrently, the evolution of the O_2 consumption was parallel to that of the shivering, but though

it was diminished by the inhalation of the carbonic gas, it never fell to basal levels (Figure 7).

Long-term Exposure to 1.5% Carbon Dioxide

An experiment was performed at New London on 23 male subjects confined in a submarine and exposed to 1.5% CO_2 in 21% O_2; the experiment was conducted over a period of 42 days, with a 9-day control period, prior and also following exposure (SCHAEFER [1961]). Oral temperature measurements were made daily at 8 A.M. They gave: 36.17 ± 0.32°C before the experiment, 36.06 ± 0.23 during days 1 to 23 of breathing 1.5% CO_2 (uncompensated respiratory acidosis), 36.08 ± 0.19 during the days 24 to 42 of 1.50% CO_2 inhalation (compensated acidosis), and 36.13 ± 0.08 during the 9 days recovery period of breathing air. The small lowering of oral temperature did not appear to be statistically significant.

Discussion

From this quite heterogeneous accumulation of experiments and observations, the following points are going to be examined in the order outlined below.

(1) Is it possible to unify the effects of CO_2 on the various mammals in which experiments have been reported?

(2) Can the discrepancies of effects of CO_2 on temperature regulation in these different mammals be explained by peculiarities of their temperature regulations? Consequently, is it possible to extrapolate the experimental results to men?

(3) After this analytic approach, a synthesis will be attempted concerning the possibilities of the action of H_2CO_3 gas on the principal mechanisms of the temperature regulation, divided into temperature deperdition and temperature production.

(1) Comparison of the Effects of Carbon Dioxide According to the Various Mammals on Which Its Action on Temperature Regulation has been studied

The first main thing to be brought out of the previously reported results and observations is that temperature regulation can be peremptorily inhibited by only high concentrations of CO_2, e.g. 10% and above. For these concentrations, experiments are only possible in animals, for they will look dangerous for man, on which however a few observations were made during accidental hypercapnia.

The best known physiological actions of CO_2 are the respiratory modifications that it provokes in practically all animal species. However, the elicited response is not unique but depends on the concentration, as shown by results of studies made in man by Haldane and Smith [1893], E. W. Brown [1930], Consolazio et al. [1947], Schaefer et al. [1963]. An increase in respiratory volume is obtained only for a concentration of CO_2 superior to 3%, and concentrations above 10% decrease the ventilation. The curve reported by Comroe [1965], which includes many subjects (DRIPPS and COMROE [1947]), shows the same general pattern as the curve of the variations of the respiratory rate of rats in relation to different concentrations of CO_2 (STUPFEL [1960]). In other words, though the respiratory rate is but a crude index of the ventilation, a similarity appears in the respiratory responses of rat and man to inhalation of different concentrations of CO_2. Nevertheless, interspecies variations must exist; for instance, according to Chapin [1954], the variations of the respiratory volume of the unanesthetized hamster are maximum for 20% CO_2, 20% O_2, and 60% N_2.

Another general effect of high concentration of CO_2 is its hypoxic action, resulting from the Bohr effect, which is a displacement toward the right of the oxyhemoglobin dissociation curve by an increase of the blood P_{CO_2}. However the consequences of the Bohr effect are not the same for all mammals, as a consequence of the discrepancies between their HbO_2 dissociation curves (BARTELS et al. [1963]). For example, according to Jones, Maegraith, and Schulthorpe [1950], the rat's oxyhemoglobin dissociation curve is more to the left than those of man and other mammals (cat, dog, rabbit, guinea pig, cow, goat, and horse). From this, it follows that the rat should be more sensitive to hypoxia; for instance, for a P_{O_2} of 50 torr for man and dog, hemoglobin should be saturated at 85% and for rat, at only 52%. In spite of that, maybe as a consequence of the hyperventilation due to the increase of P_{CO_2}, the augmentation of the O_2 content of the CO_2 mixtures did not change the cooling effect of different concentrations of CO_2, as was reported in rats (STUPFEL [1960]), and in rabbits (REPIN [1959]).

Though it is difficult to be quite positive, it would seem reasonable when reading the literature (ROUGIER [1947]; SOLLMANN [1964]) to establish a certain uniformity of actions in different kinds of mammals for different concentrations of CO_2. These might include the increase of the pulmonary ventilation for 4% to 6%; culmination of respiratory stimulation for 10% to 15%; depressive ataxia (or narcosis?) for 25% to 30%, coma and death for 40% to 50%. The work of Stupfel and Bouley [1971] concerning acute toxicity will serve as an example. Using young Sprague Dawley and Wistar rats as well as CF_1 mice, at environmental temperatures of 20°C to 25°C they brought about death in about 50% of the animals in 1 to 4 hours for concentrations of 30% to 40% CO_2, with no difference relating to species or to sex.

To conclude this part of the discussion, if there is a gross similarity between the physiological and toxicological effects of CO_2 in the different kinds of mammals on which an effect on temperature regulation was demonstrated, still, as in the case of the Bohr effect, there could be obvious differences. So extrapolation to man of toxicological actions, especially concerning effects on the central nervous system, is quite dubious.

(2) Particularities of the Temperature Regulation Mechanisms of the Mammals for Which Carbon Dioxide Action on Homeothermia has Been Investigated

The results exposed above concerned mainly rats; some findings have been reported on rabbits, cats, and dogs, and the observations on men are infrequent.

The rat, though it is a nocturnal animal, has been used as a "model" for many physiological researches, but concerning its temperature regulation, it has many particularities. First it is very small—200 g compared to a man of 70 kg is a 1/350 part. If the temperature regulation processes are ignored and if the volume alone is considered, a body of 200 ml is much easier to cool or to warm than a body of 70 l. For this reason, the rat has a relatively high metabolic rate, as it results from the relations between weight, surface, body size, and heat production (BRODY [1954]; KAYSER [1963]; PROSSER and

BROWN [1966]). The maintenance of homeothermia in such a small animal which, as a consequence of its tiny size, cools and warms quickly, requires an almost instantaneous trigger release of heat production on heat deperdition, for small variations of environmental temperatures. Secondarily, the rat appears to be more able to protect itself against cold than against warmth. The albino rat on which the experiment was done has a nice thick fur entrapping an air layer from 0.3 cm to 0.8 cm. In addition, a thick skin reinforced by a good layer of fat augments its body insulation against cold. To combat heat its defences are not as good. Its aprocine sudation is apparently devoid of thermoregulatory significance, but, is one of its sexual secondary characters (KUNO [1934]), and the sweating exocrine glands are rare (RÖMER [1896]; HIERONYMI [1931]; TENNENT [1945]; RING and RANDALL [1947]). At high temperatures, ordinarily no panting appears in the rats, but water losses through the skin and the upper airways increase. Sometimes, too, when the rat is licking its fur with its saliva—hypersalivation—could be considered a means of thermodeperdition (HAINSWORTH and STRICKER [1969]).

Other possibilities of temperature regulation in such an animal covered with a thick fur coat are provided by the naked appendages of its tail (KNOPPERS [1942]; CHEVILLARD, ARNAL, and GIONO [1958]) and paws, which realize efficient heat exchanging organs. Their colorations vary from purple to red when the ambient temperature varies from cold to warm. High doses of CO_2 stops the circulation in these different appendages and make them appear cold and cyanotic.

In small mammals, pulmonary hyperventilation can play a particular role in their temperature regulation, either in the warmth, in helping to augment the caloric deperdition, or in the cold, in permitting the increase of the O_2 consumption. Chapin [1954] observed that in a wake hamster, respiratory volume is two times greater either at 22°C or 30°C than at 27°C to 28°C. The measurements of Schmidt-Nielsen [1952], as well as those of

Stupfel, give 24°C for the rat's intranasal temperature. In a warm environment, the gradient of humidity between inspired and expired air gets a determining role in the evaporative water losses. Besides, the smaller the animal the greater is its O_2 consumption and, consequently, the greater must be its ventilation in order to bring it a sufficient quantity of O_2. In his thesis, inspired by Bargeton, Chassain [1959] noted that when cold, the rat increases its ventilation at the same time as its O_2 consumption, and he proposed that in small mammals this hyperactivity of the respiratory muscles can be considered a process of defense against cold as well as an increase of the muscular tone or of shivering.

The other animals—rabbits, dogs, and cats—in which the temperature reactions towards CO_2 were studied have, as the rats, no sweat glands.

However, the most conspicuous peculiarity of dogs is the hyperventilation provoked by heat which permits it, when it pants, to augment its heat deperdition by cooling its tongue. As it has been seen previously, the way in which the thermal polypnea of this animal is modified by CO_2 is difficult to interpret. Cats and rabbits also present a thermal polypnea of a thermolytic significance, and CO_2 also makes them hyperventilate. However, to be efficient to remove an excess of calories, such increased ventilation should be quite shallow and must not involve deep respiratory movements; otherwise oxygen consumption would augment (FINDLAY [1957]).

Under conditions of cold, the numerous arteriovenous anastomoses of the ears of the rabbit, widely influenced by temperature as Grant et al. pointed out [1932], present episodic periods of vasoconstriction and vasodilation called "hunting phenomenon," which have an important temperature regulatory significance and which are quite similar to what was depicted by Repin, as it has been previously discussed.

In man, other considerations must not be forgotten concerning the variations observed in subjects from different origins, races, and countries, for in a general way, man, instead of getting acclimatized to adverse environments, succeeds always to avoid them by clothing and housing processes. To take him out of his well protected microclimate, without any training, and to put him in a climatic stress, aggravated by a gaseous intoxication, could have more serious consequences than it could be presumed.

(3) Carbon Dioxide and the Different Mechanisms of Temperature Regulation

In an homeothermic animal, temperature regulation is the sum of the mechanisms which keep its temperature constant as it is subjected often to wide variations of the ambient temperature. For that, at every moment an equilibrium between thermogenesis and thermolysis must be maintained; otherwise homeothermia would not be preserved. The modifications of thermolysis, which are operated through purely physical processes and are physiologically obtained by vasodilation, vasoconstriction, and water evaporation through the skin or the superior respiratory airways, constitute the physical temperature regulation. The modifications of thermogenesis, which consist in increases of the intensity of the oxidations above the basal metabolic rate, are the support of the chemical temperature regulation. So now, in an attempt to get to a synthetic approach, the possible effects of CO_2 on these various temperature regulatory mechanisms will be discussed.

Action of Carbon Dioxide on the Physiological Thermolytic Mechanisms

Heat deperdition results from physical factors: radiation, convection, conduction, and evaporation. Among these factors which depend primarily on the thermal, hygrometric, and anemometric conditions of the environment and of the surface exposure of the animals, conduction only can be physically modified by CO_2. The thermoconductibility of pure CO_2 is less than the thermoconductibility of air. According to Fritz (HENNING [1938]) CO_2: ct at $0°C = 1.23$ and at $50°C = 1.23$; air: ct at $0°C = 2.07$ and at $50°C = 2.35 \times 10^{-2}$ K cal/m h °C, so that hypercapnic mixtures should, in a cold environment, prevent the cooling and in a hot environment prevent the warming up.

These physical exchanges of temperature depend on the body surface of the animal, in other words, on its size, also in addition to its position, they depend on postural changes, such as curling in cold to reduce body surface (BARGETON [1954, 1955]). Consequently, radiative losses are indirectly influenced by concentrations of CO_2 above 20% that decrease motility and so impede the way in which the living mammal can modify its radiating surface.

CO_2 acts also on the physiological reactions which determine that physical thermolysis and which are the peripheral vasomotor reactions, mostly cutaneous, the cardiovascular reactions conditioning them, the water shifts in the different compartments of the body, and the water losses.

Action of Carbon Dioxide on the Chemical and Physiological Mechanisms of Heat Production

At thermoneutrality (critical temperature), the O_2 consumption of a homeothermic mammal is at its minimum, which corresponds to its basal metabolic rate and which is controlled by the obligatory thermogenesis. To resist to cold, the mammal increases its O_2 consumption to enhance its oxidations. This corresponds to the chemical temperature regulation (defined by Rubner [1902] as an augmentation of heat production) in the animal at rest and exposed to cold. This chemical temperature regulation, also called regulatory thermogenesis, can be decomposed in shivering thermogenesis and in non-shivering thermogenesis (CARLSON and HSIEH [1970]).

So we will examine, in the following order, the action of CO_2 on the *O_2 consumption*, on the participation of muscles in temperature regulation, on the *cellular oxidations*, and its effect on the *endocrines* which control these chemical thermoregulatory processes.

Oxygen Consumption

At environmental temperature, below thermoneutrality CO_2, for concentrations between 3% and 10%, increases the O_2 consumption, mostly as a consequence of the hyperventilation it causes. More precisely, man breathing 3% to 5% CO_2 enhances his metabolism by an augmentation of the work of his respiratory muscles and an increase of his cardiac output (SHEPHARD [1955]). It has previously been reported that, for the rat, at thermoneutrality ($27°C$ to $29°C$), 8.5% CO_2 did not change the value of the O_2 consumption, i.e. of the basal metabolic rate. But, if the hyperventilation provoked by these small concentrations of CO_2 is abolished, as can be done by suppressing the central nervous system, it could be expected that CO_2 by itself decreases the O_2 consumption. For example, according to Cordier, Magne and Mayer [1927], in the curarized and artificially ventilated rabbit, with a section of the medulla oblongata, 4.21% CO_2 in 21% O_2 diminishes the O_2 consumption by 14%. In other words, it can be supposed that, at small doses, CO_2 conceals its inhibiting effect on O_2 consumption by the increase in pulmonary ventilation which it provokes.

For environmental temperatures inferior to thermoneutrality, it has been reported, in rats, that 8.8% CO_2 inhibits the augmentation of metabolism provoked by their exposure to cold, i.e., it inhibits the chemical temperature regulation as defined by Rubner [1902]; on the contrary, for temperatures superior to that thermoneutrality, this same concentration tends to increase the metabolism. Chevillard [1935], in mice breathing 10% to 15% CO_2, noted a decrease of 30% to 65% of their respiratory exchanges with disturbances of their body temperatures. He found also, in these same animals, that hypoxia, resulting from the inhalation of 8%

O_2, diminishes their O_2 consumption from 40%, which results in hypothermia.

Higher concentrations of CO_2 (20% to 30%) lowered, in cold and even once in a warm environment, the O_2 consumption of rats below the basal metabolic rate. Chapin and Edgar [1963], in 4 rats breathing 30% CO_2, also obtained, at an ambient temperature of 28°C, a decrease of more than 50% of their basal metabolic rate. In the experimental conditions that have just been described, Cordier, Magne and Mayer [1927] got a decrease of 60% in the O_2 consumption of rabbits inhaling 18.93% CO_2.

Muscles have a great place in the reflex thermogenesis, represented by increase of muscular tone and shivering when the ambient temperature is below thermoneutrality. The inhibition of shivering by CO_2 results from the experiments of Repin [1959] with rabbits breathing concentrations of 15% to 20% CO_2, of Good and Sellers [1957] in anesthetized dogs inhaling 4% CO_2, of Chapot [1967] in anesthetized cats artificially ventilated with a mixture containing 6% CO_2, and of Bullard and Crise [1961] in men inspiring 6% of the gas. The decrease of shivering or muscular tone by CO_2 can be interpreted either as a direct action on muscular contraction or as a nervous inhibition. In favor of the first hypothesis, Haywood [1927] reported that the contraction of the muscle cutaneous pectoris of the frog, immersed in Ringer, is inhibited by CO_2, and not by anoxia or by its acidification with chlorhydric acid. Biochemically, that would correspond to an action of CO_2 on the ATPase and on the contractile proteins of the muscle, which are the supposed factor of the muscular tone and shivering. The second hypothesis should show a direct action of CO_2 on the peripheral receptors, which would produce the disappearance of the sensation of cold (Dodt [1956]; Boman, Hensel, and Witt [1957]), or at high doses, where there would be a possible effect on the medullary (Besson, Benoist, and Aleonard [1971]) and/or hypothalamic centers. To explain the overcoming of shivering by 6% CO_2, which

they have demonstrated in man, Bullard and Crise [1961] suggest that after a period of inhibition, which lowers heat production and increases respiratory heat loss, the total thermal drivers are increased so that the hypothalamic thermostat is once more activated.

Cellular Oxidations

The similitude observed by Stupfel [1960], on the rats' metabolism, of the effects of a 9.0% CO_2 and of a 11% O_2 atmosphere induces one to advance that, in both cases, the suppression of the increase of the O_2 consumption with cold is related to a diminution of the oxidation and/or other biochemical-related processes which produce caloric energy. Besides, the - hypothermic effect of hypoxia on different mammals at a temperature below thermoneutrality is a well established fact (Béhague, Garsaux, Richet [1927]; Mayer [1931]; Chevillard [1935]; Gellhorn and Janus [1936]; Giaja [1940]; Kottke et al. [1948]; Blood and Glover [1949]; Hemingway and Nahas [1952]; Cheymol and Levassort [1956]; Chanel [1956]; Hill [1959]; Van Liere and Stickney [1963]; Bhatia, Georges, and Rao [1969]).

Though it is not our purpose to investigate here the biochemical aspect of the CO_2 effects on the temperature regulation processes, it can be supposed that three mechanisms can be chemically involved: the Krebs cycle, the Bohr effect, and modifications by pH changes or enzymatic activities to which nerve cells are particularly sensitive.

Endocrinal Controls of the Chemical Temperature Regulation

The adrenal medulla is the chief gland defending homeothermia against cold, especially by releasing norepinephrine, which increases metabolism and has a possible indirect action on cyclic AMP. Thibault (1946, 1948, 1949), evaluates at 40% its part in the cold thermogenesis of the rat. Concerning this gland, it has been known for a long time that H_2CO_3 gas directly excites the sympathoadrenal system, both via nervous system pathways and by a less important direct action on the adrenalin secretion centers (CANNON and HOSKINS [1911]; ANREP [1912]; TOURNADE and MALMEJAC [1934]; SCHAEFER et al. [1955]; TENNEY [1956, 1960]). As cold also increases the secretion of epinephrine, it would be suspected that CO_2 and cold would, in a general way, add their action on the sympathetic system. Binet and Burstein [1949], reporting on the dog's leg perfused with a constant flow, said that a concentration of 10% CO_2 reinforced the vasoconstriction provoked by epinephrine, if the blood vessels are normally innervated as well as if they are disconnected from the central nervous system. But, according to Tenney [1956], the hypertension following an injection of epinephrine is diminished by carbon dioxide and the response of the nictating membrane to epinephrine is inhibited by CO_2 concentrations between 3% and 15%. In the rat breathing 10% CO_2 at three different temperatures, Stupfel and Roffi [1960] observed at 23°C a decrease of the content of the catecholamines of the suprarenals with a simultaneous increase of their levels in the blood. At 10°C (where an hypothermia of -6.7°C was obtained) and at 32°C, the abovementioned concentration of CO_2 suppressed the catecholamines variations in the plasma, but not those in the suprarenals. In man, inhalation of 7% to 15% CO_2 caused elevations both in epinephrine and norepinephrine concentrations (PRICE [1960]).

The adrenal cortex have a secondary role in the defense against cold, mostly in the adaptating processes to cold. Experiments on rats have shown, once more, that opposite results can be obtained for different concentrations of carbonic acid gas. When inferior to 5%, they protect against the stresses of exposures to 3°C or to 36°C to 37°C, stresses which are demonstrated by a depletion of the adrenal cortex in ascorbic acid and in cholesterol (LANGLEY and KILGORE [1955]). On the contrary, in rats, a 15% CO_2 and 19% O_2 atmosphere results in an hyperplasia of the suprarenal cortex and in an involution of the lymphatic tissue

(FORTIER [1949]), and for concentrations between 10% and 30% CO_2, the adrenal cortex is depleted of its ascorbic acid and cholesterol content (LANGLEY and KILGORE [1955]). In the guinea pig, according to Schaefer, King, and Williams [1955], a mixture of 30% CO_2 in air should provoke, in a delay of 10 to 60 min, an increase of the weight of the suprarenals, an augmentation of the blood eosinophils and a diminution of the cholesterol of the suprarenals. The direct measurement by Richards and Stein [1957] of the 17-hydroxycorticosteroids in the blood of the suprarenal vein of the anesthetized dog, shows that, for CO_2 concentrations between 2% and 30%, the response of the adrenal cortex is directly related to the CO_2 percentage. Besides, for 20%, a marked increase of the 17-hydroxycorticosteroids is observed in the 15 first minutes. As the augmentation of these corticosteroids is suppressed by hypophysectomy, Richards and Stein conclude that this secretion is controlled by ACTH. These same authors insist on the role of the carbon dioxide acidosis (arterial pH of 7.00 and below, P_{CO_2} of 100 torr) on these endocrinal reactions. Besides, Nahas [1957], experimentating on the heart lung preparation, recommends the injection of hydrocortisone to prevent the cardiovascular collapse resulting from an exposure to 5% to 20% CO_2.

Apparently, the action of carbon dioxide on other endocrine glands that, such as thyroid, can modify the temperature regulation is not known.

Action of Carbon Dioxide on the General Control of Temperature Regulation by Nervous System

It is impossible, with the actual lack of experimental data, to have a clear knowledge how CO_2 can influence the control of temperature regulation through its action on the central nervous system. Nevertheless, many informations show the great influence that hypercapnia has on different formations of this system: brain, medulla oblongata, and even peripheral thermal receptors. Here again, it will be tried to relate, when possible, the physiological actions to different concentrations of CO_2.

Concerning the nervous centers of the brain, CO_2 at concentrations of 5% to 7%, increases the cerebral circulation (WOLF et al. [1930], COBB and FREMONT-SMITH [1931], IRVING and WELSCH [1936], BOUCKAERT and JOURDAN [1936], KETY and SCHMIDT [1948], PATTERSON et al. [1955], SOKOLOFF [1960]) and the oxygenation of the cortex (CLARK, MISRAHY, and FOX [1958]) provokes an excitation of the subcortical formation, particularly of the hypothalamus (GELLHORN [1953]), of the reticular activator system (DELL and BONVALLET [1954]), while it depresses, in a general way, the activity of the cerebral cortex (BROWN [1930], GELLHORN and FRENCH [1953]). Two general studies of the effects of higher concentrations of carbon dioxide on the central nervous system according to its concentration were performed, one on monkey by Carey, Schaefer, and Delgado [1955], and one on rat by Woodbury et al. [1958]. On monkeys, the inhalation of 10%, 15%, and 30% CO_2 diminished the threshold of the electrical stimulation of the hypothalamus and of the reticular substance. In rat, concentrations, varying from 5 to 20% CO_2, increased the cerebral excitability, while 40% decreased it and brought general anesthesia. To get "carbonarcosis" in man (LOEVENHART, LORENZ, and WATERS [1929]), a concentration of 30% CO_2 in O_2 is necessary. Golodof [1946] thought that the mechanisms of the hypothermia produced by these high doses of CO_2 depends from a complete depression of the central nervous system, for he reported that the cooling of the body is similar in decerebrated rabbits and in rabbits breathing 30% CO_2.

Conclusions

From experiments on more than 500 rats it was found that concentrations of 8% to 10% CO_2 are required to disturb their temperature regulation. For these euthermic mammals, easy to cool and easy to warm, as a consequence of their tiny size, at an ambient temperature of 24°C, there is a good relationship between CO_2 concentration and the rate of cooling.

At high concentrations, CO_2 directly decreases thermoconductibility and modifies the physiological processes of physical temperature regulation. In rats, at cold, an atmosphere containing more than 10% CO_2 diminishes their cutaneous convective and radiative heat losses by a peripheral vasoconstriction, and also the blood shifts conditioning the core to shell thermal conduction. Panting, resulting from hypercapnia, increases the work of the respiratory muscles and also the thermolysis by the respiratory upper ways. At ambient temperatures between 26°C and 33°C, 10% CO_2 augments the evaporative heat losses by perspiration as well as by hyperventilation. However, above 29°C, which is the rats' thermoneutrality (or critical temperature), 10% CO_2 provokes hyperthermia and panting, and above the colic temperature of 43°C death occurs. On man, it has been observed that 6% CO_2 provokes a transitive sweating reaction at ambient temperatures above 27°C.

In regard to thermogenesis, it is established that in most mammals oxygen consumption is increased for CO_2 concentrations between 3% and 10%. From an experimentation on rats, it is shown that 9% CO_2, preventing the increase of the O_2 consumption, for exposure at an ambient temperature below 29°C (thermoneutrality) induces hypothermia; at ambient temperatures above 29°C, hypercapnia enhances O_2 consumption which, with the prevention of an efficient thermolysis as was described previously, provokes hyperthermia. Suppression of shivering was proved in man inhaling 6% CO_2 at a temperature of 5°C and in refrigerated rabbits breathing 15% to 20% CO_2. In rats it was observed that the effects of CO_2 on temperature regulation were obtained only if the animals breathe CO_2 and not when their bodies are plunged into a 8% CO_2 atmosphere, their heads being out of the hypercapnic environment. However, for higher concentrations it is possible that CO_2 could penetrate inside the organism.

The mechanism of action of CO_2 on temperature regulation appears to be complex, as the gas influences most of the physiological functions. Related to its thermal effects, many possible sites are defined: The peripheral cutaneous thermoreceptors; the adrenal medulla, through sympathetic innervation or through catecholamines release: and the adrenal cortex on which hypercapnia, associated to adverse environmental temperatures would act as a stress factor. At concentrations above 20 %, CO_2 has a generalized depressive effect on the medullary centers and principally on the cortex, with ataxia and a kind of narcosis as consequences, presumably on the hypothalamic centers of temperature regulation and, in addition, on the cardiovascular system, resulting in cardiovascular collapse.

The importance of an eventual direct action on the chemical processes of temperature regulation must not be dismissed. The analogy of effects on rats' colic temperature between the inhalation of 9 % CO_2 and 11 % O_2 makes us consider the possibility, at the cell level, of a decrease of the oxidations by a diminution of the Po_2 resulting either from a direct effect on the oxidation of the carbon molecule, either indirect through the Bohr effect. Experiments on rats and rabbits permit us to eliminate that last possibility, without knowing if it is not concealed by a compensating hyperventilatory reaction. But it is also permissible to consider the physico-chemical consequences of the modification of the acid-base balance on the enzymatic systems which condition all the cellular vital processes such as respiration or permeability.

Measurements of blood gases prove that the elimination of CO_2 is immediate as soon as the body is taken out of the hypercapnic atmosphere—the return to normothermy, like the rate of cooling or of warming, being longer and depending chiefly on the size of the body.

Animal experiments demonstrate that the danger of CO_2, in cold and especially in hot environments, must be considered each time that such an association is possible; yet, concerning man, nothing definite is known.

Bibliography

Adachi, J., *J. Orient. Med., Dairen,* 25:97 (1936).

Andjus, R. K., and Smith, A. U., *J. Physiol.,* 128:446 (1955).

Anrep, G. V., *J. Physiol.* 45:307–18 (1912–1913).

———, and Hammouda, M. *J. Physiol.,* 77:16–34 (1932).

Barbour, J. H. and Seevers, M. H. *J. Pharmacol. Exper. Therap.* 78:11–21 (1943).

———, and Seevers, M. H. *J. Pharmacol. Exper. Therap.,* 78:296–303 (1943).

Bargeton, D. *Rev. Path. Gén. Comparée.* 669: 915–19 (1955).

———, Eon, M., Krumm-Heller, C., Libermann, C., and Masson, J. *J. Physiol.* 46:845–60 (1954).

Bartels, H., Hilpert, P., Barbey, K., Betke, K., Riegel, K., Lang, E. M., and Metcalfe, J. *Am. J. Physiol.* 205:331–36 (1963).

Béhague, P., Garsaux, and Richet, C., *C.R. Soc. Biol.* 96:766–768 (1927).

Bert, P. *C.R. Soc. Biol.* 5:156–58 (1873).

Besson, J. M., Benoist, J. M., and Aleonard, P. *Intern. J. Neuroscience,* 1:319–26 (1971).

Bhatia, B., Georges, S., and Rao, T. L. *J. Appl. Physiol.,* 27:583–86 (1969).

Binet, L. and Burstein, M. *C.R. Soc. Biol.* 143: 239 (1949).

Blood, F. R., Glover, R. M., Henderson, J. B., and D'Amour, F. E. *Am. J. Physiol.,* 156:62–66 (1949).

Boman, K., Hensel, H., and Witt, I. *Pflüg. Arch. Physiol.,* 264:107–12 (1957).

Bouckaert, J. J. and Jourdan, F. *Arch. Intern. Pharmacodyn. Thérap.,* 54:155–62 (1936).

Boussingault, R. *C.R. Ac. Sc.,* 40:1006–09 (1855).

Brody, S. *Bionergetics and Growth.* New York: Reinhold (1945).

Broom, B. *Nature,* 193:1262–63 (1962).

Brown, E. B., Jr. School of Aviation Medicine, USAF Report 56–81, Randolph AFB, Texas (1956).

Brown, E. W. *U.S. Naval Med. Bull.,* 28:721–34 (1930).

Bullard, R. W. *J. Appl. Physiol.,* 19:137–41 (1964).

Bullard, R. W., and Crise, J. R. *J. Appl. Physiol.*, 16: 633–38 (1961).

Burton, A. C. and Bazett, H. C. *Am. J. Physiol.*, 117:36–54 (1936).

Cannon, W. B. and Hoskins, R. G. *Am. J. Physiol.*, 29:274–79 (1911).

Carey, C. R., Schaefer, K. E., and Delgado, J. M. R., *Fed. Proc.*, 14:25 (1955).

Carlson, L. D. and Hsieh, A. C. L. *Control of energy exchange.* New York: Macmillan (1970).

Chanel, J. Sciences Thesis, Lyon (1956).

Chapin, J. L. *Am. J. Physiol.*, 179:146–48 (1954).

———, Edgar, J. L. R. *Am. J. Physiol.*, 204: 723–26 (1963).

Chapot, G. *J. Physiol.*, 58:491–92 (1966).

———. *La température du corps est réglée par la respiration.* Paris: Arnette publ. (1967).

———. *C.R. Soc. Biol.*, 164:282–84 (1970).

Chassain, A. P. Medicine Thesis, Paris (1959).

Chevillard, L. *Ann. Physiol. Physico-Chimie Biol.*, 11:461–532 (1935a).

———. *Ann. Physiol. Physico-Chimie Biol.*, 11: 1015–88 (1935b).

———, Arnal, M. C., and Giono, H. *C.R. Soc. Biol.*, 152:303 (1958).

Cheymol, J. and Levassort, C. *C.R. Soc. Biol.*, 150:2106 (1956).

Clark, L. C., Jr., Misrahy, G., and Fox, R. P., *J. Appl. Physiol.*, 13:85–91 (1958).

Cobb, S. and Fremont-Smith, F. *Arch. Neurol. Psychiat.*, 26:731–36 (1931).

Comroe, J. H., Jr., Forster, R. E., Dubois, A. B., Briscoe, W. A., and Carlsen, E. *The lung.* Chicago: Year Book Medical Publ. (1965).

Consolazio, W. V., Fisher, M. B., Pace, N., Pecora, L. J., Pitts, G. C., and Behnke, A. R. *Am. J. Physiol.*, 151:479–503 (1947).

Cordier, D., Magne, H., and Mayer, A. *Ann. Physiol. Physio-Chimie Biol.*, 3:791–817 (1927).

Dell, P. and Bonvallet, M. *C.R. Soc. Biol.*, 148: 855–58 (1954).

Dodt, E. *Pflüg. Arch. Physiol.*, 263:188–200 (1956).

Dripps, R. D. and Comroe, J. H., Jr. *Am. J. Physiol.*, 149:43–51 (1947).

Dubois, R. *C.R. Soc. Biol.*, 10:814–15 (1895).

———. *Physiologie comparée de la Marmotte.* Paris: Masson Publ. (1896).

Du Bois-Reymond, R. *Arch. Anat. Physiol.*, 187–90 (1893).

Findlay, J. D. *J. Physiol.*, 136:300–09 (1957).

Fortier, C. L. *Proc. Soc. Exper. Biol. Med.*, 70:76–8 (1949).

Friedlander, C. and Herter, E., *Z. Physiol. Chem.* 2:97–176 (1878–1879).

Garrelon, L. and Langlois, J. P. *J. Physiol. Path, Gén.*, 9:640–52 (1907).

———, and Langlois, J. P. *J. Physiol. Path. Gén.*, 9:948–56 (1907).

Gellhorn, E. *Am. J. Physiol.*, 120:189–94 (1937).

———. *J. Ment. Sci.*, 99:357 (1953).

———, and French, L. A. *Arch. Internat. Pharmacodyn.*, 93:427–33 (1953).

———, and Janus, A. *Am. J. Physiol.*, 116:321 (1936).

Genaud, P. and Gros, J. *Ann. Médecine Légale Criminologie* 34:104–08 (1954).

Giaja, J. *C.R. Ac. Sc.*, 210:80–82 (1940).

———. *Biol. Méd.*, 42:545–80 (1953).

Goldscheider, A. *Arch. Anat. Physiol.*, 575–80 (1887).

———, and Ehrmann, R. *Pflüg. Arch. Physiol.*, 206:303–07 (1924).

Gollwitzer-Meier, K. *Klin. Wochensch.*, 2:1418–21 (1937).

Golodof, I. I. *The effect of high concentrations of carbonic gas in organism (experimental investigation).* (In Russian.) Leningrad (1946) quoted by Repin.

Good, A. L. and Sellers, A. F. *Am. J. Physiol.*, 188:451–55 (1957).

Grant, R. T., Bland, E. F., and Camp, P. D. *Heart*, 16:69–101 (1932).

Hainsworth, F. R. and Stricker, E. M. *Am. J. Physiol.*, 217:494–97 (1969).

Haldane, J. and Smith, J. L. *J. Path. Bact.*, 1: 168–86 (1893).

Haywood, C. *Am. J. Physiol.*, 82:241 (1927).

Hemingway, A. and Nahas, G. G. *Am. J. Physiol.*, 170:426–33 (1952).

Henning, F. *Wärmetechnische Richtwerte*, Berlin: V.D.I. Publ. (1938).

Hensel, H. *Arch. Physiol.*, 252:107–10 (1949).

Hieronymi, E. In R. Jaffe. *Anatomie und Pathologie.* Berlin: Julius Springer (1931).

Hill, J. R. *J. Physiol.*, 149:346–73 (1959).

Houdas, Y. Personal communication (1971).

Irving, L. and Welsch, M. S. *Quart. J. Physiol.*, 25:121 (1936).

Jones, E. S., Meagraith, B. G., and Sculthorpe, H. H., *Ann. Trop. M. Parasit., Liverp.*, 44: 168–86 (1950).

Kayser, C. *Ann. Physiol. Physicochim. Biol.*, 15:1087 (1939).

Kayser, C. *The physiology of natural hibernation.* Oxford: Pergamon Press (1961).

———. *Physiologie.* Paris: Editions Méd. Flammarion (1963).

Kety, S. S. and Schmidt, C. F. *J. Clin. Investigation,* 27:484–92 (1948).

Knoppers, A. T. *Arch. Néerl.,* 26:364–406 (1942).

Kottke, F. J., Phalen, J. S., Taylor, C. B., Visscher, M. B., and Evans, G. T. *Am. J. Physiol.,* 153:10–15 (1948).

Kramer, K. and Sarre, H. *Arch. Exp. Path. Berlin,* 180:545–56 (1935–36).

Kuno, Y. *The physiology of human perspiration,* London: Churchill (1934).

Langley, L. L. and Kilgore, W. G. *Am. J. Physiol.,* 180:277–78 (1955).

Liljestrand, G. and Magnus, R. *Pflüger's Arch. Physiol.,* 193:527–54 (1922).

Loevenhart, A. S., Lorenz, W. F., and Waters, R. M. *J.A.M.A.,* 92:880 (1929).

Lyman, C. P. and Chatfield, P. O. *Physiol. Rev.,* 35:403–25 (1955).

———, and Hastings, A. B. *Am. J. Physiol.,* 167:633 (1951).

Mayer, A. *Exposés des travaux scientifiques d'André Mayer, Professeur de Physiologie à la Faculté de Médecine de Strasbourg.* Paris: Hermann et Cie (1922).

———. *Bull. Acad. Méd.,* 105: No. 4:127–30 (1931).

Molnar, G. W., Hurley, H. J., Jr., and Ford, R. Army Medical Res. Lab. Fort Knox., Ky. Rep. No. 147 (June 21, 1954).

Nahas, G. G. *Circulation Research,* 5:489 (1957).

———. *J. Physiol.,* 49:323 (1957).

———, and Cavert, M. H. *Federation Proc.,* 10: No. 1:92 (1957).

Niazi, S. A. and Lewis, F. J. *J. Appl. Physiol.* 10:137–38 (1957).

Ozanam, C. *C.R. Ac. Sci.,* 54:1154–55 (1862).

Patterson, J. L., Heyman, A., Battey, L. L., and Ferguson, R. W., *J. Clin. Invest.,* 34:1857–64 (1955).

Price, H. L. *Anesthesiology,* 21:652–63 (1960).

Prosser, L. C. and Brown, F. A., Jr., *Comparative animal physiology.* Philadelphia: Saunders (1965).

Repin, I. S. *Pat. Fiziol. Eksp. Ther.,* 3:48–56 (1959).

Richard, J. and Stein, S. N. *Am. J. Physiol.,* 188:1–6 (1957).

Ring, J. R. and Randall, W. C. *Anat. Rec.,* 99: 7–19 (1947).

Römer, F. *Jenaische Z.f. Nat.,* 30:604–22 (1896).

Rougier, G. *C.R. Soc. Biol.,* 151:78 (1947).

Rubner, M. *Die Gesetze des Energieverbrauchs.* Leipzig and Vienna (1902).

Schaefer, K. E. *J. Appl. Physiol.,* 13:1–14 (1958).

———. *Aerospace Med.,* 32:197–204 (1961).

———, Hastings, B. J., Carey, C. R., and Nichols, G., *J. Appl. Physiol.,* 18: 1071–78 (1963).

———, King, C. T. G., Mego, J. L., and Williams, E. E., *Am. J. Physiol.,* 183:53–62 (1955).

Schindewolf, G. and Weigmann, R. *Klin. Wochensch,* 30:547–51 (1952).

Schmidt-Nielsen, K. and Schmidt-Nielsen, B. *Physiol. Rev.,* 32:135–66 (1952).

Shaw, L. A. and Messer, A. C. *Am. J. Physiol.,* 98:92 (1931).

Shephard, R. J. *J. Physiol.,* 129:393–407 (1955).

Sokoloff, L. *Anesthesiology,* 21:664–73 (1960).

Sollmann, T. *A manual of Pharmacology,* 8th ed. Philadelphia: Saunders (1964).

Stupfel, M. *J. Physiol.,* 52:575–606 (1960).

———. *J. Physiol.,* 52:673–725 (1960).

———, and Bouley, G. *The 2nd Internat. Clean Air Cong., Proceedings Digest,* Washington D.C. (Dec. 6–11, 1970).

——— and Geloso, J. P. *C.R. Ac. Sci.,* 248: 740–42 (1959).

———, and Geloso, J. P. *J. Physiol.,* 51:568–69 (1959).

———, and Roffi, J., *C.R. Soc. Biol.,* 154:1387–90 (1960).

———, Jouany, J. M., and Jaulmes, C., *C.R. Soc. Biol.,* 151:2045–49 (1957a).

———, Servant, P., and Jouany, J. M. *C.R. Soc. Biol.,* 151:874–78 (1957b).

———, Servant, P., and Jouany, J. M. *C.R. Soc. Biol.,* 151:1337–41 (1957c).

Tennent, D. M. *Am. J. Physiol.,* 145:436–39 (1945–46).

Tenney, S. M. *Am. J. Physiol.,* 187:341 (1956).

———. *Anesthesiology,* 21:674–85 (1960).

Thibault, O. *C.R. Soc. Biol.,* 140:940–42 (1946).

———. *Ann. Nutrit. Aliment.,* 2:89–157 (1948).

———. *Revue Canad. Biol.,* 8:3–131 (1949).

Tournade, A. and Malmejac, M. J. *C.R. Soc. Biol.,* 115:1106 (1934).

Van Liere, E. J. and Stickney, C. J. *Hypoxia.* Chicago: University of Chicago Press (1963).

Veselkin, N. V. Doctoral Thesis, Saint Petersburg (1913).

Weigmann, R. and Schindewolf, G., *Pflüg. Arch. Physiol.,* 258:315–23 (1954).

Wolff, H. G., Lennox, W. G., and Allen, M. B. *Arch. Neurol. Psych.*, 23:1097–1120 (1930).

Woodbury, D. M., Rollins, L. T., Gardner, M. D., Hirschi, W. L., Hogan, J. R., Rallison, M. L., Tanner, G. S., and Brodie, D. A. *Am. J. Physiol.*, 192:79–90 (1958).

Stupfel Discussion

LOESCHKE: Dr. Stupfel, I think that you mainly put your weight on the metabolic effects, on the heat production as a factor of thermal regulation, and I therefore want to ask you two questions: First, are they merely physical effects? For example, what is the specific heat of CO_2 as gas? Is the transport by the gas better, or worse? And second, you didn't say much about the circulation of the skin which would play a big role in the temperature regulation, and what does CO_2 on that in this case?

STUPFEL: CO_2 has an effect on the physical conductivity of air (F. Henning, 1938). But at the concentration of 10% used in our experiments, it is not very great, but at higher concentrations it could have an effect. I did not get, sir, your second question about the skin.

LOESCHKE: The skin circulation, blood flow in the skin.

STUPFEL: There are many data in the literature about the effect of carbon gas and they are done in the aqueous water medium. I made measurements on the skin of rats. After exposure to 10 to 30% CO_2 I always found a decrease of the skin temperature.

SCHAEFER: I can, perhaps, answer this. During exposure to 15% CO_2 for one hour the skin blood content of guinea pigs is increased 75% and falls below initial levels after three days of exposure, when a physiological adaptation has been reached. However, there is an additional point. Under such conditions the blood vessels cannot respond to cold, they stay open.

NAHAS: I would like to ask three questions: (1) Does high CO_2 actually inhibit non-shivering thermogenesis? (2) What happens to the turnover rate of free fatty acids and glycerol under those conditions of high CO_2? Isn't there any evidence that such a turnover rate is inhibited and this might be a mechanism of the decrease of temperature under these conditions? And (3) what happens to the turnover rate of the catechol amines, especially in the adrenal gland and peripherally, under those conditions of associated hypercapnia and hypothermia, because these two conditions separately imposed on animals produced an increased turnover rate of catechol amines as shown by Steinsland and Nahas [1968].

STUPFEL: The difficulty with CO_2 is that it has many side effects. It has effects on catechol amine in blood and tissues, and it also affects the thermoreceptors and the cutaneous circulation, which I showed you in studies about the ear of the rabbit. Often it is very difficult to relate all those phenomena together.

Bibliography

Nahas, G. G. and Steinsland, O. S. "Increased rate of catechol amines during respiratory acidosis." *Resp. Physiol.*, 5:108–17 (1968).

Part IV

Carbon Dioxide and Regulation of
Organ Function

1. Bone Carbon Dioxide Stores and Acid-Base Regulation

Dominique Bursaux and Claude Poyart

Institut d'Anesthesie
Université de Paris, Faculté de Médecine
121 Rue de l'Ecole de Médecine
Paris VIe, France

The physiological function of bone carbon dioxide is a puzzling problem.

It has been known for a long time that bone contains a very large amount of carbon dioxide, as compared to the rest of the body. The physico-chemical processes by which carbon dioxide and electrolytes accumulate in certain structures seems to occur frequently in nature. It occurs in bones, it occurs in the shell of eggs, it occurs in the formation of rocks and seashells (GODDARD [1960]). It has recently been shown to occur also in the mitochondria (LEHNINGER [1965]).

The problem of bone carbon dioxide is of major importance in physiology for several reasons:

(1) Bone constitutes a carbon dioxide sink, which complicates the interpretation of metabolic oxydation studies (STEELE [1955]).
(2) It interferes with the dynamics of whole body carbon dioxide stores (LONGOBARDO et al. [1967]).
(3) It plays a major role in the maintenance of a normal acid-base status.

Figure 1, issued from Professor Rahn's work, shows that bone is by far the major site of carbon dioxide storage in the whole body. Bone is also a major reservoir for electrolytes, such as calcium, phosphorus, magnesium, sodium, and potassium.

We have developed in our laboratory a method which permits the measurement of all these parameters on fresh bone (Figure 2). Fresh rat femurs and tibia are rapidly weighed and introduced, as shown in the figure, in a known amount of 5 N hydrochloric acid. The gas phase of the system is re-circulated for 18 hours, and bone carbon dioxide is trapped in a known amount of sodium hydroxide 5 N. Sodium hydroxide is then back titrated to measure the exact

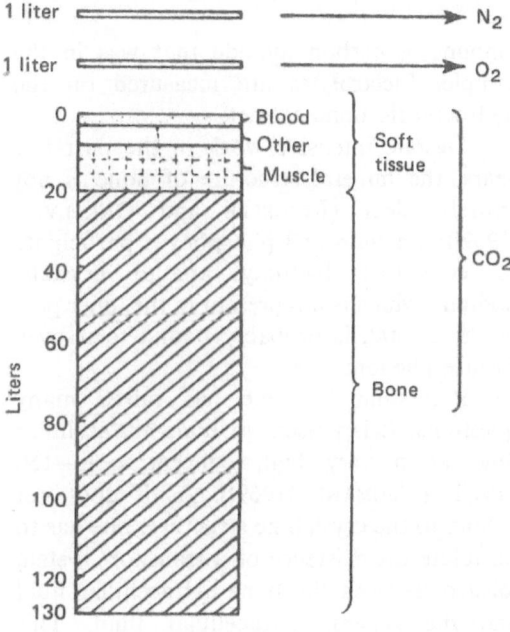

Fig. 1. Estimated total gas stores of the human body.

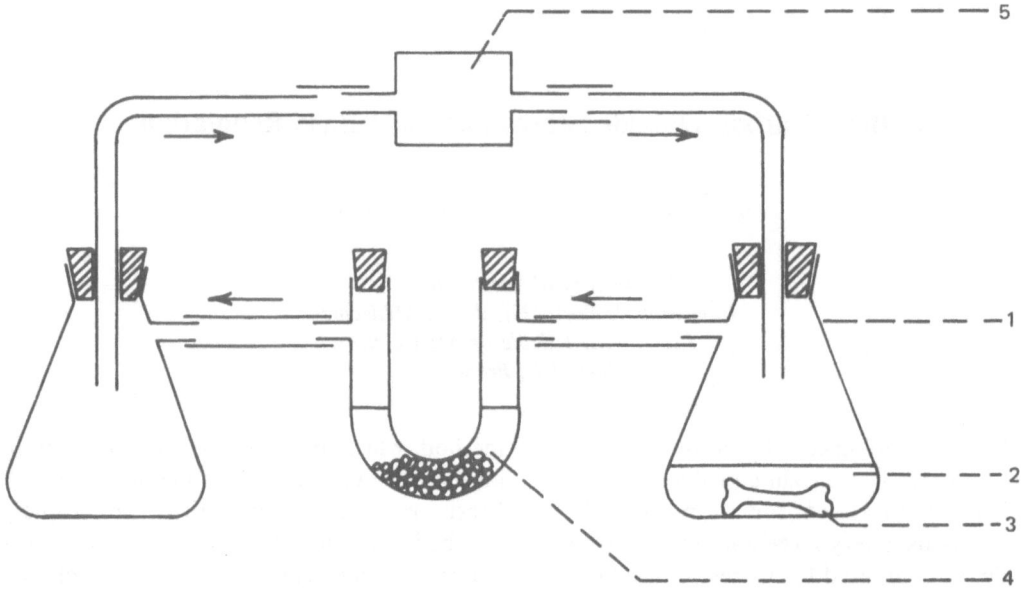

Fig. 2. Apparatus for measurement of bone carbon dioxide and electrolytes.
1   flask
2   HCl, 5 N
3   bone sample
4   NaOH, 5 N
5   circulating pump

amount of carbon dioxide that was in the sample. Electrolytes are measured on the hydrochloric bone extract.

Despite intensive work in the past few years, the mineral structure of bone is not entirely clear (RICHELLE and ONKELYNX [1969]): Calcium and phosphorus participate to constitute hydroxy apatite crystals. Sodium, which is not present in the inner part of the crystal, is probably bound to it by a surface phenomenon.

Potassium in bone has raised many questions. It is present in bone extracellular fluid at a very high concentration—150 meq/1. (NEUMANN [1969]). As it does not belong to the crystalline structure, one has to postulate the existence of a transport system located between the bone extracellular fluid and the general extracellular fluid. This hypothesis may also apply to part of the bone carbon dioxide.

Several attempts have been made to clarify the physico-chemical status of carbon

dioxide in bone: For a long time it has been admitted that bone carbon dioxide was present only as fixed carbonates and participated in long-term exchange processes such as those occurring in chronic metabolic acidosis.

Then, many authors using X-ray diffraction studies showed that bone carbon dioxide cannot be substituted as carbonates within the crystal lattice, except for a very small amount (POSHER [1969]).

Beebe and coworkers, on the basis of their experiments, have suggested that some carbon dioxide in bone may be adsorbed on the surface of the crystals. So far this has not been satisfactorily documented.

Neuman and coworkers have had a very interesting approach to the problem of bone carbon dioxide physical chemistry. They showed first that a significant amount of bone carbon dioxide could be released simply by heating at 150°C for a few hours (NEUMANN and MUTRYAN [1967]). Figure 3 shows that

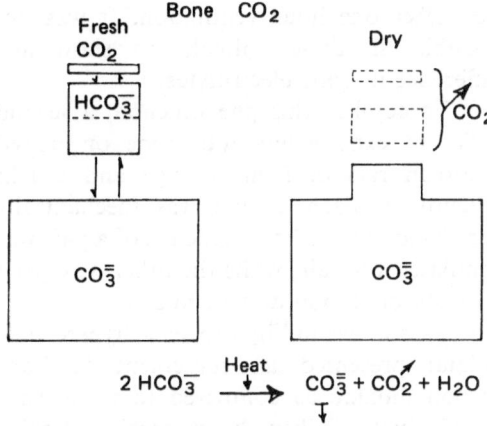

$$2 \, HCO_3^- \xrightarrow{\text{Heat}} CO_3^= + CO_2 \nearrow + H_2O$$

Fig. 3. The bottom of the figure shows the reaction which occurs on heating HCO_3. The upper part is a theoretical representation of bone carbon dioxide pools.

bicarbonate ions can be dehydrated by heating at such a temperature.

Heating two molecules of bicarbonate gives rise to one molecule of gaseous carbon dioxide and one molecule of carbonate, which stays in the reaction medium. The mechanism of the reaction is: One molecule of bicarbonate takes an H ion from the other, and thus can dissociate in water and carbon dioxide. If this reaction, and only this reaction, takes place upon heating bone, it becomes possible, by measuring the amount of carbon dioxide lost on heating, to calculate the quantity of bicarbonate that was originally present in fresh bone.

We applied this method to paired rat femurs in order to measure their bicarbonate content. One of the samples was analyzed fresh, while the other was oven-dried for 18 hours at 150°C before carbon dioxide measurement.

The difference in carbon dioxide content between fresh and dried sample was taken as half of the bicarbonate originally present. In this way we found that femurs of young rats contained 450 to 500 μ moles of carbon dioxide per gram of fresh weight, 40 to 50% of which was bicarbonate. This figure is close to that obtained by Neumann and Mulryan [1967].

Thereafter it was tempting to represent bone carbon dioxide as it is in Figure 3. That is a large pool of carbonates, a pool of bicarbonates averaging 40% of the total, and a negligible fraction of dissolved carbon dioxide. The next problem is to determine if this representation of bone carbon dioxide has any physiological meaning.

It is surprising to see how quickly radioactive bicarbonate injected intravenously reaches the bone mineral. Investigating this problem in rats, Neumann showed that the bulk of radioactivity trapped in bone was located in the heat labile carbon dioxide fraction. After a single ^{14}C bicarbonate injection, he found that the specific activity of carbon dioxide lost on heating the bones was more than twice that of the remaining carbon dioxide. He concluded that the rapidly exchangeable bone carbon dioxide pool was mainly represented by bicarbonates.

Our first approach to this problem was slightly different. To measure the exchangeability of bone carbon dioxide, fresh rat femurs were placed in an atmosphere containing a known amount of radioactive ^{14}C O_2. The accumulation of radioactivity was measured as a function of time. The results obtained in this type of experiment showed that most of the activity accumulates in the heat labile fraction of bone carbon dioxide. This, again, is in favor of a rapidly exchangeable pool of bicarbonate in bone (Figure 6).

The exchangeability between blood and bone bicarbonate led us to reinvestigate the short-term participation of bone to respiratory changes in whole-body carbon dioxide stores.

In 1953 Professor W. O. Fenn studied in rats the effects of chronic hyper- and hypocapnia. He concluded that bone carbon dioxide could increase significantly after chronic exposure to carbon dioxide and that this increment was accompanied by an increment in bone calcium and phosphorus (FREEMAN and FENN [1953]).

In 1958 Nichols [1958] studied the effects of acute hypercapnia on bone carbon dioxide. He found, on the basis of a few experiments, that bone carbon dioxide would decrease in hypercapnic acidosis. He concluded that bone carbon dioxide was in equilibrium with blood carbonate. However, in these experiments carbon dioxide was measured on dried bone samples. Therefore, he could not demonstrate a possible change occurring in bone bicarbonate.

To see whether or not bone carbon dioxide would be influenced by respiratory changes in the acid-base status, we used a different experimental procedure. Sherman rats were anesthetized, and mechanically ventilated for one hour at constant rate and respiratory volume. The gas mixtures used for ventilation contained variable amounts of carbon dioxide. In this way were realized hypo- and hypercapnia of one hour duration.

At the end of the experimental period both femurs and tibias of each rat were rapidly retrieved and assayed for carbon dioxide and electrolytes.

Figure 4 shows the results obtained in this experiment. There is a good correlation between bone carbon dioxide and mixed venous blood P_{CO_2} obtained by catheteriza-

tion after one hour ventilation. It was not possible, in these animals, to show any difference in bone electrolytes.

To confirm this phenomenon, a second series of experiments was done on paired Sherman rats of identical age and weight (Figure 5). Each animal was mechanically ventilated for one hour. One rat of a pair was ventilated with air, while the other was given 4 to 6% of carbon dioxide in air.

As is shown in Figure 5, each hypercapnic animal presented an increment in bone carbon dioxide as compared to its normocapnic mate. When bone carbon dioxide content was correlated with mixed venous blood P_{CO_2}, the average slope obtained was

1. 27 mM CO_2/kg/bone/torr.

These results demonstrate the existence of bone carbon dioxide changes in acute hypercapnic acidosis.

However, many questions remain unsolved. We were not able to show any changes in bone electrolytes during these experiments, and this has to be further documented. The

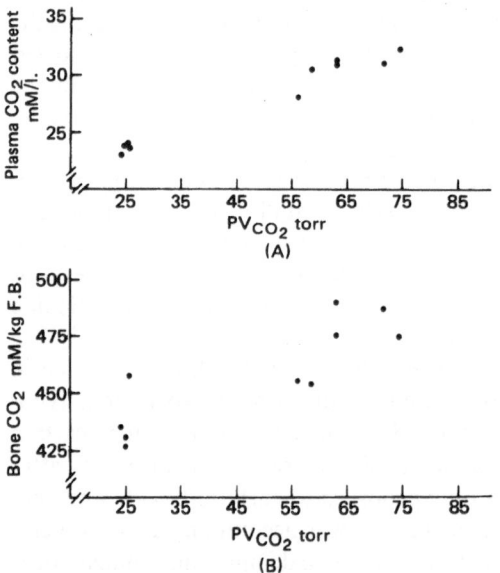

Fig. 4. This figure shows the relationship between $P\bar{v}_{CO_2}$ and bone CO_2 of anesthetized and mechanically ventilated rats.

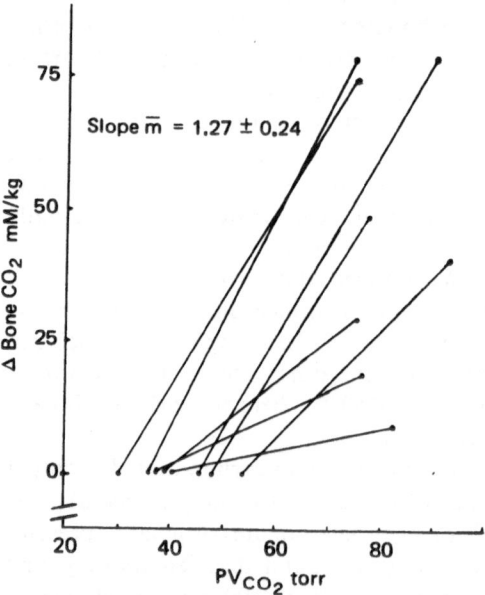

Fig. 5. Each line of the figure represents a pair of rats. One of them is normally ventilated (low $P\bar{v}_{CO_2}$), while the other is made hypercapnic.

use of radioactive carbon dioxide and electrolytes in the forthcoming experiments will help us to answer this problem, and also

(1) to identify the bone carbon dioxide pool which is concerned with these acute changes, and
(2) to investigate the dynamics of bone carbon dioxide during metabolic acid base disorders.

Bibliography

Freeman, F. H. and Fenn, W. O., "Changes in carbon dioxide stores of rats due to atmospheres low in oxygen or high in carbon dioxide." *Am. J. Physiol.* 174:422 (1953).

Goddard, D. R., "The biological role of carbon dioxide." *Anesthesiology,* 21:587 (1960).

Lehninger, A. L., *The Mitochondrion.* New York: W. A. Benjamin, Inc.

Longobardo, G. S., Cherniack, N. S., and Staw, I., "Transients in carbon dioxide stores." *IEEE Trans. Bio. Med. Ing.* BME 14:182 (1967).

Neumann, W. F., "The milieu intérieur of bone: Claude Bernard revisited." *Fed. Proc.* 28: 1846 (1969).

———, and Mulryan, B. J., "Synthetic hydroxy-apatite cristal, III: The carbonate system." *Calc. Tis. Res.* 1:94 (1967).

Nichols, G., Jr., "Serial changes in tissue carbon dioxide content during acute respiratory acidosis." *J. Clin. Invest.* 37:1111 (1958).

Posner, A. S., "Crystal chemistry of bone mineral." *Physiological rev.* 49:760 (1969).

Richelle, L. F. and Onkelynx, C., "Recent advances in the physical biology of bone and other hard tissues." In *Mineral Metabolism.* C. L. Comar and L. Bronner, eds. New York: Academic Press.

Steele, R., "The retention of metabolic radioactive carbonate." *Biochemical J.,* 6:447 (1955).

Bursaux Discussion

RAHN: I would also like to join you. I would like to commend you upon this very nice work but I think it's a real breakthrough for physiologists like myself. When I talk to bone people they always throw so many complicated equations and functions at me that I don't know how to translate it, but I think what you have provided now is an access for a simple biologist like myself who visualizes bone as a compartment that can be analyzed in terms of acute changes. Can you tell me again, approximately, what the bicarbonate—I think it's an important distinction you have drawn, at least for me, of the bicarbonate pool versus a carbonate pool—can you give me approximately the percentage dimensions?

BURSAUX: Well on the basis of our figures, bicarbonate should represent in the normal state about 40% of the total carbon dioxide in bone. However, I must say that there is a criticism on our theory which is as follows: If any hydrogen ions can be liberated on heating the bone, then our estimation of bicarbonate would not be true because if you provide hydrogen ions to carbonate, then it will go off as gaseous carbon dioxide. However, the examination of the pK's of the different compounds being presented at bone structures leads us to believe that it's very unlikely that H ions can be liberated on heating.

RAHN: And the other question—how much of this bicarbonate pool do you think was available in terms of your acute experiment? That is, can you estimate it at all? Is it 10%, 20%?

BURSAUX: I am, myself, afraid by the steepness of the slope that we found in acute experiments, but we have not done yet the experiments measuring at the same time total carbon dioxide and bicarbonate, but I believe that the fraction that moves is bicarbonate and that about 10% of bone carbon dioxide can be acutely mobilized in hypercapnia.

RAHN: And could one make electron microscope pictures, not electron microscope pictures—I'm talking about radiographic pictures—to show *where* the carbon dioxide is exchanging?

BURSAUX: Newman has made that type of work and shown very nice autoradiographies locating the radioactive carbon dioxide on the periphery of bone. That's all I know for the present time.

COURNAND: I should like to ask Dr. Bursaux, he has—or maybe ask you also as a physiologist—whether you have an idea what is the slope to the skeleton as a whole? Well, someone may have read a paper of Hardin Jones which goes back to, I think, 1945 or 1946, where he estimated the various blood flow rates in the organs, including the skeleton. I have a faint recollection that the total flow of the bone of the skeleton was something of the order of 10%, at most, with an extraordinarily slow turnover.

BURSAUX: I think you're right, Dr. Cournand, and moreover I think that Dr. Rahn has issued a slide in *Handbook of Physiology* which shows the relative carbon dioxide and blood flow for all the organs and shows especially that blood flow to bone is very high.

RAHN: If I did, I'm sure I took it from somebody else's notes, but I was wondering if you could not, from your slope dynamic characteristics, make assumptions of the accumulation of carbon dioxide in bone, and estimate the blood flow by this means? It would be rough, but it gives you an order of magnitude.

BURSAUX: As we don't know yet the exact mechanism as to how carbon dioxide accumulates in bone, it prevents us from making any assumption on blood flow and so on.

RAHN: But if you have some data, it's worthwhile trying different parameters to see if something fits the 10%.

COURNAND: May I mention one more fact which may be of interest to you eventually? In certain bone diseases such as Recklinghausen disease or Paget's disease, it has been found that the total cardiac output is enormously increased. That has been found around 1945 or 1946, and now we think that this case might be of consequent interest to find out what is a pool and what is a turnover.

NAHAS: The fraction of total blood flow going to bones is a function of age. It is high in the younger, growing people where it might reach 10% of cardiac output, but in the adults the figure which is given in the literature, (1971), is between 6 and 9%.

SEVERINGHAUS: What fraction of the bone you have been studying is watery tissue? That is, not calcium carbonate, histologically, perhaps? Or how much water can you drive off when you dry a bone? I was just wondering because it's probably that in that water component are the proteins which could, to

some extent, donate hydrogen on and free carbon dioxide from the calcium carbonate and therefore look like bicarbonate.

BURSAUX: We studied whole bones with their marrow, but on drying they lose at the most about 30 to 35% of their weight. Is that the answer to your question?

SEVERINGHAUS: Yes, perhaps. Do you know whether there's water in the solid matrix of the bone?

BURSAUX: There is 20% water in the solid matrix of the bone. That is, if you isolate a part of cortical bone and oven dry it, you find that it loses 20% weight, which has to be water, because carbon dioxide amounts for a very small amount in weight loss, and that water seems to be located first in the cells, and second in a space enclosed between the bone cell on one side and the bone crystal on the other. Otherwise it seems as if the bone possessed a special extracellular fluid which was located behind the cellular barrier and in between the bone cell and the bone crystal.

SEVERINGHAUS: Does each bone crystal have its own bone cell?

BURSAUX: If I can, I will be glad to try and draw you a schematic representation of bone unit on the blackboard (Figure 7).

If you have followed the work of Rasmussen and the literature, it shows more and more, nowadays, that just as you can identify the nephrons in the kidney, you can schematically represent a unit bone structure which is constructed as follows: Here you have the bone cell, here you have the blood vessel, and here you have the crystalline structure of bone, and in between the cell and the crystalline structure there's a quite large amount of liquid phase, which actually must contain all the electrolytes that do not have place in the bone crystals, that is 150 milliequivalent of potassium/liter, a lot of sodium, and probably the bulk of bone bicarbonate. Any substance that is present in this compartment has to go through the transport system of the bone cell to reach the general extracellular fluid. And, moreover, this barrier is a real one, because bone cells reach each other through their expansions. This way no substance can cross the barrier without going through the cell or one of its expansions. It has been proposed on biochemical and histological grounds.

———: I think we can't do this comparison because the carbon dioxide with bicarbonate of sodium in the blood is unstable but carbonate sodium of the bone is stable. To liberate carbon dioxide of the bone we need a strong acid, but for the blood we don't need this, because the composition is not stable and it always changes. So it is difficult to make any comparison of carbon dioxide in the bone with carbon dioxide in the blood.

BURSAUX: Well, part of it seems to be unstable because it's able to change with respiratory influence. I don't have any idea whether bicarbonate in bone is bound to a cation or free and ionized the medium, but it seems to be able to move back and forth with the change in P_{CO_2} and pH.

RAHN: I would just like to urge you to put this picture in your paper so that I can see what a bone cell looks like. I appreciate this picture very much.

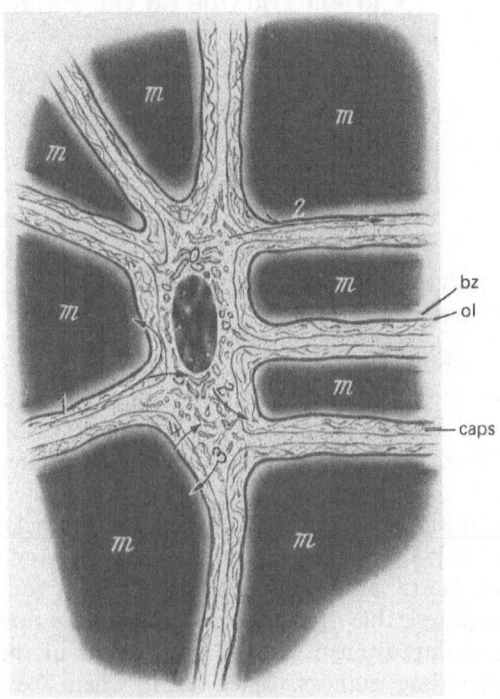

Fig. 7. Representation of the electon microscope of an osteocyte in its lacuna (taken from WASSERMAN, F. and YAEGER, J. A., "Fine Structure of the Osteocyte Capsule and the Wall of the Lacuna in the Bone," Z. Zellforsh Mikroskop. Anat. 67, 636-442, 1965). Note the capsule (caps) surrounding the cell process (which afford a fluid and fibrous extracellular medium for ion transfer) and the matrix (m). Arrows indicate possible pathways for ion transfer between blood and matrix.

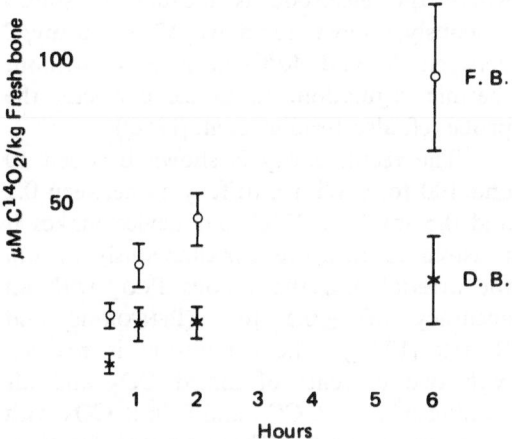

Fig. 6. Uptake of $C_{14}O_2$ by fresh bone (F.B.) and dry bone (D.B.). (From NAHAS, G. G. and SCHWARTZ, I. Unpublished data.)

2. Continuous Control of Intravascular P_{CO_2} and Reflexogenic Effects of Carbon Dioxide on the Pulmo-Cardio-Vascular System *in situ*

Boris Rybak

Zoophysiologie, Faculté des Sciences
Université de Caen
France

Three Generations of pH and P_{CO_2} Catheterizable Probes*

For the realization of the P_{CO_2} probes we took the greatest account of the concepts and macro-electrodes of Dole [1952], Severinghaus and Bradley [1958], Bates [1961], Stow and Randall [1954], Stow, Baer, and Randall [1957], and Gertz and Loeschcke [1958]; and of the medium size P_{CO_2} electrode of Hertz and Siesjö [1959]. In fact our catheterizable probes are miniaturization and improvements of the realizations of the preceding authors. Since 1954, when Stow and Randall gave the principle of measuring P_{CO_2} with a pH electrode using a selective membrane for gases (rubber), and since 1957, when Stow, Baer, and Randall built the first macro-P_{CO_2} electrode in which the reference electrode was a wire of chloridized silver, and since Gertz and Loeschcke in 1958 used a polyethylene membrane instead of the rubber membrane of Stow and collaborators, we moved from an electrode of 2-cm outer diameter to our probe of 1.5-mm outer diameter, and from unstable measurements with a response time lying between 3 and 5 min to the catheterizable P_{CO_2} probes which show the following performances:

Our probe of the second generation is largely insensitive to temperature change between 20 and 40°C; the probe of the third generation *is* sensitive to temperature change, *but* because of the rectilinearity: Millivoltage *versus* Celsius (where ΔE belongs to the Ag/AgCl electrode)—if the local temperature, where the electrode is located, is simultaneously known, for a $\Delta E/\Delta T \sim 0.6$ mv/C between 20 and 40°C—it is easy without thermic regulation, to utilize correctly the probe (cf. also Bradley et al. [1956]).

The rectilinearity is shown between 10 and 100 torr. With a drift lying between 0.2 and 0.5 mv/h at 37°C, our device makes it possible to measure simultaneously *in situ* the arterial and the venous P_{CO_2} with an accuracy of ± 0.5 torr (Penfornis and Rybak [1971]). The calibration is realized with two currents of mixed CO_2 and air loading of 5.31 % CO_2 and 9.56 % CO_2 with an error of ± 0.03. These percentages were chosen following the point of Siemon [1967], according to whom the error on the blood P_{CO_2} is higher when the P_{CO_2} of the reference gases are far from the blood P_{CO_2}. The calibration mixtures run at 1.5 to 3 l./h in a thermostated humidificator, $P_{CO_2} = \%$ CO_2 $(Pb - P_{H_2O})$ torr at a definite temperature, where Pb = barometric pressure (to accomplish this one uses the Scholander apparatus).

As for the response time—which is dependent on numerous factors such as the concavity of the pH-sensitive glass (Siesjö [1961]) and the fixation of membranes—one may say that at 37°C, using the two quoted concentrations of CO_2 (corresponding

---

* Rybak et al. [1968], Rybak and Penfornis [1969], Penfornis and Rybak [1971], and Rybak [1971].

approximately to a ΔP_{CO_2} of 30 torr), 95% of the full response is given in 1 min 30 sec— 3 min when P_{CO_2} increases and 2 to 4 min when P_{CO_2} decreases.

The time constant of the response (by definition 63% of the full response) is between 20 and 30 sec (if this value is more than 50 sec, the "membranes" have to be changed). The membranes system is inspired by the device proposed by Severinghaus and Bradley: A water solution of NaCl 0.1 M + HNaCO$_3$ 0.01 M bathing the active part of the glass sphere and reference arrangement and, between the internal part of the outer selective teflon membrane (6 μ thickness) and the glass diaphragm, a lattice of nylon ("10 deniers") is fixed to stabilize mechanically the solution. The thickness of the solution will be minimized to improve the response time.

Presently aging of the electrode is insignificant, even after many months.

In order to eliminate the artifact of anesthesia and promote what I called the *physiological physiology* (RYBAK [1969]), we used a radio-telemetering device to measure pH and P_{CO_2} (RYBAK and DEDIEU). We are then able to work with freely moving, unanesthetized animals, adding some new dimension for exploring the life systems, a dimension which is inaccessible by the mass spectrograph and the other macrodevices.

Certainly for pH measurements— which are faster with our probes than P_{CO_2} measurements—the question of a protein deposit upon the surface of the glass has to be considered. But if one adopts the solution proposed by Staehelin and collaborators (STAEHELIN et al. [1968])—an indwelling catheterizable pH electrode—or if one lets a protein layer itself play the role of a hydrophilic membrane, it is possible to reasonably overcome this difficulty. In any case the preparation has to be under anti-blood clotting treatment. Presently with anesthetized dogs we obtain different results and mainly we see that a nasal inhalation of a relatively large amount of oxygen provokes a rise in the blood P_{CO_2} and a corresponding lowering of pH, hypercapnaemia which confirms the results of Meyer, Gotoh, and Tasaki [1961] experimenting with Macaques and using a by-passing device. The reaction, which is more pronounced in the arterial than in the venous blood, can be due to the Haldane effect. In addition, it could be a washout of the CO_2 stored in tissues in the venous side.

Carbon Dioxide as a Vegetative Reflexogenic Compound: A Further Step

With the discovery of the aortic chemoceptors by Heymans and Heymans [1927] and the carotic body chemoceptors by Heymans, Bouckaert and Dautrebande [1930], following the independent suggestion of de Castro, an impressive series of publications arose giving some invaluable results —sometimes with a number of rather unexpected processes (LEUSEN [1950]). But the question is not exhausted. Using the original P_{O_2} catheterizable probes (RYBAK [1964], and RYBAK and LE CAMUS [1966]), I found a reflex induced by a transient nasal stream of CO_2. The polyphasic P_{O_2} sequence [baseline-downward (the heart becomes frequently cyanotic)—upward overshoot, (heart again vermillion)]—is an indication of the reflex.

It is noticeable that similar polyphasic reactions occur as well when the apnea is induced by blowing CO_2 ($\dot{V} \sim 2$ l./min) through the nasal pathway or when there is no apnea at all by giving the CO_2 blown (same $\dot{V}$) through the sublaryngeal pathway. However, the morphology of the two processes is not exactly the same, the downward and upward events differing by the intensivity and by the duration of the deflections. The explanation is that when a sudden apnea is provoked, only a small amount of exogenous CO_2 penetrates inside the ventilatory tractus, but a profound transient hypoxia and an arrest of CO_2 elimination are produced. Then the accumulated *endogenous* CO_2 activates the ventilatory sensitive nervous zones. But when a nonnegligible amount (same $\dot{V}$) of exogenous CO_2 is blown directly inside the alveolar system, the blood P_{CO_2} increases for a transitory period because the inhaled P_{O_2} decreases, followed by hyperventilation due chiefly to the *exogenous* CO_2 which may be acting primarily upon the neural system of the lungs. The changes in the arterial and venous sides during this sublaryngeal insufflation could be the consequence of some rough acid-basic and electrolytic intercompartmental translocations. These observations support the conclusion of W. O. Fenn founded on rest and exercise behavior of CO_2 (FENN [1963]): "that endogenous or metabolic CO_2 is handled differently from inhaled or exogenous CO_2." It should be noted that the internal tracheobronchic receptors of Widdicombe may be involved here.

The interval between the two homologous peaks of the arterial and the venous polyphasic waves defines the circulation time.

That the trigeminal nerve of the nasal mucosa may be specifically involved in the apneal part of the CO_2 reflex is actually shown [I never severed the Vth nerve (WALL and PRIBRAM [1950])] in two ways. (1) Considering the P_{O_2} monophasic wave—and the following process—obtained only when clamping the superior trachea and placing an intratracheal canula of appropriate length to obtain about the same "dead space," the CO_2 streams being given through nasal pathway, one must conclude that under these conditions, related with a transient bradypnea, it should be a small amount of accumulated endogenous CO_2, (2) Because the mechanical stimulation of the nasal pathway —even by a $\dot{V}$ 9 l./min stream of air—is ineffective, one can tentatively suppose that the nasal "roots" of the trigeminal nerve act as chemoceptors which could be nociceptors (by irritation), the whole being presumably a kind of "chemoreflex" (DEJOURS [1962], and COMROE [1967]). This CO_2 reflex is independent of a double Vagotomy.

While the arterial pressure and P_{O_2}/P_{CO_2}

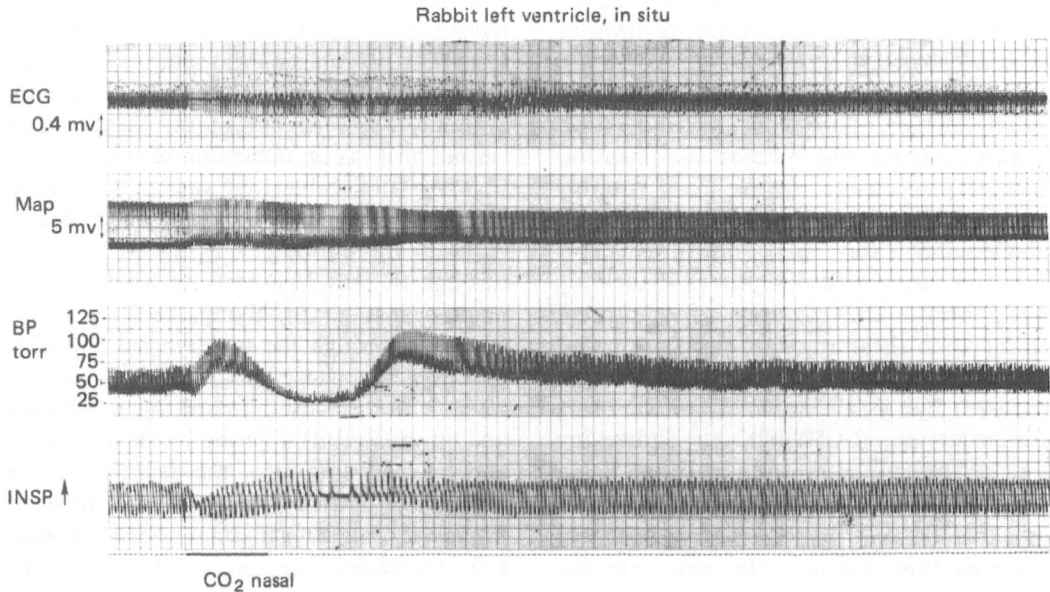

Rabbit left ventricle, in situ

ECG 0.4 mv

Map 5 mv

BP torr 125 100 75 50 25

INSP

CO_2 nasal

Fig. 1. This figure shows simultaneous four channels chart recording of the CO_2 reflex (global electrocardiogram recorded with needle-leads inserted in the right and left anterior limbs, monophasic action potential with a suction electrode, arterial pressure with a Statham P23AA strain gauge, ventilatory process recorded at the epidiaphragmatic level with a transducer Grass FT-10C, time base delivering the second).

are linked, since the time courses for blood pressure and P_{O_2} are different, it does not seem that these two processes are superimposed.

Thanks to the left thoractomy technique (RYBAK [1964]) it was possible to reach directly *in situ* the epicardium of the rabbit heart itself. Figure 1 (RYBAK et al. [1971]) gives the simultaneous four channels chart recording of the CO_2 reflex (global electrocardiogram recorded with needle-leads inserted in the right and left anterior limbs, monophasic action potential with a suction electrode, arterial pressure with a Statham P23AA strain gauge, ventilatory process recorded at the epidiaphragmatic level with a transducer Grass FT-10 C, time base delivering the second). It is to underline that a strong bradycardia happens during the blood vasotensive events. The monophasic action potential of both ventricles becomes a biphasic action potential during the hypertensive period of the CO_2 reflex; this quite entirely reversible patterning is comparable when CO_2 or small intravenous doses (9

μg/kg) of epinephrin are given to the preparation (the mechanocardiogram has often been picked up by placing a hook connected to a "Grass" transducer through a hole made in the left diaphragm at the ventricular apex); Figure 2.

Now, using the combined fluorometer-reflectometer (RYBAK et al. [1970]), focusing attention on liver, kidney and—with the possibilities offered by the left thoracotomized rabbit—on the external side of a mammal heart *in situ*, the heme pigments (haemoglobin and myoglobin of the cardiac ventricle mainly) were estimated in function of their oxygenation by evaluating the difference in optical density between $\lambda_1 = 543$ nm and $\lambda_2 = 615$ nm. The fluorometric estimations of $NADH_2$ were quasi-simultaneously recorded by exciting with $\lambda_3 = 365$ nm the fluorescence at 450 nm of the reduced co-enzyme I. The successive λ_1, λ_2, λ_3 were collected with the same photomultiplier in darkness.

Figure 3 shows the polyphasic reaction displayed at the epiventricular level *in situ*,

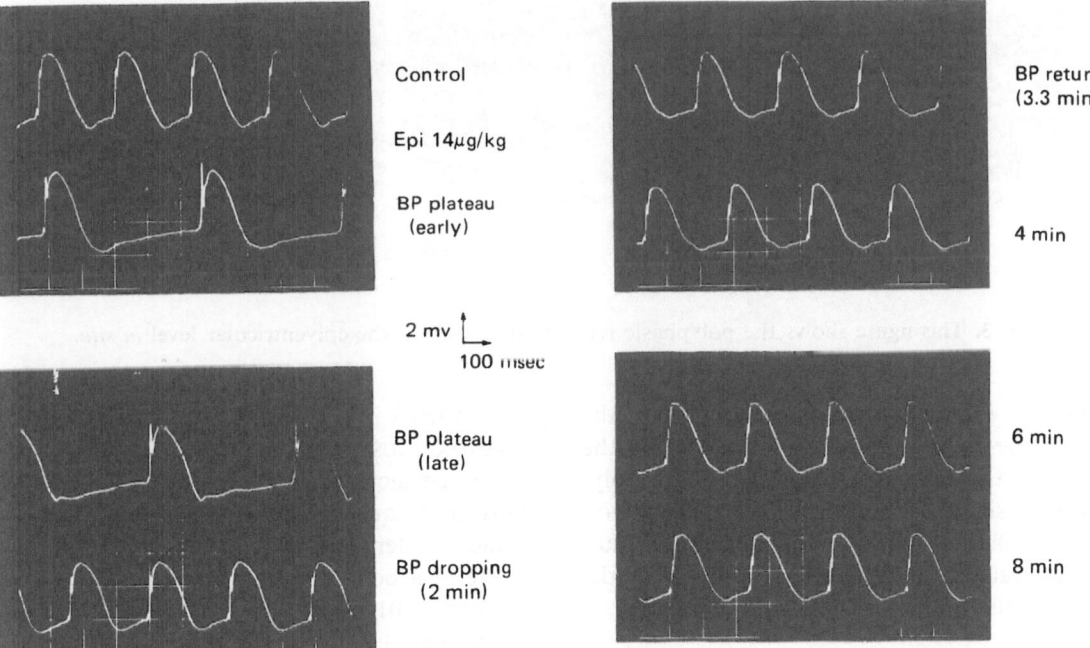

Fig. 2. Rabbit right ventricle, *in situ*.

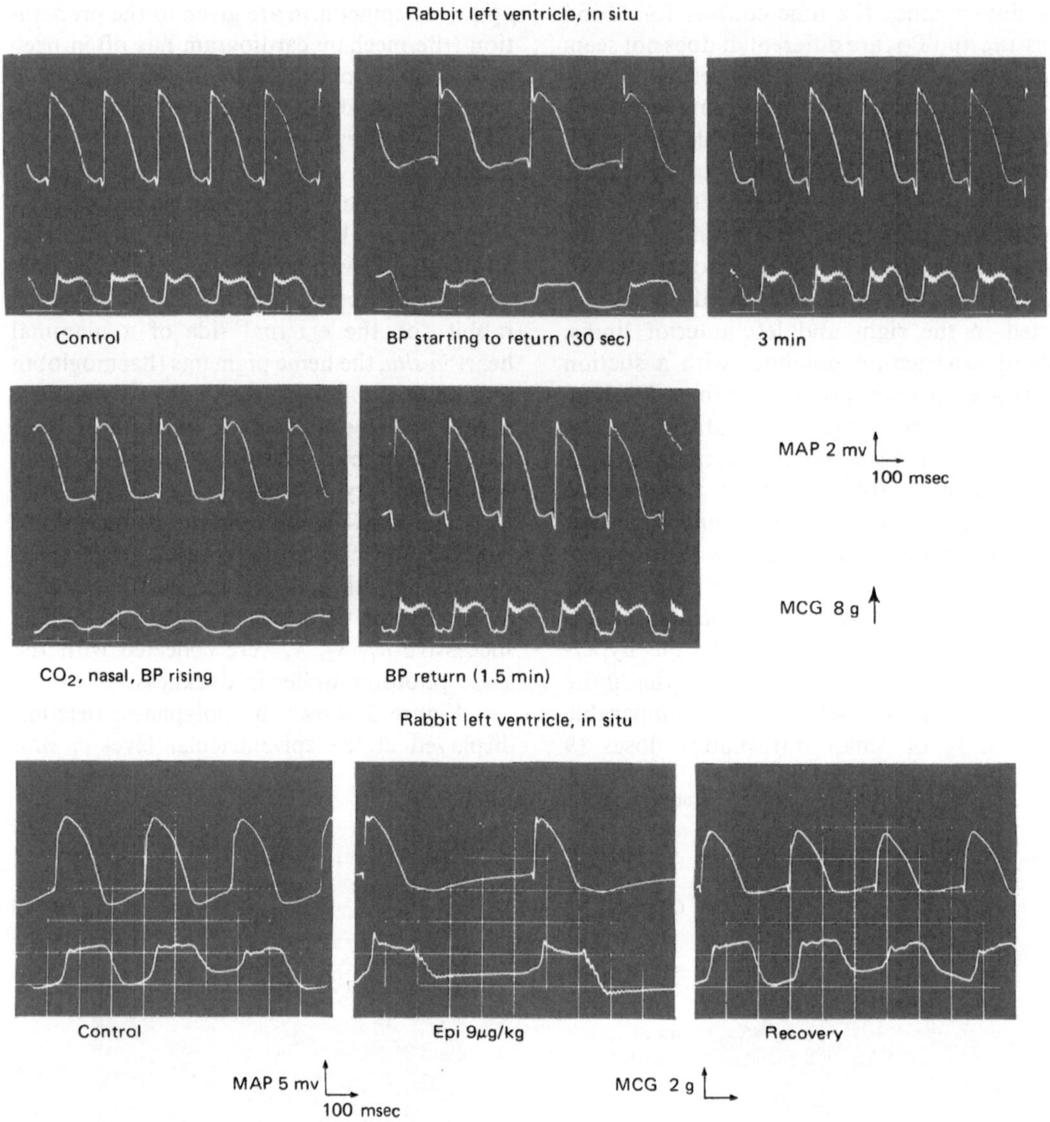

Rabbit left ventricle, in situ

Control

BP starting to return (30 sec)

3 min

MAP 2 mv

100 msec

MCG 8 g

CO_2, nasal, BP rising

BP return (1.5 min)

Rabbit left ventricle, in situ

Control

Epi 9µg/kg

Recovery

MAP 5 mv

100 msec

MCG 2 g

Fig. 3. This figure shows the polyphasic reaction displayed at the epiventricular level *in situ.*

i.e., a fluorescent reaction in which the pyridine-nucleotides are involved during the nasal CO_2 reflex, the organ giving also polyphasic signals according to the heme blood and muscular pigments. This demonstrates the existence of intracellular reflexes at the metabolic level (RYBAK et al. [1970]).

Discussion

The sensitivity of the P_{CO_2} probes

$[S = \Delta pH / \Delta \log P_{CO_2}$ according to SEVERINGHAUS and BRADLEY [1958]] can indeed be increased by working out a standard technique of positioning the "membranes" system and by reducing the thickness of the bicarbonate layer. In any case, as far as Corning 015 glass type is utilized, it seems to me that the use of the catheterizable pH probes during a rather deep hibernation ($T < 15°C$) is theoretically limited, since the more the temperature is decreasing, the greater the electrical resistance of the electrode and the greater its response time becomes.

As for the nervous impact of the CO_2 reflex, it seems that the brain stem reticular system is directly involved (DELL [1957]), considering that the ventilatory rate changes during the events as well as the pressure processes; this does not eliminate the possible role of the hippocampus (PASSOUANT and PTERNITIS [1967]). In any case, biogenic amines, and more specifically the catecholamines, seem to be involved, but the pharmacologic examination of the nasal CO_2 reflex remains to be done.

The decoupling of the MAP during the CO_2 reaction demonstrates the compound structure of this "monophasic" outlined graph. If such separation happens in the poikilothermic heart ventricle (GOTO and BROOKS [1969]), it is under quite different conditions and particularly in a rather abnormal treatment with hypertonic Ringer solutions containing glycerol and Mn^{++}. The glycerinated cardiac fibers are not, of course, in the same situation as that of the classical psoa muscle glycerinated preparation of Szent-Gyorgyï but they are certainly under osmotic stress (BOZLER and BOZLER [1967]). In the rabbit heart one can consider that the transit of micro-ions is modified and that mainly Ca^{++} could intervene when the cardiac tonus increases (KUNZE et al. [1961]) by forming a strong troponin-Ca^{++} compound (RYBAK et al. [1970]).

During the CO_2 reflex, as the fluorescent polyphasic signal demonstrates, important metabolic perturbations are manifested inside the heart cells notably. Therein it is possible that during the hypoxic phase of the reflex, lactic acid is produced in the heart muscle, after which the reverse reactions can occur when the hyperoxic phase exists, the net result being an absence of energetic hysteresis, of metabolic memory, when the reversibility of the reflex is total, as happens with a healthy animal. It is a matter of fact that by observing a reasonable relaxation time, the CO_2 reflex

may be produced several times, even with the left thoracotomized preparation. But, when the reversibility is not total, the preparation is suffering and the biochemical reactions operate in the most entropic direction; an imperfect recovery occurs, indicated by the fact that the trace is not returning to the baseline. Then for any process involved as a living process—and indeed the whole organism itself—the regulation capacity can be considered as an extended formulation of the buffer capacity. What the term *buffer* is mediating is not only a "purely" chemical fact but also an energetic one, since a buffer stabilizes concomitant acidic and alkaline processes, oxidation and reduction processes, etc. It corresponds to the law of mass action. Thus, as for the carbonic system in water

$$CO_2 + H_2O \rightleftharpoons H_2CO_3 \rightleftharpoons H^+ + HCO_3^- \quad (1)$$

in which the most probable (= the most entropic state = the lowest energy level) is located at the left side of the equilibrium reaction; i.e., CO_2 and H_2O (RIEGEL [1965]).

Now, the respiration *per se* can be schematized as follows:

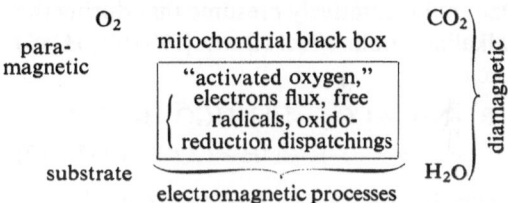

This system is not an entropic disaster because of ATP formation, the energy-coupling mechanism controlling the rate of electron transfer into cytochrom c by a control ratio of over tenfold (LEE and ERNSTER [1957]). The moderative effect of ATP can even induce a reversal of electron transfer in the respiratory chain for adequate ATP/ADP-P_i ratio (CHANCE [1962]). Uncoupling oxidative-phosphorylation could not be afforded for a too long time. Then ATP formation is not only an energy saving-process but a regulatory one; the electrons flux control the ATP formation and, by a feedback process, the ATP formed controls the electrons flux.

I would like to emphasize that the paramagnetism and the diamagnetism of the components of the systems are also fundamental; pointing out that χ = mass or specific magnetic susceptibility = volumic magnetic susceptibility K (unitless)/density in g/cm^3 of the substance, for the respiratory input–output molecules at $20°C$ $\chi_{O_2} = +3,449.0 \cdot 10^{-6}$ cgs, $\chi_{air} = +24.16 \cdot 10^{-6}$ cgs (with $\chi_{N_2} = -12.0 \cdot 10^{-6}$ cgs, $\chi_{H_2O} = -12.97 \cdot 10^{-6}$ cgs, $\chi_{CO_2} = -21.0 \cdot 10^{-6}$ cgs) (WEAST and SELBY [1967]). The oxygen in the triplet state with its two unpaired electrons is the form which combines with the haemoglobin and myoglobin. According to Perutz [1970], "the oxygen-free form is constrained in salt-bridges which are broken by the energy of haem-haem interaction with a release of H^+," and, "the α-amino-groups of valine 1 α and the imidazole groups of histidine 146 β are free in oxyhaemoglobin, but come close to carboxyl groups in the deoxy form; the imidazole groups of histidine 122 α approach guanidium groups in the oxy and carboxyl groups in the deoxy form." One could tentatively presume that during the "alkaline" Bohr effect (BOHR [1904]) (pH $\geqslant$ 6) when

$$R-NH_2+CO_2 \rightleftharpoons HbNHCO_2H \rightleftharpoons$$
$$R-NH-COO^-+H^+ \quad (2)$$

occurs [as for the bicarbonate equilibrium, (eq. 1), increasing entropy is to the left] the Fe (II)-carbamino-haemoglobin χ should shift from χ_{HHb} or from χ_{HbO_2} values (the carbamino-compounds having a pK < 6 being in any way completely ionized at the normal pH of the blood). Then, during the twofold process characterizing the CO_2 reflex (hypercapnaemia phase followed by a hyperoxemic phase), the electromagnetic properties of the blood are changing extensively and reversibly, as they should at the level of the mitochondrial respiratory chain.

As an additional point in connection with the blood gases transfer, it could be that when using inert gases (notably xenon), the so-called "inert" gases are not so inert. To support this statement we have the observation of Maio and Nelville [1970] that tissue oxygen consumption decreases in the presence of inert gases. This xenon's paradox can be explained by considering that xenon binding to the hydrophobic part of the molecules causes conformational disturbances of myoglobin (SCHOENBORN [1968]) and changes its reactivity, especially toward cyanide (MILDVAN et al. [1968]). I just would like to draw the attention to the fact that all these "inert" gases show χ 10^{-6} cgs *negative* values—are diamagnetic—listing at ordinary temperature: -1.88 for helium, -6.74 for neon, -19.6 for argon, -28.8 for krypton, and -43.9 for xenon. Under hyperbaric conditions the ligand binding should more strongly change the conformation of the pigments carrying gases and, it might be, of the metallo-porphyrins carrying electrons.

Bibliography

Bates, R. G., in *Reference electrodes, theory and practice.* D. J. G. Ives and G. J. Hanz, eds. New York: Academic Press (1961).

Bohr, Ch., Hasselbach, K., and Krogh, A., *Skand. Arch. Physiol.* 16:402 (1904).

Bozler, E., and Bozler, H. M., *Am. J. Physiol.* 213:1317 (1967).

Bradley, A. F., Stupfel, M., and Severinghaus, J. W., *J. Appl. Physiol.* 9:201 (1956).

Castro, F. de, quoted in C. Heymans, and E. Neil, *Reflexogenic areas of the cardiovascular system.* London: Churchill (1958).

Chance, B., *J. Gen. Physiol.* 45:595A (1962).

———, Legallais, V., and Schoener, B., *Rev. Sci. Instrum.* 34:1307 (1963).

Comroe, J. H., *Physiologie de la respiration,* translated by J. Gontier. Paris: Masson (1971).

Dejours, P., *Physiol. Rev.* 42:335 (1962).

Dell, P. C., in "Reticular formation of the brain," *Henry Ford Hosp. Internat. Symp.* (Detroit, 1957), London: Churchill.

Dole, M., *L'électrode en verre,* translated by L. Giraut-Erler. Paris: Dunod (1952).

Fenn, W. O., in "Regulation of respiration." G. G. Nahas, consulting ed. *Ann. New York Acad. Sci.,* art. 2:415 (1963).

Gertz, K. H., and Loeschcke, H. H., *Naturwiss.* 45:160 (1958).

Goto, M., and Brooks, C. McC, *Proc. Soc. Exptl. Biol. Med.* 131:1427 (1969).

Hertz, G. H., and Siesjö, B., *Acta Physiol. Scand.* 47:115 (1959).

Heymans, C., Bouckaert, J. J., and Dautrebande, L., *Arch. Int. Pharmacodyn.* 39:400 (1930).

Heymans, J. F., and Heymans, C., *Arch. Int. Pharmacodyn.* 33:272 (1927).

Kunze, K., Lübbers, D. W., and Rybak, B., *C.R. Acad. Sci.* 253:904 (1961).

Lee, C. P., and Ernster, L., *Fed. Proc.* 26:610 (1957).

Leusen, I. R., *Experientia* 6:272 (1950).

Maio, D. A., and Neville, J. R., quoted in W. H. Koch and D. Hershey, "Blood Oxygenation" (D. Hershey, ed.) New York: Plenum Press (1970), p. 222.

Meyer, J. S., Gotoh, F., and Tazaki, Y., *J. Appl. Physiol.* 16:96 (1961).

Mildvan, A. S., Rumen, N., and Chance, B., in Abstracts, Division of Biological Chemistry, American Chemical Society 32 (1968).

Passouant, P., and Pternitis, C., in *Progress in brain research*, W. Ross Adey and T. Tokizane, eds. Vol. 27 ("Structure and function of the limbic system.") Amsterdam: Elsevier (1967).

Penfornis, H., and Rybak, B., *J. Physiol.* 63: 149 A (1971)

Perutz, M. F., *Nature* (*London*), 228:732 (1970).

Riegel, J. A., *Energy, life and animal organisation.* London: The English University Press (1965).

Rybak, B., (a) *Life Sci.* 3:725–36 (1964); (b) *Proc. Can. Fed. Biol. Soc.* 10:27 (1967).

———, *Life Sci.* 3:1123 (1964).

———, (a) *Rev. Ens. Sup.* 1:81 (1966); (b) *Coopération techn.* 54 (1969).

———, Transactions of the New York Academy of Science 33:11, 44, 371 (1971).

———, and Le Camus, L., *Life Sci.* 5:1097 (1966).

———, and Dedieu, J. M., (a) *Life Sci.* 6:1417 (1967); (b) *Bordeaux Médical* 1366 (juillet 1968).

———, Boivinet, P., and Penfornis, H., *Experientia* 24:102 (1968).

———, and Penfornis, H., *J. Physiol.* 394 (1969).

———, Chance, B., Paddle, B., and Kaplan, A., *Life Sci.* 9, part 1:557 (1970).

———, Gretenstein, M., Suckling, E. E., and Brooks, C. McC, *J. Physiol.* 62: suppl. 3, 444 (1970).

———, Gretenstein, M., and Suckling, E. E., *J. Electrocardiology* 4:153 (1971).

Schoenborn, B. P., in *Abstracts, Division of Biological Chemistry.* American Chemical Society 30 (1968).

Severinghaus, J. W., and Bradley, A. F., *J. Appl. Physiol.* 13:515 (1958).

Siemen, G., *Ges. Exp. Medizin* 142:33 (1967).

Siesjö, B. K., *Acta Physiol. Scand.* 51:297 (1961).

Staehelin, H. B., Carlsen, E. N., Hinshaw, D. B., and Smith, L. L., *Am. J. Sur.* 116:280 (1968).

Stow, R. W., and Randall, B. F., *Am. J. Physiol.* 179:678 (1954).

Stow, R. W., Baer, R. F., and Randall, B. F., *Arch. Phys. Med. Rehabil.* 38:646 (1957).

Wall, P. D., and Pribram, K. H., *J. Neurophysiol.* 13:409 (1950).

Weast, R. C., and Selby, S. M., eds. *Handbook of chemistry and physics.* Cleveland, Ohio: The Chemical Rubber Co. (1967).

3. The Effects of Carbon Dioxide and pH on the Regulation of the Pulmonary Circulation*

Yale Enson†

*Department of Medicine,
College of Physicians and Surgeons,
Columbia University
630 West 168th Street,
New York, New York 10032*

The pulmonary vasculature is unique among the various regional circulations in that it must accommodate the entire cardiac output. Unfortunately, precisely the same factors that make this possible—the highly compliant vessels, their scant smooth musculature, the paucity of nervous control, and the consequent low intravascular pressures—also render the evaluation of pulmonary vasomotion difficult. The bed is so distensible that blood flow normally ceases at the end of diastole (MORKIN et al. [1965], KARATZAS and LEE [1969], and GABE et al. [1969]); nor is there a pressure gradient across the bed at that time. The use of mean pressure and mean flow for calculating resistance to pulmonary blood flow, in order to assess the effects of physiologic stimuli or pharmacologic agents, may lead, for these reasons, to conclusions which are quite inappropriate (HARVEY and ENSON [1969]).

This brief consideration of the effect of carbon dioxide and pH on the pulmonary circulation will begin, therefore, with a review of the determinants of pulmonary arterial pressure in normal subjects, and in patients with commonly encountered forms of pulmonary hypertension, in an effort to provide some logical framework within which to assess the response of the bed to these agents. Then we will examine the response of the pulmonary circulation to naturally occurring alterations in alveolar carbon dioxide tension and blood pH, using chronic obstructive lung disease as a model. Finally we will discuss the effect of these stimuli in some other conditions.

Studies in animals (HAMILTON et al. [1939], CARLILL and DUKE [1956]) and in patients without significant pulmonary vascular or mitral valvular disease (KALTMAN et al. [1966]) have shown that the pressure in the pulmonary artery is the same as that in the left heart at the end of diastole. It is possible to extend these observations to a wide range of normal activities by substituting the mean pulmonary "wedge" pressure for the left ventricular end-diastolic pressure, since the latter has not been studied extensively in normal man. Pulmonary arterial diastolic and mean "wedge" pressures at rest and during strenuous exercise reported in the Swedish literature (HOLMGREN et al. [1957], BEVEGARD et al. [1963], GRANATH and STRANDELL [1964]) are presented in Figure 1. Cardiac output varied from 4 to 28 liters

* Supported in part by grants HE-05741-09 and HE-02001-15 from the National Heart Institute, and by a grant-in-aid from the New York Heart Association.
† Recipient of an investigatorship of the Health Research Council of the City of New York under contract I-176.

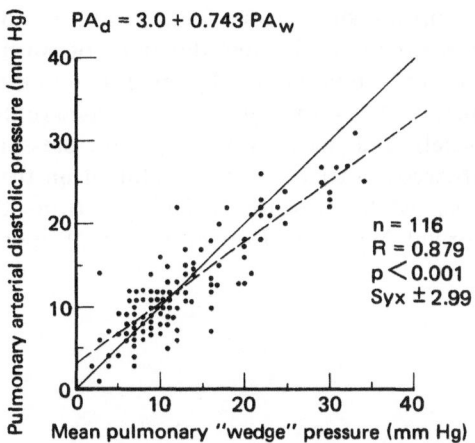

$$PA_d = 3.0 + 0.743\ PA_w$$

n = 116
R = 0.879
p < 0.001
Syx ± 2.99

Fig. 1. Graphic representation of the relation between pulmonary arterial diastolic (PA_d) and "wedge" (PA_w) pressures. One hundred and sixteen observations in 44 normal subjects are included. The lines of identity (continuous) and regression (interrupted) are included. For discussion see text. (STOLLERMAN [1969]).

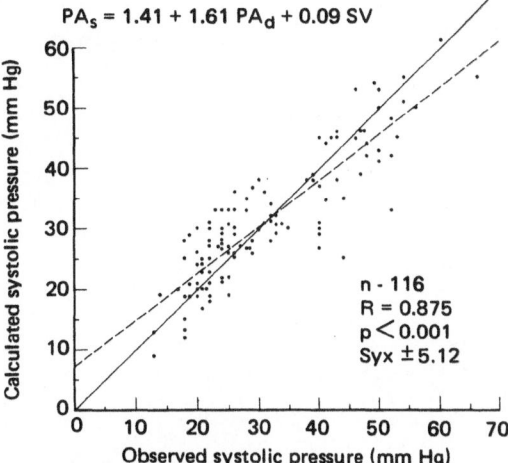

$$PA_s = 1.41 + 1.61\ PA_d + 0.09\ SV$$

n - 116
R = 0.875
p < 0.001
Syx ± 5.12

Fig. 2. Graphic representation of the relation between pulmonary arterial systolic pressure (PA_s) observed in normal subjects and that calculated from the equation indicated above. The lines of identity (continuous) and regression (interrupted) are included. For discussion see text. (STOLLERMAN [1969]).

per minute and stroke volume from 60 to 190 ml. Values of "wedge" pressure, on the *x* axis, as high as 34 mm Hg were encountered during severe exertion. The interrupted line is the regression, while the solid line represents the line of identity. The close relation between the two levels of pressure is apparent. The pulmonary artery diastolic pressure in normal man reflects the pressure at the end of diastole in the left heart. The identity of these pressures indicates that stroke volume and blood flow have no detectable effect on the level of pulmonary arterial diastolic pressure.

The systolic pressure reflects the contribution of the stroke volume to the volume of blood already distending the elastic arteries at the end of diastole. It should be possible, then, to predict the systolic pressure from the stroke volume and diastolic pressure if they are indeed its sole determinants. Utilizing the same Swedish data, the equation relating systolic and diastolic pressures and the stroke volume, indicated at the top of Figure 2, was solved. Pressures calculated on this basis are plotted on the *y* axis; observed pressures, on the *x* axis. The regres-

sion line and the line of identity are again included, and do not differ significantly from each other.

The determinants of normal pulmonary arterial pressures are summarised schematically in Figure 3. Elevation of the left heart filling pressure causes a rise in pulmonary arterial diastolic pressure of the same magnitude. The systolic and mean pressures also rise, but to a greater extent. This presumably reflects diminishing compliance of the elastic arteries in the face of an increasing pulmonary blood volume. Right ventricular stroke volume has no discernible effect on diastolic pressure, but at any given level of diastolic pressure, the larger the stroke volume, the greater will be the systolic and mean pressures. This effect of stroke volume is not great: an increase of 50 ml in stroke volume produces only a 4-mm rise in systolic pressure. It is apparent that changes in left heart pressure induce greater changes in pulmonary blood volume and in systolic and mean pressure than do changes in stroke volume. The pulse pressure depends on the volume of blood ejected into the elastic vessels beat by beat, and not on the level of

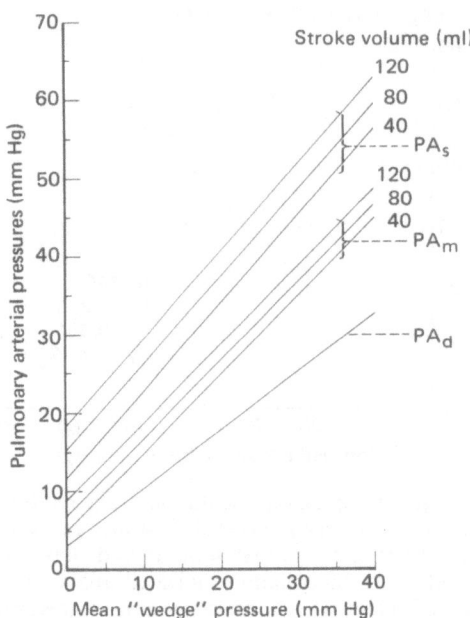

Fig. 3. Schematic representation of the effect of the left heart filling pressure and stroke volume on pulmonary arterial systolic (PA_s), mean (PA_m), and diastolic (PA_d) pressures in normal subjects. (STOLLERMAN [1969]).

mean flow. The normal pulmonary circulation is more appropriately characterized as a volume-regulated bed rather than as a flow-sensitive one.

Let us consider, now, the pulmonary circulation in disease. Since pulmonary hypertension is a frequent occurrence in patients with left ventricular disease, with mitral stenosis, and with chronic obstructive lung disease, I have chosen large groups of patients representing each of these entities to illustrate various mechanisms which participate in the evolution of pulmonary hypertension.

First we shall examine the compliance of the elastic pulmonary arteries in these three groups of patients. Although atherosclerosis of the large vessels is encountered in the disease states under consideration, it is rarely extensive. The compliance of these vessels, then, should be normal; stroke volume should have no greater effect on the systolic pressure than it does in normal subjects. The relation between systolic (and

mean) pressure, stroke volume and diastolic pressure derived from the data of normal subjects should be equally applicable to these disease states. In Figure 4 the systolic (upper panel) and mean (lower panel) pressures observed in each group are plotted on the x axis, while pressures calculated from the normal regression (top of Figure 2) appear

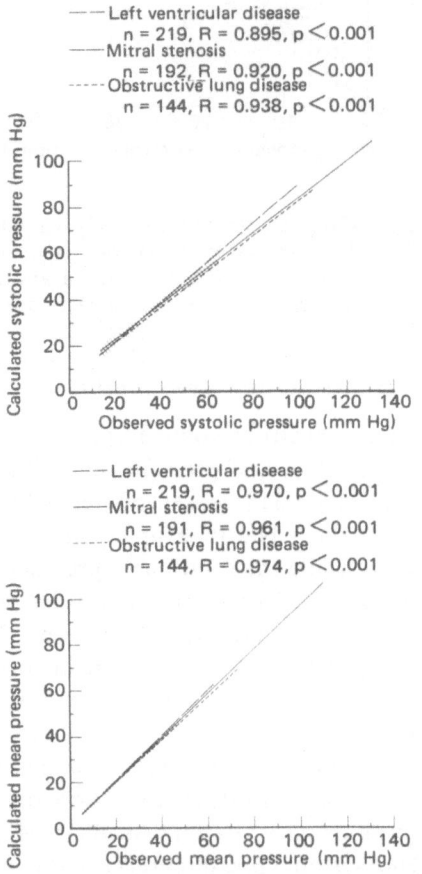

Fig. 4. Graphic representation of the relation between pulmonary arterial systolic (PA_s, upper panel) or mean (PA_m, lower panel) pressures in three groups of patients with those calculated from equations derived from normal subjects. In each panel the dashed line represents the regression for patients with left ventricular disease, the solid line the regression for patients with mitral stenosis, and the dotted line the regression for patients with chronic obstructive lung disease. The length of each regression indicates the range of observations in each group. The shaded area indicates one standard deviation about the regression calculated for normal subjects. (STOLLERMAN [1969]).

on the *y* axis. The coarsely dashed line in each panel represents the regression calculated for patients with left ventricular disease (VARNAUSKAS [1955], SELZER and MALMBORG [1962], MALMBORG [1965]), the solid line represents the regression calculated for patients with mitral stenosis (ELIASCH [1952], WERKO et al. [1953], YU et al. [1954], DICKENS et al. [1957]) and the finely dashed line the regression for patients with chronic obstructive lung disease drawn from our own data. The shaded area indicates one standard deviation about the regression calculated for normal subjects.

The systolic and mean pressures of these patients with acquired heart disease are predicted with the same degree of accuracy as they were in normal subjects. It would appear then, that in these patients compliance of the arteries is normal. When pulmonary hypertension is encountered in these disease states, we must turn to a consideration of the factors regulating the level of the diastolic pressure to understand its genesis.

In Figure 5 are plotted the relation between pulmonary arterial diastolic and the mean wedge pressures observed in the same patients with left ventricular disease (panel A), with mitral stenosis (panel B), and with chronic obstructive lung disease (panel C). The solid line in each panel is the regression; and the dashed lines, one standard deviation. The shaded areas indicate one standard deviation about the regression calculated for normal subjects.

A highly significant relationship exists in each group: the higher the wedge pressure, the higher will be the diastolic pressure. The slopes of the regressions vary markedly, however, from one group to another. In the case of patients with left ventricular disease (panel A), it is apparent that the level of the pulmonary arterial diastolic .pressure may result solely from elevation of pressure within the left heart, in a fashion similar to normal subjects. In some cases, however, indicated by the area which does not overlap the normal range, the diastolic exceeds the wedge pressure

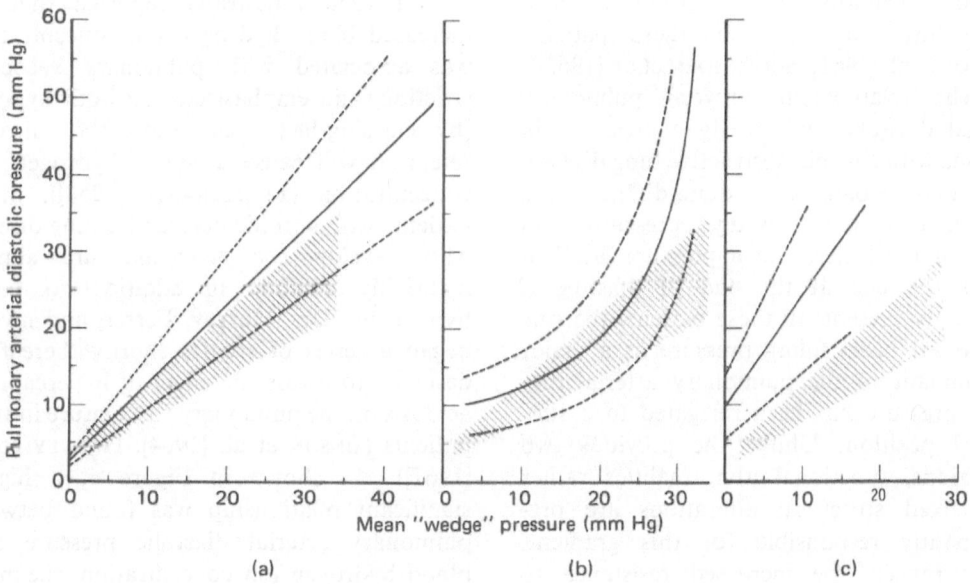

(a)   (b)   (c)

Fig. 5. Graphic representation of the relationship between pulmonary arterial diastolic and "wedge" pressures in patients with left ventricular disease (panel A), mitral stenosis (panel B), and chronic obstructive lung disease (panel C). The regressions (continuous) and one standard deviation (interrupted) are included. The shaded area indicates one standard deviation about the regression calculated for normal subjects. (STOLLERMAN [1969]).

and a gradient exists across the lung which is largest at higher levels of mean wedge pressure: other factors have been superimposed on the left heart pressure in the regulation of pressure in this bed. This gradient, indicative of increased resistance to pulmonary blood flow, is best ascribed to structural changes in the muscular arteries (SMITH et al. [1954]), which presumably arise as a consequence of prolonged pulmonary hypertension, and which, in turn, contribute to it.

The effect of left atrial pressure is also apparent in patients with mitral stenosis (panel B). Pulmonary hypertension in some of these patients is a passive consequence of elevation of the left atrial pressure. However, at levels of "wedge" pressure in excess of 20 mm Hg the diastolic pressure is disproportionately increased with respect to the "wedge." The diastolic gradient in these patients has been ascribed to marked structural changes in the muscular arteries, although vasoconstriction secondary to low alveolar oxygen tension resulting from disturbed distribution of ventilation has also been shown to occur in these patients (BISHOP et al. [1961], SODERHOLM et al. [1962]).

The relationship between pulmonary arterial diastolic and "wedge" pressures in patients with chronic obstructive lung disease, illustrated in panel C, is quite different: the diastolic exceeds the "wedge" pressure at all levels of the latter, and a pressure gradient across the bed at the end of diastole is constantly present. In these patients the role of the left heart filling pressure as a major determinant of the pulmonary arterial diastolic pressure has been relegated to a subsidiary position. Unlike the previous two conditions, functional abnormalities rather than fixed structural alterations are predominantly responsible for this gradient, which reflects the increased resistance to pulmonary blood flow that is characteristic of these patients. This conclusion is based upon two sets of observations. First, pulmonary hypertension is reversible in these patients when disturbed gas exchange is corrected by therapeutic measures. Second, at necropsy there is no correlation between the degree of anatomic disruption of the bed and the degree of right ventricular hypertrophy and dilatation that coexist (CROMIE et al. [1961], DUNHILL [1965]).

Let us turn now, to a consideration of the role of hypercapnia and acidosis in the generation of this abnormal pressure gradient. While it is well established that hypoxia plays a major role in the evolution of pulmonary hypertension in patients with chronic obstructive lung disease (EULER and LILJESTRAND [1946], MOTLEY [1947], HARVEY et al. [1951]), several lines of evidence indicate that other factors must also be implicated. On the basis of statistical considerations, hypoxia accounts for only 50% of the variation in pulmonary artery pressure observed in such patients. Further, the imposition of a hypoxic stimulus in a patient previously in cardiorespiratory failure and optimally treated fails to reproduce the level of pulmonary arterial pressure found in that subject soon after his admission to the hospital.

In 1958 Liljestrand reported that an increased blood hydrogen ion concentration was associated with pulmonary vasoconstriction, and emphasized that both hypoxia (by releasing lactic acid) and carbon dioxide retention will cause a rise in hydrogen ion concentration (LILJESTRAND [1958]). Since patients with chronic obstructive lung disease who develop *cor pulmonale* are almost invariably acidotic in addition to being hypoxemic, Drs. Harvey, Ferrer, and myself began a series of studies shortly thereafter, designed to assess the effect of hypercapneic acidosis on the pulmonary vasculature in such patients (ENSON et al. [1964], HARVEY et al. [1967]). As shown in Figure 6, a highly significant relationship was found between pulmonary arterial diastolic pressure and blood hydrogen ion concentration: the more acidotic the blood, the higher is the diastolic pressure. A similar relationship was also found between the diastolic pressure and the arterial carbon dioxide tension.

Since such correlations do not establish

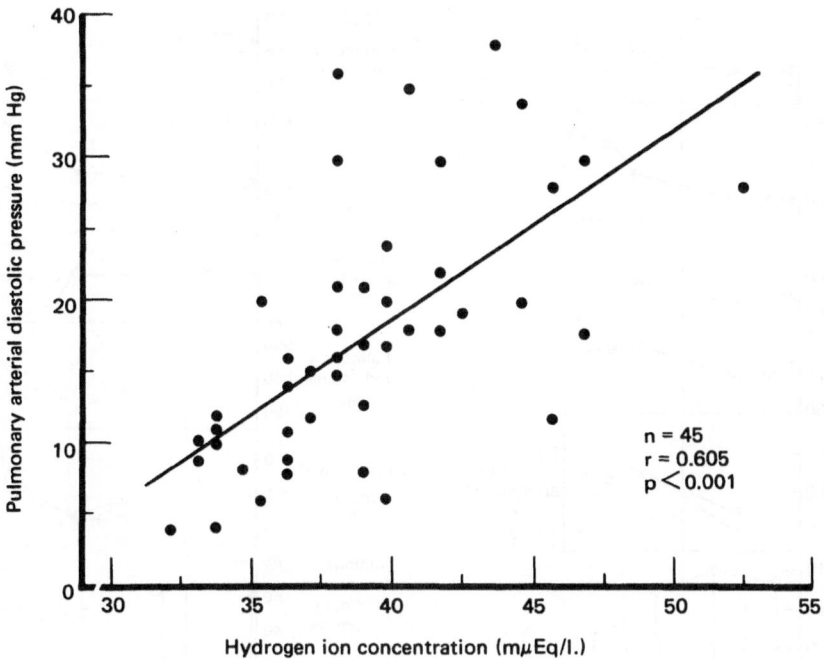

Fig. 6. Graphic representation of the relationship between pulmonary arterial diastolic pressure and blood hydrogen ion concentration in 45 patients with chronic obstructive lung disease. (From HARVEY, ENSON, and FERRER. [1971]).

a causal relationship between pH or carbon dioxide tension and pressure, acute alterations of pH were produced by intravenous infusion of sodium bicarbonate, the amine buffer THAM, and hydrochloric acid. The effect of bicarbonate infusion is illustrated in Figure 7: blood pH, arterial carbon dioxide tension, and pulmonary blood flow rose during the infusion, while pressures fell as the result of vasodilatation. In Figure 8 we see the effect of an infusion of THAM: again pH and blood flow rose, but arterial carbon dioxide tension was unaltered, minute venilation fell, and arterial oxygen saturation fell strikingly. Despite these changes, pulmonary artery pressures fell and pulmonary blood volume rose, again indicating vasodilatation. Consistent with this pressure response to alkalosis is the response to acidosis produced by the infusion of hydrochloric acid, shown in Figure 9: pulmonary arterial diastolic pressure rose (without a change in the wedge pressure) as the pH fell, indicating a vasoconstrictive response on the part of the

precapillary pulmonary vessels. These studies are summarized in Figure 10. The various agents employed produced dichotomous changes between hydrogen ion concentration and carbon dioxide tension. In each case the pulmonary artery diastolic pressure followed the direction of change in hydrogen ion concentration. This indicates that the vasoconstrictor effect of carbon dioxide is mediated solely through its effect on hydrogen ion concentration. Indeed, Viles and Shepherd have indicated that carbon dioxide, per se, may well be a pulmonary vasodilator (VILES and SHEPHERD [1968]).

Alveolar oxygen tension and hydrogen ion concentration appear to be interacting stimuli which are the main determinants of the pulmonary artery diastolic pressure in patients with chronic obstructive lung disease, accounting for about 75% of the variance in observed values of that parameter. The level of the one either augments or attenuates the effect of the other. All available evidence indicates that their site of action is at the

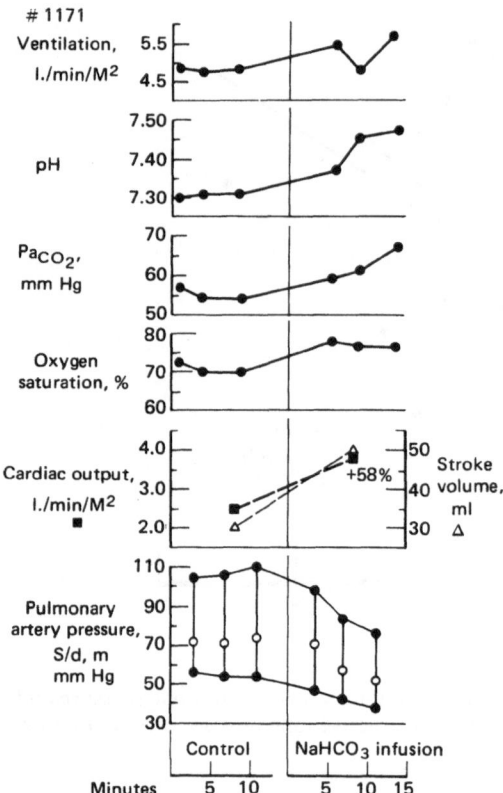

Fig. 7. Graphic representation of the effects of sodium bicarbonate infusion in a patient with chronic obstructive lung disease. The increases in arterial pH and carbon dioxide tension were accompanied by an elevation of cardiac output and a fall in pulmonary artery pressure (reproduced by permission of the Journal of Clinical Investigation). (From ENSON et al. [1964]).

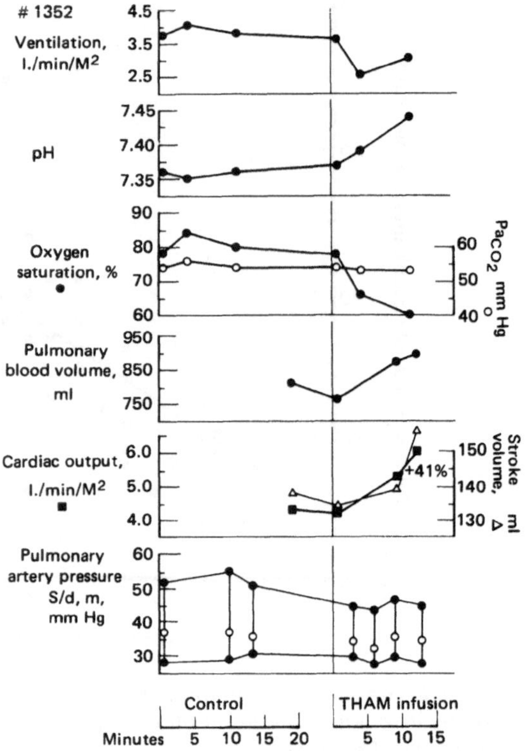

Fig. 8. Graphic representation of the effects of THAM infusion in a patient with chronic obstructive lung disease. The rise in arterial pH was accompanied by hypoventilation, arterial oxygen unsaturation, and increased cardiac output. Pulmonary artery pressure fell (reproduced by permission of the Journal of Clinical Investigation). (From ENSON et al. [1964]).

level of the most muscular pulmonary arteries which have a diameter of approximately 100 to 400 micra. Such vessels are immediately accessible to alveolar gas tension, and several studies indicate that alveolar gases diffuse through their walls (STAUB [1961], JAMESON [1963], ENSON and COURNAND [1963]). While the intimate mechanism by which these agents alter vasomotor tone is unknown, the studies of Bergofsky indicate that hypoxia is associated with partial depolarization of the smooth muscle membrane, a potassium flux, and increased contractility (BERGOFSKY [1966]).

Similar data on the effect of acidosis

and on the interaction of acidosis and hypoxia have been reported by a number of investigators both in man and in a wide variety of animal preparations. Data published by Vogel, shown in Figure 11, illustrate the interplay of hypoxia and hypercapneic acidosis in obesity hypoventilation (VOGEL and BLOUNT [1965]). Correction of only hypoxia (with 100% oxygen) or only of acidosis (with THAM or voluntary hyperventilation) results in an incomplete reduction in pulmonary artery pressure. The simultaneous correction of acidosis and hypoxia, however, effected a maximal fall in pressure. (The values in parentheses next to each pH indicate the

	Control	Hydrochloric acid
Cardiac output (l./min/m²)	3.08	3.22
Stroke volume (ml)	69	69
Sa_{O_2} (%)	84	86
pH_a	7.42	7.34

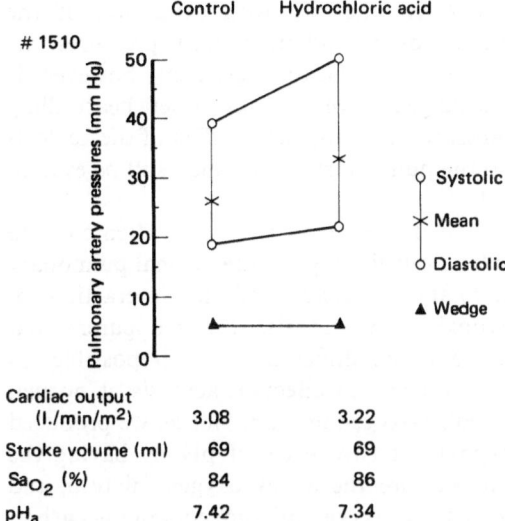

Fig. 9. Graphic representation of the hemodynamic response to an infusion of hydrochloric acid. (From Harvey, Enson, and Ferrer [1971]).

	P_{PA_D}	$[H]^+$	Pa_{CO_2}
Bicarbonate	↓	↓	↑
THAM -----	↓	↓	nc
HCl -------	↑	↑	nc

Fig. 10. Summary of the effects of bicarbonate, THAM, and hydrochloric acid infusions on pulmonary arterial diastolic pressure in patients with chronic obstructive lung disease. For discussion see text.

arterial carbon dioxide tension.)

Several workers have been unable to confirm the vasoconstrictive effect of acidosis. In some instances one suspects that the alveolar oxygen tension was sufficiently high as to attenuate the effect of increased hydrogen ion concentration. In others the reason is unknown, although the differences reported may be related to the manner in which the acid stimulus was imposed on the bed (Daly and Hebb [1966]). One finding merits special consideration, since it affords some insight into yet another effect of acidosis on the

	P_{PA_m} (mm Hg)	pH	Sa_{O_2} %
Control ------------	48	7.32 (54)	84
100% O_2 -----------	42	7.31 (56)	100
THAM -------------	30	7.50	90
Hyperventilation ----	26	7.50 (28)	97
Hyperventilation + O_2	23	7.51 (29)	100

Fig. 11. Summary of the effects on pulmonary arterial pressure of altering alveolar oxygen tension and blood hydrogen ion concentration in a patient with obesity hypoventilation. Adapted from Vogel and Blount [1965].

lesser circulation. Both Moret [1962] and Daum et al. [1970] have indicated that acute acidosis produced a rise in left heart filling pressure, and, apparently, only a passive rise in pulmonary arterial pressure. I say "apparently" because only mean pressure, rather than diastolic pressure was reported, and the presence or absence of a diastolic gradient could not be evaluated. Our study of the effects of acidosis in asiatic cholera may have some bearing on these results (Harvey et al. [1966]). We found that blood pH is a major determinant of the distribution of the circulating blood volume in patients with this disease. In Figure 12 hydrogen ion concentration is shown on the *x* axis and the fraction of the total blood volume held in the central circulation on the *y* axis. At normal pH some 20% of the total blood volume is held in the central circulation, while at pH 7.0 this value rises to 30%—an increase of some 50%. The best explanation for this phenomenon is that acidosis causes peripheral venoconstriction with a decrease in the capacity of the venous reservoirs and an increase in venous return to the central circulation. This volume expension, then, may increase the left heart filling pressure and passively raise the pulmonary arterial pressure. An experimental model of this series of events in patients with chronic obstructive

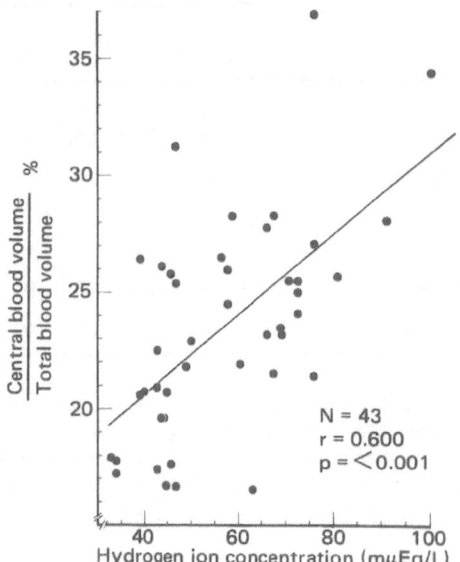

Fig. 12. Graphic representation of the relationship between hydrogen ion concentration and the ratio of central blood volume to total blood volume in patients with cholera. Forty-three observations were made in 23 subjects. For discussion see text. (Reproduced by permission of the Transactions of the Association of American Physicians.)

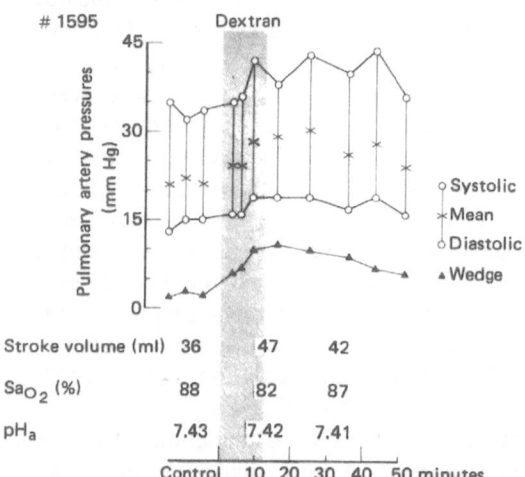

Fig. 13. Graphic representation of the effects of a rapid infusion of 500 ml Dextran in a patient with obstructive lung disease. For discussion see text. (From HARVEY, ENSON, and FERRER [1967]).

lung disease, produced by the infusion of dextran (HARVEY et al. [1967]), is illustrated in Figure 13. As the "wedge" pressure and

stroke volume rise with expansion of the blood volume, all pulmonary pressures rise as well. The diastolic gradient, however, is unchanged by the increase in left heart filling pressures, and any direct effect of the acidosis on the pulmonary vessels may still be evaluated.

More recently we have attempted to extend our findings to the normal pulmonary circulation. Because of the interaction of hypoxia and acidosis, it was apparent that it would be difficult, if not impossible, to demonstrate an effect of acidosis at normal alveolar oxygen tension. Hence, we produced hypoxia at two levels of pH by having the subjects breathe a low oxygen mixture, and then a low oxygen mixture containing carbon dioxide. In Figure 14 the average slopes of pressure on saturation for both stimuli are indicated. Hypoxia in the presence of carbon dioxide, which prevents respiratory alkalosis, is accompanied by a more pronounced rise in pressure than is hypoxia alone at pH 7.47. As in the abnormal bed, the pulmonary pressor effect of hypoxia is augmented by an increased hydrogen ion concentration. Pulmonary vasoconstriction with acidosis alone has not yet been reported in the normal human. It is not likely that alkalosis alone

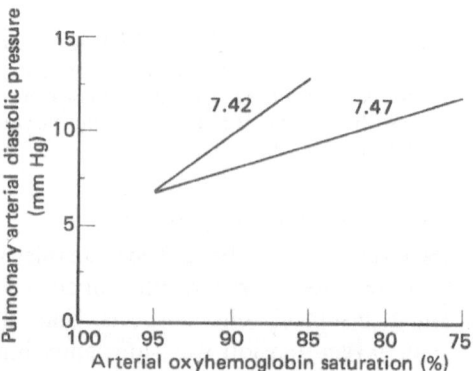

Fig. 14. Graphic representation of the relation between arterial oxyhemoglobin saturation and pulmonary arterial diastolic pressure in normal subjects breathing a low oxygen mixture and a low oxygen mixture containing carbon dioxide. The levels of pH indicated are the average values observed at the end of each test period. For discussion see text.

can produce vasodilatation in this highly compliant bed.

In summary, the normal pulmonary circulation is passively regulated by the activities of the right and left hearts through their influence on the pulmonary blood volume. In disease, increased resistance to pulmonary blood flow may occur as the result of structural changes in the muscular pulmonary arteries, or of active vasoconstriction of these vessels. While the contributions of the right and left heart continue, the bed begins to resemble the systemic circulation more closely, and a pressure gradient develops across the bed at the end of diastole, which indicates the presence of increased resistance to flow. Acutely induced changes in the level of this gradient denote vasomotion. In a wide variety of human and animal studies alkalosis is reported to produce pulmonary vasodilatation, while acidosis evokes a vasoconstrictive response. The bed is relatively insensitive to this phenomenon in the presence of a normal alveolar oxygen tension, while it is extremely sensitive when the alveolar oxygen tension is reduced. In this manner the distribution of pulmonary blood flow is regulated to maintain ventilation-perfusion ratios as high as possible.

Bibliography

Bergofsky, E. H., "Ions and membrane permeability in the regulation of the pulmonary circulation" in *The pulmonary circulation and interstitial space.* A. P. Fishman and H. H. Hecht, eds. Chicago: The University of Chicago (1966).

Bevegard, S., Holmgren, A., and Jonsson, B., "Circulatory studies in well trained athletes at rest and during heavy exercise, with special reference to stroke volume and influence of body position." *Acta Physiol. Scand.* 57:26 (1963).

Bishop, J. M., Harris, P., Bateman, M., and Davidson, L. A. G., "The effect of acetylcholine upon respiratory gas exchange in mitral stenosis." *J. Clin. Invest.* 40:105 (1961).

Carlill, S. D., and Duke, H. N., "Pulmonary vascular changes in response to variations in left auricular pressure." *J. Physiol.* 133: 275 (1956).

Cromie, J. B., "Correlation of anatomic pulmonary emphysema and right ventricular hypertrophy." *Am. Rev. Resp. Dis.* 84:657 (1961).

Daly, I. de B., and Hebb, C., *Pulmonary and bronchial vascular systems.* London: Edward Arnold, Ltd. (1966).

Daum, S., Krofta, K., Jahn, E., Nikoymová, L., and Švorcik, Č., "Effect of carbon dioxide on the pulmonary capillary circulation in acute experiments." In *Progress in respiration research.* Vol. 5. J. Widimsky, S. Daum, and H. Herzog, eds. Basel: S. Karger (1970).

Dickens, J., Villaca, L., Waldow, A., and Goldberg, H., "The haemodynamics of mitral stenosis before and after commissurotomy." *Brit. Heart J.* 19:419 (1957).

Dunill, M. S., "Quantitative observations on the anatomy of chronic non-specific lung disease." *Med. Thorac.* 22:261 (1965).

Eliasch, H., "The pulmonary circulation at rest and on effort in mitral stenosis." *Scand. J. Clin. Lab. Invest.*, vol. 4, suppl. 4 (1952).

Enson, Y., and Cournand, A., "Respiratory variation in blood oxygen saturation within the great veins, right heart, and pulmonary artery." *Fed. Proc.* 22:516 (1963).

Enson, Y., Guintini, C., Lewis, M. L., Morris, T. Q., Ferrer, M. I., and Harvey, R. M., "The influence of hydrogen ion concentration and hypoxia on the pulmonary circulation." *J. Clin. Invest.* 43:1146 (1964).

Euler, U. S. von, and Liljestrand, G., "Observations on the pulmonary arterial blood pressure in the cat." *Acta Physiol. Scand.* 12:301 (1946).

Gabe, I. T., Gault, J. H., Ross, J., Jr., et al., "Measurement of instantaneous blood flow velocity and pressure in conscious man with a catheter-tip velocity probe." *Circulation* 40:603 (1969).

Granath, A., and Strandell, T., "Relationships between cardiac output, stroke volume and intracardiac pressures at rest and during exercise in supine position and some authropometric data in healthy old men." *Acta Med. Scand.* 174:447 (1964).

Hamilton, W. F., Woodbury, R. A., and Vogt, E., "Differential pressures in the lesser circulation of unanesthetized dog." *Am. J. Physiol.* 125:130 (1939).

Harvey, R. M., Ferrer, M. I., Richards, D. W., Jr., and Cournand, A., "Influence of chronic pulmonary disease on the heart and circulation." *Am. J. Med.* 10:719 (1951).

———, Enson, Y., Lewis, M. L., "Hemodynamic effects of dehydration and metabolic acidosis in asiatic cholera." *Trans. A. Am. Physicians* 79:177 (1966).

———, Enson, Y., Betti, R., Lewis, M. L., Rochester, D. F., and Ferrer, I. M., "Further observations on the effect of hydrogen ion on the pulmonary circulation." *Circulation* 35:1019 (1967).

———, Enson, Y., and Ferrer, M. I., "Further considerations of the causes of pulmonary hypertension in cor pulmonale." *Bull. Physio-Path. Resp.* 3:624 (1967).

———, and Enson, Y., "Pulmonary vascular resistance," in *Advances in internal medicine.* Vol. 15. G. H. Stollerman, ed. Chicago: Year Book Medical Publishers, Inc. (1969).

———, Enson, Y., and Ferrer, M. I., *Chest* 59:82 (1971).

Holmgren, A., Jonsson, B., Levander, M., et al., "Low physical working capacity in suspected heart cases due to inadequate adjustment of peripheral blood flow (vasoregulatory asthena)." *Acta Med. Scand.* 158:413 (1957).

Jameson, A. G., "Diffusion of gases from alveolus to precapillary arteries." *Science* 139:826 (1963).

Kaltman, A. J., Herbert, W. H., Conroy, R. J., et al., "The gradient in pressure across the pulmonary vascular bed during diastole." *Circulation* 34:377 (1966).

Liljestrand, G., "Chemical control of the distribution of the pulmonary blood flow." *Acta Physiol. Scand.* 44:216 (1958).

Karatzas, N. B., and Lee, G. de J., "Propagation of blood flow pulse in the normal human arterial system." *Circ. Res.* 25:11 (1969).

Malmborg, R. O., "A clinical and hemodynamic analysis of factors limiting the cardiac performance in patients with coronary heart disease." *Acta Med. Scand.*, vol. 117, suppl. 426 (1965).

Moret, P. R., "Circulation pulmonaire. Influence du debit cardiaque, de l'anoxie et de l'hypercapnie sur les pressions et resistances pulmonaires." *Cardiologia* 40:207 (1962).

Morkin, E., Collins, J. A., Goldman, H. S., et al., "Pattern of blood flow in the pulmonary veins of the dog." *J. Appl. Physiol.* 20:118 (1965).

Motley, H. L., Cournand, A., Werko, L., Himmelstein, A., and Dresdale, D., "The influence of short periods of induced acute anoxia upon pulmonary artery pressures in man." *Am. J. Physiol.* 150:315 (1947).

Selzer, A., and Malmborg, R. O., "Hemodynamic effects of digoxin in latent cardiac failure." *Circulation* 25:695 (1962).

Smith, R. C., Burchell, H. B., and Edwards, J. E., "Pathology of the pulmonary vascular tree." IV. Structural changes in the pulmonary vessels in chronic left ventricular failure. *Circulation* 10:801 (1954).

Soderholm, B., Werko, L., and Widimsky, J., "The effect of acetylcholine on pulmonary circulation and gas exchange in cases of mitral stenosis." *Acta Med. Scand.* 172:95 (1962).

Staub, N. C., "Gas exchange vessels in the cat lung." *Fed. Proc.* 20:107 (1961).

Stollerman, G. E., et al., eds. *Advances in internal medicine.* Vol. 15. Year Book Medical Publishers (1969).

Vogel, J. H. K., and Blount, S. G., Jr., "The role of hydrogen ion concentration in the regulation of pulmonary artery pressure: observations in a patient with hypoventilation and obesity." *Circulation* 32:788 (1965).

Varnauskas, E., "Studies in hypertensive cardiovascular disease with special reference to cardiac function." *Scand. J. Clin. Lab. Invest.* Vol. 7, suppl. 1955.

Viles, P. H., and Shepherd, J. T., "Evidence for a dilator action of carbon dioxide on the pulmonary vessels of the cat." *Circ. Res.* 22:325 (1968).

Werko, L., Biorck, G., Grawford, C., Wulff, H., Krook, H., and Eliasch, H., "Pulmonary circulatory dynamics in mitral stenosis before and after commissurotomy." *Am. Heart J.* 45:477 (1953).

Yu, P. N. G., Simpson, J. H., Lovejoy, F. W., Jr., Joos, H. A., and Nye, R. E., Jr., "Studies of pulmonary hypertension." IV. Pulmonary circulatory dynamics in patients with mitral stenosis at rest. *Am. Heart J.* 47:330 (1954).

Enson Discussion

———: Dr. Enson, apparently in the isolated heart-lung preparation it's possible to show an effect of acidosis on myocardial contractility. In your studies is it possible to attribute any of your changes to alteration of myocardial function, or do you feel that all of this is secondary to peripheral veno-constriction?

ENSON: You're talking now about the cholera study? Yes. Well, I have to describe the way this information was obtained for you to get the full flavor of it. What we did was to examine a series of patients who were in severe vascular collapse, with hypovolemic shock, a little bit different from blood loss shock, but in some ways, at least, comparable. They were brought to normal levels of pressure and flow with a saline transfusion. At this point we corrected the blood pH, and the only way one can assess myocardial contractility, I think, in this rather chaotic series of events, was that when we corrected the pH from acid to alkaline, the cardiac output fell and the central blood volume fell, despite the fact that the total circulating blood volume continued to increase. I certainly think that Downing's studies in which the perfusion of papillary muscles has been maintained intact, have indicated that you have to get the Po_2 down to a desperately low level in the perfusate before the contractility of the papillary muscle begins to deteriorate with an acidotic stimulus, be it a hypercapneic stimulus or a metabolic acidosis. And I think that one of the things that this data indicates, to me at least, is that much of the work in the literature at the present time was done on extraordinarily hypoxic myocardia.

————: On one slide we could see an increased central blood volume, and this increased central blood volume may have evoked the Gauer-Henry reflex and effects on the kidney. Did you observe an increased diuresis?

ENSON: These patients started out with a pH someplace between 6.9 and 7.0. They were anuric. The fascinating thing to me was that restoration of cardiac output and repletion of circulating blood volume did not change renal function. There was no urinary output. But correction of pH, up to a level let's say about 7.22 or 7.24, often resulted in a very prompt diuresis and, although we were not studying renal function in this group of patients (I believe the Johns Hopkins group

in Calcutta was, at the relatively same time), these people could pass 2 to 300 ml of highly concentrated urine, beginning at a pH of 7.24 (this is arterial pH), and with the passage of the urine their pH would be 7.36 or 7.37.

NAHAS: Dr. Truino informed me that inactivation of angiotensin occurred actually in the lung, inasmuch as I think 80% was in one circulation. So it occurs, it is possible that alterations in the internal environment of the lung, whether a decrease in Po_2 or an alteration in pH, might also change some of the activity of the neurotransmitters such as angiotensin or prostaglandins, and this might be one of the fundamental mechanisms by which alterations in H^+ or Po_2 could act on the vasculature of the lung, and I wonder if Dr. Turino, who must be here somewhere, could comment on this point?

TURINO: It's hard to know just how applicable these considerations are to the observations that Dr. Enson has reported, but I think information that has been coming forth in the last three or four years, much of it from Vane's work in England [1969], does suggest that pulmonary tissue and we don't know exactly where in pulmonary tissue—it may be in the intimal lining cells, it may be in alveolar macrophage cells—that there is a capacity in the lung to perform rapid chemical changes on vasoactive substances and you mentioned Angiotensin I which is changed to Angiotensin II in the lung, in large part. Prostaglandins are also inactivated and bradykinine, and probably other kinines which we at present do not recognize, and it's conceivable that part of the change in distribution of blood volumes which you observed between the central circulation and peripheral circulation could be mediated by substances like this which are being metabolized abnormally because of either pH effects primarily, or distribution of blood flow.

ENSON: Yes. In this connection I think we're just beginning a new era with respect to humeral influences on the pulmonary vessels. There is a recent paper in the JCI by Hyman [1971], in Tulane, who in a rather unusual preparation was able to activate some form of vaso-active substance with acid infusions, and showed that if blood was bypassed around the lung, it had a constrictive effect on the systemic circulation; if it's passed through the lung it has a constrictive effect on the pulmonary circulation, but then is metabolized and is inactive in the systemic circulation. I don't know, again, how applicable this is, but I think it denotes the direction in which this field is going next. It's rather provocative work.

Bibliography

Hyman, A. L., Woolverton, W. C., Guth, P. S,. and Ichinoze, H., "The pulmonary vasopressor response to decreases in blood pH in intact dogs." *J. Clin. Invest.* 50:1028 (1971).

Vane, T. R., "The release and fate of vasoactive hormones in the circulation." *Brit. J. Pharmacology* 35:209 (1969).

4. Carbon Dioxide and the Kidney*

Floyd C. Rector, Jr.

Department of Internal Medicine,
The University of Texas Southwestern Medical School,
5323 Harry Hines
Dallas, Texas 75235

The kidney participates in acid-base homeostasis by regulating the concentration of bicarbonate in extracellular fluid. If plasma P_{CO_2} is maintained at a normal level by respiratory mechanisms, then the kidney will maintain plasma bicarbonate concentration in the range of 25 to 28 meq/l., despite the continual accession of metabolic acids and bases into the extracellular fluid. If plasma P_{CO_2} is altered in either an upward or downward direction as a result of abnormal respiratory function, plasma bicarbonate concentrations will be appropriately re-adjusted by resetting the renal mechanisms.

Two processes are involved in the renal control of plasma bicarbonate concentration. *First*, bicarbonate in the glomerular filtrate is reabsorbed by the tubules. When plasma bicarbonate concentration is below a critical threshold level reabsorption is complete, preventing loss into the urine. When plasma bicarbonate concentration rises above this threshold level, tubular reabsorption becomes incomplete and the excess filtered bicarbonate is excreted into the urine. *Second*, the kidney regenerates that bicarbonate which was consumed by the buffering of metabolic acids entering extracellular fluid. This is accomplished by excreting hydrogen into the urine bound to either filtered buffers (as titratable acid) or newly formed buffer (as NH_4^+). For each hydrogen excreted into the urine in this fashion, a newly formed bicarbonate is added to renal venous blood.

Studies on the mechanism of urinary acidification indicate that H^+ secretion plays a major role in both bicarbonate reabsorption and formulation of titratable acid and ammonium. The theoretical basis of these studies is shown in Figure 1. As shown in the left-hand panel, if bicarbonate reabsorption were mediated by H^+ secretion, carbonic acid would be generated in tubular fluid. If the carbonic acid did not diffuse out of the lumen and if the tubular fluid were not in contact with carbonic anhydrase, then the concentration of carbonic acid in the tubular fluid would rise to a level sufficient to drive the uncatalyzed dehydration of carbonic acid at a rate equal to the rate of bicarbonate reabsorption. From the known rates of bicarbonate reabsorption, the predicted steady-state concentration of carbonic acid would result in the *in vivo* intratubular pH being approximately 1 pH unit more acid than estimated from the tubular fluid bicarbonate concentration and plasma P_{CO_2}.

As shown in the right-hand panel of Figure 1, excess carbonic acid would not be generated if bicarbonate ions were re-absorbed directly. In fact, if tubular fluid contained significant quantities of non-bicarbonate buffer and bicarbonate reabsorption were nearing completion, carbonic acid would be consumed and the *in vivo* intra-

* Work supported by USPHS Grant 1 POL HE-11662.

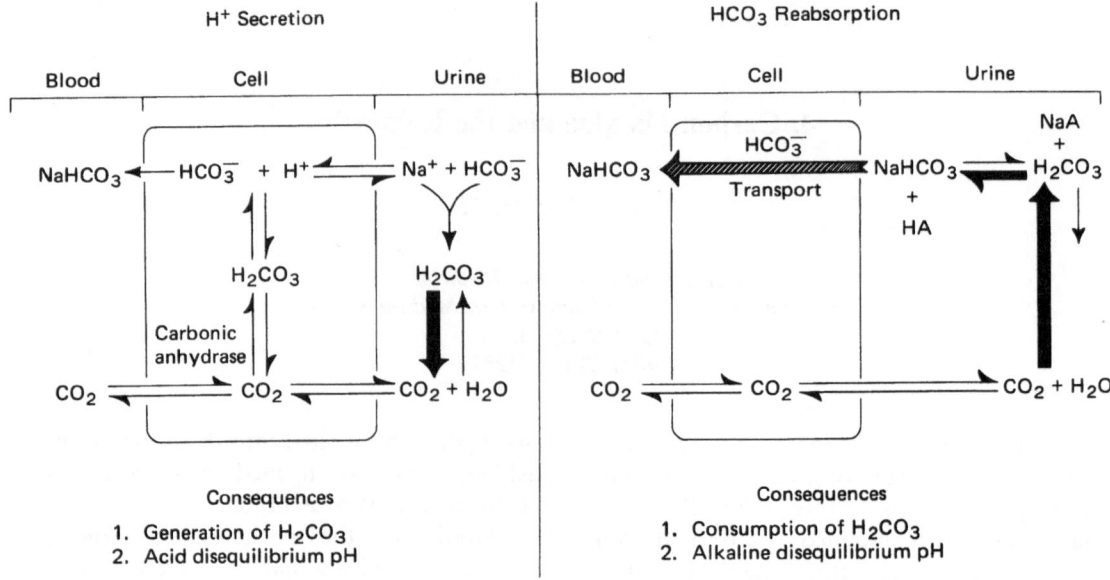

Fig. 1. The theoretical portrayal of effects of hydrogen secretion versus bicarbonate reabsorption.

tubular pH would be more alkaline than the calculated equilibrium pH.

Studies based on these theoretical considerations have been performed in our laboratory (RECTOR, CARTER and SELDIN [1965]) and by Vieira and Malnic [1968]. In a series of micropuncture studies in rats *in vivo* intratubular pH was measured with either pH-sensitive glass or antimony microelectrodes and compared with the equilibrium

pH calculated from the measured tubular fluid bicarbonate concentration and the plasma Pco_2.

The results are shown in Table 1. In the distal tubule we found the *in vivo* intratubular pH to be 0.85 units more acid than the calculated equilibrium pH during $NaHCO_3$ diuresis. The disequilibrium was obliterated by injecting carbonic anhydrase intravenously in amounts sufficient to give

Table 1. Comparison of Steady State *in vivo* Intratubular pH and *in vitro* Equilibrium pH of Distal Tubular Fluid

Investigator	Treatment	1 Intratubular pH	2 Equilibrium pH	1-2 Disequilibrium pH
Rector et al. (1965)	$NaHCO_3$ infusion	6.85	7.73	−0.85
	$NaHCO_3$ infusion + carbonic anhydrase	7.67	7.70	−0.03
Vieira and Malnic (1968)	Control	6.45	6.79	−0.34
	$NaHCO_3$ infusion	7.41	7.65	−0.24
	Acetazolamide	7.10	7.64	−0.54

measureable activity in the urine, indicating that the discrepancy was due to excess carbonic acid. These results have been confirmed by Vieira and Malnic, although they obtained a lower value for the disequilibrium pH. These results indicate that bicarbonate reabsorption in the distal tubule is mediated by hydrogen ion secretion.

The results obtained in the proximal tubule are shown in Table 2. In normal hydropenic rats, in rats infused with NaH_2PO_4, and in rats undergoing sodium bicarbonate diuresis, the measured intratubular pH was equal to the calculated equilibrium pH. After inhibition of carbonic anhydrase with benzolamide, however, the *in vivo* intratubular pH became 0.8 pH units more acid than the calculated equilibrium pH. These results have also been confirmed by Vieira and Malnic, but as in the case of the distal tubule, their value for the disequilibrium pH of 0.4 is less than the value we obtained. Nevertheless, both sets of data indicate that bicarbonate reabsorption in the proximal, as well as the distal, tubule is mediated by hydrogen ion secretion.

However, as shown in Figure 2, the hydrogen ion secretory systems in the proximal and distules differ markedly with respect to the role of carbonic anhydrase. In both areas of the nephron carbonic anhydrase probably plays a cellular role in maintaining an intracellular supply of H_2CO_3 and H^+ by catalyzing the hydration of CO_2. In addition, carbonic anhydrase subserves an additional function in the proximal tubule. The enzyme appears to be in functional contact with proximal tubular fluid so that H_2CO_3 formed by the reaction of secreted H^+ with filtered bicarbonate is rapidly broken down to CO_2 and H_2O. Carbonic anhydrase, presumably located in the luminal membrane, prevents the accumulation of excess H_2CO_3. As a result of this action, the steady-state intratubular pH is approximately 1.0 pH units higher than it would be if carbonic anhydrase were not present in the luminal membrane. In the proximal tubule, therefore, carbonic anhydrase facilitates the transport of large quantities of H^+ by both furnishing an intracellular supply of H^+ and preventing steep pH gradients. In contrast, the distal tubule does not contain carbonic anhydrase in its luminal membrane and must always secrete H^+ against a concentration gradient, even in the presence of high bicarbonate concentrations.

The data showing an acid disequilibrium

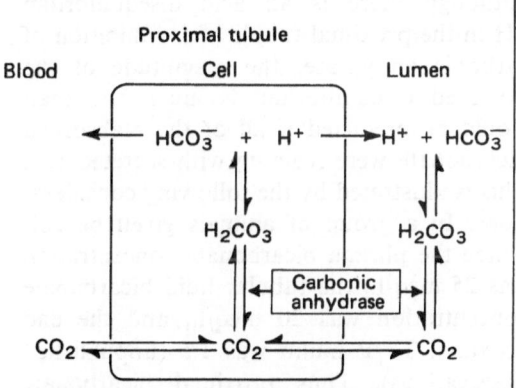

1. Cytoplasmic carbonic anhydrase (C.A.)
Accelerates intracellular H^+ formation

2. Luminal membrane C.A.
Catalyzes H_2CO_3 breakdown and prevents generation of pH gradients

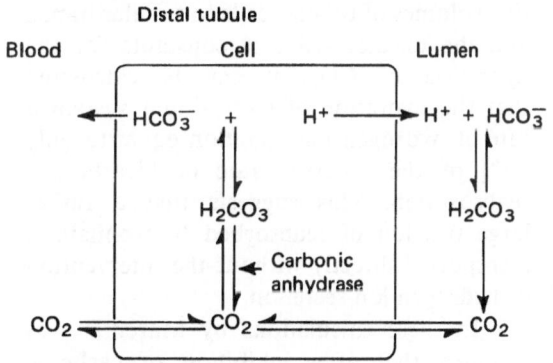

1. Cytoplasmic C.A.
Accelerates intracellular H^+ formation

2. Luminal membrane C. A.
Absent

Fig. 2. Role of carbonic anhydrase in facilitating hydrogen secretion in proximal and distal tubules.

Table 2. Comparison of Steady State *in vivo* Intratubular pH and *in vitro* Equilibrium pH of Proximal Tubular Fluid

Investigator	Treatment	1 Intratubular pH	2 Equilibrium pH	1-2 Disequilibrium pH
Rector et al. (1965)	None	6.82	6.88	−0.06
	Na_2HPO_4 infusion	6.87	6.82	+0.05
	$NaHCO_3$ infusion	7.53	7.49	−0.04
	$NaHCO_3$ infusion + benzolamide	6.71	7.56	−0.85
Vieira and Malnic (1968)	Control	6.70	6.84	−0.14
	$NaHCO_3$ infusion	7.35	7.42	−0.07
	Acetzolamide	6.67	7.08	−0.41

pH in tubular fluid establishes that hydrogen ion secretion plays an important role in bicarbonate reabsorption; however, it does not exclude the possibility of direct transport of bicarbonate ions per se. Maren [1968] has pointed out that in the presence of complete inhibition of carbonic anhydrase, the uncatalyzed hydration of CO_2 in the cell is not sufficient to account for the observed rates of bicarbonate reabsorption. From the relative volumes of tubular cells to tubular lumen and the uncatalyzed rate constants for the hydration of CO_2, it can be calculated that the hydration of CO_2 would sustain a rate of hydrogen ion secretion equal to only 20% of the observed rate of bicarbonate reabsorption. This suggests that a rather large fraction of reabsorbed bicarbonate is transported directly without the intervention of hydrogen ion secretion.

In these calculations by Maren it was assumed that after inhibition of carbonic anhydrase the intracellular hydration of CO_2 would proceed at the known rates for the completely uncatalyzed reaction. It is known, however, that many substances other than carbonic anhydrase catalyze the hydration of CO_2. Some of these, such as phosphate and organic anions, may be present in cells in fairly high concentrations. Therefore, it is probable that even in the complete absence of carbonic anhydrase the intracellular hydration of CO_2 might proceed at a rate several times greater than the simple uncatalyzed rate.

There is yet another problem in attempting to explain all bicarbonate reabsorption on the basis of hydrogen ion secretion. Although there is an acid disequilibrium pH in the proximal tubule after inhibition of carbonic anhydrase, the magnitude of the observed disequilibrium is much less than would be predicted if all of the reabsorbed bicarbonate were reacting with secreted H^+. This is illustrated by the following considerations. In a group of animals given benzolamide the plasma bicarbonate concentration was 25 meq/l., the tubular fluid bicarbonate concentration was 20 meq/l., and the end proximal TF/P inulin was 1.5 (unpublished observations). Thus proximal bicarbonate reabsorption after inhibition of carbonic anhydrase was approximately 10 meq/l. filtrate. This is approximately 40% of the control hydropenic value. The transit time through the proximal tubule under these conditions was 10 sec. Therefore the rate at which carbonic acid would be generated in tubular fluid if all bicarbonate reabsorption were mediated by hydrogen ion secretion is 1.07 meq/l./sec. From this rate of carbonic acid generation it can be calculated that the *in vivo* intratubular pH would be 1.17 pH units more acid than the calculated equilibrium pH. In contrast, the 0.8 acid disequilibrium pH which we found is equivalent to a rate of 0.55 meq/l./sec, while the disequilibrium of 0.41 obtained by Vieira and Malnic is equivalent to a rate of only 0.25 meq/l./sec. Thus the magnitude of the measured disequilibrium pH is compatible with 50 to 75% of bicarbonate reabsorption occurring via some mechanism which does not generate excess carbonic acid, such as direct transport of bicarbonate ions per se.

Thus it is possible that there are two processes contributing to bicarbonate reabsorption after inhibition of carbonic anhydrase: hydrogen ion secretion, accounting for approximately 30%, and direct bicarbonate transport, accounting for 70% of the total reabsorption.

There is evidence against this view, however. The experiment presented in Table 3 demonstrates the marked sensitivity of bicarbonate reabsorption to changes in P_{CO_2} following the administration of acetazolamide. At a plasma P_{CO_2} of 50 mm Hg bicarbonate reabsorption was 12 meq/l. If only 30% of this were due to hydrogen ion secretion, maintained by the uncatalyzed hydration of CO_2, and the remaining 70% were due to direct transport of bicarbonate ions, then only that small portion mediated by H^+ secretion would respond to changes

in P_{CO_2}, while the much larger fraction mediated by bicarbonate transport would be relatively constant at all CO_2 tensions. In this instance doubling P_{CO_2} would be expected to increase the H^+ secretory component from 3.6 to 7.2 meq/l. GFR and not change the 8.4 meq/l. GFR due to bicarbonate transport; total bicarbonate reabsorption would be expected to rise from 12 to 15.6 meq/l. GFR. In contrast to these predicted results, total bicarbonate reabsorption doubled, rising from 12 to 23.4 meq/l. GFR when P_{CO_2} was elevated from 50 to 99 mm Hg. These results indicate that, following inhibition of carbonic anhydrase, virtually all of the remaining bicarbonate reabsorption is dependent on P_{CO_2}. This suggests that direct transport of bicarbonate ions contribute very little to overall bicarbonate reabsorption.

It is possible to explain the discrepancies between the observed rate of bicarbonate reabsorption, the calculated rate of intracellular hydration of CO_2, and the observed acid disequilibrium pH, as well as the marked dependence on P_{CO_2}, by a single hydrogen ion secretory system as shown in Figure 3. Within the cell the hydration of CO_2 generates H_2CO_3. The hydrogen ion secretory system consumes the intracellular H_2CO_3, while at the same time generating H_2CO_3 in the lumen. In the presence of carbonic anhydrase the reactions between CO_2 and H_2CO_3 in both cell and lumen are in equilibrium. Following inhibition of both cytoplasmic and luminal membrane carbonic anhydrase, the equilibrium between CO_2

Table 3. Effect of P_{CO_2} on Bicarbonate Reabsorptive Capacity after Acetazolamide

Plasma P_{CO_2}	Observed	Bicarbonate reabsorption		
		Predicted		
		H^+ Secretion	HCO_3^- Trans.	Total
mm Hg		meq/l. GFR		
50	12.0	3.6	8.4	12.0
100	23.4	7.2	8.4	15.6

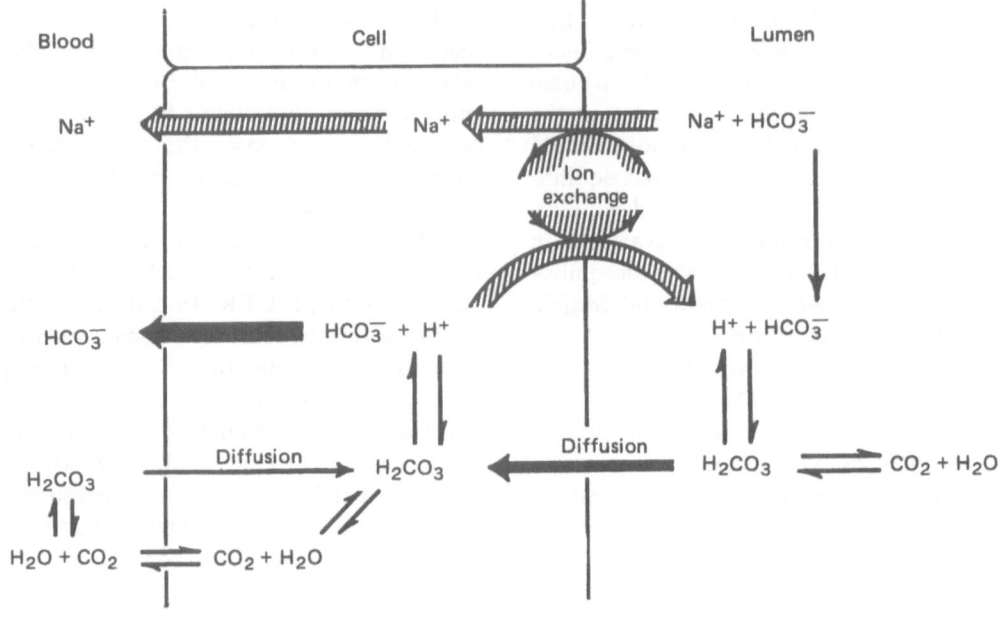

Fig. 3. The role of the back diffusion of H_2CO_3 in meditating bicarbonate reabsorption via hydrogen secretion.

and H_2CO_3 no longer exists; intracellular H_2CO_3 is reduced, while luminal H_2CO_3 is markedly elevated. As a result of this steep concentration gradient non-ionized H_2CO_3 will diffuse out of the lumen back into the cell. This will have two consequences. First, it will maintain the intracellular supply of H_2CO_3 necessary for continued H^+ secretion. In a cyclic process such as this the rate at which new H_2CO_3 must be produced by intracellular hydration of CO_2 needs to be only as great as the rate at which H_2CO_3 is lost from the cycle by decomposition to CO_2 in the tubular lumen. The second consequence of this model is that the magnitude of the disequilibrium pH would be less than predicted if all of the generated H_2CO_3 remained in the lumen, and decomposed to CO_2. In the example cited earlier the rate of hydrogen ion secretion was 1.07 meq/l./sec and the calculated disequilibrium pH was 1.16. However, if 50% of the H_2CO_3 generated by hydrogen ion secretion were recycled into the cell and 50% were retained in the lumen, then the predicted disequilibrium pH would be 0.8 units, a value very close to that

observed by us. Finally, according to this model the rate at which the overall cycle operates would be critically dependent on P_{CO_2}.

With this model as a background it is of interest to examine the relative contributions of CO_2 tension and carbonic anhydrase activity to the maximal H^+ secretory capacity. These results are shown in Figure 4 (taken from RECTOR et al. [1960]). In normal dogs infused with hypertonic $NaHCO_3$ the maximal rate of bicarbonate reabsorption (bicarbonate Tm) is approximately 2.8 meq/100 ml GFR at a P_{CO_2} of 40 mm Hg. The bicarbonate Tm falls to 1.5 meq/100 ml GFR when P_{CO_2} is reduced to 10 mm Hg and increases progressively, although not in a linear fashion, when P_{CO_2} is elevated to very high levels. The failure of the bicarbonate Tm to increase proportionately as P_{CO_2} is raised may be due to partial saturation of the hydrogen transport system at higher CO_2 tensions. However, since the measurement of the bicarbonate Tm during severe hypercapnia requires very high plasma concentrations of bicarbonate, the curvilinear character of the

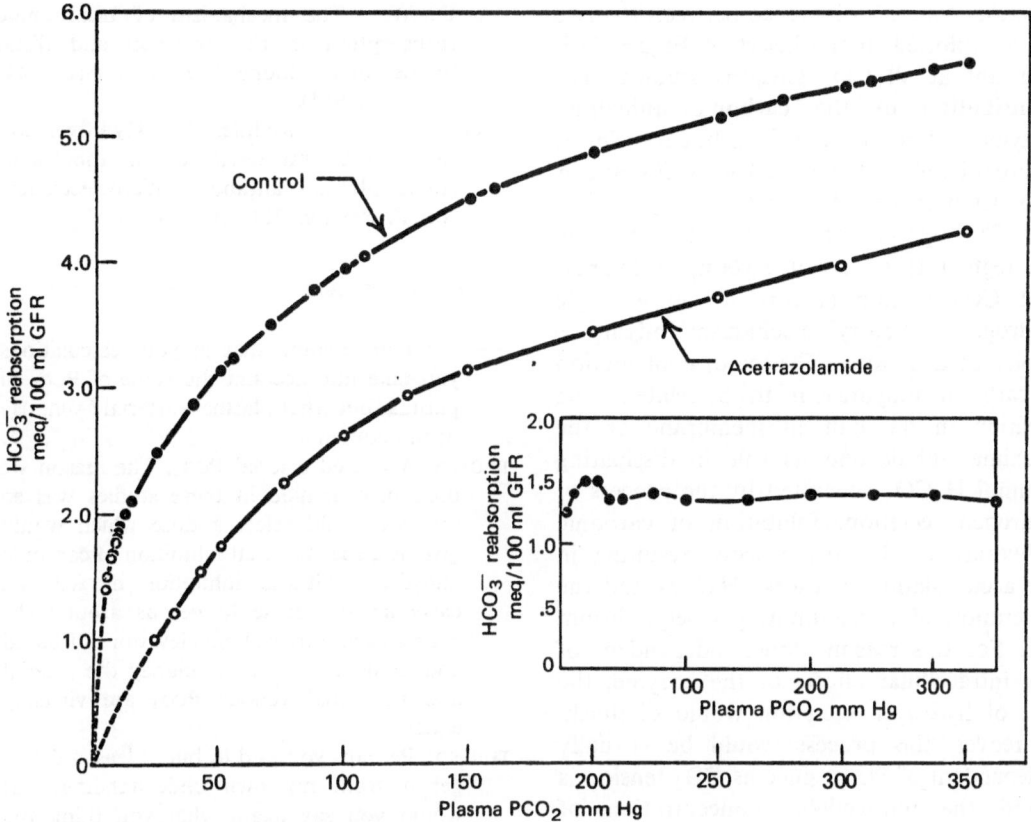

Fig. 4. Comparison of the relation between bicarbonate reabsorption and plasma P_{CO_2} with and without acetazolamide. The contribution of the carbonic anhydrase enzyme system at all levels of plasma P_{CO_2} is plotted in the inset as the difference between the upper and lower curves. (RECTOR. *et al.* [1960]).

curve in Figure 4 may reflect in part the superimposed effects of ECF volume expansion rather than the intrinsic kinetics of the hydrogen secretory system.

Plasma P_{CO_2} is thought to influence bicarbonate reabsorption through its effects on the intracellular concentration of hydrogen ions, either by furnishing a plentiful supply of H_2CO_3 to the hydrogen transport system or by neutralizing hydroxyl ions generated by the pumping of hydrogen out of the cell. Both of these reactions are dependent on the enzyme carbonic anhydrase; thus it might be predicted that the sensitivity of the system to P_{CO_2} would be severely restricted following the inhibition of carbonic anhydrase. As shown by the lower curve in Figure 4, this is

clearly not the case; the hydrogen secretory mechanism is just as sensitive to P_{CO_2} following the administration of a large dose of acetazolamide (20 mg/kg) as in the presence of an intact carbonic anhydrase enzyme system. It appears, therefore, that the regulatory effect of P_{CO_2} on the capacity to reabsorb bicarbonate is independent of carbonic anhydrase.

In contrast, the contribution of carbonic anhydrase activity to the bicarbonate Tm appears to be completely independent of P_{CO_2}, at least over the range examined. A comparison of the relationship between the bicarbonate Tm and plasma P_{CO_2} in the presence and absence of carbonic anhydrase activity (upper and lower curves of Figure 4) discloses that the difference between the two values (plotted in the insert of Figure 4) is constant at all CO_2 tensions studied. The contribution of the carbonic anhydrase enzyme system to the bicarbonate Tm is approximately 1.4 meq/100 ml GFR and is completely independent of P_{CO_2}.

The apparent lack of interaction between the regulatory effects of carbonic anhydrase and CO_2 tension (Figure 4) on a single hydrogen secretory mechanism might be explained as follows. The major contribution of carbonic anhydrase might be related to its location in the luminal membrane of the proximal tubule and its role in dissipating luminol H_2CO_3 generated by the process of hydrogen secretion. Inhibition of carbonic anhydrase blocks this process, resulting in the accumulation of excess H_2CO_3 and the generation of a rate-limiting disequilibrium pH. For this reason alone, independent of any intracellular effects of the enzyme, the rate of hydrogen secretion would diminish. Moreover, this process would be virtually independent of P_{CO_2}, since as CO_2 tension is raised the intracellular concentration of H_2CO_3, the rate of luminal generation of H_2CO_3 and the luminal concentration of H_2CO_3 would all increase more or less proportionately; the limiting pH gradient imposed by the disequilibrium in the luminal fluid would be approximately the same at all CO_2 tensions. Thus, if the major contribution of carbonic anhydrase to the system were its luminal action, this fraction of the bicarbonate Tm would be P_{CO_2}-independent.

Bibliography

Maren, T. H., "Renal carbonic anhydrase and the pharmacology of sulfonamide inhibitors." In *Handbook of experimental pharmacology*. Diuretics, Heidelberg: Springer (1968).

Rector, F. C., Jr., Seldin, D. W., Roberts, A. D., Jr., and Smith, J. S., "The role of plasma CO_2 tension and carbonic anhydrase activity in the renal reabsorption of bicarbonate." *J. Clin. Invest.* 39: 1706–1721 (1960).

Rector, F. C., Jr., Carter, N. W., and Seldin, D. W., "The mechanism of bicarbonate reabsorption in the proximal and distal tubules of the kidney." *J. Clin. Invest.* 44: 278–290 (1965).

Vieira, F. L., and Malnic, G., "Hydrogen ion secretion by rat renal cortical tubules as studied by an antimony microelectrode." *Am. J. Physiol.* 214:710–718 (1968).

Rector Discussion

———: I understand that in your calculations you take into account the value of P_{CO_2} in plasma, but what plasma—arterial? venous? or in between?

RECTOR: We used arterial P_{CO_2}. The reason we used benzolamide in these studies was so that we could select a dose which would give us a specific renal inhibition of carbonic anhydrase without inhibition of red cell carbonic anhydrase to get us around the problems and thus avoid elevations of blood and tissue P_{CO_2}. In the kidney the arterial and the renal venous P_{CO_2} are virtually equal.

TURINO: Perhaps you said it, but at least I didn't get it from my own understanding, but would you say again what you think the mechanisms involved are for this reabsorption of bicarbonate in the absence of carbonic anhydrase. In other words, what is the pump?

RECTOR: I think it's all hydrogen secretion, no bicarbonate transport, and that the discrepancies in the system as far as the intracellular hydration of CO_2 and the breakdown of carbonic acid in the lumen are all accounted for by the recycling of carbonic acid between lumen and cell. The primary mechanism is hydrogen secretion.

TURINO: And you think this takes place over the whole tubule or just in a proximate tubule?

RECTOR: Both the proximal and distal tubules.

SEVERINGHAUS: With benzolamide do you assume that the drug gets into the renal tubular cell or only in the lumen?

RECTOR: It is assumed that it gets into the renal tubular cell. The whole basis of the pharmacology of benzolamide is that it contains a strong sulfonic group which increases its uptake by the renal tubule cell.

———: At what P_{CO_2} is the transport mechanism working at its maximum capacity?

RECTOR: That's very difficult to say. We have examined the so-called bicarbonate transport capacity up to a P_{CO_2} of 400 mm of mercury and it increases without ever completely saturating, but it's curvilinear. I'm not certain whether the curvalinear characteristics of this relation represent saturation of the hydrogen secretory system or is simply related to the fact that in order to examine the system at these P_{CO_2}'s you must have a very high bicarbonate concentration and therefore must infuse large amounts of fluid with hypertonic salt. As a result there is superimposed volume expansion which suppresses proximal reabsorption of sodium chloride, bicarbonate, and water.

5. Scanning Electron Microscopy of the Urinary Pole of the Distal Tubule Cells in the Rat Subjected to Respiratory Acidosis and to Metabolic Alkalosis

Jacqueline Hagège and Gabriel Richet

Service de Nephrologie
Hopital Tenon,
4 Rue de la Chine
Paris XXᵉ, France

In previous publications (RICHET et al. [1970], and HAGÈGE and RICHET [1970]) we have shown that in the rat, metabolic alkalosis, and especially respiratory acidosis, induce some modifications of the distal tubule cells, clearly demonstrated by the mitochondrial techniques (RICHET et al. [1970]). The changes observed consisted of an increase in the number of dark cells. Moreover, characters peculiar to dark cells appeared in most of the light cells, leading to an increase in the intermediary states. From these facts, together with the results of other experiments reported in the same publications, we have concluded that the light and dark cells are merely two functional aspects of the same line of tubular cells.

By scanning electron microscopy, we have shown that the light cells have a smooth surface in the supranuclear zone, with small microvilli at the periphery, and that the dark cells have an irregular surface made up of tangled and confluent leaflets separated by deep breaches (HAGÈGE and RICHET [1970]). Between these two extremes are seen types differing in the number and dimension of the irregularities of relief, especially in the downstream part of the distal convoluted tubule and in the cortical part of the collecting duct. Indeed these appearances confirm and complete those described in transmission

electron microscopy (ROULLIER and MULLER [1969], and GRIFFITH et al. [1968]). The present study was undertaken to follow the variations in tubular relief in rats subjected to either a dose of $NaHCO_3$ or to a respiratory acidosis. The regions examined were restricted to the distal convoluted tubule and cortical part of the collecting duct.

Male Sprague-Dawley rats of 200 to 250 g were subjected either to intravenous infusion of 1.4% $NaHCO_3$ at a dose of 25 $\mu l/min$ for $4\frac{1}{2}$ to 3 hours, or to a respiratory acidosis by inhalation of a 90% O_2, 10% CO_2 mixture for $2\frac{1}{2}$ to 3 hours. The kidneys of the experimental and of the control animals, the latter with or without intravenous infusion of 0.9% NaCl at a dose of 25 $\mu l/min$, were fixed *in vivo* by intra-aortic perfusion (pressure 150 mm Hg) of a buffered solution of glutaraldehyde. Fragments were ringed and processed in a 1% solution of phosphotungstic acid in NHCl for an hour, dehydrated, coated with copper and observed in a stereoscan. The arterial pH was measured in all animals at the end of the experiment.

In the experimental animals, unlike the controls (Figures 1, 3, and 5), the *apical* pole of the tubular cells was very often convex (Figure 6), the supranuclear region was never smooth (Figure 2) and the relief of all the cells was extremely irregular. The microvilli

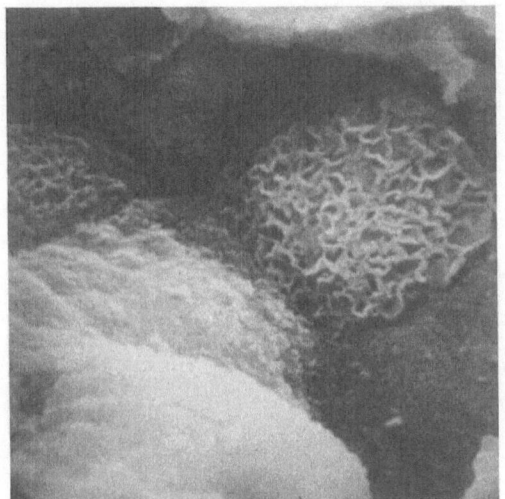

Fig. 1. Urinary poles of five distal convoluted tubular cells from a control rat: Two dark cells with microleaflets, three light cells with few microvilli (× 4700).

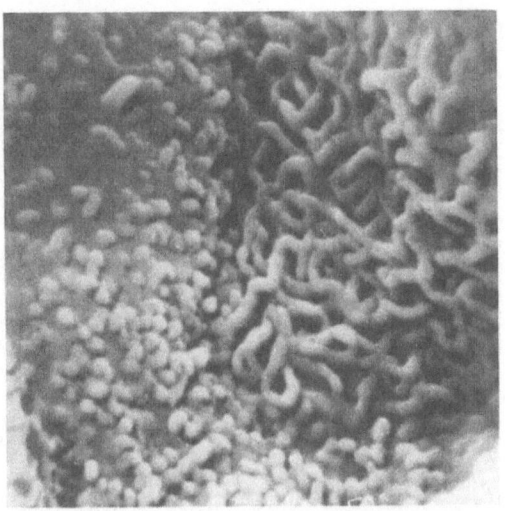

Fig. 3. Two distal convoluted tubular cells from a control rat: A light cell with microvilli, a dark cell with microleaflets (× 9300).

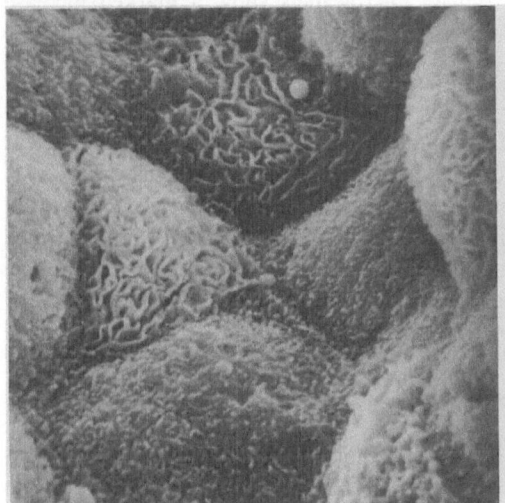

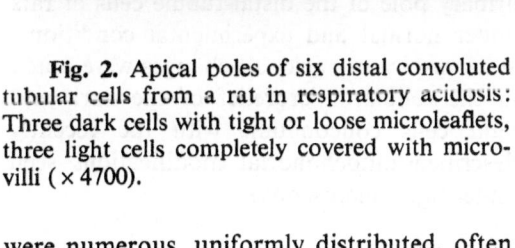

Fig. 2. Apical poles of six distal convoluted tubular cells from a rat in respiratory acidosis: Three dark cells with tight or loose microleaflets, three light cells completely covered with microvilli (× 4700).

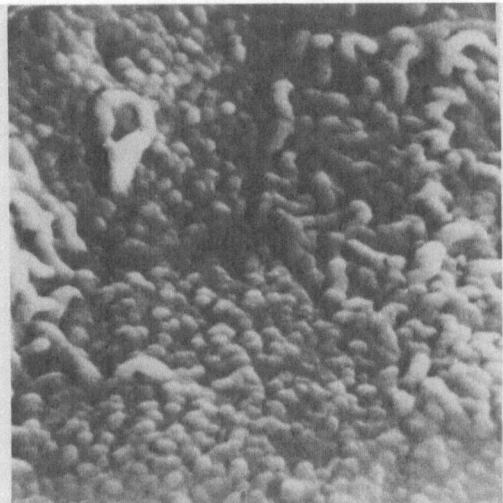

Fig. 4. Distal convoluted tubular cells from a rat under respiratory acidosis and with an oral supplement of bicarbonate: Two light cells with numerous microvilli; to the right, an intermediary cell with microleaflets, mixed with microvilli (× 9300).

were numerous, uniformly distributed, often coming in contact with one another (Figures 4 and 6). The leaflets were either tightly or loosely packed, thick or thin, and the protuberances were strongly contrasted with

the hollows (Figures 2, 4, and 6). Some forms intermediate between these two appearances were frequently seen (Figure 4). Although the leaflet-covered cells could not be counted by this technique, they were obviously more

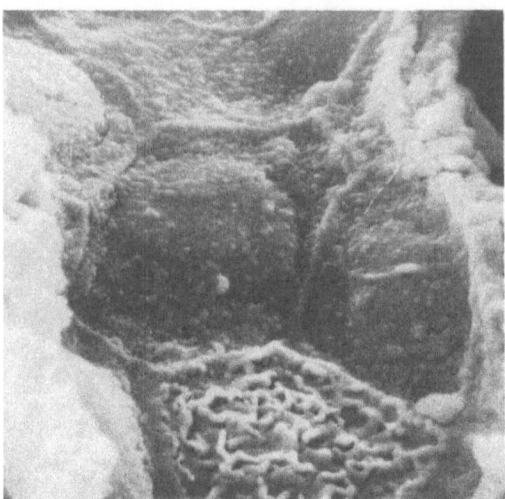

Fig. 5. Four light cells and one dark cell from a collecting duct of a control rat (× 5250).

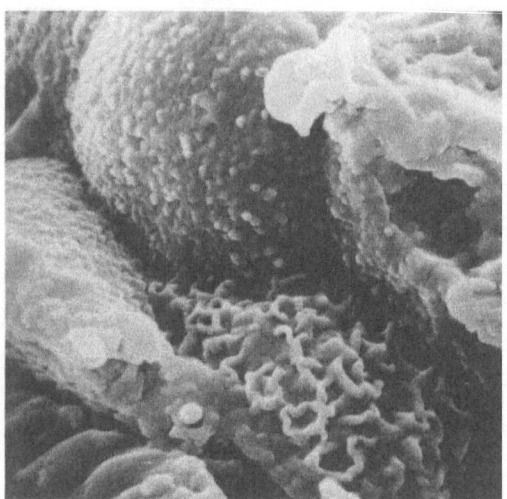

Fig. 6. Four cells from a collecting duct of a rat under respiratory acidosis: Three light cells, of which one is very swollen, with numerous microvilli, and one dark cell in which the loosely arranged microleaflets show a marked increase in brilliance (× 5230).

numerous than in the controls. All those modifications were more marked in the respiratory acidotic animals than in those receiving an infusion of $NaHCO_3$.

The changes in relief of the urinary pole correspond to the mitochondrial modifications with increase in number of the dark cells observed in rats subjected to identical experimental conditions (RICHET et al. [1970]). The membrane surface is increased, not only by the increase in number of microvilli on the surface of the light cells but also by the increase in the number and depth of the leaflets of the dark cells. Processing with phosphotungstic acid produces, in both the control and experimental animals, a distinct difference in brilliance between protuberances and hollows. This reaction at low pH, insofar as it is specific (PEASE [1970], and SCOTT and GLICK [1971]), could be taken to reveal the presence of mucopolysaccharides in the cell coat (MARTINEZ–PALOMO [1970]). Thus the observed differences in brilliance would then indicate variations in the mucopolysaccharide content of the cell coat. Also the large quantity of mucopolysaccharides found at the urinary pole of the dark cells (GRIFFITH et al. [1968]) would be explained by the fact that the microvilli are more numerous there.

The observed morphological modifications could be linked to the two physiological responses created by the respiratory acidosis and the metabolic alkalosis. There exists only one point in common between each of those metabolic situations, the increase in the reabsorption and/or tubular production of bicarbonates.

Summary

The present scanning electron microscopy study affords a comparison between the urinary pole of the distal tubule cells of rats under normal and experimental conditions. With respiratory acidosis changes were noted in the cellular microrelief of the dark and light cells concomitant with the recently described mitochondrial modifications seen under light microscopy.

Bibliography

Ericsson, J. L. R., and Trump, B. F., *Electron microscopy of the uriniferous tubules in the kidney*. Vol. 1. C. Roullier and A. F. Muller, eds. New York and London: Academic Press (1969).

Griffith, L. D., Bulger, R. E., and Trump, B. J., *Anat. Rec.* 160:643 (1968).

Hagège, J., and Richet, G., *C.R. Acad. Sc., série D*, Paris 271:331 (1970).

Martinez-Palomo, A., *Int. Rev. Cytol.* 19:29 (1970).

Pease, D. C., *J. Histochem. Cytochem.* 18:455 (1970).

Richet, C., Hagège, J., and Case, M., *Nephron* 7:413 (1970).

Scott, J. E., and Glick, D., *J. Histochem. Cytochem.* 19:63 (1971).

6. Carbon Dioxide in Cerebral Extracellular Fluids

Vladimir Fencl

Department of Physiology
Harvard Medical School
25 Shattuck Street, Boston, Massachusetts 02115

The extravascular extracellular compartment of the cerebral fluids consists of the cerebral interstitial fluid (cISF) and of the cerebrospinal fluid (CSF). Both these fluids are continuously formed from, and returned to, the blood plasma (DAVSON [1967]). The rate of formation and bulk absorption of CSF is slow, about 0.5% of its total volume per minute (HEISEY et al. [1962]). In cISF the turnover is probably faster (FENCL et al. [1966]). CSF in the ventricles is separated from cISF by the ependyma; on the outer surface of the brain the separation between CSF and cISF is formed by pia-glia. Both these boundaries permit exchange by free diffusion of even large molecules, between cISF and the CSF in large cerebral cavities (BRIGHTMAN et al. [1970]).

The concentration of protein in CSF is only about 25 mg%, and buffering for CO_2 is very poor as compared with blood. There is an electric potential between CSF and blood; normally CSF is 4 to 5 mv positive, and the potential increases with increasing acidity of blood (HELD et al. [1964]). Most of the ions in CSF, including HCO_3^- and H^+, are in electrochemical disequilibrium with plasma (HELD et al. [1964], and SEVERINGHAUS [1965]). In the normal acid-base balance, CSF is more acid than arterial plasma. In chronic acid-base disturbances, surprisingly enough, pH in the poorly buffered CSF is more stable than pH in blood (MITCHELL et al. [1965]).

pH in CSF and in cISF follows the ratio of the local bicarbonate concentration to the local P_{CO_2}. The mean cerebral-tissue P_{CO_2} ($Pc.t._{CO_2}$) can be derived as

$$Pc.t._{CO_2} = Pa_{CO_2} + \Delta P_{CO_2},$$

where Pa_{CO_2} relates to the concentration of molecular CO_2 in the arterial blood, and ΔP_{CO_2} is the increment in the partial pressure, going from the incoming arterial blood to the tissue level. ΔP_{CO_2} is indirectly proportional to the cerebral blood flow (CBF), and directly proportional to the CO_2 production by the brain which, under most conditions, remains constant. Cisternal P_{CO_2} is considered by most investigators to represent the mean P_{CO_2} in the cerebral tissue (PONTÉN and SIESJÖ [1966]).

The concentration of bicarbonate in CSF varies with systemic acid-base disturbances, and so does the distribution of this ion between blood and CSF. In all mammalian species, in the normal acid-base balance $[HCO_3^-]_{CSF}$ is lower than what would correspond to the ultrafiltrate of plasma. In steady metabolic acidosis and alkalosis the change in the steady-state bicarbonate concentration in CSF is only 30 to 40% of its change in arterial plasma. The range given reflects the differences between the various mammalian species that have been studied. In the "respiratory" acid-base disturbances CSF bicarbonate follows more closely the changes in plasma bicarbonate concentration: In hypercapnic dogs the change in $[HCO_3^-]_{pl}$. is almost completely reflected in CSF; in humans with chronic CO_2 retention almost $\frac{2}{3}$ of the increase in plasma bicarbonate occurs in CSF (see Fencl [1971] for references). This variable distribution of bicarbonate between plasma and CSF in stable acid-base disorders of various origin is attributed to the "blood-brain barrier." The detailed mechanisms involved in the "barrier" are poorly understood (active transport of ions? (HELD et al. [1964], and SEVERINGHAUS [1965]), effect of the variable electric potential between CSF and blood? (SIESJÖ and KJÄLLQUIST [1969]), variable production of lactate by the brain? (MINES and SØRENSEN [1971])).

In the steady state of a given acid-base condition the ionic composition of CSF is the same as in cISF (FENCL et al. [1966]). On the other hand, in transients of acid-base disturbances the change in composition of the large-cavity fluid (CSF) lags behind that occurring in cISF, due to the difference in turnover rate of the two compartments. Under these transient conditions concentration gradients for HCO_3^-, Cl^-, and H^+ must exist between CSF and cISF, with functional implications for those regulatory mechanisms that are related to the acidity of cISF (FENCL et al. [1966]).

In terms of functional adaptations, the content of CO_2 and the acidity in cerebral fluids relate to the following:

(a) the ratio of the CO_2 production in the whole body ($\dot{V}CO_2$) to the effective ventilation of the lungs ($\dot{V}A$):$\dot{V}CO_2/\dot{V}A$, which determines Pa_{CO_2};

(b) the cerebral blood flow which, at the constant CO_2 production by the brain, determines the increment in PCO_2 between arterial blood and the brain tissue;

(c) the poorly defined mechanisms at the "blood-brain barrier" which, at a given $[HCO_3^-]$ in plasma determine $[HCO_3^-]$ in CSF.

In acid-base disturbances of "metabolic" origin, both the pulmonary ventilation and CBF can be presented as a single function of the acidity in cISF (FENCL et al. [1969]). Thus two interrelated regulatory loops of negative feedback are constituted, one for the adaptation of the resting $\dot{V}A$, the other for the regulation of CBF. These two regulatory systems, in combination with the mechanisms that create the "blood-brain barrier" for bicarbonate, act to reduce the variation in acidity of the cerebral fluids, as compared with the variation produced in blood pH in steady metabolic acidosis or alkalosis. Thus in humans it has been estimated that the change in cerebral fluid $[H^+]$ is only one-tenth of that occurring simultaneously in arterial blood with chronic metabolic acidosis or alkalosis (FENCL et al. [1969]). Nevertheless, the small variation in cISF pH serves as the signal for the regulation of CBF and $\dot{V}A$. It is probable that in acid-base disturbances of "respiratory" origin, especially in chronic CO_2 retention, the efficiency of this homeostatic system is hampered by extraneous factors that affect the rate of CO_2 elimination by the lungs.

Bibliography

Brightman, M. W., Reese, T. S., and Feder, N., "Assessment with the electronmicroscope of the permeability to peroxidases of cerebral endothelium and epithelium in mice and sharks." In *Capillary permeability*. C. Crone and N. A. Lassen, eds. Copenhagen: Munksgaard (1970).

Davson, H., *Physiology of the cerebrospinal fluid*. London: J. A. Churchill (1967).

Fencl, V., "Distribution of H^+ and HCO_3^- in cerebral fluids." In *Ion homeostasis of the brain*. B. K. Siesjö and S. C. Sørensen, eds. Copenhagen: Munksgaard (1971).

———, Miller, T. B., and Pappenheimer, J. R. "Studies on the respiratory response to disturbances of acid-base balance, with deductions concerning the ionic composition of cerebral interstitial fluid." *Am. J. Physiol.* 210:459–72 (1966).

———, Vale, J. R., and Broch, J. A. "Respiration

and cerebral blood flow in metabolic acidosis and alkalosis in humans." *J. Appl. Physiol.* 27:67–76 (1969).

Heisey, R. S., Held, D., and Pappenheimer, J. R. "Bulk flow and diffusion in the cerebrospinal fluid system of the goat." *Am. J. Physiol.* 203:775–781 (1962).

Held, D., Fencl., V., and Pappenheimer, J. R. "Electrical potential of cerebrospinal fluid." *J. Neurophysiol.* 27:942–59 (1964).

Mines, A. H., and Sørensen, S. C. "Changes in the electrochemical potential difference for HCO_3^- between blood and cerebrospinal fluid, and in cerebrospinal fluid lactate concentration during isocarbic hypoxia." *Acta Physiol. Scand.* 81:225–33 (1971).

Mitchell, R. A., Carman, C. T., Severinghaus, J. W., Richardson, B. W., Singer, M. M., and Shnider, S. "Stability of cerebrospinal fluid pH in chronic acid-base disturbances in blood." *J. Appl. Physiol.* 20:443–52 (1965).

Pontén, U., and Siesjö, B. K. "Gradients of CO_2 tensions in the brain." *Acta Physiol. Scand.* 67:129–40 (1966).

Severinghaus, J. W. "Electrochemical gradients for hydrogen and bicarbonate ions across the blood-CSF barrier in response to acid-base balance changes. In *Cerebrospinal fluid and the regulation of ventilation.* C. McC. Brooks, F. F. Kao, and B. B. Lloyd, eds. Oxford: Blackwell (1965).

Siesjö, B. K., and Kjällquist, Å. "A new theory for the regulation of the extracellular pH in the brain." *Scand. J. Clin. Lab. Med.* 24:1–9 (1969).

7. Acid-Base and Energy Metabolism of the Brain in Hypercapnia and Hypocapnia

Bo K. Siesjö, Jaroslava Folbergrová,* and Kenneth Messeter

The Brain Research Laboratory
E-Blocket, University Hospital
Lund, Sweden

Introduction

The metabolism of brain tissue shows some characteristic and specific features (for details and further references, see MCILWAIN [1966], BACHELARD and MCILWAIN [1969], BALACZ [1970]). Thus the organ is active continuously, and in spite of its small weight it is responsible for about 20% of the resting oxygen consumption of the body. Further, although isolated brain tissues can oxidize a variety of substrates *in vitro*, only glucose can normally pass the blood-brain barrier with sufficient speed to maintain the energy requirements *in vivo*. Measurements of arteriovenous differences for glucose, oxygen, and carbon dioxide show that the respiratory quotient is close to unity, thus confirming that glucose is the sole substrate. These measurements show that about 95% of the glucose consumed is oxidized to carbon dioxide. The rest of the glucose (about 5%) appears as an arteriovenous difference for lactate (see COHEN [1971]). However, the arteriovenous balance does not reveal the rapid interconversion of glucose carbon between the tricarboxylic acid cycle and the glutamate group of amino acids. In fact, as much as 30% of the ^{14}C administered in radioactive glucose may label these acids (aspartate, glutamate, glutamine, and γ-aminobutyrate), but since an equivalent

amount of amino acid carbon is fed into the Krebs cycle the end result is compatible with simple glucose oxidation (ROBERTS et al. [1959], VRBA [1962], see also TOWER [1960], BACHELARD [1965]). The rapid turnover of the glutamate group of amino acids, which is partly specific for the brain, may be related to the fact that some of the acids function as excitatory or inhibitory transmittors.

Most of the metabolic carbon dioxide in the brain is formed during the decarboxylations of pyruvate, isocitrate, and succinate, associated with the Krebs cycle, but a substantial amount may also be formed through decarboxylation of γ-aminobutyrate in the GABA shunt pathway. Some carbon dioxide may also be formed in the pentose shunt, but the enzymes involved in this anaerobic carbon dioxide-producing pathway occur in rather low concentrations, and it is usually assumed that only a minor fraction of the metabolic carbon dioxide of the mature brain emanates from these reactions (BACHELARD and MCILWAIN [1969], BALACZ [1970]).

Most of the oxidative reactions which lead to carbon dioxide formation occur with such a large negative free energy change that they may be considered irreversible (KREBS and KORNBERG [1957], LEHNINGER [1970]). Therefore, we cannot expect that variations in the carbon dioxide tension should significantly influence the rate of decarboxylations in the

---

* On leave of absence from the Institute of Physiology, Czechoslovak Academy of Sciences, Prague.

tissue. It seems more probable that the concentration of molecular carbon dioxide has an influence on the rate of carbon dioxide fixation reactions. However, although it has been shown that there is a rapid incorporation of $^{14}C - CO_2$ at the malate-oxaloacetate sites with extensive labeling of the glutamate group of amino acids (BERL et al. [1962], WAELSCH et al [1964], BERL et al [1964]), neither the physiological role of the carbon dioxide fixation reactions nor the net fixation rate of carbon dioxide seems clarified. It appears probable that the reactions may be operative in replenishing Krebs cycle intermediates which are drained off for synthetic purposes, but it remains to be shown how the carbon dioxide tension or the bicarbonate concentration enter as regulatory parameters.

The lack of knowledge on the direct effects of carbon dioxide upon brain metabolism is somewhat unexpected when one considers that carbon dioxide has effects on brain function which range from seizure activity to narcosis (WOODBURY and KARLER [1960], WYKE [1963]). However, most of the effects exerted by carbon dioxide may be elicited by the secondary changes in intracellular pH which occur during hyper- and hypocapnia. The present communication discusses how changes in the carbon dioxide tension affect the intracellular pH of brain cells. It will be demonstrated that pH$'_i$ in the brain is remarkably well regulated and that this regulation seems to involve metabolic adjustments with production or consumption of metabolic acids. It will then be discussed how hypercapnia may influence the energy state of the tissue. The results presented will show that the intracellular acidosis has marked effects on the creatine phosphokinase and the lactate dehydrogenase equilibria and that it also can affect the cytoplasmic NADH/NAD$^+$ ratio. However, the results did not indicate that carbon dioxide inhibited brain metabolism to such an extent that the energy state was affected, at least not during the periods studied (15 min to 72 hr).

The Regulation of Intracellular pH' in Hyper- and Hypocapnia

The Validity of a Derived Intracellular pH

In tissues like the brain in which direct intracellular pH measurements cannot readily be performed, the pH$'_i$ must be calculated from the distribution of weak acids such as H_2CO_2 (DANIELSSON and HASTINGS [1939], WALLACE and HASTINGS [1942]) or DMO (WADDELL and BUTLER [1959]). Such calculations have been applied to a variety of tissue, and they have almost invariably given pH$'_i$ values close to 7.0 (see CALDWELL [1956], WADDELL and BATES [1969], ROBSON et al. [1968]). This pH value is far in excess of that which would fit a passive distribution of H$^+$ across the cell membranes. Thus at an extracellular pH of 7.4 and with the transmembrane potentials observed in muscle and nerve tissues (-80 to -90 mv) a passive distribution of H$^+$ would require an intracellular pH of close to 6.0. It is therefore natural that the pH values calculated for these tissues have been interpreted to indicate the presence of an active transport of H$^+$ from the cells, the actual pH observed being set by the balance between active extrusion of H$^+$ and the passive influx of H$^+$ along the electrochemical gradient. However, since transport of H$^+$ in one direction is synonymous with transport of HCO$^-_3$ in the reverse direction, the ion species treated by the transport system is not specified.

Although the pH values calculated for muscle and brain have been corroborated by direct electrometric pH measurements in large muscle and nerve cells (CALDWELL [1958], KOSTYUK and SOROKINA [1961]), there have been conflicting reports which have indicated pH$'_i$ values in muscle tissue of close to 6.0, thus fitting a Donnan equilibrium for H$^+$. Conway and his associates (CONWAY and FEARON [1944], CONWAY [1957]) maintained that since a large part of the total CO$_2$ of muscle was not precipitated by barium at an alkaline pH, it did not represent HCO$^-_3$, and when the authors corrected for the nonbicarbonate CO$_2$ they arrived at a pH'_i of close to 6.0. CARTER et al. [1967] obtained similar values by inserting pH electrodes of ultramicro size into muscle cells. Not only did the authors measure a pH of close to 6.0 in the resting control state, but they also found that variations of the membrane potential gave rise to almost instantaneous changes in pH'_i, so that the electrochemical potential difference for H^+ always remained close to zero. In order to explain the divergence between their own results and previous ones, CARTER et al. [1967] had to assume that the CO_2 and the DMO measurements, as well as previous direct pH measurements, were in error. In addition, and in order to explain the extremely fast adjustments of pH'_i after changes in the membrane potential, the authors had to assume that the flux of H^+ (or HCO^-_3) across the membranes resembled superconductance in ice-like structures. All these assumptions made a rather weak case for an equilibrium distribution of H^+, and it has recently been reported that if electrodes of the type used by Carter and his associates are inserted well into the muscle cells, the results give values closer to 7.0 than to 6.0 (PAILLARD et al. [1971]). Furthermore, since the barium-soluble CO_2 fraction of Conway now seems adequately explained (BUTLER et al. [1967]), there appear to be few reasons to question the nonequilibrium distribution of H^+ across muscle and nerve cell membranes, or the validity of the pH'_i values calculated from the distribution of CO_2 or DMO. There may remain some uncertainty as to the interpretation of the pH'_i values in terms of compartmentation within the tissue or within the cells of a tissue, but this uncertainty also pertains to the meaning of the tissue concentration of ions in general or to metabolites of other kinds. However, although the pH calculated for the intracellular space of a tissue like the brain may come close to that existing in the cytoplasmic phase, it nevertheless represents an idealized parameter in a nonhomogenous system. It therefore seems appropriate to name it an "equivalent intracellular pH" (pH'_i), i.e., the pH of a homogenous system which has the same carbon dioxide tension and the same bicarbonate concentration as the corresponding *mean* values derived for the tissue (see SIESJÖ and MESSETER [1971]).

The Derivation of Intracellular pH' *in the Brain*

In calculating brain intracellular pH' we have followed the classical procedure of Hastings and collaborators (DANIELSON and HASTINGS [1939], WALLACE and HASTINGS [1947]), who measured the total CO_2 content of muscle tissue and derived the intracellular HCO^-_3 concentration after correcting for the extracellular bicarbonate. In calculating pH'_i, the authors used an assumed solubility coefficient (S) and a pK'_1 for carbonic acid measured on muscle tissue homogenates (DANIELSON et al. [1939]). As applied to brain tissue the derivation is as follows

$$(HCO^-_3)_i = \frac{TCO_2 - P_tCO_2 \cdot S_1 - (HCO^-_3)_{Bl} \cdot V_{Bl} - (HCO^-_3)_{CSF} \cdot V_{ECF}}{V_i} \quad (1)$$

$$pH'_i = pK'_1 + \log \frac{(HCO^-_3)_i}{P_tCO_2 \cdot S_2} \quad (2)$$

In these equations the symbols have the following meaning:

$(HCO^-_3)_i$ = mean i.c. HCO^-_3 concentration in meq/kg of i.c. water

TCO_2 = tissue CO_2 content in mmoles/ kg of wet tissue

P_tCO_2 = mean tissue CO_2 tension in mm Hg

$S_1(0.0292)$ = CO_2 solubility in total tissue in mmoles/kg wet tissue × mm Hg

$S_2(0.0314)$ = CO_2 solubility in i.c. water in mmoles/kg i.c. water × mm Hg

$(HCO^-_3)_{Bl}$ = HCO^-_3 concentration in whole blood in meq/kg

V_{Bl} = volume of blood in tissue as g blood/g tissue

$(HCO^-_3)_{CSF}$ = HCO^-_3 concentration in cisternal CSF in meq/kg

V_{ECF} = volume of extracellular water as g ECF/g tissue

V_i = volume of intracellular water as g i.c. H_2O/g tissue

pK'_1 = first apparent pK of carbonic acid in cell water.

The following experimental procedures are routinely used in the laboratory for the derivation of pH'_i. The animals are lightly anesthetized with halothane or nitrous oxide, immobilized with tubocurarine chloride, artificially ventilated and maintained at a body temperature of close to 37°C. When a respiratory steady state is obtained, defined as a maximal variation in Pa_{CO_2} of 10% between two consecutive blood samples taken at an interval of 10 to 15 min, 50 to 100 μ1 of cisternal CSF is sampled for immediate analysis of either the total CO_2 content (SIESJÖ [1962a]) or the P_{CO_2} (PONTÉN and SIESJÖ [1966], BRZEZINSKI et al. [1967]). Immediately after the CSF sampling, the tissue is frozen *in situ* for subsequent measurement of the total CO_2 content (PONTÉN and SIESJÖ [1964]). The tissue CO_2 tension is then either equated with the CSF CO_2 tension or is calculated from the arterial CO_2 tension using a standard relation between the two as determined in control experiments (c.f. PONTÉN and SIESJÖ [1966], BRZEZINSKI et al. [1967]). The CSF HCO^-_3 concentration is calculated from the total CO_2 content, using the P_tCO_2 and a solubility factor of 0.0314 mmoles/kg · mm Hg (SIESJÖ [1962a]), and the blood HCO^-_3 concentration is derived from the Pa_{CO_2}, the plasma pH and the blood hemoglobin content. The S values (SIESJÖ [1962a]) and the pK'_1 value (SIESJÖ [1962b]) have previously been determined on tissue homogenates. The determination of the pK'_1 value indicated that the tissue does not contain significant amounts of nonbicarbonate CO_2 such as carbamino-CO_2 (see SIESJÖ [1962b]).

The blood volume of brain tissue is close to 3% of the tissue weight (EVERETT et al. [1956]), and since the correction for the bicarbonate contained in the blood of the tissue is a small one, it will not matter if the blood volume changes moderately during the experiments. The correction for the extracellular bicarbonate is more critical. Recent results have shown that the extracellular volume of brain tissue is close to 15% (WOODWARD et al. [1967], RALL and FENSTERMACHER [1971]) and that it does not change even in extreme hypercapnia (CAMERON et al. [1970]). It has further been shown that the HCO^-_3 concentrations in CSF and in true interstitial fluid are identical at steady-state conditions (FENCL et al. [1966]). In non-steady-state conditions deviations may occur, and the calculation of the extracellular HCO^-_3 content introduces an uncertainty.

The pH'_i of Brain Cells

When the physiological state of the experimental animals is adequately controlled, and with the methods used, the intracellular pH'_i can be derived with a standard error which is usually not greater than that obtained for plasma pH (MESSETER and SIESJÖ [1971b]). However, the absolute pH'_i obtained depends on the assumption regarding the size of the extracellular space. Table 1 compares the acid-base parameters in cisternal CSF (MESSETER and SIESJÖ [1971a]) with the corresponding intracellular parameters,

Table 1. Acid-base relations in arterial blood, cisternal cerebrospinal fluid, and brain intracellular fluid of rats under control conditions.

Compartment	P_{CO_2}, mm Hg	[HCO^-_3], meq/kg	pH
Blood	38	26.3*	7.42
CSF	44	28.3	7.43
I.c. fluid			
10% ECV	44	13.3	7.11
15% ECV	—	12.0	7.06
20% ECV	—	10.6	7.00

* Calculated per kilogram of plasma water.

calculated for ECF volumes of 10, 15, and 20%, respectively (data from MESSETER and SIESJÖ [1971b]). It is seen that the mean intracellular HCO^-_3 concentration is less than half the extracellular concentration, and the pH'_i is 0.3 to 0.4 units lower than pH_{ECF}.

The Regulation of pH'_i in Hyper- and Hypocapnia

In order to study the regulation of brain intracellular pH' in hyper- and hypocapnia, we have induced wide variations in the carbon dioxide tension for 45 min, and also exposed animals to carbon dioxide (10 to 12%) for periods ranging from 5 min to 72 hr. Most of the results have been published previously (KJÄLLQUIST et al. [1969], SIESJÖ and MESSETER [1971], MESSETER and SIESJÖ [1971a, b]), but a preliminary account will be given of some recent experiments in which animals were exposed to 20, 30, and 40% CO_2, respectively.

At least three mechanisms may contribute to the pH'_i regulation in hyper- and hypocapnia, *viz.* (1) physicochemical buffering, (2) production or consumption of metabolic acids, and (3) transmembrane fluxes of H^+ and HCO^-_3 (SIESJÖ and MESSETER [1971]). Titrations with CO_2 *in vitro* have indicated that brain tissue has a physicochemical buffer capacity, defined as $\Delta \log P_{CO_2}/\Delta pH$, of about 1.6 (SIESJÖ and MESSETER [1971]). This buffer capacity, which is similar to that of whole blood *in vitro*, requires the presence of a buffer concentration of about 40 mmoles/l. (*c.f.* EDSALL and WYMAN [1958]). The acid-base relations in a system with this buffer capacity can be calculated from an equation which relates the P_{CO_2}, the pH, the buffer base concentration (BB), the concentration of the nonbicarbonate buffer acid and the pK of the buffer acid. However, in order to simulate physiological conditions, we have divided the concentration of the buffer acid into five acids with equal concentrations (C_1 to C_5) with pK_{Ha} values covering the physiological range (pK = 6.5,

6.8, 7.1, 7.4, and 7.7, respectively). The general equation then becomes

$$BB = \frac{P_{CO_2} \cdot S \cdot K_{H_2CO_3}}{(H^+)}\left[1 + \frac{2 \cdot K_{HCO^-_3}}{(H^+)}\right]$$
$$+ \frac{K'_1 \cdot C_1}{K'_1 + (H^+)} + \cdots \frac{K'_n \cdot C_n}{K'_n + (H^+)} \quad (3)$$

where *BB* is the sum of the total buffer anion concentration and *C* the concentration of nonbicarbonate buffer acids (see SIESJÖ and MESSETER [1971]).

Figure 1 shows the relation between the tissue carbon dioxide tension (log scale) and the pH'_i in animals that were either mechanically hyperventilated during 45 min or exposed to various carbon dioxide concentrations for an equally long period (see KJÄLLQUIST et al. [1969], MESSETER and SIESJÖ [1971a, b]). The figure compares the pH values which would be expected if only physico-chemical buffering were regulating the pH'_i (stippled line) with those actually derived. The curve representing physicochemical buffering was calculated from equation (3), using a total buffer concentration of 0.040 moles/kg ($C_1 = C_2 = C_3 = C_4 = C_5 = 0.008$ moles/kg). In moderate hypercapnia ($P_{CO_2} < 100$ mm Hg) and in hypocapnia the regulation of pH'_i was far better than what the physico-chemical buffer capacity would predict. In fact, in extreme hypocapnia the intracellular space behaved almost as an isohydric system; i.e., the pH'_i remained essentially constant when the P_{CO_2} was changed. However, in extreme hypercapnia ($P_{CO_2} > 100$ mm Hg) the variation of pH'_i with the carbon dioxide tension was closer to that corresponding to the physico-chemical buffer capacity (*c.f.* slope of lines).

The fact that the pH'_i in hyper- and hypocapnia does not vary according to the buffer line of Figure 1 implies that the intracellular buffer base concentration changes. Thus hypocapnia must be associated with a decrease in buffer base (release of

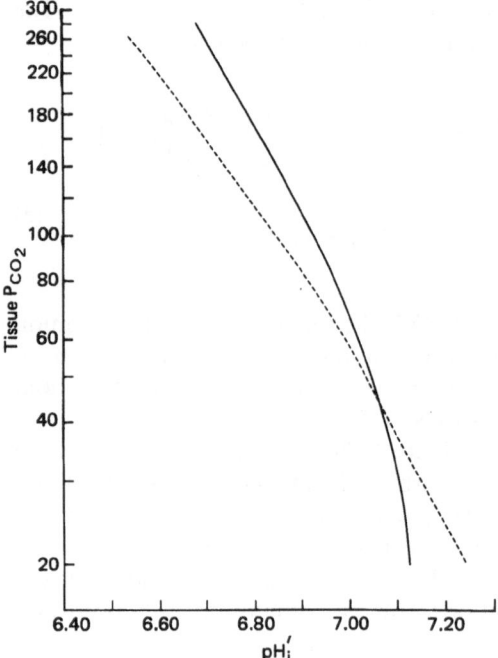

Fig. 1. The relationship between the tissue carbon dioxide tension and the intracellular pH' in the brain of rats which were either hyperventilated or were exposed to various carbon dioxide tensions for 45 min. The solid line was drawn as the best visual fit to values calculated on the assumption of a 15% extracellular volume from the results published by KJÄLLQUIST et al. [1969] and by MESSETER and SIESJÖ [1971b], as well as from results recently obtained in animals exposed to 20, 30, and 40% CO_2, respectively. The interrupted line is the P_{CO_2}/pH relationship which would be expected if only physico-chemical buffering were regulating the pH'_i during hyper- and hypocapnia. Note that the regulation of pH'_i was far in excess of that corresponding to the physico-chemical buffer capacity, especially in hypocapnia and in moderate hypercapnia.

acids) and hypercapnia with an increase in the buffer base concentration (disappearance of acid). The variations in buffer base during hyper- and hypocapnia may be due either to consumption and production of acids, respectively, or to net fluxes of H^+ and HCO^-_3 between the intra- and extracellular fluids (see above). However, since 45 min may be too short a time to permit transmembrane fluxes of sufficient magnitude to account for

the buffer base changes, we may look for variations in the steady-state concentrations of nonvolatile acids. It has been known for a time that hypo- and hypercapnia are associated with increases and decreases, respectively, of the tissue concentrations of lactate and pyruvate (BAIN and KLEIN [1949], LEUSEN and DEMEESTER [1966], GRANHOLM and SIESJÖ [1969], KJÄLLQUIST et al. [1969]), and it has recently been shown that there are similar variations in α-ketoglutarate and glutamate (SIESJÖ and MESSETER [1971], MESSETER and SIESJÖ [1971c]). Figure 2 shows how the tissue concentrations of these four meta-

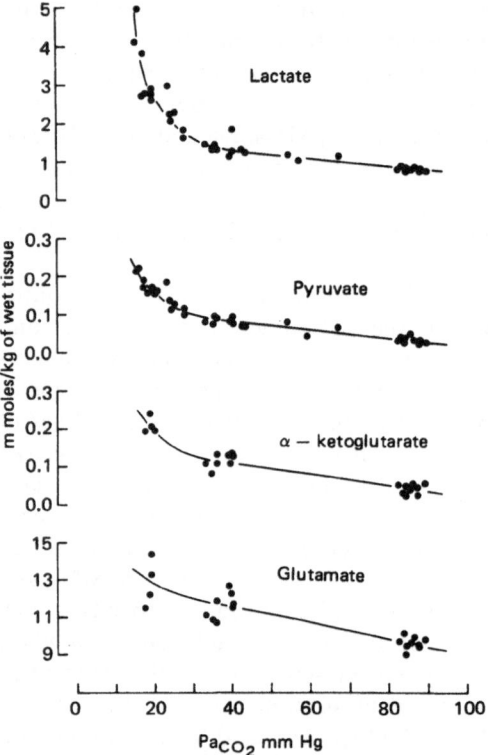

Fig. 2. The influence of changes in the tissue carbon dioxide tension (45 min of hyper- or hypocapnia) upon the brain tissue concentrations of lactate, pyruvate, α-ketoglutarate, and glutamate. Most of the values were replotted from previous reports (KJÄLLQUIST et al. [1969], SIESJÖ and MESSETER [1971], SIESJÖ et al. [1971]a, MESSETER and SIESJÖ [1971c]). The concentrations of all metabolites were markedly dependent upon the carbon dioxide tension.

bolites vary with the tissue carbon dioxide tension during acute (45 min) hyper- and hypocapnia. The results demonstrate that hypercapnia is associated with decreases in the concentration of all four acids, while hypocapnia gives the reverse. In extreme hypocapnia there is a steep increase in the intracellular lactate concentration, which in individual animals may exceed 5 mmoles/kg of i.c. water.

It appears probable that the metabolic changes in hypo- and hypercapnia are caused by a pH-dependent activation and inhibition, respectively, of a rate limiting glycolytic step, e.g. the phosphofructokinase reaction (LOWRY and PASSONNEAU [1966]), which gives rise to an increase and a decrease, respectively, of the steady-state levels of substrates distal to that step. Since these substrates are the anions of acids with relatively low pK values (see EDSALL and WYMAN [1958]), a decrease in the concentrations of the acids should be associated with a stoichiometrical disappearance of H^+ ions, and an increase should lead to a corresponding release of H^+. In other words, the metabolic changes induced by the pH changes could by themselves function as important pH-regulating mechanisms which serve to reduce the acid shift in pH during hypercapnia and which seem able to keep pH'_i within a few hundredths of a pH unit from the normocapnic value during extreme hyperventilation.

Experiments with continuous exposure of animals to about 11% CO_2 for periods of up to 72 hr have shown that there is a further regulation of pH'_i during the first 3 hr which brings the pH'_i back to within a few hundredths of a pH unit of the normocapnic pH in spite of the continuous hypercapnia (MESSETER and SIESJÖ [1970, 1971b]). Figure 3 shows the regulation of pH'_i with time during the continuous hypercapnia. In the figure the pH'_i at each exposure period (unfilled circles) was calculated for three different extracellular volumes (10, 15, and 20%, respectively). For comparison, the pH'_i values derived were compared to two different theoretical pH values. The first of these is the

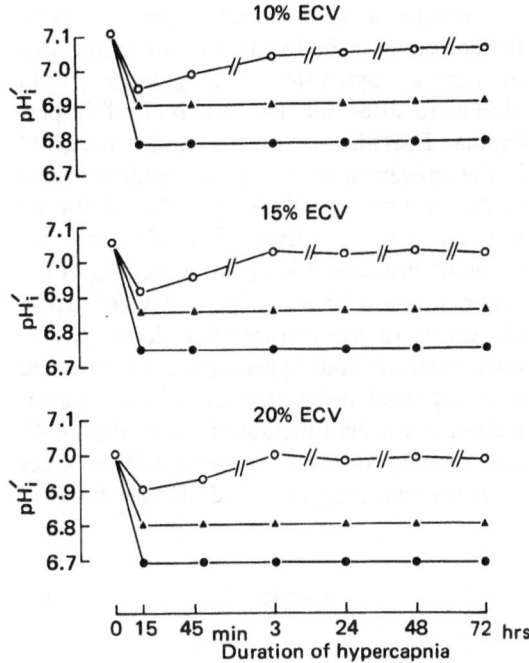

Fig. 3. The regulation of intracellular pH' in the brain during continuous hypercapnia (Pa_{CO_2} about 85 mm Hg.) The pH'_i was calculated for extracellular volumes of 10, 15, and 20%, respectively (open circles), and compared to the pH which would result if no pH regulating mechanisms were present, i.e., if the HCO_3^- content had remained constant during the hypercapnia (filled circles), as well as to the pH which would result if only physio-chemical buffering were regulating the pH' (triangles). Note that physico-chemical buffering could explain only about a third of the total pH regulation in sustained hypercapnia.

pH which would result if no pH regulatory mechanisms were present, i.e., if the carbon dioxide tension would be increased to the given value at an unchanged HCO^-_3 concentration (closed circles). The second is the pH which would result if physico-chemical buffering were the only mechanism regulating pH (triangles). The figure shows that irrespective of the assumption regarding the size of the extracellular space, it may be concluded that there is an extensive regulation of pH'_i during the first 3-hr period, only a third of which may be explained by physico-chemical buffering.

Figure 4 shows that there were no further changes in the tissue concentrations of lactate, pyruvate, α-ketoglutarate, and glutamate after the first 45 min of hypercapnia. Provided that no changes occurred in the concentrations of other, undetermined acids, we must conclude that the additional accumulation of bicarbonate observed between 45 min and 3 hrs (3 to 4 meq/kg of i.c. water) was due to an influx of HCO_3^- from the extra- to the intracellular fluids. Moreover, since chronic hypercapnia is associated with a partial normalization of the concentration of the acid metabolites (see Figure 4), the net influx of bicarbonate should be larger than the increase observed in the HCO_3^-

concentration between 45 min and 3 hr.

The net influx of bicarbonate from the extracellular to the intracellular fluids during the hypercapnia does not seem to depend passively upon the extracellular HCO_3^- concentration. Figure 5 compares the percentage pH regulation in extra- and intracellular fluids, the latter being calculated for three extracellular volumes. The percentage pH regulation, which expresses the total pH regulation irrespective of its mechanisms, can be calculated from the equation

$$\% \ pH \ regulation =$$

$$100 \cdot \frac{\log (HCO_3^-)'' - \log (HCO_3^-)'}{\log Pco_2'' - \log Pco_2'} \quad (4)$$

where the superscripts (") and (') stand for

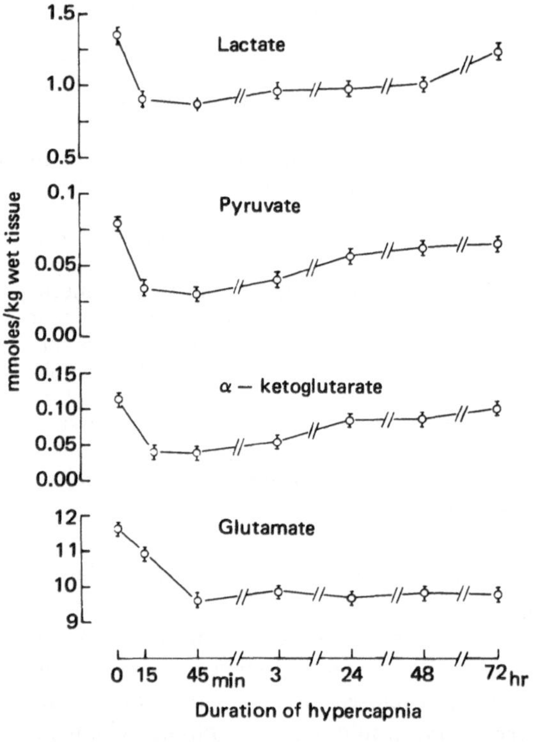

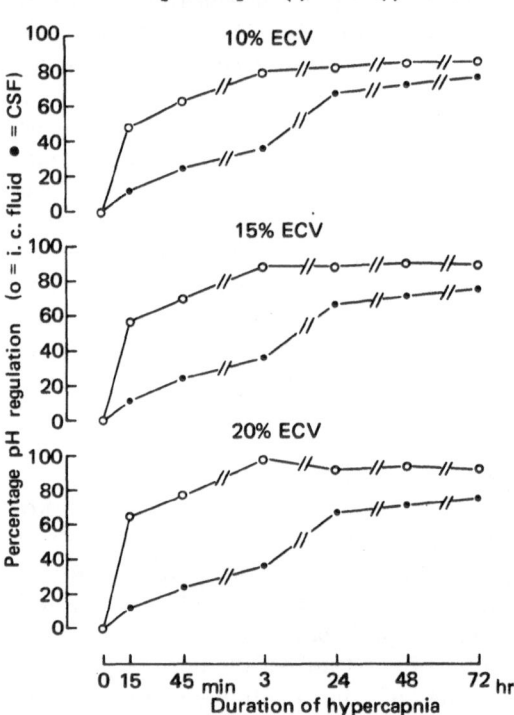

Fig. 4. Time-dependent changes in the brain tissue concentrations of lactate, pyruvate, α-ketoglutarate, and glutamate during continuous hypercapnia (Paco$_2$ about 85 mm Hg). The values (means $\pm$ s.e.) were taken from a recent publication (MESSETER and SIESJÖ [1971c]). There was a partial normalization of the concentrations of all metabolites except glutamate in sustained hypercapnia.

Fig. 5. Percentage pH regulation (see text) in CSF and in brain intracellular water during continuous hypercapnia (Paco$_2$ about 85 mm Hg). The regulation of pH$'_i$ was calculated assuming extracellular volumes of 10, 15, and 20%, respectively. There was a more efficient pH regulation in the intra- than in the extracellular space, and maximal regulation was achieved much faster intracellularly.

the hypercapnic and normocapnic situations, respectively (SIESJÖ [1971]). The figure shows that the regulation of intracellular pH' was more rapid and more efficient than that of the extracellular pH.

The question of whether or not the net flux of HCO^-_3 from extra- to intracellular fluids is passive or active can only be answered by a determination of the work of transport of HCO^-_3 (or H^+) across the membranes. A tentative calculation of the transport work, assuming constant membrane potentials, suggests that the accumulation of HCO^-_3 intracellularly in sustained hypercapnia could be due either to a decreased membrane permeability to HCO^-_3 (or H^+) at constant transport power or to an increased transport power at an unchanged membrane permeability (SIESJÖ and MESSETER [1971]). With the latter alternative we would have to assume that the hypercapnic brain has to use more energy to transport HCO^-_3 (or H^+) than the normocapnic brain.

The Influence of Hypo- and Hypercapnia upon the Energy State of the Brain

In evaluating effects of low and high carbon dioxide tensions upon the energy metabolism of the tissue, the oxygen or glucose consumption, as measured from arteriovenous differences, will not give decisive information, nor is the lactate production of the tissue unequivocally informative. This is because the substrate and oxygen utilization always must be related to the (unknown) energy requirement of the tissue (see HUCKABEE [1965], SIESJÖ et al. [1971b]) and that an increased lactate production may be due to intracellular alkalosis in the absence of an inhibition of energy production (DOMONKOS and HUSZÁK [1959], DELCHER and SHIPP [1966], SHEUER and BERRY [1967]). It therefore seems appropriate to consider parameters which reflect the balance between the energy production and the energy utilization. One such parameter is the energy charge potential of the adenine nucleotide pool (ECP) as described by Atkinson [1968].

$$ECP = \frac{ATP + 0.5\,ADP}{ATP + ADP + AMP} \quad (5)$$

This term, which has been shown to be a regulatory parameter in both energy-yielding and energy-utilizing reactions, may be expected to be decreased in all situations in which the energy production falls short of the energy demand (see also LEHNINGER [1970]). However, it is usually considered that the creatine phosphokinase reaction acts as an ATP buffer and that, therefore, a fall in the phosphocreatine (PCr) concentration is an earlier sign of energy depletion than a fall in ATP. Although this may often be the case, the pH dependence of the reaction (KUBY and NOLTMANN [1962]) suggests that acidosis by itself may lead to a decreased phosphocreatine/creatine ratio in the absence of charges in ATP and ADP.

$$\frac{PCr}{Cr} = \frac{ATP}{ADP} \cdot \frac{K'}{H^+} \quad (6)$$

An additional parameter which may be useful for evaluating the energy state of the tissue is the cytoplasmatic $NADH/NAD^+$ ratio which can be calculated from the intracellular lactate/pyruvate ratio and from pH'_i (BÜCHER and KLINGENBERG [1958], HOHORST et al. [1959], WILLIAMSON et al. [1967]; see also GRANHOLM and SIESJÖ [1969], NILSSON and SIESJÖ [1971]). There is, though, no straightforward way of interpreting cytoplasmic $NADH/NAD^+$ ratios, since they only indirectly reflect mitochondrial redox events (see below).

Marked *hypocapnia* has been shown to decrease the oxygen consumption of the intact brain (ALEXANDER et al. [1968]), and to increase the intracellular concentration of lactate (LEUSEN and DEMEESTER [1966], LEUSEN et al. [1967], PLUM and POSNER [1967], WEYNE and LEUSEN [1971]) as well as the lactate/pyruvate and $NADH/NAD^+$ ratios (GRANHOLM and SIESJÖ [1969, 1971]). These findings suggest that hypocapnia interferes with energy production in the tissue. However, the effect is not due to the decreased carbon dioxide tension as such, but to a fall in cerebral blood flow and therefore to a restriction of the oxygen supply to the tissue. Thus, when vigorous hyperventilation is performed under hyperbaric conditions, some of the signs of hypoxia are abolished (REIVICH et al. [1968], PLUM et al. [1968]).

The results obtained by different investigators indicate that part of the lactate accumulation during hyperventilation is due to hypoxia. However, since neither the PCr concentration nor the concentrations of ATP, ADP, or AMP are significantly affected by vigorous hyperventilation (GRANHOLM and SIESJÖ [1969, 1971], SIESJÖ et al. [1971a]) any hypoxia present must be moderate. The increase in the $NADH/NAD^+$ ratio in the absence of changes in the high-energy phosphates is not necessarily inconsistent, since the redox state of the tissue may change before the rate of phosphorylation of ATP declines. Moreover, it has to be explored if an *unchanged* PCr concentration during hyperventilation does not imply a shift in the CPK equilibrium due to energy depletion. Thus, the intracellular alkalosis accompanying hyperventilation should by itself shift the equilibrium in favor of an *increased* PCr concentration.

The Effect of Hypercapnia upon the Energy State of the Brain

Although measurements of the overall oxygen consumption of the intact brain have failed to show any significant changes during acute, moderate hypercapnia (KETY and SCHMIDT [1948]), there are other reports which indicate that CO_2 may inhibit the energy metabolism of tissues. Thus, CO_2 has been found to affect oxidative phosphorylation in isolated liver mitochondria, an effect which has been alternatively interpreted as an uncoupling (FANESTIL et al. [1963]) or as an inhibition of succinate oxidation (KASBEKAR [1966]). Furthermore, chronic hypercapnia has been reported to be associated with a decrease in the ATP content of brain tissue (NAVON and AGREST [1963]).

Finally, hypercapnia seems to increase the susceptibility of the brain to ischemia (SIESJÖ et al. [1971b]).

In order to study the effect of CO_2 upon the energy state of the tissue, we have recently analyzed labile phosphates in brains of animals exposed to about 11% CO_2 for periods of 15 min to 5 days. Table 2 demonstrates the tissue concentrations of PCr, ATP, ADP, AMP, and inorganic P. Acute hypercapnia (15 and 45 min) was associated with a decrease in the PCr content, which was approximately in accordance with a pH-dependent shift in the CPK equilibrium (MESSETER and SIESJÖ [1971c]), and there was a stoichiometrical increase in the P_i concentration. However, the PCr concentration did not normalize when pH'_i returned toward normal in sustained hypercapnia. In the absence of information about the creatine concentration, the somewhat low PCr concentrations in sustained hypercapnia are difficult to interpret.

It can be concluded from Table 2 that the energy charge potential (ECP) of the adenine nucleotide pool remained constant during acute and sustained hypercapnia. There was thus no indication that the hypercapnia interfered with the energy metabolism in such a way that the energy state of the tissue was affected. However, since Navon and Agrest [1964] found a decreased ATP content of the brain first after several days of hypercapnia, it remains to be studied whether or not a prolongation of the hypercapnia may change the energy charge potential.

We have recently demonstrated that the calculated intracellular lactate/pyruvate ratio increases during acute hypercapnia and that it returns to normal, or subnormal, values in sustained hypercapnia (MESSETER and SIESJÖ [1971b], see also GRANHOLM and SIESJÖ [1969], KJÄLLQUIST et al. [1969]). These changes are qualitatively in accordance with a pH effect on the lactate dehydrogenase equilibrium. However, no quantitative agreement was obtained if the predicted changes were calculated according to the equation

Table 2. Effect of continuous exposure to CO_2 (about 11 %) upon labile phosphates in rat brain.

Exposure period	PCr	ATP	ADP	AMP	P_i
		(mmoles/kg of wet tissue)			
Control	5.07	2.82	0.37	0.04	1.87
(4)	± 0.07	± 0.02	± 0.01	± 0.00	± 0.10
15 min	4.34	2.83	0.37	0.02	2.44
(10)	± 0.05	± 0.03	± 0.02	± 0.00	± 0.13
45 min	4.36	2.83	0.37	0.03	2.55
(9)	± 0.08	± 0.04	± 0.01	± 0.01	± 0.27
3 hrs	4.25	2.84	0.37	0.04	2.42
(9)	± 0.05	± 0.05	± 0.01	± 0.01	± 0.24
24 hrs	4.46	2.72	0.38	0.02	1.72
(7)	± 0.06	± 0.05	± 0.01	± 0.00	± 0.11
48 hr	4.58	2.72	0.38	0.02	1.42
(8)	± 0.08	± 0.03	± 0.02	± 0.01	± 0.11
72 hr	4.31	2.64	0.38	0.04	1.50
(8)	± 0.05	± 0.04	± 0.01	± 0.01	± 0.10

$$\frac{lactate}{pyruvate} = \frac{NADH}{NAD^+} \cdot \frac{[H^+]}{K'}$$

on the assumption of an unchanged $NADH/NAD^+$ ratio. Thus, the results indicated that the $NADH/NAD^+$ ratio remained increased during the first 3 hr of hypercapnia and that it decreased to subnormal values during sustained hypercapnia. However, these results should be interpreted with great caution. Thus, the very low pyruvate concentrations encountered in hypercapnia are difficult to measure accurately with the enzymatic spectrophotometric techniques employed, and enough CSF and blood samples were not obtained to permit rigid conclusions regarding intracellular lactate and pyruvate concentrations. Therefore, and until further information is available, it can only be concluded that hypercapnia changes the intracellular lactate/pyruvate ratio in a way which is grossly in accordance with a pH-dependent shift in the LDH equilibrium.

Summary

A short review is given of the effects of hypercapnia and hypocapnia upon the energy and the acid-base metabolism of the brain. The following conclusions are drawn. When the tissue carbon dioxide tension is acutely altered, the intracellular pH' varies much less than what could be expected on the basis of the physico-chemical buffer capacity of the intracellular space. In hypocapnia the marked regulation of pH' seems to depend on increased production of metabolic acids, particularly lactic acid, induced by means of a pH-dependent activation of glycolysis. In acute hypercapnia consumption of acids with a decrease in the steady-state concentrations of metabolic acids may contribute to the regulation of pH'$_i$. However, in sustained hypercapnia, which is associated with a 80 to 90 % regulation of pH'$_i$, an influx of HCO^-_3 from the extra- to the intracellular fluids probably plays a significant role. It is possible that this accumulation of HCO^-_3 in the cells during sustained hypercapnia requires an increased expenditure of energy.

It is concluded that extreme hypocapnia induces moderate tissue hypoxia due to a drastic fall in the cerebral blood flow, but this hypoxia is not sufficiently severe to affect the phosphorylation state of the adenine nucleotides of the tissue. Neither acute nor sustained hypercapnia was found to affect the energy state of the tissue, as judged from the energy charge potential of the adenine nucleotide pool of the tissue. However, acute hypercapnia caused a shift in the creatine phosphokinase equilibrium, with a resultant decrease in the phosphocreatine concentration and a secondary rise in inorganic P. The increase in the intracellular lactate/pyruvate ratio, which is observed in acute hypercapnia, is largely due to a pH-dependent shift in the lactate dehydrogenase equilibrium, but it remains to be shown whether or not there is also a change in the cytoplasmatic NADH/NAD$^+$ ratio.

Acknowledgments   The work reported was supported by grants from the Swedish Medical Research Council (Project No. B71–14X–263–07A and B71–14X–2179–03), from the Swedish Bank Tercentenary Fund, and by U.S. PHS grant No. 5 RO1 NS 07838–11 from NIH.

Bibliography

Atkinson, D. E., "The energy charge of the adenylate pool as a regulatory parameter. Interaction with feedback modifiers." *Biochem.* 7:4030–34 (1968).

Alexander, S. C., Smith, T. C., Strobel, G., Stephen, G. W., and Wollman, H., "Cerebral carbohydrate metabolism of man during respiratory and metabolic alkalosis." *J. Appl. Physiol.* 24:66–72.

Bachelard, H. S., "Glucose metabolism and α-keto-acids in rat brain and liver in vivo." *Nature* 205:903–04 (1965).

———, and McIlwain, H., "Carbohydrate and oxidative metabolism in neural systems." In *Comprehensive biochemistry.* Vol. 17. M. Florkin and E. H. Stotz, eds. Amsterdam: Elsevier (1969).

Bain, J. A., and Klein, J. R., "Effect of carbon dioxide on brain glucose, lactate, pyruvate and phosphates." *Am. J. Physiol.* 158:478–84 (1949).

Balacz, R., "Carbohydrate metabolism." In *Handbook of neurochemistry.* A. Lajtha, ed. New York: Plenum Press (1970).

Berl, S., Takagaki, G., Clarke, D. D., and Waelsch, H., "Carbon dioxide fixation in the brain." *J. Biol. Chem.* 237:2570–73 (1962).

———, Cheng, S.-C., and Waelsch, H., "Carbon dioxide fixation in vertebrate and invertebrate nervous tissue. In *Comparative Neurochemistry.* D. Richter, ed. New York: Pergamon Press (1964).

Brzezinski, J., Kjällquist, Å., and Siesjö, B. K., "Mean carbon dioxide tension in the brain after carbonic anhydrase inhibition." *J. Physiol.* (London) 188:12–23.

Butler, T. C., Waddell, W. J., and Poole, D. T., "Intracellular pH based on the distribution of electrolytes." *Federation Proc.* 26:1327–32 (1967).

Bücher, T. H., and Klingenberg, M., "Wege des Wasserstoffs in der lebendigen Organisation." *Angew. Chem.* 70:552–70 (1958).

Cameron, I. R., Davson, H., and Segal, M. B., "The effect of hypercapnia on the blood-brain barrier permeability to sucrose in the rabbit." *Yale J. Biol. Med.* 42:241–47 (1970).

Caldwell, P. C., "Intracellular pH." *Intern. Rev. Cytol.* 5:229–77 (1956).

———, "Studies on the internal pH of large muscle and nerve fibres." *J. Physiol.* (London) 142:22–62 (1958).

Carter, N. W., Rector, F. C., Jr., and Seldin, D. W., "Measurement of intracellular pH of skeletal muscle with pH sensitive glass microelectrodes." *J. Clin. Invest.* 46:920–33 (1967).

Cohen, P. J., "Energy metabolism of the human brain." In *Ion homeostasis of the brain.* B. K. Siesjö and S. C. Sørensen, eds. Copenhagen: Munksgaard (1971).

Conway, E. J., and Fearon, P. J., "The acid-labile CO_2 in mammalian muscle and the pH of the muscle fibre." *J. Physiol.* (London) 103:274–89 (1944).

———. "Nature and significance of concentration relations of potassium and sodium ions in skeletal muscle." *Physiol. Rev.* 37:84–132 (1957).

Danielson, I. S., Chu, H. I., and Hastings, A. B., "The pK′ of carbonic acid in concentrated protein solutions and muscle." *J. Biol. Chem.* 131:243–57 (1939).

———, and Hastings, A. B., "A method for determining carbon dioxide." *J. Biol. Chem.* 130:349–56 (1939).

Delcher, H. K., and Shipp, J. C., "Effect of pH, P_{CO_2} and bicarbonate on metabolism of glucose by perfused rat heart." *Biochim. Biophys. Acta* 121:250–60 (1966).

Domonkos, J., and Huszák, I., "Effect of hydrogen ion concentration on the carbohydrate metabolism of brain tissue." *J. Neurochem.* 4:238–43 (1959).

Edsall, J. T., and Wyman, J., *Biophysical Chemistry*, Vol. 1. New York: Academic Press (1958).

Everett, N. B., Simmons, B., and Lasher, E. P., "Distribution of blood (Fe^{59}) and plasma volumes of rats determined by liquid nitrogen freezing." *Circulat. Res.* 4:419–24 (1956).

Fanestil, D. D., Hastings, A. B., and Mahowald, T. A., "Environmental CO_2 stimulation of mitochondrial adenosine triphosphate activity." *J. Biol. Chem.* 238:836–40 (1963).

Fencl, V., Miller, T. B., and Pappenheimer, J. R., "Studies on the respiratory response to disturbances of acid-base balance, with deductions concerning the ionic composition of cerebral interstitial fluid." *Am. J. Physiol.* 210:459–72 (1966).

Geiger, A., "Metabolism and function in the brain." In *Neurochemistry*. K. A. C. Elliot, I. H. Page, and J. H. Quastel, eds. Springfield: Charles C. Thomas (1962).

Granholm, L., and Siesjö, B. K., "The effects of hypercapnia and hypocapnia upon the cerebrospinal fluid lactate and pyruvate concentrations and upon the lactate, pyruvate, ATP, ADP, phosphocreatine and creatine concentrations of cat brain tissue." *Acta Physiol. Scand.* 75:257–66 (1969).

———, and Siesjö, B. K., "The effect of combined respiratory and nonrespiratory alkalosis on energy metabolites and acid-base parameters in the rat brain." *Acta Physiol. Scand.* 81:307–14 (1971).

Hohorst, H. J., Kreuz, F. H., and Bücher, T., "Uber Metabolitgehalte und Metabolit-Konzentrationen in der Leber der Ratte." *Biochem. Z.* 332:18–46 (1959).

Huckabee, W. E., In *Effects of Anesthesia on metabolism and cellular functions*. J. P. Bunker and L. D. Vandam, eds. *Pharmacol. Rev.* 17:183, pp. 247–52 (1965).

Kasbekar, D. K., "Effect of carbon dioxide-bicarbonate mixtures on rat liver mitochondrial oxidative phosphorylation." *Biochim. Biophys. Acta*, 128:205–08 (1966).

Kety, S. S., and Schmidt, C. F., "The effects of altered arterial tensions of carbon dioxide and oxygen on cerebral blood flow and cerebral oxygen consumption of normal young men." *J. Clin. Invest.* 27:484–91 (1948).

Kjällquist, Å., Nardini, M., and Siesjö, B. K., "The regulation of extra- and intracellular acid-base parameters in the rat brain during hyper- and hypocapnia. *Acta Physiol. Scand.* 76:485–94 (1969).

Kostyuk, P. G., and Sorokina, Z. A., "On the mechanism of hydrogen ion distribution between cell protoplasm and the medium." *Membrane Proc. Symp., Prague.* New York: Academic Press (1961).

Krebs, H. A., and Kornberg, H. L., *Energy transformation in living matter*. Berlin: Springer Verlag (1957).

Kuby, S. A., and Noltmann, E. A., "ATP-creatine transphosphorylase." In *The enzymes*, Vol. 6. New York: Academic Press (1962).

Lehninger, A. L., *Biochemistry*. New York: Worth Publishers (1970).

Leusen, I., Lacroix, E., and Demeester, G., "Lactate and pyruvate in the brain of rats during changes in acid-base balance." *Arch. Internat. Physiol. Biochem.* 75:310–24 (1967).

———, and Demeester, G., "Lactate and pyruvate in the brain of rats during hyperventilation." *Arch. Internat. Physiol. Biochem.* 74:25–34 (1966).

Lowry, O. H., and Passonneau, J. V., "Kinetic evidence for multiple binding sites on phosphofructokinase." *J. Biol. Chem.* 241:2268–79 (1966).

McIlwain, H., *Biochemistry and the central nervous system*. London: J. & A. Churchill Ltd. (1966).

Messeter, K., and Siesjö, B. K., "Regulation of intracellular pH in the rat brain in chronic hypercapnia." *Acta Physiol. Scand.* 79:136–38 (1970).

———, and Siesjö, B. K., "Regulation of the CSF pH in acute and sustained respiratory acidosis." *Acta Physiol. Scand.* 83:21–30 (1971).

———, and Siesjö, B. K., "The intracellular pH' in the brain in acute and sustained hypercapnia. *Acta Physiol. Scand.* 83:210–219 (1971).

———, and Siesjö, B. K., "The effect of acute and chronic hypercapnia upon the lactate, pyruvate, α-ketoglutarate, and glutamate contents of the rat brain." *Acta Physiol. Scand.* 83:344–351 (1971).

Navon, S., and Agrest, A., "ATP content in the central nervous system of rats exposed to chronic hypercapnia." *Am. J. Physiol.* 205:957–58 (1963).

Nilsson, L., and Siesjö, B. K., "The effect of hypoxia upon labile substrates and upon acid-base parameters in the brain." In *Ion homeostasis of the brain.* B. K. Siesjö and S. C. Sørensen, eds. Copenhagen: Munksgaard (1971).

Paillard, M., Sraer, J. D., and Leviel, J. D., Direct measurement of intracellular pH in rat and crab muscle in vitro. Abstract, Fifth Annual Meeting, European Society for Clinical Investigation. April 1971.

Plum, F., and Posner, J. B., "Blood and cerebrospinal fluid lactate during hyperventilation." *Am. J. Physiol.* 212:864–70 (1967).

———, Posner, J. B., and Smith, W. W., "Effect of hyperbaric-hyperoxic hyperventilation on blood, brain, and CSF lactate." *Am. J. Physiol.* 215:1240–44 (1968).

Pontén, U., and Siesjö, B. K., "A method for the determination of the total carbon dioxide content of frozen tissues." *Acta Physiol. Scand.* 60:297–308 (1964).

———, and Siesjö, B. K., "Gradients of CO_2 tension in the brain." *Acta Physiol. Scand.* 68:152–63 (1966).

Rall, D. P., and Fenstermacher, J. D., "Volume of cerebral extracellular fluids." In *Ion homeostasis of the brain.* B. K. Siesjö and S. C. Sørensen, eds. Copenhagen: Munksgaard (1971).

Roberts, R. B., Flexner, J. B., and Flexner, L. B., "Biochemical and physiological differentiation during morphogenesis—XXIII." *J. Neurochem.* 4:78–99 (1959).

Robson, J. S., Bone, J. M., and Lambie, A. T., "Intracellular pH." In *Advances in clinical chemistry.* Vol. 2. O. Bodansky and C. P. Stewart, eds. New York: Academic Press (1968).

Reivich, M., Dickson, J., Clark, J., Hedden, M., and Lambertsen, C. J., "Role of hypoxia in cerebral circulatory and metabolic changes during hypocarbia in man: studies in hyperbaric milieu." In *CBF & CSF.* D. H. Ingvar, N. A. Lassen, B. K. Siesjö, and E. Skinhøj, eds. *Scand. J. Clin. Lab. Invest.* Suppl. 102. IV:B (1968).

Scheuer, J., and Berry, M. N., "Effect of alkalosis on glycolysis in the isolated rat heart." *Am. J. Physiol.* 213:1143–48 (1967).

Siesjö, B. K., "The solubility of carbon dioxide in cerebral cortical tissue of cats. With a note on the solubility of carbon dioxide in water, 0.16 M NaCl and cerebrospinal fluid." *Acta Physiol. Scand.* 55:325–41 (1962a).

———. "The bicarbonate/carbonic acid buffer system of the cerebral cortex of cats as studied in tissue homogenates. 2. The pK'_1 of carbonic acid at 37.5°C, and the relation between carbon dioxide tension and pH." *Acta Neurol. Scand.* 38:121–41 (1962b).

———. "Quantification of pH regulation in hypercapnia and hypocapnia." *Scand. J. Clin. Lab. Invest.* 28:113–119 (1971).

———, and Messeter, K., "Factors determining intracellular pH." In *Ion homeostasis of the brain.* B. K. Siesjö and S. C. Sørensen, eds. Copenhagen: Munksgaard (1971).

———, Nilsson, L., Rokeach, M., and Zwetnow, N. N., "Energy metabolism of the brain at reduced cerebral perfusion pressures and in arterial hypoxemia." In *Brain hypoxia.* J. B. Brierley, ed. Heinemann Medical (1971b).

Tower, D. B., *Neurochemistry of epilepsy.* Springfield Ill.: Thomas (1960).

Vrba, R., "Glucose metabolism in rat brain in vivo." *Nature* (London). 195:663–65 (1962).

Waddell, W. J., and Butler, T. C., "Calculation of intracellular pH from the distribution of 5.5-dimethyl-2.4-oxazolidinedione (DMO). Application to skeletal muscle of the dog." *J. Clin. Invest.* 38:720–29 (1959).

———, and Bates, R. G., "Intracellular pH." *Physiol. Rev.* 49:285–329 (1969).

Waelsch, H., Berl, S., Rossi, C. A., Clarke, D. D., and Purpura, D. P., "Quantitative aspects of CO_2 fixation in mammalian brain in vivo." *J. Neurochem.* 11:717–28 (1964).

Wallace, W. M., and Hastings, A. B., "The distribution of the bicarbonate ion in mammalian muscle." *J. Biol. Chem.* 144:637–49 (1942).

Weyne, J., and Leusen, I., "Bicarbonate, chloride and lactate in brain during acid-base alterations." In *Ion homeostasis of the brain.* B. K. Siesjö and S. C. Sørensen, eds. Copenhagen: Munksgaard (1971).

Williamson, D. H., Lund, P., and Krebs, H. A., "The redox state of free nicotinamide-adenine dinucleotide in the cytoplasm and mitochondria of rat liver." *Biochem. J.* 103:514–27 (1967).

Woodbury, D. M., and Karler, R., "The role of carbon dioxide in the nervous system." *Anesthesiology*. 21:686–703 (1960).

Woodward, D. L., Reed, D. J., and Woodbury, D. M., "Extracellular space of rat cerebral cortex." *Am. J. Physiol.* 212:367–70 (1967).

Wyke, B., *Brain function and metabolic disorders.* London: Butterworths (1963).

Siesjö Discussion

GORTNER: Thank you. I'd like to make a comment on Dr. Siesjö's comment, since he quite unfairly said that the high P_{CO_2} in our experiments was due to bad treatment. First of all, I'd like to ask him how he could explain the concentration of these weak acids by bad treatment; secondly, how he can explain the measurements Pierce in these cholera patients where only an arterial puncture was done and a lumbar needle was put in and they found the P_{CO_2} averaged 19 mm higher in the cerebrospinal fluid than in the arterial blood? These are patients with acidosis, a similar condition where we found very large P_{CO_2} differences. And also a second comment, from your papers your brain surface measurements seem—at least it seems to us —that they are measurements of pia P_{CO_2}. Now when we did this with our mass spectrometer we found results very similar to yours, that the pia measurements—what you would call brain surface measurements— were very similar to blood. Now the pia is a very vascular organ and I suspect that in these large vessels with slow flow through them this measurement is actually very close to a blood measurement and, at least it's our feeling, that this does not represent cerebrospinal fluid nor does it represent brain tissue P_{CO_2} which we think is also high.

SIESJÖ: I am sorry if my remarks sounded rather rude. What I said was that in our experiments, when we treated the animals rather badly, then we got the same results you are getting now. This, of course, implied that you could have the same error. But I seriously think you may be in trouble if you don't sample cerebral venous blood from

the same parts of the brain which are in equilibrium with the cerebrospinal fluid on which you are measuring. And I don't think you should put any confidence in the P_{CO_2} gradients measured when you compare arterial and cerebral venous blood with lumbar CSF. It's a very long distance between the cistern and the side ventricle and lumbar CSF, and in severely ill patients I am quite sure you can get large gradients that way. I think you are right when you are saying that the tissue electrode may measure something else than the mean tissue carbon dioxide tension. To us it was an empirical measurement; we said that probably this is a mean tissue carbon dioxide tension. We applied the Krogh diffusion model, using the arterial and venous values, and I measured together with Thews the diffusion coefficient for carbon dioxide in the tissue (SIESJÖ and THEWS [1962]). We calculated the expected mean tissue carbon dioxide tension, being then a carbon dioxide tension integrated across the length of the capillary and across the cross-section of the tissue cylinder. We put the carbon dioxide electrode on top of the tissue, or we took CSF samples, and in all circumstances the values agreed with those calculated. So we felt rather confident that we measured a mean tissue carbon dioxide tension which had some quantitative meaning, but we have not studied metabolic acidosis.

FENCL: I think Dr. Siesjö has covered most of it, but I would add to those patients in cholera that the high bicarbonates you are referring to in the spinal fluid are hardly steady-state distribution of the ion, and it takes some 10 hr in man to reach a steady-state distribution after establishing a situation in the blood.

GORTNER: These were 24 hr; cholera, Pierce's paper.

FENCL: Right. But to reach the steady-state distribution of bicarbonate as showing on those steady-state data you have to maintain a given composition of blood for 10 hr, in man, and at that time it's seen in the cistern. I'm not sure how it's going to be in the lumbar sac, and all those regulations of cerebral blood flow related to the acid base disturbances do influence the P_{CO_2} in the intercranial CSF. I don't think they are going to have anything to do with the P_{CO_2} in the lumbar region. There, the field equilibrates with the local tissue P_{CO_2} which has nothing to do with those strange regulations of cerebral blood flow.

SEVERINGHAUS: I'd like to suggest, though, that perhaps we go a little bit cautious on saying that you disagree entirely with Dr. Gortner because I, too, have some tissue surface measurements which in general at normal P_{CO_2} have agreed quite well, mine with venous blood a little higher than yours, but I found a very strange thing—and that is that during hypercapnia the tissue P_{CO_2} was far higher than the venous or the arterial blood. I never could understand that and I always mistrusted the electrodes and I've never published it, but it does accord with what Dr. Gortner's saying.

SIESJÖ: We had exactly the same observations, but we found that these observations were obtained when we could see that the tissue was in a way traumatized, with bleeding under the electrode (PONTÉN and SIESJÖ [1966]). If we had to put another burr hole into the skull or if we had to have the electrode sit for long periods, then the tissue carbon dioxide tension went above the venous carbon dioxide tension, but I don't think that is representative for a normal, untraumatized tissue.

SEVERINGHAUS: Well, in mine it was just a burr hole and it was reversible; that is, we could go up and down and at normal levels the P_{CO_2}'s agreed and at hypercapnia they didn't.

SIESJÖ: We don't find that.

SCHAEFER: You know there are changes in the apparent space of extracellular or intracellular volume under carbon dioxide in different organs. You assumed a constant value of extracellular space. Did you have any measurements of the extracellular space in brain?

SIESJÖ: That is extremely difficult to measure since you need a long, steady-state period with ventriculocisternal perfusion of inulin. We have not measured it. We have tried to calculate what a certain change could make for our calculations, and if there are reasonable changes, say within plus-minus 5% of the tissue weight, the effect is small. I cannot agree with you that it is well known that the

space changes due to hypercapnia. The only measurement that exists in the literature, as far as I know, is that of Cameron et al. [1970], who studied the cerebral extracellular volume, and they found no change whatsoever in hypercapnia.

TURINO: With regard to utilization of organic acids by brain tissue, during chronic hypercapnia and acidosis is the production of these organic acids increased, perhaps as a function of the increased blood flow to the brain?

SIESJÖ: Normally, 5% of the glucose consumed is utilized anaerobically and is released as lactic acid, but that is dependent on the blood concentration. No one knows how it is in hypercapnia, and it's very difficult to measure. You have a very high blood flow and very small arteriovenous differences, but I would not assume that there is a change in the production of the organic acids.

RECTOR: I say, briefly, in your calculation of the redox potential you make a correction for hydrogen ion concentration. Assuming that your changes are directionally correct, how critical is the absolute value for your hydrogen ion in those calculations?

SIESJÖ: I'm not quite sure about that because I haven't done the calculations at an intracellular pH of around 6, but we always compare our values with those for the normal control state, so the changes should be, I think, approximately the same even if the intracellular pH would be very much lower.

RECTOR: Well, I'm not even certain that the value of 6 is the crucial value, even if the electrodes were correct, because the local pH in a gel-sol solution around charged macromolecules can be quite different than in the aqueous solution and, as you know, it's possible to shift pH optimum of enzymes as much as one pH unit by adsorbing onto charged macromolecules, so that in these localized regions which may be in a quasi-equilibrium, you may have quite different hydrogen or hydroxyl ion concentrations that could influence these ratios. I just wondered had you given any thought to this possibility?

SIESJÖ: I think we have a kind of disagreement there, but where is the bicarbonate then in the tissue?

RECTOR: I think it may be around macromolecules plus in trapped compartments.

SIESJÖ: Anyhow, it's reached by lactic acid since it is blown off in cerebral hypoxia.

RECTOR: Yes, I think it's accessible for buffering.

Bibliography

Cameron, I. R., Davson, H., and Segal, M. B., "The effect of hypercapnia on the blood-brain barrier permeability to sucrose in the rabbit." *Yale J. Biol. Med.* 42:241–47 (1970).

Ponten, U., and Siesjö, B. K., "Gradients of CO_2 tension in the brain." *Acta Physiol. Scand.* 67:129–40 (1966).

Siesjö, B., and Thews, G., "Ein Verfahren zur Bestimmung der CO_2-leitfähigkeit, der CO_2-diffusionskoeffizienten und des scheinbaren CO_2-löslichkeitskoefficienten im Gehirngewebe." *Pflüg. Arch.* 276:192–210 (1962).

Part V

Adaptation to Carbon Dioxide

1. Metabolic Aspects of Adaptation to Carbon Dioxide

Karl E. Schaefer

Chief Biomedical Sciences Division
Submarine Medical Research Laboratory
United States Naval Submarine Medical Research Laboratory
Groton, Connecticut 06340

Acute hypercapnia has been shown to result in an inhibition of glycolysis, lipolysis, and cyclic AMP formation by Nahas and his coworkers (NAHAS, POYART, and TRINER [1968], POYART and NAHAS [1968a], NAHAS and STEINSLAND [1968b], NAHAS [1971]). We were interested in studying adaptation of metabolic functions in chronic hypercapnia following the depression induced during the acute phase of hypercapnia. Guinea pigs and rats were used during prolonged exposure to 15% CO_2. Under these conditions we observed biphasic changes, an initial transitory depression of functions followed by a recovery and a return to control levels or near control levels associated with the biphasic changes in pH. The concentration of 15% CO_2 was chosen for these studies because it is high enough to cause during the acute phase a sufficiently large fall in pH (7.4 to 7.0) so as to affect pH-dependent enzymes. During the subsequent adaptation to respiratory acidosis the pH rises again above the level at which most of the pH-dependent enzymes are inhibited (SCHAEFER, MESSIER, and MORGAN [1970]). Under these conditions we observed a transient pH-dependent inhibition and subsequent recovery of red-cell glycolysis (JACEY and SCHAEFER [1971]) which was associated with a biphasic shift in the oxygen dissociation curve (SCHAEFER, MESSIER, and MORGAN [1970]) and pH-dependent changes in red cell 2,3-diphosphoglycerate (MESSIER and SCHAEFER [1971]).

The second form of metabolic adaptation studied under identical experimental conditions was the pH-dependent inhibition of fibrinolytical activity in the lungs developed with the appearance of hyaline membranes, loss of surfactant and alteration in lamellar bodies of granular pneumocytes. The subsequent rise in pH resulted in a recovery of all these functions and a disappearance of hyaline membranes, (NIEMOELLER and SCHAEFER [1962]; SCHAEFER, AVERY, and BENSCH [1964], SCHAEFER [1968a]).

The third form of metabolic adaptation discussed in this report is the pH-dependent fall and recovery of body temperature associated with a transitory inhibition of energy metabolism (SCHAEFER, MORGAN, and MESSIER [1972]). During exposure to 15% CO_2 inhibition of lipolysis occurred as indicated in the failure of glycerol and triglycerides to rise during the initial three-day stress period during which corticosterone levels rose and adrenal epinephrine release increased (SCHAEFER, McCABE, and WITHERS [1968b]).

The 15% CO_2 experiment provides a biological model which gives a great deal of information. Although the initial fall of pH is outside the physiological range, the level of pH reached in the later phase after seven days corresponds with the initial fall of pH produced by exposure to 3% CO_2 and is within the pH range encountered under clinical conditions.

The Effect of Chronic Respiratory Acidosis on Oxygen Affinity, Red-Cell Cation Exchange, and Red-Cell Metabolism

Figure 1 shows the shift of the oxygen dissociation curve to the left after one day of exposure and a return to near control level after seven days of exposure. The dependence of the displacement of the oxygen dissociation curve on the acid base status of the blood is clearly expressed in Figure 2, showing the parallel time course of intracellular pH of red cells and P 50 values (O_2 affinity). The P 50 values for red cells (lower curve) was calculated using Dill's factor and the differ-

ence between the pH of whole blood and red-cell hemolysate.

The cation concentrations of red cells have also biphasic pH-dependent changes consisting in a large fall of potassium concentration during the initial phase of respiratory acidosis associated with a slight rise in sodium concentration. After three days these changes subsided without reaching the initial levels of red cell sodium and potassium.

As shown in Figure 3, the ratio erythrocyte cations/HB used by Waldeck and Zander [1969] shows an excellent correlation with the P 50 values ($r = 0.96$). This linear relationship does not, however, prove the existence of a causal relationship between intracellular cations and oxygen affinity, although it has been known for a long time that intracellular cations influence oxygen

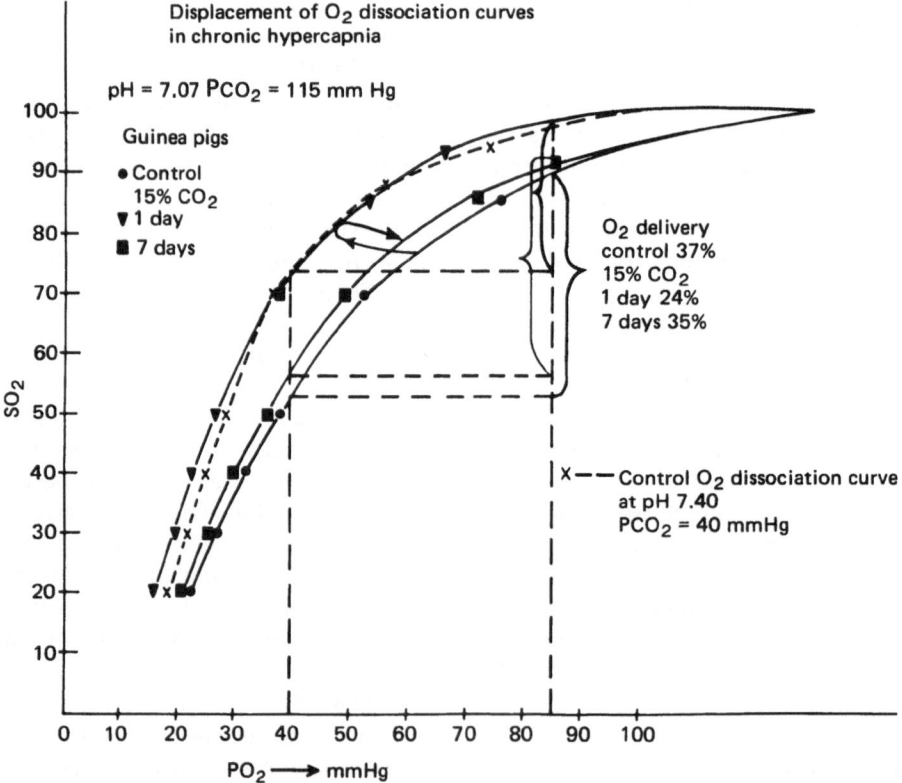

Fig. 1. Displacement of oxygen dissociation curves of guinea pigs in chronic hypercapnia (15% CO_2). Equilibration of blood samples obtained under control conditions (B), and following exposure to 15% CO_2 with gas mixtures at a P_{CO_2} of 115 mm Hg corresponding to the partial pressure of a 15% CO_2 gas mixture. (A) Blood samples of control animals equilibrated at a P_{CO_2} of 40 mm Hg.

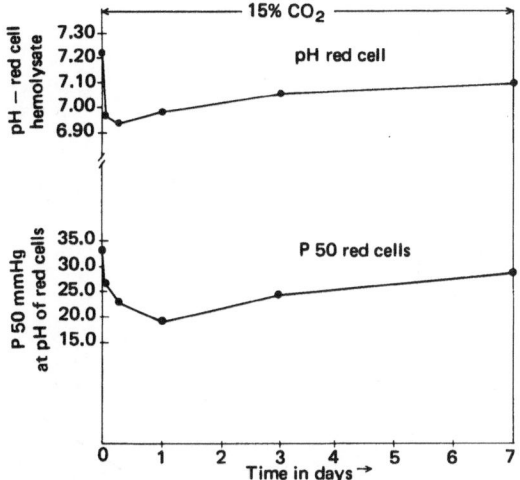

Fig. 2. Time course of red-cell pH and half-saturation pressure (P 50) of guinea pigs during chronic hypercapnia (15% CO_2). Blood samples were equilibrated with gas mixtures of varying oxygen tensions, but constant Pco_2 of 40 mm Hg. Red-cell P 50 was calculated using Dill's factor and the difference between whole-blood and red-cell hemolysate.

affinity. There is, however, another mechanism which is pH-dependent and influences oxygen affinity and cation exchange. This is 2,3-diphosphoglycerate. Figure 4 shows the 2,3-diphosphoglycerate values obtained under these experimental conditions plotted against the P 50 values. The correlation coefficient is 0.93 (MESSIER and SCHAEFER [1971]). The decrease in red-cell potassium and increase in red-cell sodium are obviously an expression of an inhibition of active transport through which sodium is pumped out of the cell and potassium pumped into the cell against a gradient. The energy for this work is derived from glycolysis. We therefore studied certain aspects of red-cell glycolysis.

Investigations of blood sugar, lactate, and pyruvate during chronic hypercapnia showed an inhibition of glucose utilization during the first phase of respiratory acidosis. As shown in Figure 5, blood sugar is greatly elevated, and returns after three days to control levels. Both lactate and pyruvate decline during exposure for 1 and 6 hr. After

one day lactate returns nearly to initial values while pyruvate increases strongly, resulting in a decrease of the lactate pyruvate ratio. The results show that the initial fall in pH to 7.0 and 6.96 causes an inhibition of glycolysis.

The lactate/pyruvate ratio has been shown to be related to the redox state of free cytoplasmatic nicotin amide-adenine dinucleotide couplet. $NAD^+/NADH$. The ratio $NAD^+/NADH$ can be calculated from the lactate pyruvate ratios, pH and the known equilibrium constants (HOHORST et al. [1965], BÜCHER and RÜSSMANN [1963], WILLIAMSON, LUND, and KREBS [1967], JACEY and SCHAEFER [1971]). $NAD^+/NADH$ ratios of blood of guinea pigs exposed to 15% CO_2 are presented in Table 1. During the acute period of hypercapnia, the $NAD^+/NADH$ ratio rises steadily, reaching the highest value at one day. This change reflects a shift toward a more oxidized state. During the subsequent period, during which a partial compensation of the respiratory acidosis is attained, the $NAD^+/NADH$ ratio shows a decline toward normal values, which indicates a return to the initial redox state.

Since regulation of glycolysis depends on the phosphofructokinase system, measurements of phosphofructokinase were carried out and are presented in Figure 6. Phosphofructokinase activity shows biphasic changes paralleling those of pH and lactate. During the acute phase of respiratory acidosis associated with maximal extracellular acidosis, phosphofructokinase activity shows a maximal reduction (55%). With increasing compensation of the respiratory acidosis during the chronic phase enzyme activity correspondingly increases, but neither pH nor phosphofructokinase activity reach control values during the seven-day exposure to 15% CO_2.

ATP, ADP, and AMP were not affected by chronic hypercapnia (Figure 6 and Table 1) (with the exception of a transient rise in ADP and AMP on the third day). The latter change is probably related to a group of animals which are unable to adapt to acidosis

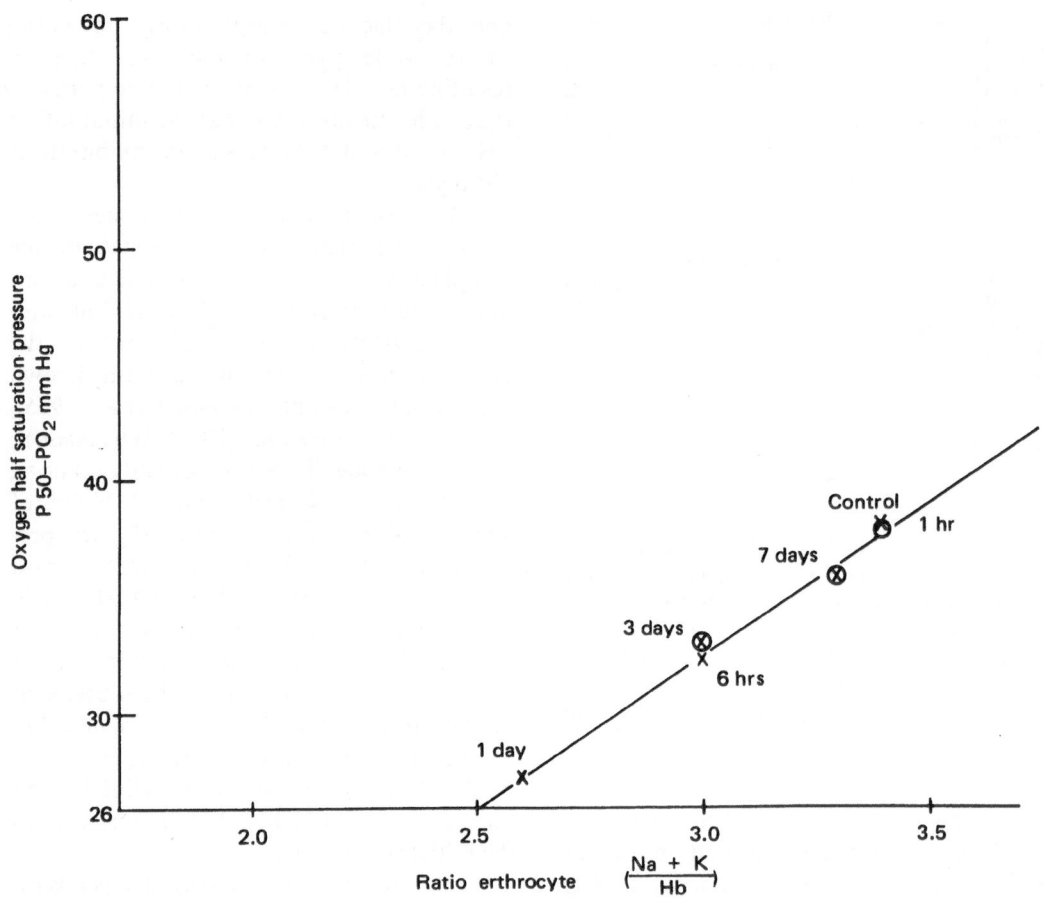

Fig. 3. Oxygen half-saturation pressure (P 50) versus ratio of erythrocyte (Na + K)/Hb. Points marked by X = uncompensated phase of respiratory acidosis. Points marked by ⊗ = compensated phase of respiratory acidosis.

and succumb usually at the third day (SCHAEFER et al. [1972]). Granholm and Siesjö [1969] observed no changes in tissue ATP, ADP, and AMP levels in the brain of cats acutely exposed to various concentrations of CO_2. In more recent studies (SIESJÖ [1971], this monograph) similar findings were obtained in the brain of rats exposed for 72 hours to 11 % CO_2, which is in line with our observations.

The energy charge of the adenylate system has been introduced by Atkinson and Walton (1967) as fundamental control parameters of metabolism. The energy charge was calculated according to Atkinson and Walton [1967] as the Energy Charge Poten-

tial (ECP) = (ATP + 0.5 ADP)/(ATP + ADP + AMP) and is listed in Table 1. No changes were observed. The constancy of the ECP values and the corresponding findings of Tappan [1971], who did not observe any significant changes in muscle creatine phosphate under the same conditions of 15 % CO_2 exposure, seems to indicate that hypercapnia is characterized by conservation of high-energy phosphate.

The strongest inhibition of red-cell glycolysis occurs after 1-hr exposure to 15 % CO_2, while the maximal decline of 2,3-diphosphoglycerate and of the cation concentrations is seen after one day. These findings suggest that changes of both 2,3-

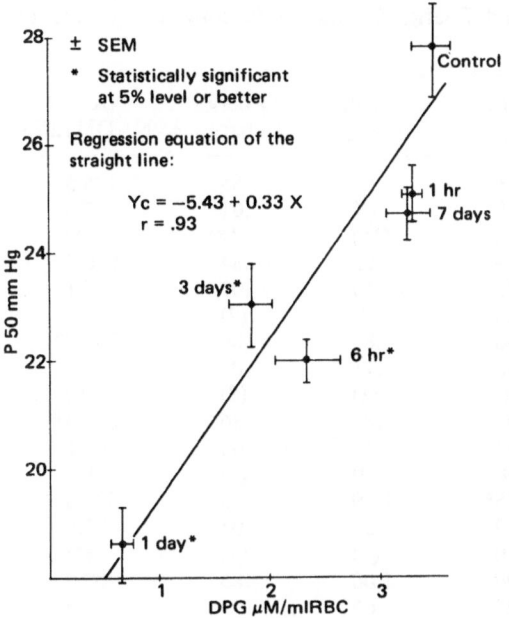

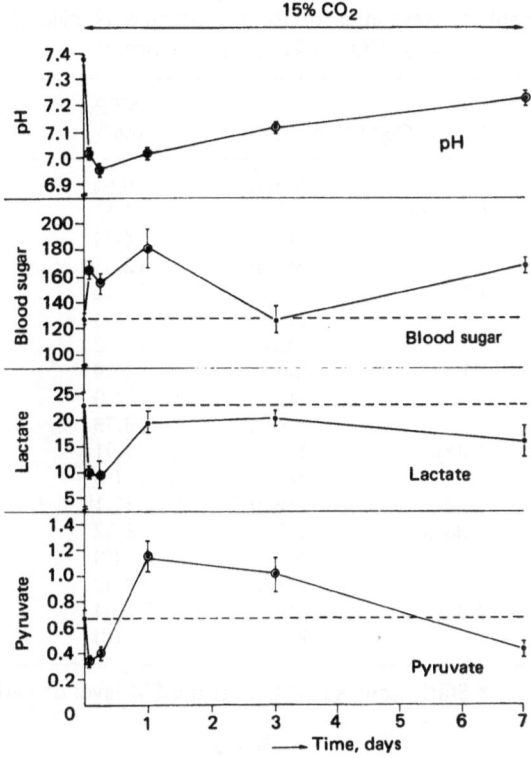

Fig. 4. Relation between half-saturation pressure (P 50) of whole blood and concentration of 2, 3-DPG (diphosphoglycerate) in chronic hypercapnia. Correlation coefficient, $r = 0.93$.

Fig. 5. Effect of prolonged exposure to 15% CO_2 on blood pH, blood sugar, lactate, and pyruvate. Points marked by ⊙ statistically significantly different from controls at the 5% level and better.

diphosphoglycerate as well as cation concentrations of the red cells develop as the consequence of the glycolytic inhibition. The fall in 2,3-diphosphoglycerate does therefore not appear to be the cause of the changes in cation permeability. In chronic hypercapnia produced by prolonged exposure to 15% CO_2 the effects on oxygen transport caused by transient pH-dependent fall in 2,3-DPG are compensated by the simultaneous increase in the Bohr effect (SCHAEFER and MESSIER [1970]).

To establish the ranges of the pH-dependent changes in red-cell metabolism additional experiments were carried out in which guinea pigs were exposed to 3% CO_2 for periods up to seven days. Blood lactate–pyruvate concentrations as well as the calculated redox state, $NAD^+/NADH$ ratios were virtually unaffected (Table 2). The maximal pH decrease of 0.12 units caused by exposure to 3% CO_2 was apparently too small to alter glycolytic metabolism of red cells in guinea pigs.

The Carbon Dioxide-Induced Hyaline Membrane Disease As a Biological Model for Study of Lung Cell Injury and Repair

We have previously reported that guinea pigs exposed to 15% CO_2 up to seven days show in 100% of the cases development of hyaline membranes after one day and none of the experimental animals exhibited hyaline membranes after seven days of exposure (NIEMOELLER and SCHAEFER [1962]). A parallel time course was established between changes in lung surfactant and alterations in lamellar bodies in the granular pneumocytes associated with both the occurrence and disappearance of hyaline membranes in guinea pigs exposed to 15% CO_2 for prolonged periods (SCHAEFER, AVERY, and BENSCH [1964]). Changes in the acid base status of blood and lungs during

Table 1. Responses of Blood Adenine Nucleotides and Energy Charge to Prolonged Exposure to 15% CO_2 in 21% O_2, Balance N_2

Condition		ATP, mg%	ADP, mg%	AMP, mg%	Energy charge	NAD+/ NADH ratio
Control	Mean	10.64	2.26	.80	.85	176.5
	SE	1.16	.19	.07	.01	22.3
	N	(18)	(18)	(18)	(18)	(11)
1 hr	Mean	12.83	2.99	.83	.84	570.8*
	SE	1.42	.29	.14	.01	46.1
	N	(7)	(7)	(7)	(7)	(9)
6 hr	Mean	11.12	1.90	.83	.86	739.2*
	SE	1.39	.18	.11	.02	113.0
	N	(8)	(8)	(8)	(8)	(9)
1 day	Mean	13.73	2.67	.87	.86	888.4*
	SE	1.91	.35	.18	.02	96.1
	N	(9)	(9)	(9)	(9)	(12)
3 days	Mean	11.19	4.55*	1.19*	.78*	504.3*
	SE	1.02	.19	.05	.01	71.9
	N	(9)	(9)	(9)	(9)	(6)
7 days	Mean	14.58	2.90	1.00	.85	200.0
	SE	2.04	.27	.03	.01	18.5
	N	(8)	(8)	(8)	(8)	(5)

* Statistically significant at the 5% level or better.

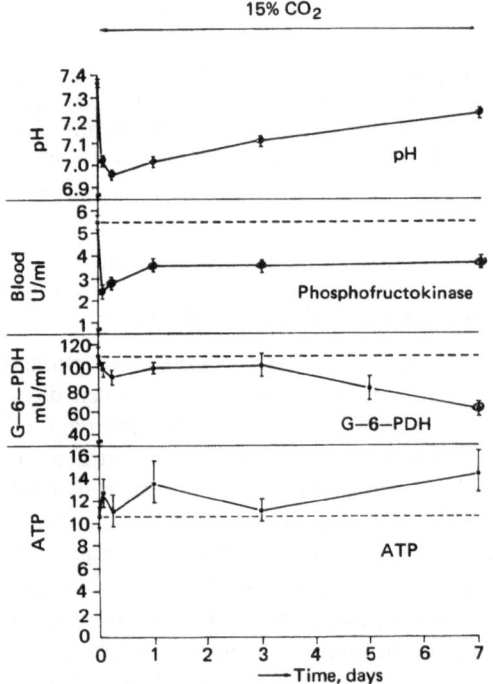

Fig. 6. Effect of prolonged exposure to 15% CO_2 on blood pH, phosphofructokinase activity, glucose-6-phosphate dehydroegenase, and blood ATP levels. Points marked by ○ statistically significant at the 5% level and better.

prolonged exposure were compared, in addition to blood pH by measuring the intracellular pH of the lungs with the CO_2 method of Fenn. Extracellular pH fell to the lowest value after 6 hr, while the maximal drop of intracellular pH of the lungs occurred after 24 hr. This large decrease of pH develops between 6 and 24 hr after a transient increase in lung pH during the period between 1 and 6 hr of exposure. Actual bicarbonate rises within 1 hr from 23.3 to 41.0 mM/L, which is followed by a transient fall at 6 hr to 36 m/m and a subsequent slow rise over the period of seven days.

The intracellular bicarbonate of the lungs also shows a steep rise in the first hour. However, there is a surprising fall in cell bicarbonate from 28 to 10 mM/L between 6 hours and one day, and subsequent recovery by three days. The time course of intracellular bicarbonate change shows clear evidence of a secondary transient intracellular metabolic acidosis. This is in line with findings of Martin et al. [1965] obtained in rats during exposure to 10% CO_2. They observed a metabolic acidosis between 8 and 48 hr in heart, muscle, liver, and brain.

Table 2. Responses of Blood Lactate, Pyruvate, and Lactate/Pyruvate Ratio and Redox State, NAD^+/ NADH Ratio to Prolonged Exposure to 3% CO_2 in 21% O_2, Balance N_2

		Control	1 hr	6 hr	1 day	3 days	7 days
Lactate mg %	Mean	20.98	19.52	23.97	24.88	22.44	23.69
	S.E.	1.47	1.69	2.38	2.20	2.19	1.98
	N	12	10	10	14	14	13
Pyruvate mg %	Mean	.65	.70	.78	.78	.95*	.75
	S.E.	.08	.09	.04	.12	.08	.10
	N	10	6	6	11	11	9
Lactate/pyruvate Ratio	Mean	25.57	28.67	30.90	31.63	23.60	35.24
	S.E.	5.08	1.60	2.20	4.88	1.11	4.15
	N	9	6	6	11	10	9
NAD^+/NADH ratio	Mean	241.3	296.2	246.4	294.0	328.4	246.9
	S.E.	37.3	23.0	38.9	34.0	21.2	35.1
	N	9	6	6	11	10	9

* Statistically significant at the 5% level or better.

A summary of the data on acid-base status of blood and lungs correlated with the measurements of lung surface tension, fibrinolytic activity, and histopathological observations on edema and hyaline membrane formation is presented in the upper part of Table 3 (NIEMOELLER and SCHAEFER [1962], SCHAEFER, AVERY, and BENSCH [1964], SCHAEFER [1967]).

Pulmonary edema is present in 100% of the animals after 1 hr of exposure. Incidence of edema remains at this level up to 24 hr, following which it steadily declines to 0% at seven days. This time course follows closely the changes in extracellular pH. This supports the notion that the edema is caused by an increased capillary permeability due to extracellular acidosis.

Hyaline membrane formation occurs with a marked time lag corresponding with the rise in minimal surface tension and the marked fall in intracellular pH and bicarbonate loss due to metabolic acidosis after 24 hr.

Data on the fibrinolysin system were obtained by Dr. Ambrus Buffalo, to whom we sent the prepared lung tissues and blood from animals. Antiplasmin and fibrinogen levels in the blood rose after 6 hr and remained increased for the rest of the exposure of seven days.

The plasminogen activator activity of the lungs disappeared after 6 hours when the edema judged by the lung weight was maximal. At the same time a plasminogen activator inhibitor was observed which was absent in the control animals. This inhibitor was limited to the first two days of exposure and can be explained as the result of the pulmonary effusion and associated transfer of higher concentrations of antiplasmin from the blood into the pulmonary tissue. With the disappearance of the pulmonary edema, the plasminogenactivator activity disappeared too, in spite of a still-increased antiplasmin level in the serum. There is a time lag between the complete loss of fibrinolytic activity in the lungs after 6 hr of exposure and the appearance of hyaline membranes after 24 hr of exposure.

These findings indicate an interplay between two processes with a faster and slower time constant: (1) the pulmonary effusion and associated depression of pulmonary fibrinolytic activity after 6 hr, (2) the development of hyaline membranes by 24 hr and the associated rise in minimal surface tension, indicating reduction in surface active material and the corresponding histopathological changes of the lamellar bodies in the large alveolar lining cells (type II granular pneumocytes).

Table 3. Metabolic adaptation during Chronic Hypercapnia in Guinea Pigs

Acid-base status and metabolic and histo-pathological processes Data comparison	Exposure to 15% CO_2 up to 7 days		
	Period 1–6 hours	Period 24–48 hours	Period 7 days
	(6 hours)	(24 hours)	(7 days)
(1) Acid-base status	Maximal extracellular acidosis	Transitory intracellular metabolic acidosis	Partial compensation of respiratory acidosis
Blood			
(1) Glycolysis	Maximal inhibition	Partial inhibition	Return to normal
(2) Phosphofruktokinase activity	55% inhibition	36% inhibition	30% inhibition
(3) Red cell K-Loss	−14.6 meq/l. R.C.	−24 meq/l. R.C.	−7 meq/l. R.C.
(4) 2,3-Diphospho-glycerate	−23%	−84%	−6%
(5) NAD/NADH ratio blood	Slightly increased	Maximal increase	Return to normal
(6) Hemolysis (fragility)	−11%	−21% (maximal)	+5%
Lungs			
(1) Fibrinolytic activity	Maximal inhibition	Maximal inhibition	Return to normal
(2) Pulmonary edema	Incidence maximal (100%)	Decrease in incidence	Return to normal Incidence 0%
(3) Surface tension	Normal	Maximal increase	Normal
(4) Hyaline membrane formation	Incidence 0%	Incidence 100%	Incidence 0%
(5) Histopathol. changes alveolar granular pneumoc.	Slight	Maximal	Return to normal
Body temperature Thermoregulat. processes	Maximal fall	Beginning recovery	Return to normal
(1) Norepin. content hypothalamus	Decrease	Maximal decrease	Return to normal
(2) 02 consumption response to cold	Complete inhibition	Complete inhibition	Normal response

Since fibrinogen has been found to be a potent inhibitor of surface activity of phospholipids *in vivo*, one should expect that the lung surface tension would be elevated after 6 hr of exposure to 15% CO_2, at which time plasminogen activator activity in the lung has disappeared and larger amounts of fibrinogen must have entered the alveoli. This is, however, not the case. One must therefore assume that the deciding factor in the change of surface activity and the development of hyaline membranes is the intracellular metabolic acidosis which develops at 24 hr. The amazing speed of recovery from hyaline membranes following the recovery from the transient metabolic acidosis gives further support to this interpretation.

Carbon Dioxide Effects on Body Temperature and Energy Production

Guinea pigs and rats exposed to 15% CO_2 for seven days showed a parallel time course of pH changes and changes in body temperature (SCHAEFER and MESSIER [1972]). The maximal drop in extracellular pH in guinea pigs exposed to 15% CO_2 occurs at

6 hr of exposure simultaneously with the maximal fall in body temperature. During the subsequent period, both pH and body temperature rise again (Table 3).

Those animals who were unable to partially compensate the respiratory acidosis by three days and elevate the pH above the low level attained at 6 hr also did not elevate the body temperature. As a matter of fact, we found that behavior of the body temperature was the best indicator of the acid-base status and adaptive potential of the animals. Similar results were obtained in rats.

Under low CO_2 (3% CO_2) body temperature did not fall; on the contrary, body temperature remained higher than under control conditions, only the data obtained after 1-hr exposure at 3% had statistical significance.

Thermoregulatory processes in the hypothalamus were affected during exposure to 15% CO_2. Norepinephrine injection in the hypothalamus of guinea pigs and rats have been found to cause a rise in body temperature, while an injection of serotonin produces a fall in body temperature. These injections also shift the threshold response for shivering (ZEISBERGER and BRUECK [1971]).

We found in both guinea pigs and rats a decrease in norepinephrine content of the hypothalamus during the first part of the exposure, reaching a maximum fall by one day. The serotonin content, on the other hand, increased slightly but not significantly during this period (SCHAEFER, MORGAN, and MESSIER [1972]).

The response of the guinea pigs to exposure to cold environment (15°C) for a period of 1 hr under control conditions and after 1 hr of exposure to 15% CO_2 were studied jointly with Dr. Wuennenberg. Both oxygen consumption and electrical activity of the muscle increased markedly during control conditions upon exposure to cold, but were both suppressed following 1 hr of exposure to 15% CO_2. After three days of exposure to 15% CO_2, both energy production and muscle activity are restored to normal in response to cold. The increase in oxygen

concentration was about 60% under normal conditions and reaches this level again after three days of exposure. In spite of the normal response of the metabolism, the fall in body temperature remains greater as under control conditions. This is most likely related to an increased heat loss due to changes of the peripheral circulation under CO_2. That means that the blood vessels in the periphery do not contract in the normal manner in response to cold.

Other studies of guinea pigs under 15% CO_2 showed a marked stress response during the first two days of exposure, as indicated in an increase in blood cortocosterone levels, a decrease in adrenal catecholamine levels, and an increase in free fatty acids (SCHAEFER, McCABE, and WITHERS [1968]). However, no significant increases in free glycerol and triglycerides were observed. The fat content of the organs such as liver, muscle, and heart increased markedly during the first three days of exposure to 15% CO_2 in guinea pigs, suggesting an inhibition of lipolysis.

The results of these studies of metabolic adaptation in chronic hypercapnia can be summarized as follows:

(1) Chronic hypercapnia produced by prolonged exposure to 15% CO_2 causes a maximal extracellular acidosis within 6 hr following which the extracellular pH rises again. At 24 hr a transitory intracellular metabolic acidosis develops in lungs, liver, and heart, which has disappeared by three days. During the period between three and seven days, partial compensation of the respiratory acidosis is accomplished.

(2) During the first phase of maximal extracellular acidosis, glycolysis and fibrinolysis are maximally inhibited. There is also a maximal fall in body temperature and inhibition of energy production and shivering response at this time. Processes depending on energy derived from the glycolytic pathways show a maximal inhibition at 24 hr, e.g., inhibition of active transport indicated in red-cell K

loss and reduction in 2,3-diphospho-glycerate.

(3) Only reduction in surfactant and hyaline membrane formation were found to be solely developed in the phase of intra-cellular metabolic acidosis.

(4) Most metabolic processes returned to near normal after partial compensation had been accomplished by seven days, and both extracellular and intracellular pH had moved out of the critical lower pH range in which enzymatic inhibition occurs.

Bibliography

Atkinson, D. E., and Walton, G. M., "Adenosin triphosphate conservation in metabolic regulation. Rat liver cleavage enzyme." *J. Biol. Chem.* 242:3239–41 (1967).

Bücher, Th., and Rüssmann, W., "Gleichgewicht und Ungleichgewicht im System der Glykolyse." *Angew. Chemie.* 75:881–93 (1963).

Granholm, L., and Siesjö, B. K., "The effects of hypercapnia and hypocapnia upon tissue levels of NADH, lactate, pyruvate, ATP, ADP phosphocreatine concentrations of cat brain tissue." *Acta Physiol. Scand.* 75: 257–76 (1969).

Hohorst, H. J., Adrese, P., Bartels, H., Stratmann, D., and Talke, H. L.(+) lactic acid and the steady state of cellular redox systems. *Ann. N.Y. Acad. Sci.* 119:974–92 (1965).

Jacey, M. J., and Schaefer, K. E., "Lactate-pyruvate and redox state responses of blood and tissue in chronic hypercapnia." *SMRL Report No. 652* (1971a).

———, and Schaefer, K. E., "The effect of chronic hypercapnia on blood phospho-fructokinase activity and the Adenine Nucleotide System." *SMRL Report No. 659* (1971b).

———, and Schaefer, K. E., "Responses of blood lactate, pyruvate and redox state to chronic exposure to 3% CO_2." *SMRL Report No. 662* (1971c).

Martin, E. C., Scamman, F. L., Attebery, B. A., and Brown, E. B., Jr., "Time-related adjustments in acid base status of extracellular and intracellular fluid in chronic respiratory acidosis." USAF School of Aerospace Med., Brooks AFB, Texas (1965).

Messier, A. A., and Schaefer, K. E., "The effect of chronic hypercapnia on oxygen affinity and 2,3-Diphosphoglycerate." *Respir. Physiol.* 12:291–96 (1971).

Nahas, G. G., and Poyart, C., Effect of arterial pH alterations on metabolic activity of norepinephrine. *Amer. J. Physiol.*, 212:765–72.

———. "Mechanisms of CO_2 and pH effects on metabolism" (this monograph).

———, and Steinsland, O. S., "Increased rate of catecholamine synthesis during respiratory acidosis." *Respir. Physiol.* 5:108–17 (1968b).

———, Poyart, C., and Triner, L., "Acid base equilibrium changes and metabolic alterations." *Ann. N.Y. Acad. Sci.* 150:562–76 (1968a).

Niemoeller, H., and Schaefer, K. E., "Development of hyaline membranes and atelectasis in experimental chronic respiratory acidosis." *Proc. Soc. Exp. Biol. (N.Y.)* 110:804 (1962).

Poyart, C. F., and Nahas, G., "Inhibition of activated lipolysis by acidosis." *Molecular Pharmacology* 4:389–401 (1968c).

Schaefer, K. E., Avery, M. E., and Bensch, K., "Time course of changes in surface tension and morphology of alveolar epthelial cells in CO_2-induced hyaline membrane disease." *J. Clin. Invest.* 43:11 (1964).

———. "The CO_2-induced hyaline membrane disease as a biological model for the study of lung cell injury and repair." *Proc. 11th Aspen Emphysema Conference*, pp. 321–22 (1968).

———, McCabe, N., and Withers, J., "Stress response in chronic hypercapnia." *Am. J. Physiol.* 214:543–48 (1968b).

———, Messier, A. A., Morgan, C. C., "Displacement of oxygen dissociation curves and red cell cation exchange in chronic hypercapnia." *Respir. Physiol.* 10:299–312 (1970).

———, and Messier, A. A., "Bohr effect in chronic hypercapnia." *Fed. Proc.* 29:476 (1970).

———, Morgan, C., and Messier, A. A., "CO_2 effects on body temperature regulation." *Fed. Proc.* 31:340 (1970).

Siesjö, K., Folbergrova, J., and Messeter, K. (this monograph). Acid-base and energy metabolism of the brain in hyper- and hypocapnia.

Stupfel, M., "Action du gaz carbonique sur la thermoregulation du rat blanc. 1. Effets de differentes concentrations de CO_2 á diverse temperatures." *J. Physiol. Paris* 52:575–606 (1960).

Tappan, D. V., "Plasma creatine phosphate and creatine phosphokinase responses to carbon dioxide." *SMRL Report* No. 661 (1971).

Waldeck, F., and Zander, R., "Displacement of the dissociation curve in response to changes in the intraerythrocytic cation and hemoglobin concentrations." Washington, D.C., *Proc. International Physiological Congress* (1968).

Williamson, D. H., Lund, P., and Krebs, H. A., "The redox state of free nicotinamide-adenine dinucleotide in the cytoplasma and mitochondria of rat liver." *Biochem. J.* 103:514–27 (1967).

Zeisberger, E., and Brück, K., "Central effects of nonadrenaline on the guinea pig." *Pflueger's Archives* 322:152–66 (1971).

Schaefer Discussion

NAHAS: This is certainly a very interesting paper. I want to ask you if during the first period of adaptation that you observed, there are any evidences of acute phase reactants in the blood? Those are the glycoproteins which are observed under conditions of severe stress, ceruloplasmin and other such compounds which are especially increased in conditions of shock. The second question I want to ask you is if there is any correlation between the weight loss that you observed and lean body mass decrement, because it seems that there are two processes which are occurring here. In the first place there is an inhibition of certain enzymes which are used for energy process such as lypolysis or glycolysis; in the second place there is a stimulation of some of the enzymes which are required for protein synthesis in certain organs, such as arginase in the kidney which actually is increased as shown by Lotspeich [1967]. He even showed that the carbon skeleton of arginine was incorporated into the tissues of kidney, accounting for the increased hypertrophy of the kidney observed during hypercapnia, and I wonder if you have observed a similar hypertrophy of the kidney? I think you did, but you didn't mention it here.

SCHAEFER: In answer to your first question, we did not study glycoproteins in hypercapnia. Organ weights obtained in animals during chronic exposure to 15% CO_2 showed a certain increase in kidney weight/body weight ratios, as did other organs such as liver. In the kidney the weight increase appeared to be related to the increased water content. Most of the organs lost water at least temporarily, with the exception of kidney, brain, and bones, which increased their water content. Water shifts occurred between organs. For instance the water content of red cells increased and that of plasma decreased, resulting in an increased osmolarity. Moreover, the liver temporarily gains water and then loses it again. There were different time courses of water shifts in various organs during chronic hypercapnia, which are probably related to the different time courses in intracellular pH and cH changes, based on different buffer capacities. In regard to your second question: During the first 24 hr the animals lose about 10% of their body weight, which appears to be related to the decreased food intake. The animals eat practically nothing for 24 hr; from the second day on they begin to eat again and then they increase in their weight. We have done studies of the urea content of the tissues, which increases during chronic hypercapnia. We considered the possibility of a kind of a chemical storage of CO_2 into urea, but we found that the increase in urea concentration in most of the tissues could be explained partly by a reduction in the urinary excretion of urea. We have not studied the enzymes of the kidney in chronic hypercapnia.

SIESJÖ: The lactate and pyruvate values you reported—were those from blood samples taken from the animals and then analyzed for it? Phosphofructokinase activity, did you measure that in the blood?

SCHAEFER: Yes, in blood samples.

SIESJÖ: Are the blood lactate levels really affected by the lactate production of the blood itself? Are they not, so to speak, a reflection of lactate production in tissues and the renewal of lactate by the liver?

SCHAEFER: We have done the measurements in tissues, too, and they follow the same pattern. The NAD^+/NADH ratio of blood and tissues shows during exposure to 15%

CO_2 an increase during the acute phase reaching a maximum at one day and subsequently declines again. By seven days the values are back to initial levels. The time course of the $NAD^+/NADH$ ratio showing a more oxidized state of blood and tissues during the acute phase of respiratory acidosis is indicative of a pH-dependent metabolic inhibition which correlates well with the transient reduction in oxygen consumption amounting to about 30% at one day. At three days the values of oxygen consumption have risen again and are not significantly different from controls. Since there is no interference with the oxygen transport, the changes in oxygen affinity are compensated by the increase in Bohr effect, the oxygen tensions in the tissues should rise. This is indeed the case as observed by van Liew [1963] under similar conditions in rats exposed to 16% CO_2.

SIESJÖ: Yes, but I was wondering if you could relate the lactate and pyruvate concentrations of the blood to the PFK in the blood, too.

SCHAEFER: Yes.

LONGMORE: I would just like to make a couple of comments. I'm very interested in your notes on the hyaline membrane. We've just gotten a good start on this ourselves, and I don't believe you've taken a look at the membrane phospholipids yet, have you? Your changes in glucose, blood glucose, and your lactate pyruvate might alter the synthesis of the lung phospholipids very rapidly, at least with the data we now have at hand. I didn't have time to present any of this, this morning. It's very interesting that these lipids that form the hyaline membrane—the phosphotidyl dioline and so on—are very sensitive to these changes. Also glucose, apparently, under certain conditions, is a very excellent precursor for the fatty acids in the lung which are also delivered back into the blood. We found some very interesting relationships between essentially free palmitate versus glucose and what the lung is using for precursors for lung lipids. So I think what you said ties in with some of the things we found. It makes more sense to me now.

SEVERINGHAUS: I, too, am interested in the pulmonary edema aspects of your results. I notice that the edema occurs about 24 hr before you see the hyaline membrane. This is also characteristic of some other forms of pulmonary edema, and it's quite consistent with the idea that the edema formation leads to protein transudation into the lung and reabsorption into the alveolar sacs of water leaving precipitated protein behind which becomes the membrane, and I don't think we need to postulate anything about changes in lipid metabolism to say that that's why there is a hyaline membrane. It may be, of course, but it—a simpler explanation is simply that there's a continuous turnover of water in the lung. I'd like to ask whether you noticed that in the early phases the edema was primarily in the perivascular or extra-interstitial space rather than in alveoli?

SCHAEFER: In the perivascular space.

COURNAND: I think that problem of relationship between metabolic acidosis and the formation of hyaline membrane is of considerable interest and I should like to ask you some questions. Would it be possible to define by what exact mechanism inhibition of, let's say, anti-oxidative enzyme the hyaline membrane formation is related? In other words, Dr. Severinghaus probably knows very well, also, that in premature children hyaline membrane is formed, and I have always wondered whether this was not related to the fact that in the premature children anti-oxidative enzymes were not already present in the lung. We are concerned by the fact, have always been puzzled by the fact, that lung tissue is the one which diffuses probably the largest amount of oxygen into the body, and yet the amount of toxicity process which is taking place is extremely small—the simple process of physical diffusion doesn't, nonetheless, explain why the oxygen molecule has absolutely no effect upon (at least that is known) the tissues themselves. Or whether it is just like a permeable thing, but nonetheless there is a molecule which in other tissues has some toxicity effect. I just wonder whether there is a way of demonstrating the inhibition of anti-oxidative enzymes, for instance in the lung, under condition of metabolic acidosis?

SCHAEFER: I have thought about this, and I had hoped to talk with Dr. Longmore about it to do the next steps. We need a biochemist to do that. So I am glad we have Dr. Longmore here and perhaps he will be able to follow this up.

We had one intriguing observation. We found an increase in fat in the lungs at the time, after three days. Electromicroscopic pictures of living tissues obtained at this time showed the fat droplets in the empty granular pneumocytes, as if the lipoproteins are separated and couldn't get together. The individual fat droplets were present. After the pH has recovered a little bit more, the lipoprotein formation seems to get going again. We have done some experiments intermittent by exposure of guinea pigs to 15% CO_2, and we were able to overload the whole lungs with fat.

SEVERINGHAUS: That is neutral fat you're talking about, or do you know whether it is neutral or is it phospholipids?

SCHAEFER: I don't know.

CALDWELL: I'd like to modify Professor Cournand's remarks to point out that we do have some information that the oxygen consumption of the lung is sensitive to oxygen tension, particularly in disease, but it's also demonstrable *in vitro* in normal lung tissue. We have looked at fatty acid incorporation in lung in relation to oxygen tension and haven't found that to be influenced in physiologic ranges of oxygen tension change.

Bibliography

Lotspeich, W. D., "Metabolic aspects of acid base change. Interrelated biochemical responses in the kidney and other organs are associated with metabolic acidosis." *Science* 155:1066–75 (1967).

van Liew, H. D., "Subcutaneous tissue pO$_2$ and pCO$_2$ of rats in a high CO_2 atmosphere." *Aerospace Med.* 34:499–500 (1963).

2. Acid-Base Equilibrium in Chronic Hypercapnia

Charles van Ypersele de Strihou

Renal Unit, Cliniques Universitaires St.-Pierre,
Louvain, Belgium

Patients with chronic respiratory acidosis are not immune to other disorders of acid-base equilibrium. As a consequence, the physician often faces a diagnostic dilemma: What in the acid-base pattern of such a patient should be attributed to hypercapnia and what is a reflection of complicating acid-base disturbances?

In patients with chronic lung insufficiency, sources of complicating metabolic alkalosis are multiple. Many of them suffer from *cor pulmonale* and are therefore likely to be treated with diuretics and a low chloride diet, a condition known to induce metabolic alkalosis. On the other hand, complicating acidosis may result from the acidifying effect of carbonic anhydrase inhibitors or from an acute superimposed respiratory insufficiency, due to an acute exacerbation of a chronic lung disease or to a drug-induced depression of the respiratory center.

How thus can one recognize whether or not the acid-base status of a patient with chronic respiratory acidosis is appropriate for the observed degree of hypercapnia? The answer to this question hinges upon the definition of what is the normal response of man to chronic hypercapnia (COHEN and SCHWARTZ [1966]).

Two approaches could be used to provide such CO_2 response curve. The first is to use normal volunteers and to put them in an environmental chamber which permits accurate and long-term control of CO_2 and O_2 tension. The alternative approach is to analyze the acid-base status of a large population of patients suffering from chronic hypercapnia.

The first approach, that of the environmental chamber, was used successfully by Schwartz and his associates (COHEN et al. [1964], and BRACKETT et al. [1965]) to define the bicarbonate response curve for acute respiratory acidosis in man and dog.

Since an acute steady state of acid-base equilibrium is established within 15 min (BRACKETT et al [1965]), short-term studies provided an excellent means of defining the *in vivo* CO_2 response curve of man. P_{CO_2} of the environmental chamber was thus raised in a stepwise fashion to approximately 80 mm of mercury (BRACKETT et al. [1965]). Simultaneously, the plasma bicarbonate concentration of the subjects rose in a curvilinear fashion (Figure 1). Despite this compensation, provided by body buffers, H^+ was not returned to normal: H^+ concentration rose in direct proportion to the degree of hypercapnia, each millimeter of P_{CO_2} rise eliciting a 0.76 nmole increment in H^+ activity (Figure 1). From their data, Brackett and coworkers [1965] provided a statistical definition of a significance band which indicates with a 95% confidence the response to be anticipated for a given degree of acute hypercapnia. Any value outside these bands points to a superimposed acid-base disorder.

The definition of the response curve for chronic hypercapnia proved more difficult.

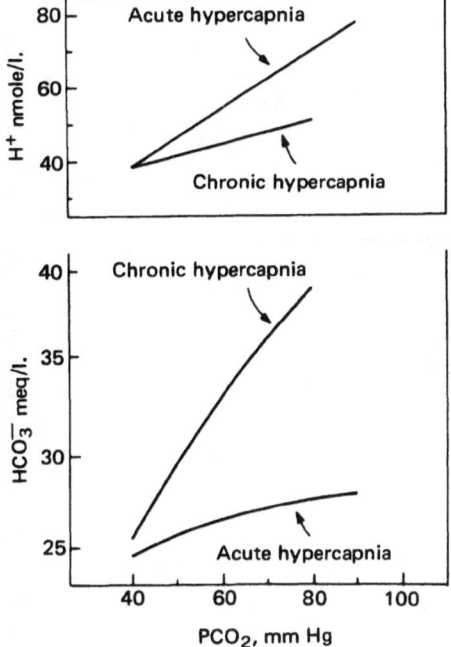

Fig. 1. Relation in man between P_{CO_2} and blood H^+ activity or plasma bicarbonate concentration in acute (BRACKETT et al. [1965]) and chronic hypercapnia (VAN YPERSELE et al. [1966]).

Whereas a steady state of acid-base equilibrium is reached within less than 15 min for acute hypercapnia, in chronic hypercapnia such a steady state is not reached before a few days, as demonstrated in Figure 2. Plasma bicarbonate concentrations were observed daily in seven dogs exposed to a 12% CO_2 atmosphere (VAN YPERSELE et al. [1962]). After an initial acute rise, plasma bicarbonate continued to increase over a period of three to four days, and stabilized only subsequently. These data demonstrate that the definition of an *in vivo* titration curve for chronic hypercapnia will require an exposure of a week at each different level of CO_2 tension, the whole study lasting several weeks. This proved to be possible for dogs but totally unbearable for human beings.

The results obtained in dogs by Schwartz et al. [1965] are represented in Figure 3. Here again P_{CO_2} of the environmental chamber is raised in a stepwise fashion to

approximately 120 mm of mercury. Adaptation was allowed at each level of P_{CO_2} for a week at least. Plasma bicarbonate concentration increased in a curvilinear fashion, this increment being markedly more important than that observed in acute hypercapnia (COHEN et al [1964]). It reflects the assistance given by the kidneys in the generation of bicarbonate. Despite this increment, however, H^+ concentration was not returned to normal. Just as in acute hypercapnia, H^+ activity increased linearly with the degree of hypercapnia. However, this increment was much smaller than that observed in acute hypercapnia since a 1 mm rise in P_{CO_2} elicited only a 0.32 nmole rise in H^+ activity versus a 0.77 nmole rise in acute hypercapnia.

Despite all that information, we are still left without answer for the definition of man's normal response to chronic hypercapnia. As mentioned earlier, it turned out that human beings were totally unable to tolerate long-term exposures to an elevated CO_2 tension in the environmental chamber. Therefore, it was necessary to turn away from physiologic studies and to resort to an analysis of patients suffering from chronic lung disease.

We analyzed the results of 781 arterial blood pH and plasma bicarbonate levels obtained in a population of patients with chronic lung disease (VAN YPERSELE et al. [1966]). Results were grouped according to increasing degrees of hypercapnia, each group encompassing a 2-mm P_{CO_2} interval. Figure 4 presents the average plasma bicarbonate concentration observed in each group: Plasma bicarbonate concentration rises in a curvilinear fashion as P_{CO_2} rises. The shape of this curve is very reminiscent of that observed in dogs (Figure 3). Here again, despite this renal compensation, H^+ concentration rises linearly with P_{CO_2}. The slope of the H^+/P_{CO_2} line is virtually identical to that observed in dogs during chronic hypercapnia (Figures 1 and 2). It must be recognized that a chronic steady state was documented in none of our patients. However, more recent evidence, published by

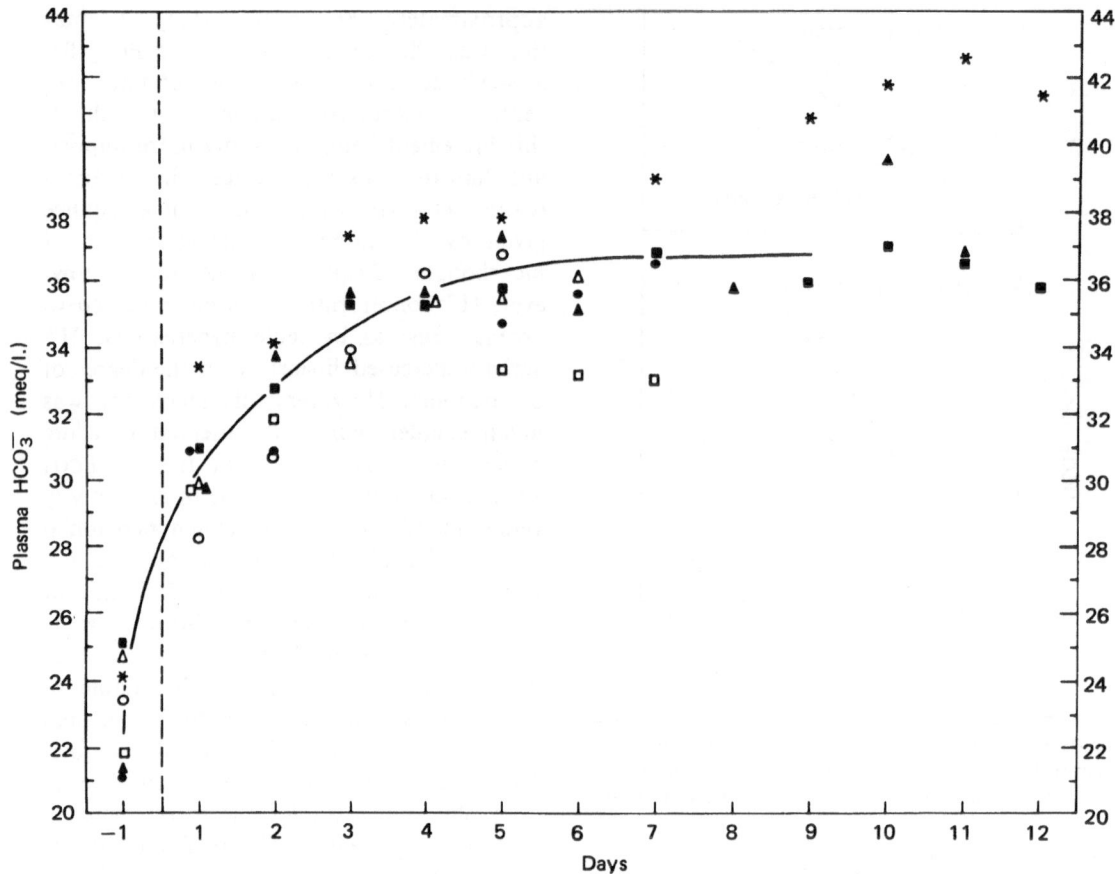

Fig. 2. Evolution of plasma bicarbonate concentration in seven dogs exposed to a 12% CO_2 atmosphere. Day -1 refers to the last day of the control period. (Reprinted from VAN YPERSELE et al. [1962]).

Brackett et al. [1969] on a few well-studied cases of patients with stable chronic hypercapnia has confirmed the validity of our data.

The acid-base behavior of man during chronic hypercapnia is thus very similar to that of dogs. From our data we calculated the 95% confidence limits of man's response to chronic hypercapnia. These values taken together with those obtained by Brackett et al. [1965] during acute hypercapnia provide a set of reference against which new observations may be evaluated (VAN YPERSELE and FRANS [1967]). Any value falling outside these bands points to a superimposed acid-base disorder. A few examples will illustrate the usefulness of the confidence bands in the analysis of mixed acid-base disorders encountered in clinical practice.

Chronic Respiratory Acidosis and Metabolic Acidosis

After a control period of 5 to 13 days, six hypercapnic patients were given 150 mg per day of a carbonic anhydrase inhibitor, dichlorphenamide. Plasma bicarbonate concentration before, during, and 5 to 7 days after treatment are plotted on the bicarbonate P_{CO_2} diagram, featuring a significance band for bicarbonate in chronic hypercapnia (Figure 5). Before dichlorphenamide all values fell within the confidence limits. The acidifying effect of the drug is evidenced by a shift of bicarbonate toward the acid side, all values leaving the band. Discontinuation of the drug returned bicarbonate values toward control levels, five values falling again within the significance band. It should be noted, incidentally, that in four of the six

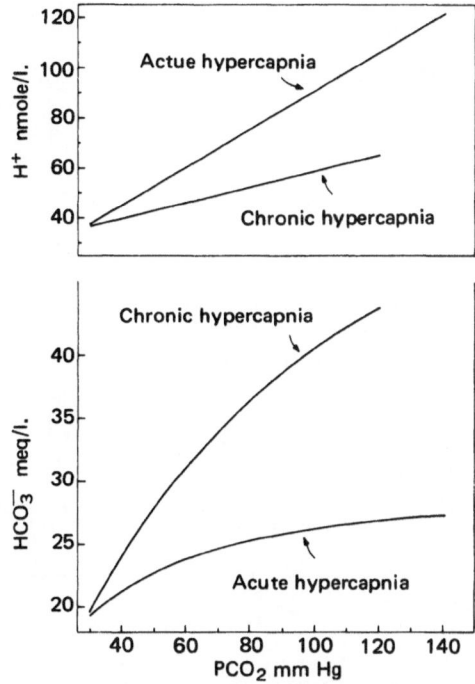

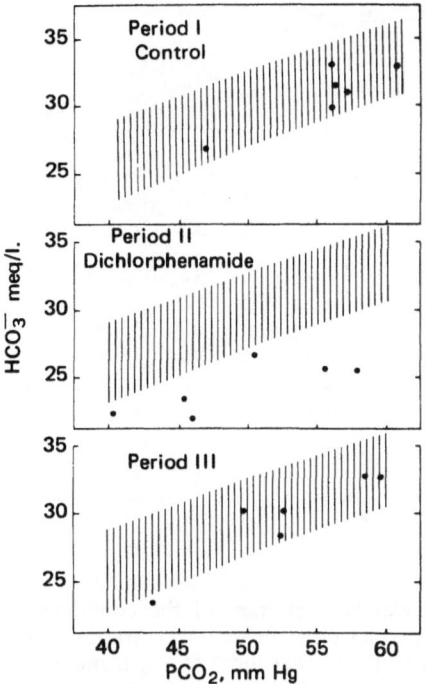

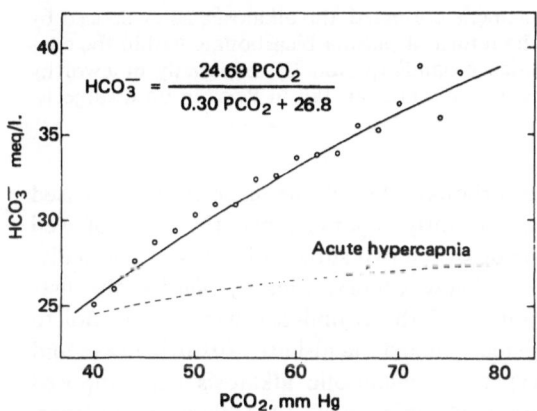

Fig. 3. Relation in dog between P_{CO_2} and blood H^+ activity or plasma bicarbonate concentration in acute (COHEN et al. [1964]) and chronic hypercapnia (SCHWARTZ et al. [1965]).

$$HCO_3^- = \frac{24.69\ PCO_2}{0.30\ PCO_2 + 26.8}$$

Fig. 4. Relation between plasma bicarbonate concentration and P_{CO_2} in a population of 420 patients with chronic lung disease. Each point represents the average of all plasma bicarbonate concentrations observed in individual groups encompassing a 2-mm Hg P_{CO_2} interval. The dotted line represents the mean bicarbonate curves observed in human volunteers in acute hypercapnia (BRACKETT et al. [1965]). (Reprinted from VAN YPERSELE et al. [1966].)

Fig. 5. Usefulness of the confidence bands for plasma bicarbonate concentration in chronic hypercapnia. Detection of superimposed metabolic acidosis (administration of dichlorphenamide). See text for further details. (Reprinted from VAN YPERSELE et al. [1966].)

patients arterial P_{CO_2} fell as a consequence of the acidification during period II.

Chronic Respiratory Acidosis and Metabolic Alkalosis

The reverse effect is illustrated in Figure 6. This patient is suffering from chronic bronchitis and *cor pulmonale*. His acid-base status on admission is plotted on the left of the same bicarbonate P_{CO_2} diagram, featuring the significance band for bicarbonate concentration. The acid-base status after three days of treatment, including large amounts of furosemide and a chloride-free diet, is depicted on the right. Bicarbonate fell within the significance band before therapy, but subsequently left the band as a result of superimposed diuretic induced metabolic alkalosis (VAN YPERSELE and MORALES-BARRIA [1969]). In contrast with the effect

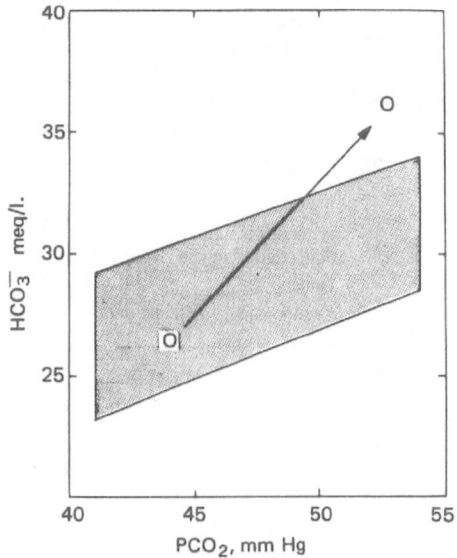

Fig. 6. Usefulness of the confidence bands for plasma bicarbonate concentration in chronic hypercapnia. Detection of superimposed metabolic alkalosis (for further details see text).

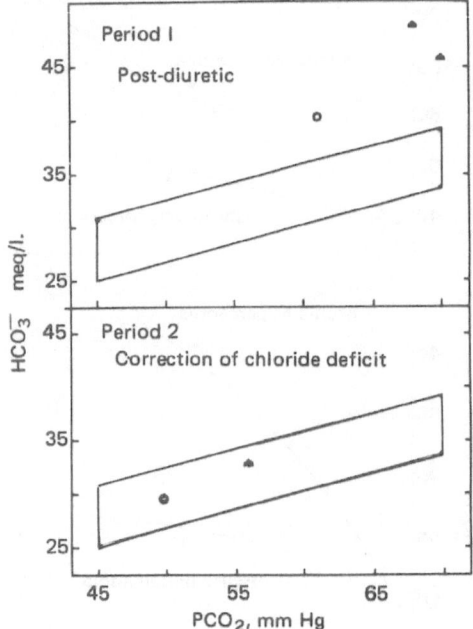

Fig. 7. Usefulness of the confidence bands for plasma bicarbonate concentration in chronic hypercapnia. A superimposed diuretic induced metabolic alkalosis was detected. A steady-state P_{CO_2} was documented in one of the two patients (period I). Administration of a chloride supplement corrected the alkalosis, as evidenced by the return of plasma bicarbonate within the confidence bands (period II). Especially noteworthy is the simultaneous fall in P_{CO_2} in both subjects.

of dichlorphenamide, the addition of metabolic alkalosis resulted in a significant increment in arterial P_{CO_2}, going from 44 to 53 mm of mercury.

The use of confidence bands has allowed the detection of a group of patients with chronic hypercapnia who fall outside the confidence bands as a consequence of superimposed metabolic alkalosis. Correction of this added disturbance may improve significantly pulmonary function by the restoration of a normal sensitivity of the respiratory center. Two such cases are illustrated in Figure 7. The first suffers from a Pickwick syndrome and the second from chronic bronchitis. Both had received prior to admission massive amounts of diuretics and a salt-free diet. Significant hypercapnia is present, and both patients are cyanotic. Superimposed metabolic alkalosis is demonstrated by the fact that bicarbonate levels are above those expected for chronic hypercapnia. Correction of the chloride deficit resulted in an impressive lowering of plasma

bicarbonate. Simultaneously, P_{CO_2} decreased significantly. Cyanosis and the sense of well being of the two subjects improved markedly.

These observations emphasize the usefulness of the confidence bands as a tool to detect mixed acid-base disturbances and especially metabolic alkalosis superimposed upon chronic respiratory acidosis. Furthermore, they underline the depressing effect of chronic metabolic alkalosis on respiration. They even suggest that metabolic alkalosis per se might be a primary cause of hypercapnia. In order to test this hypothesis and to quantitate the effect of metabolic alkalosis on respiration, we reviewed the acid-base status of 30 patients treated by repeated dialysis for chronic renal failure (VAN

YPERSELE and FRANS [1970]). A dialysate rich in acetate was used to produce a sustained elevation of plasma bicarbonate concentration. All subjects had a normal lung function. The results were grouped according to plasma bicarbonate concentration, each group encompassing a 1 meq/l. interval. Figure 8 presents the average blood PCO_2 observed in each group. PCO_2 is linearly related to bicarbonate. When plasma bicarbonate concentration exceeds 31 meq/l., arterial PCO_2 rises above 45 mm Hg, suggesting to an untrained observer a diagnosis of respiratory acidosis. The usefulness of the confidence bands for chronic hypercapnia in detecting primary metabolic alkalosis is illustrated in Figure 9. All PCO_2 values above 40 mm Hg observed in the alkalotic patients were plotted on the bicarbonate PCO_2 diagram for chronic hypercapnia. It is of interest to note that in approximately 50 % of the cases of metabolic alkalosis with compensatory hypercapnia, plasma bicarbonate values fall outside the confidence bands. For values higher than 47 mm Hg, almost all values can be distin-

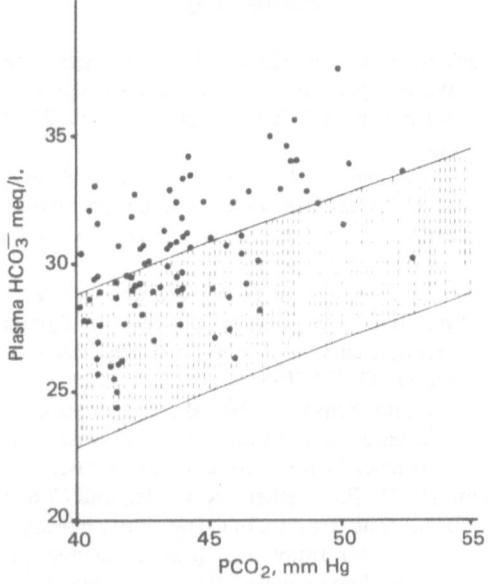

Fig. 9. Usefulness of the confidence bands for plasma bicarbonate concentration in chronic hypercapnia. Distinction between primary hypercapnia and hypercapnia compensating primary metabolic alkalosis. All the values plotted on the diagram were obtained in patients with normal lung function and primary metabolic alkalosis (for further details see text).

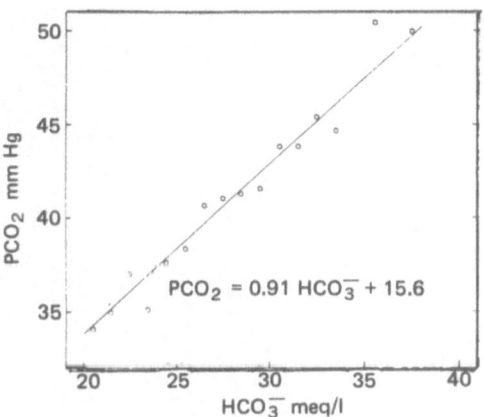

Fig. 8. Relation between arterial PCO_2 and plasma bicarbonate concentration in 48 patients undergoing chronic hemodialysis. Bicarbonate concentration was elevated by increasing the acetate content of dialysate. Blood samples were obtained only after a new dialysate had been used for a period of at least a week. Each point represents the average of all PCO_2 values observed in individual groups encompassing a 1 meq/l. bicarbonate interval.

guished from those of primary chronic hypercapnia.

To summarize, we have reviewed the physiologic data available to delineate the normal response of man to respiratory acidosis. We have shown that full acid-base compensation never occurred in chronic hypercapnia and we have presented the confidence limits of the bicarbonate level for increasing degrees of hypercapnia. Subsequently, we have illustrated the usefulness of these bands in the unravelling of mixed acid-base disorders.

Finally, we have delineated a group of hypercapnic patients in whom detection and correction of a superimposed metabolic alkalosis led to a significant improvement and even in the complete cure of chronic respiratory acidosis.

Bibliography

Brackett, N. C., Jr., Cohen, J. J., and Schwartz, W. B., "Carbon dioxide titration curve of normal man." *New Engl. J. Med.* 272:6 (1965).

———, Wingo, C. F., Muren, O., and Solano, J. T., "Acid-base response to chronic hypercapnia in man." *New Engl. J. Med.* 280:124–30 (1969).

Cohen, J. J., Brackett, N. C., Jr., and Schwartz, W. B., "The nature of carbon dioxide titration curve in the normal dog." *J. Clin. Invest.* 43:777 (1964).

———, and Schwartz, W. B., "Evaluation of acid-base equilibrium in pulmonary insufficiency." *Am. J. Med.* 41:163 (1966).

Schwartz, W. B., Brackett, N. C., Jr., and Cohen, J. J., "The response of extracellular hydrogen ion concentration to graded degrees of chronic hypercapnia: the physiologic limits of the defense of pH." *J. Clin. Invest.* 44:291 (1965).

van Ypersele de Strihou, C., Gulyassy, P. F., and Schwartz, W. B., "Effects of chronic hypercapnia on electrolyte and acid-base equilibrium. III. Characteristics of the adaptative and recovery process as evaluated by the provision of alkali." *J. Clin. Invest.* 41:2246 (1962).

———, Brasseur, L., and De Coninck, J., "The 'carbon dioxide response curve' for chronic hypercapnia in man." *New Engl. J. Med.* 275:117 (1966).

———, and Frans, A., "Les désordres acido-basiques au cours de l'insuffisance respiratoire. Un nouveau diagramme destiné à leur interprétation." *La Presse Méd.* 75:1797 (1967).

———, and Morales-Barria, J., "The influence of dietary sodium and potassium intake on the genesis of frusemide induced alkalosis." *Clin. Sci.* 37:859 (1969).

———, and Frans, A., "The respiratory compensation of metabolic alkalosis." *Proc. EDTA* 7:200 (1970).

3. The Extracellular Bicarbonate Concentration and the Regulation of Ventilation in Chronic Hypercapnia in Man*

Gerard M. Turino†, Roberta M. Goldring‡, and Henry O. Heinemann§

*From the Department of Medicine, College of Physicians and Surgeons,
Columbia University, 630 West 168th Street
New York, New York 10032,
and the
Cardiorespiratory Laboratory,
Columbia Presbyterian Hospital,
New York, New York 10032*

Introduction

Chronic hypercapnia has been associated with a change in the ventilatory responsiveness to inspired CO_2 (CHAPIN et al., and SCHAEFER et al. [1963]). States of severe chronic hypercapnia in man are usually associated with disease of the ventilatory apparatus, so that it is difficult to distinguish the limitations in ventilatory responsiveness imposed by abnormal mechanical function of the chest bellows or lungs and those imposed by changes in sensitivity to the CO_2 or H^+ stimulus (ALEXANDER et al. [1955], and CHERNIAK and SNIDAL [1956]). In this study two aspects of the ventilatory responsiveness to chronic hypercapnia were investigated: (1) the "normal" or predicted HCO_3^- P_{CO_2} relationship in individuals with chronic hypercapnia who are in normal electrolyte

balance; and (2) the effect of chloride depletion, potassium chloride replacement, and ammonium chloride acidosis on the ventilatory responsiveness to inspired CO_2. The subjects selected for study were patients with alveolar hypoventilation from long-standing chest-wall disease and included three men aged 41 to 58 years with cardiorespiratory failure secondary to kyposcoliosis and one woman aged 20 with alveolar hypoventilation secondary to skeletal muscle disease. Their level of alveolar hypoventilation was stable. The experimental design consisted of three study periods; (1) a five- to eight-day control period during which dietary sodium chloride remained restricted, as it had been for many months prior to their entering the study: (2) a five-day period of potassium chloride administration (100 mm/day) orally; and (3) a five-day period during which ammonium chloride (100 mm/day) was administered orally.

The patients were maintained on a metabolic unit where they were kept on a constant diet of low sodium chloride (less than 20 mm/day) and normal potassium (60 mm/day) during control and experimental periods. Except for mercuhydrin administration as part of the experimental protocol in two patients, no diuretics were administered. The

* Work supported in part by USPHS Grant HE-05741 and CA-11096.
† Career Investigatorship of the Health Research Council of the City of New York (I-182).
‡ Present address: Department of Medicine, New York University College of Medicine, New York, New York 10016.
§ Career Investigatorship of the Health Research Council of the City of New York (I-590).
Present address: Cornell University College of Medicine, New York, New York 10021.
Work supported in part by USPHS Grant CA-11096.

daily urinary excretion of creatinine, sodium, potassium chloride, and H^+ was measured. Serum electrolytes and arterial blood gas composition were determined at regular intervals throughout the experimental period.

Ventilatory responsiveness was determined by measuring the increment in ventilation induced by inhaling 5% CO_2 for 20 to 30 min in room air using an open circuit. Changes in respiratory quotient of less than 0.13 between control and the test run were required for inclusion in the study.

The detailed results with respect to resting ventilatory volume, arterial blood gases, urinary electrolyte concentration, and individual responses to breathing 5% CO_2 have been presented elsewhere (GOLDRING et al. [1971]). In discussing results here, data will be presented on: (1) the $HCO_3^- - P_{CO_2}$ relationship during each experimental period; (2) the effects of the administration of potassium chloride and of ammonium chloride on serum electrolytes and blood gas composition; and (3) the changes in ventilatory responsiveness induced by the changing state of electrolyte and acid-base relationships in each experimental period.

The Effect of Chloride Deficiency and Potassium Chloride Administration

The $HCO_3^- - P_{CO_2}$ relationship before and after potassium chloride administration is plotted in Figures 1A and 1B. The blood HCO_3^- and P_{CO_2} values obtained during the control period (all patients were sodium chloride depleted during this experimental period) and values obtained in 14 normal subjects are shown in Figure 1A. The dotted line is shown for reference and was obtained from the data of Schwartz et al. [1965] during the development of uncomplicated chronic respiratory acidosis in dogs on controlled electrolyte intake. The patients with chronic hypercapnia fall above this line. The normal subjects, however, fall on the line. Following the administration of potassium chloride to those same subjects in the next experimental period (Figure 1B), the values for HCO_3^- concentration now fall on the reference line

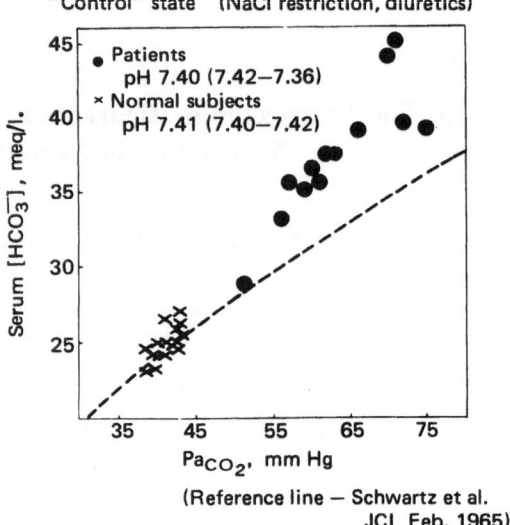

"Control" state   (NaCl restriction, diuretics)

● Patients
   pH 7.40 (7.42–7.36)
× Normal subjects
   pH 7.41 (7.40–7.42)

(Reference line — Schwartz et al. JCI, Feb. 1965)

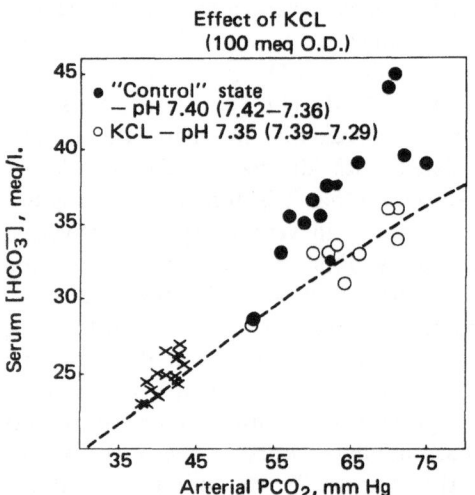

Effect of KCL
(100 meq O.D.)

● "Control" state
   — pH 7.40 (7.42–7.36)
○ KCL — pH 7.35 (7.39–7.29)

Fig. 1(A) shows the $HCO_3^- - P_{CO_2}$ relationship in arterial blood in subjects during the "control" period when they were undergoing dietary salt restriction and while receiving diuretics. The crosses indicate subjects with normal blood gas composition without disease of the ventilatory apparatus. The dotted line indicates the $HCO_3^- - P_{CO_2}$ relationship obtained by Schwartz [1965] et al. during the development of uncomplicated chronic respiratory acidosis in dogs. The values in the patients of the study were generally above this line and fell on the reference line (Figure 1B) after the administration of oral potassium chloride (100 mm/day). (From TURINO et al. [1970].)

derived for dogs. All patients maintained their new HCO_3^-–P_{CO_2} relationship despite continued administration of potassium chloride in this dose indicating that no additional reduction of bicarbonate occurred after chloride was replenished.

With regard to the changes in serum electrolytes and blood gas composition after the administration of potassium chloride, the HCO_3^- concentration decreased and the serum chloride concentration increased in each subject. In one subject with the greatest drop in HCO_3^-, the P_{CO_2} also decreased. Figure 2 shows balance studies in subject (W.D.). It can be seen that a prompt HCO_3^- diuresis and a lowered total H^+ excretion occurred during the first two days of potassium chloride administration. During this time chloride retention occurred, while potassium excretion was increased.

As shown in Figures 1A and B, the pH decreased in all subjects except one whose pH was not initially elevated and who was thought to have only minor degrees of chloride depletion.

Also in the three patients who had the most marked chloride depletion, the administration of KCl induced a HCO_3^- diuresis during the first two days. There was also a decrease in ammonium and titratable acid output and therefore a reduction in total hydrogen excretion in three of the four individuals. Potassium excretion rose promptly in all subjects, indicating little pre-existing potassium deficiency; chloride excretion, on the other hand, rose more slowly so that by the end of the observation period of five days, three of the four individuals who where chloride depleted continued to retain chloride as evidence of pre-existing chloride deficiency.

The changes in ventilatory responsiveness after KCl administration are presented below. Estimation of the amount of HCO_3^- lost from extracellular fluid revealed losses ranging from 14 to 102 mm over five days. A fraction approximating 50% of this HCO_3^- loss in extracellular fluid was recovered in the urine.

The Effect of Ammonium Chloride Administration

A second control period lasting for five to seven days preceded the administration of ammonium chloride. The same low sodium chloride and constant potassium diet was administered. These data comprise a total of five studies since one subject was studied on two occasions six months apart.

The serum chloride concentration increased slightly in four of the five studies, while the serum HCO_3^- concentration decreased in all studies. Serum sodium and potassium ion concentrations, however, did not show consistent changes. On this dose of ammonium chloride both the patients and normal subjects showed minor reduction in resting arterial P_{CO_2} despite a consistent decrease in serum HCO_3^- and pH. Changes in arterial P_{CO_2} were minor and usually

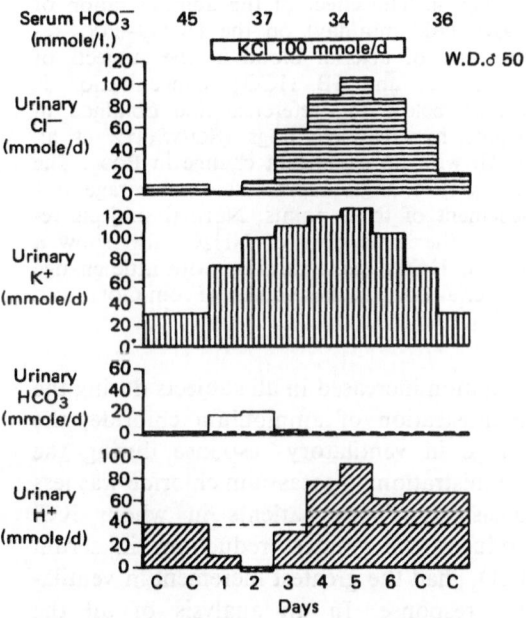

Fig. 2. The effect of KCl (100 mm/day) administration on urinary excretion of Cl^-, K^+, HCO_3^- and H^+ after repletion of Cl^- as KCl in subject W. D. Note the HCO_3^- diuresis, the prompt increase in potassium excretion, and the lagging Cl excretion (see text).

increased 2 to 3 mm Hg, except in one patient who experienced tachypnea, feelings of breathlessness, and a reduction in arterial P_{CO_2} (see Figure 3.)

As shown in Figure 4, the $HCO_3^- - P_{CO_2}$ relationship of these subjects while on ammonium chloride now falls below the reference line for dogs and the line for these same subjects when chloride was repleted. The reduction in serum bicarbonate was more marked than the reduction in arterial P_{CO_2}.

As expected, urinary excretion of chloride, total hydrogen, and ammonium ion increased during the administration of ammonium chloride in all subjects.

Ventilatory Response to Inhalation of 5 Percent Carbon Dioxide in Room Air Following Administration of Potassium Chloride or Ammonium Chloride

In all subjects the response to 5% CO_2 was assessed on several occasions before and after administration of either potassium chloride or ammonium chloride.

While the ventilatory response to CO_2

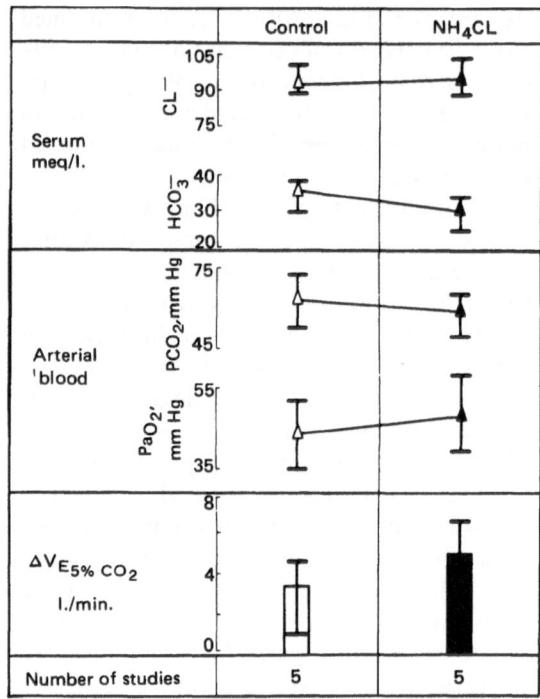

Fig. 4. The effect of the administration of NH_4Cl (100 mm/day) on the $HCO_3^- - P_{CO_2}$ relationship of arterial blood in the subjects of Figures 1A and 1B. HCO_3^- concentration is lowered below the reference line obtained in chronic hypercapneic dogs (Schwartz et al. [1965]) with no significant change in P_{CO_2}. The light grey triangle represents the average displacement of these points. Normal subjects receiving the same dose of NH_4Cl also show a reduced HCO_3^- concentration with little change in arterial P_{CO_2} at these doses. (From Goldring et al. [1971].)

inhalation increased in all subjects during the administration of ammonium chloride, the change in ventilatory response during the administration of potassium chloride was less consistent. Those patients in whom KCl produced the greatest reductions in serum HCO_3^- had the greatest increment in ventilatory response. In an analysis of all the ventilatory response measurements observed during chloride depletion, potassium chloride, and ammonium chloride administration, there is an exponential and inverse relationship between the increments in ventilation and the serum HCO_3^- concentration des-

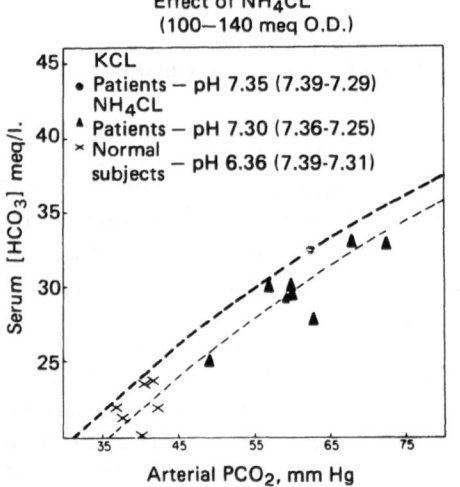

Fig. 3. The effects of oral NH_4Cl (100 mm/day) in the four subjects studied. The height of the bar indicates the average values measured, and the brackets the range. Reductions in serum bicarbonate and increases in ventilatory responses to 5% CO_2 were more consistent, while changes in P_{CO_2} were slight (see text).

cribed by the equation $y = 309.5e - 0.021x$ (Figure 5).

An attempt to relate the ventilatory response to 5% CO_2 inhalation to the H^+ concentration of arterial blood obtained prior to CO_2 inhalation during each of the experimental periods showed no significant correlation. However, when the ventilatory response to breathing 5% CO_2 is considered as a function of the increase in extracellular H^+ concentration induced by breathing 5% CO_2 and plotted against the level of serum HCO_3^-, the increment in ventilation per increment in H^+ concentration is constant over the wide range of HCO_3^- concentration studied in these patients. A corollary of this observation is that the ventilatory stimulus to breathing 5% CO_2 is higher at the lower level of serum HCO_3^- concentration than at the upper level as demonstrated in Figure 4.

Discussion

This study demonstrates that deviations from a specific HCO_3^-–Pco_2 relationship determined by underlying ventilatory insufficiency and/or alterations in serum HCO_3^- concentration induced by chloride deficiency or the administration of H^+, are associated with alterations in the ventilatory

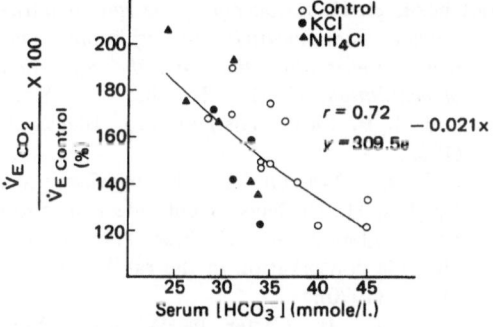

Fig. 5. The relationship between the serum HCO_3^- concentration and the ventilatory response to breathing 5% CO_2 in subjects during the "control" state and after the administration of KCL and NH_4Cl. Administration of either agent resulted in a rise in ventilatory response which was exponentially related to the increment in ventilatory response to 5% CO_2. (From GOLD-RING et al. [1971].)

responsiveness which are exponentially related to the extracellular HCO_3^- concentration and not to the level of extracellular H^+ activity existing prior to the CO_2 breathing.

Several studies have analyzed the metabolic acid-base disorders in patients with chronic hypercapnia (ROBIN [1963], BRACKETT et al. [1969], VAN YPERSELE DE STRIHOU et al. [1966], REFSUM [1964], ENGEL et al. [1968], COHEN and SCHWARTZ [1966]). Some studies have indicated that the reduced ventilatory response to CO_2 may be related to abnormal ventilatory mechanics as well as to altered sensitivity of the central respiratory control mechanism (ALEXANDER et al. [1955], and CHERNIAK and SNIDAL [1956]). In this study, patients were without airway obstruction and their mechanical ventilatory limitation during the periods of study was stable, so that the observed effects of an altered acid-base status could be ascribed to changes in central ventilatory control.

The good correlation between the serum HCO_3^- concentration and increments in ventilation in response to breathing 5% CO_2 suggests that HCO_3^- in the extracellular fluid may be the critical controlling factor in setting the sensitivity of the ventilatory control mechanism to the natural CO_2 stimulus. Such a concept was originally proposed by Scott [1920]. If it is accepted that the H^+ concentration within or in the vicinity of the cells of the respiratory center is the ultimate effective stimulus to ventilation while breathing CO_2 (WINTERSTEIN [1956], LEUSEN [1965], and LOESCHCKE [1965]) then an increased HCO_3^- pool by limiting the increase in H^+ concentration for a given change in Pco_2 provides a mechanism for the observed alterations in ventilatory responsiveness in this study. Thus, the HCO_3^- concentration would be the regulator of the change in H^+ concentration and the H^+ activity the crucial determinant of the ventilatory response to CO_2. The results of the present study are consistent with the data of FENCL et al. [1966]), in which a direct relationship was shown between the ventilatory response to altered acid-base relationships in goats and the changes in serum HCO_3^- concentration. In the experiments cited, the serum HCO_3^- concentration bore a fixed relationship to changes in cerebrospinal fluid pH and presumably the pH of the interstitial central nervous system perfusate.

The data of this study also demonstrates that chloride deficiency in patients with chronic hypercapnia leads to distortion of the serum HCO_3^-–P_{CO_2} relationship so that the subjects have a normal or alkaline pH instead of an acidotic level of H^+ as occurred after chloride replacement. The urinary data in these patients supports the concept that serum HCO_3^- excess following the induction of chloride loss is maintained by continued increased sodium for H^+ exchange sustaining an elevated renal HCO_3^- threshold.

It remains unclear why an inappropriately elevated HCO_3^- concentration following chloride loss is not accompanied by a reduction in alveolar ventilation and an increase in arterial P_{CO_2} with a return to a low pH value. A role for hypoxemia to sustain this lower P_{CO_2} could not be demonstrated in this study and it has not been demonstrated by Sapir et al. [1967]. This heightened activity of ventilatory control with respect to the predicted HCO_3^-–P_{CO_2} relationship is sustained by additional, and as yet unrecognized variables, which may be intracellular and not reflected in the extracellular fluid.

Bibliography

Alexander, J. K., West, J. R., Wood, J. A., and Richards, D. W., "Analysis of the respiratory responses to carbon dioxide inhalation in varying clinical states of hypercapnia, anoxia and acid-base derangement." *J. Clin. Invest.* 34:511 (1955).

Brackett, N. C., Wingo, C. F., Muren, O., and Solano, J. T., "Acid-base response to chronic hypercapnia in man." *N. Eng. J. Med.* 280:124 (1969).

Chapin, J. L., Otis, A. B., and Rahn, H., "Changes in sensitivity of the respiratory center in man after prolonged exposure to 3% CO_2." U.S. Air Force Wright Field Development Technical Report WADC No. 55–357.

Cherniack, R. M., and Snidal, D. P., "The effect of obstruction to breathing on the ventilatory response to CO_2 inhalation." *J. Clin. Invest.* 35:1286 (1956).

Cohen, J., and Schwartz, W. B., "Evaluation of acid-base equilibrium in pulmonary insufficiency (Editorial)." *Am. J. Med.* 41:163 (1966).

Engel, K., Dell, R. B., Rahill, W. J., Denning, C. R., and Winters, R. W., "Quantitative displacement of acid-base equilibrium in chronic respiratory acidosis." *J. Appl. Physiol.* 24:288 (1968).

Fencl, V., Miller, J. B., and Pappenheimer, J. R., "Studies on the respiratory response to disturbances of acid-base balance, with deductions concerning the ionic composition of cerebral interstitial fluid." *Am. J. Physiol.* 210:459 (1966).

Goldring, R. M., Turino, G. M., and Heinemann, H. O., "Respiratory-renal adjustments in chronic hypercapnia in man: Extracellular bicarbonate concentration and the regulation of ventilation." *Am. J. Med.* 51:772 (1971).

Leusen, I. R. *Aspects of acid-base balance between blood and cerebrospinal fluid. Cerebrospinal fluid and the regulation of ventilation.* (C. McC. Brooks, F. F. Kao, and B. B. Lloyd, eds.) Oxford: Blackwell (1965).

Loeschcke, H. H. *A concept of the role of intracranial chemosensitivity in respiratory control. Cerebrospinal fluid and the regulation of ventilation.* (C. McC. Brooks, F. F. Kao, and B. B. Lloyd, eds.) Oxford: Blackwell (1965).

Luke, R. G., Warren, Y., Kashgarian, M., Levitan, H., "Effects of chloride restriction and depletion on acid-base balance and chloride conservation in the rat." *Clin. Sci.* 38:385 (1970).

Rector, F. C., Jr., Carter, N. W., and Seldin, D. W., "The mechanism of bicarbonate reabsorption in the proximal and distal tubules of the kidney." *J. Clin. Invest.* 44:278 (1965).

Refsum, H. E., "Acid-base status in patients with chronic hypercapnia and hypoxemia." *Clin. Sci.* 27:407 (1964).

Robin, E. D., "Abnormalities of acid-base regulation in chronic pulmonary disease with special reference to hypercapnia and extracellular alkalosis." *N. Eng. J. Med.* 268:917 (1963).

Sapir, D. G., Levine, D. Z., and Schwartz, W. B., "The effects of chronic hypokalemia on electrolyte and acid-base equilibrium: An examination of normocapneic hypoxemia and of the influence of hypoxemia on the adaptation to chronic hypercapnia." *J. Clin. Invest.* 46:369 (1967).

Schaefer, K. E., Hastings, B. J., Carey, C. R., and Nichols, G., Jr., "Respiratory acclimatization to carbon dioxide." *J. Appl. Physiol.* 18:1071 (1963).

Schwartz, W. B., Hays, R. M., Polak, A., and Haynie, G. D., "Effects of chronic hypercapnia on electrolyte and acid-base equilibrium. II. Recovery with special reference to influence of chloride intake." *J. Clin. Invest.* 40:1238 (1961).

Schwartz, W. B., Brackett, N. C., Jr., and Cohen, J., "The response of extracellular hydrogen ion concentration to graded degrees of chronic hypercapnia, the physiologic limits of the defense of pH." *J. Clin. Invest.* 41:291 (1965).

Scott, R. W., "Observations on the pathologic physiology of chronic pulmonary emphysema." *Arch. Int. Med.* 26:544 (1920).

Turino, G. M., Goldring, R. M., and Heinemann, H. O., "Water, electrolytes and acid-base relationships in chronic cor pulmonale." *Prog. Cardiovascular Dis.* 12:467 (1970).

Van Ypersele de Strihou, C., Brasseur, B., and Deconinck, J., " 'Carbon dioxide response curve' for chronic hypercapnia in man." *N. Eng. J. Med.* 275:117 (1966).

Winterstein, H., "Chemical control of pulmonary ventilation. III. The 'reaction theory' of respiratory control." *N. Eng. J. Med.* 255: 331 (1956).

Turino and Ypersele Discussion

SEVERINGHAUS: Both of these papers are very interesting, I'm sure to many of us, and deserve a lot of comment which we won't have time for. I'm particularly interested in the slope of the CO_2 response curve during hypercapnia, for which you presented some data. You did not show us whether there was any relationship between the ventilatory response to CO_2 and the level of P_{CO_2}. You plotted it against H^+ and bicarbonate and you showed us that when the bicarbonate was reduced, the slope was steeper, but when the hydrogen was, I didn't see that. So can you tell us, does the slope get steeper when the P_{CO_2} comes down. That question is particularly relevant since I think you showed us that giving potassium chloride to these subjects lowered their bicarbonate without having much effect on P_{CO_2}. That is, you converted them from patients to dogs and lowered their pH from normal to an acid level, but you didn't say that they felt any better nor did they breathe any better. I would like to know whether the response was steeper at the same P_{CO_2}?

TURINO: When the ventilatory response to breathing 5% CO_2 in air is plotted against the arterial P_{CO_2}, there is an increase in slope of the ventilatory response as the bicarbonate concentrations are lowered. That is, the ratio of the increment in ventilation to the increment in arterial P_{CO_2} is greater as the bicarbonate is lowered by either the administration of potassium chloride or the administration of ammonium chloride.

SEVERINGHAUS: Do you have spinal fluid pH's on some of these?

TURINO: We did not measure cerebrospinal fluid pH in these patients. In view of the length of these studies and the frequent arterial blood sampling, we did not wish to subject them to repeated lumbar punctures.

SEVERINGHAUS: Do they feel better, or worse?

TURINO: We could not detect any real change in clinical well-being of the patients when their bicarbonates were lowered by either potassium chloride or ammonium chloride over the usual day-to-day variation, even though the resting arterial P_{O_2} tended to be from 2 to 5 mm Hg higher. One of the subjects with severe kyphoscoliosis had some tachypnea and increased dyspnea while taking ammonium chloride, but we could not rule out some mild intercurrent pulmonary infection.

FRUMIN: The increase in P_{O_2} with potassium chloride—was this a simple relationship in the alveolar equation as the CO_2 dropped or is there some other explanation for the rise in P_{O_2}?

TURINO: Total minute volumes at rest were not significantly increased in these subjects when either potassium chloride or ammonium chloride was administered, even though responsiveness to breathing 5% CO_2 was increased and the resting alveolar ventilation must have increased to lower the resting arterial P_{CO_2}. In addition to an increase in alveolar P_{O_2} as a cause of the rise in arterial P_{O_2}, there could be subtle changes in ventilation-perfusion relationships as well as the change in the oxyhemoglobin dissociation curve which shifts to the right as the pH is lowered.

SEVERINGHAUS: A rise in R.Q. will also raise the alveolar P_{O_2}.

———: I would like to ask Dr. Van Ypersele a question. You showed in your last slide high P_{CO_2} values in metabolic alkalosis of more than 55 mm mercury. Were these patients without any lung disease or were they chronic bronchitis patients?

VAN YPERSELE: All the patients we showed with chronic metabolic alkalosis on the last slide were all patients with normal lung function and evaluated by chest X-rays, by arterial P_{O_2}, when they had a normal plasma bicarbonate concentration.

———: Don't you think it's a rather high level of P_{CO_2} for a compensation?

VAN YPERSELE: Well, these patients had arterial plasma bicarbonate concentration around 40 meq/l. with a pH around 7.49.

FENCL: May I ask a question, Dr. Van Ypersele? Some time ago, Refsum from Oslo published some data of patients with CO_2 tension, and he claims that the buildup of bicarbonate by the renal mechanism has a ceiling at the P_{CO_2} of around 65 to 70 mm of mercury, so I believe, if I remember correctly. He presented the data in the pH bicarbonate plot, and he shows a very steep buildup of bicarbonate. When you reach the 65 or 70 isobar of P_{CO_2}, then it levels off and for some reasons which I don't know—nobody has ever explained—goes parallel with what looks like the buffer line for the extracellular space. How would your data, at that level of P_{CO_2}, look in this relationship? Perhaps another question for Dr. Rector: Could he tell us what is known about the ceilings of the renal mechanisms for building up bicarbonate, and whether this suggestion that Refsum made was true?

VAN YPERSELE: In answer to your question about Refsum's data, we do not have data above 70 mm (at least good data above 70 mm),

and it's very difficult to get chronic steady-state patients without superimposed acid base disturbance. I am not quite sure that Refsum's data are unequivocal. What is certainly true is that in dogs, at least, plasma bicarbonate concentration still goes up and there is no breaking of the curve around 70 mm of mercury. Now it's possible that man is different from dog, but it would be amazing that he behaves almost identically up to 70 mm of mercury and then that around 70 mm of mercury he would behave differently.

OTIS: Some years ago Hobson and I made some observations on the acid-base status of patients with rather large right-to-left circulatory shunts, and I was wondering if either of the speakers had studied this type of patient? I would like to see you do a more complete job than we did. It's quite a complex situation.

ENSON: Both speakers have quite appropriately concerned themselves with the effect of sodium and potassium repletion on central nervous system sensitivity. I wonder if they might make any comment on the effects on respiratory muscle function?

TURINO: In the experimental circumstances reported we were not dealing with profound degrees of acidosis and the patients did not manifest any awareness of much weakness. While more marked acidosis may interfere with skeletal muscle function as it does for cardiac muscle, I am not aware of data on muscle function *in vivo* with the arterial pH lowered to this degree. In this regard it is of interest that despite musculoskeletal abnormalities and increased work of breathing, they fall on the $HCO_3^- - P_{CO_2}$ relationship predicted for normal dogs.

———: Am I correct in understanding Dr. Turino's data insofar as he suggests that potassium chloride lowering of bicarbonate is more efficient in stimulating respiration in these chronic patients than an equivalent lowering of plasma bicarbonate with ammonium chloride?

TURINO: That is an important question. From the data I would say "no" and that the results demonstrate the opposite—that is, actually greater increases in ventilatory responsiveness and lowering of serum bicarbonate with the administration of ammonium chloride. To go along with that result, the administration of ammonium chloride resulted in a greater amount of hydrogen retained than when potassium chloride was administered. In these experiments potassium chloride was being administered to reverse a deficiency state for chloride and hydrogen, which when corrected did not result in further lowering of HCO_3^- despite continued intake of potassium chloride supplements. However, with ammonium chloride administration there was greater retention of H^+ and decrease in serum HCO_3^- concentration to levels lower than those obtained after potassium chloride alone.

4. Respiratory Gas Exchange, Acid-Base Balance, and Electrolytes during and after Maximal Work Breathing 15 mm Hg PI$_{CO_2}$

Ulrich C. Luft, S. Finkelstein, and J. C. Elliott

Physiology Department, Lovelace Foundation,
Albuquerque, New Mexico 87108

Introduction

It is generally accepted on the basis of practical experience in submarines and other confined spaces that accumulation of CO_2 in the inspired air amounting to a partial pressure of 15 mm Hg is subjectively acceptable—if even noticeable—and compatible with ordinary physical and mental activities. Nevertheless, measurable changes in ventilation and alveolar PCO_2 have been reported by Lambertsen [1960] in resting subjects at 15 mm Hg PCO_2 and in light exercise by Froeb [1960]. Schaefer and his associates [1963] have described alterations in respiration, acid-base, and electrolyte balance in the course of acclimatization and de-acclimatization to an environment with a PI$_{CO_2}$ of 11 mm Hg. Relatively little factual information exists, however, on the effects of CO_2 under conditions of strenuous exertion verging on the limits of work capacity as might be encountered in emergency situations in space operations, in submarines, or in diving activities. An excellent investigation by Menn, Sinclair, and Welch [1970] with inspired CO_2 tensions ranging from 8 to 30 mm Hg revealed a consistent and proportionate increase in ventilation, but reduced CO_2 output and respiratory exchange ratio (R.E.R.) in submaximal exercise. In exhausting exercise, with PI$_{CO_2}$ 21 mm Hg ventilation was not significantly different from the controls, while maximal O_2 intake was only slightly less. But there was a highly significant reduction in CO_2 output. These authors concluded that strenuous exercise with exogenous hypercapnia leads to CO_2 retention, adding respiratory acidosis to the metabolic one, thus forcing the respiratory system to its limits.

The following experiments were designed to further explore the interaction of hypercapnia and exercise with a PI$_{CO_2}$ of 15 mm Hg, which is the highest acceptable level for emergencies in spacecraft, by following the respiratory and circulatory responses to graded exercise including maximal work capacity and the alterations in acid-base balance, blood gases, and electrolytes at the breaking point and during recovery.

Methods and Procedures

The study consisted of two series of experiments. The first was focused primarily on exercise tolerance in terms of maximal aerobic power with and without added CO_2 and the course of respiratory and cardiovascular adjustments under increasing work loads. Twelve subjects participated in this series working on a bicycle ergometer at an initial brake load of 300 kpm/min at 50 rpm for the first three minutes. Subsequently the brake load was increased by 75 kpm/min every minute until the subject was unable to maintain the pedaling rhythm given by a metronome. Each subject was his own control with one test on air and the other with a mixture producing a PI_{CO_2} of 15 ± 2 mm Hg in random sequence. With the exception of the technician operating the gas supply, neither the subject nor the investigators monitoring the test were aware which gas was being administered. Both gases were supplied from pressure tanks through a large humidifying bottle and buffer bag with wide-bore tubing (i.d. 3.4 cm) to a low-resistance unidirectional breathing valve (Lloyd). The total resistance of the valve and collecting tubing was 2.5 cm H_2O at a flow rate of 5 l./sec. Heart rate and blood pressure were recorded each minute, and ventilation and gas exchange were derived from expired air collected at regular intervals in neoprene bags and analyzed immediately by the Scholander technique. With two exceptions, the subjects were not habitually active physically. Their mean age was 26.5 years, mean height 179 cm, mean weight 75.9 kg, and mean body surface area 1.93 m². Subjective sensations during tests with CO_2 elicited after both tests had been performed varied from no difference to a feeling of acute suffocation at the end point.

In the second series of tests on 10 subjects main attention was directed toward the interactions between respiratory gas exchange with arterial blood gases, acid-base balance, and electrolytes at peak performance and during 30 min of recovery. The exercise protocol was similar to the one followed in the first series, with the difference that an attempt was made to equalize the duration of exercise by imposing a handicap on the stronger subjects by increasing the brake load by 150 instead of 75 kpm/min during the first few minutes of the test so that the average duration to exhaustion was 14 min.

Prior to the exercise data were obtained at supine rest for 10 to 15 min after an indwelling Teflon catheter had been inserted into a brachial artery under local anesthesia. Blood was drawn simultaneously with respiratory measurements for blood gases and pH and the determination of sodium, chloride, potassium, calcium, phosphorus,

total plasma protein, hemoglobin, cholesterol, and lactic dehydrogenase. The subject then mounted the bicycle and began the exercise program. Ventilation measurements were made during the last two minutes of exercise and in an uninterrupted sequence for the first seven minutes of recovery sitting on the bicycle. During the eighth minute the subject moved to an adjacent couch and expired air was collected in the 8–10th, 11–14th, 15–18th, 19–22nd, 23–26th, and 27–30th minutes. Arterial samples were drawn during the last minute of exercise, from 30–60 seconds after ceasing work, then in the 4th, 10th, 20th, and 30th minutes of recovery. Blood gases and pH were measured immediately with a Corning Model 16 electrode system, plasma bicarbonate and base deficit were derived according to Sigaard-Anderson whereby no correction was made for actual body temperature which was not measured. Analyses for calcium, phosphorus, total protein, cholesterol, and LDH were performed on a sequential auto analyzer (Technicon 12/30). Sodium, potassium, and chloride were measured with a four-channel electrolyte analyzer (Technicon). Hemoglobin determinations were made on samples at rest before exercise, in the first minute after and after 30 minutes using the cyanmethemoglobin method.

Results

I.

Table 1 presents circulatory data at three ascending work loads and at the end point. At all submaximal work loads the mean heart rate was consistently slightly higher in the runs with CO_2 than in the controls. However, the difference was not statistically significant. At the end point heart rate was always lower in the experimental tests than in the control, as if other than cardiovascular factors prevented the subjects from reaching their maximal frequencies. Systolic blood pressure was regularly higher on the average at all work

Table 1. Cardiovascular Parameters, Mean Values for 12 Subjects

| | 300 kpm/min | | 600 kpm/min | | 900 kpm/min | | End point | |
	Control	Exper.	Control	Exper.	Control	Exper.	Control	Exper.
Heart rate	111	114	128	131	152	155	185	180
Systolic blood pressure	143	150	159	167	181	188	204	211
Oxygen pulse	8.2	8.3	10.5	10.3	13.0	12.8	16.8	15.1

loads, including the maximal level with CO_2 without this being statistically significant. It was also noted that the O_2 pulse (product of stroke volume and arteriovenous O_2 difference) was less at end point with CO_2 than on air, while there was little difference under submaximal work conditions.

The respiratory data shown on Table 2 shows the expected excess ventilation caused by CO_2 at the lower and submaximal work loads, where the difference was 40 to 50% and statistically highly significant. At maximal work, however, the difference was only 2% and not significant.

Mean O_2 consumption was consistently slightly higher in the experimental runs at the intermediate work levels, possibly reflecting the increased energy cost of breathing. On the other hand, the significantly lower maximum O_2 uptake (-13%) is due to the fact that the subjects could not perform as much work under the effect of added CO_2. On the other hand, CO_2 elimination was consistently lower on the experimental mixture at comparable work levels, and the tendency for CO_2 loading is also apparent from the lower respiratory exchange ratios as seen on the last line of Table 2.

The hypothesis for this study had postulated on the basis of the alveolar equation (7) modified for CO_2 in the inspirate that in order to maintain the same P_{CO_2} and pH for a given CO_2 output with $PI_{CO_2} = 15$ mm Hg, total ventilation would have to increase by more than 60%. The results in Table 3 show that the average increase in ventilation was actually only 48% at 300, 47% at 600, and 43% at 900 kpm/min, whereas at the end point ventilation was only 2% more on CO_2 than in the controls. The implications are that while a moderate degree of hypercapnia must be already present during submaximal exercise with CO_2, CO_2 loading must assume drastic proportions during maximal exertion where further increase in ventilation is no longer possible leading to acute respiratory acidosis at a point where metabolic acidosis is rapidly building up. The second series of experiments was to substantiate this contention.

Gas Exchange
II

As pointed out earlier, in the second series respiratory measurements were made at recumbent rest before exercise, during the

Table 2. Ventilation and Gas Exchange, Mean Values for 12 Subjects

| | 300 kpm/min | | 600 kpm/min | | 900 kpm/min | | End point | |
	Control	Exper.	Control	Exper.	Control	Exper.	Control	Exper.
VI BTPS	27.67	41.04	40.0	58.7	62.66	89.45	139.4	142.2
V_{O_2} STPD	.89	.93	1.31	1.329	1.95	1.97	3.10	2.69
V_{CO_2} STPD	.84	.66	1.22	1.094	1.94	1.84	3.44	2.84
R.E.R.	.94	.71	.93	.82	.99	.94	1.11	1.06

Table 3. Ventilation and Respiratory Gas Exchange, Mean Values and Standard Deviations

	l./min. (BTPS)		l./min. (STPD)		l./min. (STPD)					
	Ventilation		O_2 uptake		CO_2 output		Resp. Exch. R.		Ventil. Equiv. for O_2	
$n = 10$	$\bar{c}\ CO_2$	Air	$\bar{c}\ CO_2$	Air	$\bar{c}\ CO_2$	Air	$\bar{c}\ CO_2$	Air	$\bar{c}\ CO_2$	Air
Rest	9.23	9.23	.274	.291	.249	.243	.910	.835	33.7	31.7
	2.90	2.34	.032	.029	.050	.035	—	—	—	—
Exercise,	126.09	121.17	2.923	3.112	2.989	3.392	1.023	1.090	43.1	38.9
2nd last'	20.57	25.30	.305	.389	.475	.492	—	—	—	—
Exercise,	133.05	125.93	3.179	3.279	3.202	3.558	1.007	1.085	41.8	38.4
last'	18.61	23.38	.275	.432	.339	.479	—	—	—	—
Recovery,	117.04	109.14	2.116	2.217	2.483	2.790	1.173	1.258	55.3	49.2
1'	12.46	17.56	.285	.304	.271	.377	—	—	—	—
2–3'	82.52	61.95	.937	.902	1.301	1.339	1.388	1.484	88.1	68.7
	21.69	11.68	.152	.129	.287	.178	—	—	—	—
4–5'	53.85	38.06	.616	.629	.739	.764	1.120	1.215	87.4	60.5
	8.76	6.44	.092	.084	.144	.092	—	—	—	—
6–7'	48.81	34.67	.581	.616	.593	.660	1.021	1.071	84.0	63.8
	9.55	9.70	.113	.112	.113	.093	—	—	—	—
9–10'	43.36	26.39	.618	.632	.580	.589	.939	.967	70.0	41.8
	12.05	5.16	.116	.087	.151	.082	—	—	—	—
12–14'	30.47	18.58	.423	.432	.362	.373	.856	.863	72.0	43.0
	6.17	2.94	.055	.052	.085	.055	—	—	—	—
16–18'	24.96	15.76	.400	.395	.297	.307	.743	.777	74.9	39.9
	4.92	2.68	.075	.061	.065	.044	—	—	—	—
20–22'	20.65	13.30	.343	.373	.243	.273	.711	.732	60.2	35.7
	4.53	2.05	.064	.042	.062	.059	—	—	—	—
24–26'	18.90	12.82	.341	.364	.221	.243	.648	.669	55.4	35.3
	3.49	2.21	.052	.051	.045	.040	—	—	—	—
28–30'	17.40	11.25	.335	.338	.208	.217	.621	.642	51.9	33.2
	1.72	1.49	.055	.042	.016	.018	—	—	—	—

Note: All values given for "Rest" in Tables 2 through 6 were obtained breathing air.

last two minutes of maximal exercise and during recovery. Figure 1 shows O_2 intake in black with 15 mm Hg $P_{I_{CO_2}}$ and cross-hatched for the controls on air. Consistent with the observations in the first series, oxygen consumption and maximum work was less with CO_2 in the last two minutes at work and during the first minute of recovery. For the following 30 min there was no appreciable difference and the cumulative O_2 consumption for this period was not significantly different being 14.9 l. with CO_2 and 15.3 l. on air. In ventilation also (Figure 2) there was not much difference between the experimental runs and the controls in the last two minutes at maximal work and the first minute of recovery. It will be noted that during that time ventilation was well over 100 l./min. But already in the 2 to 3 min, and for each sample period, ventilation was significantly greater with added CO_2, as more ventilatory reserve became available. This sequence of events is also reflected in the CO_2 output (Figure 3), which was significantly less (statistically) only during the last two minutes of exercise and the first minute of recovery. Thereafter the difference was consistently present over the 30 min but was no longer significant. The respiratory exchange ratio (R.E.R.) plotted in Figure 4 indicates that while under experimental and control conditions much more CO_2 was discharged than O_2 taken up (particularly during the first few minutes of recovery) the

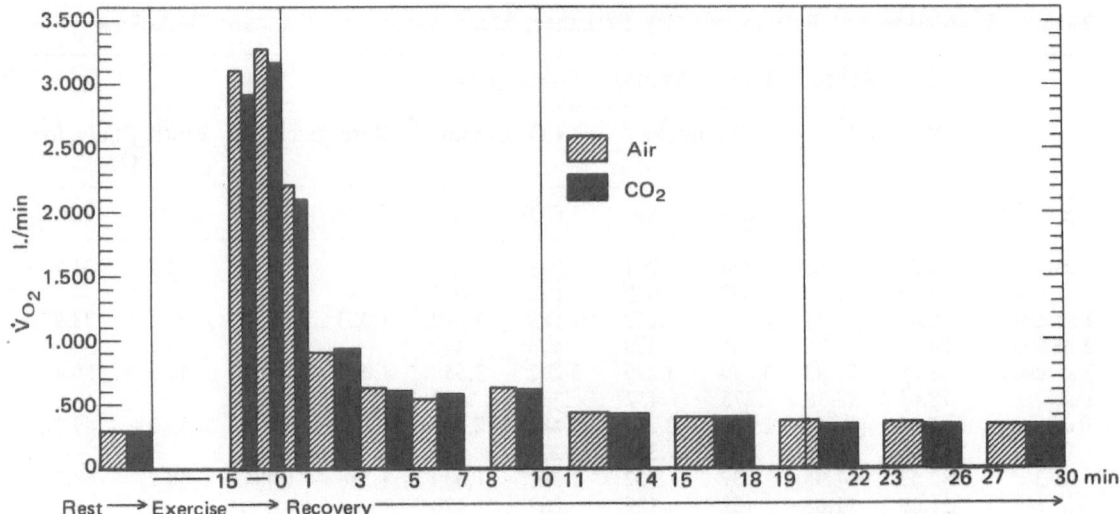

Fig. 1. Oxygen intake at rest before, during the last two minutes of exercise and for 30 min recovery.

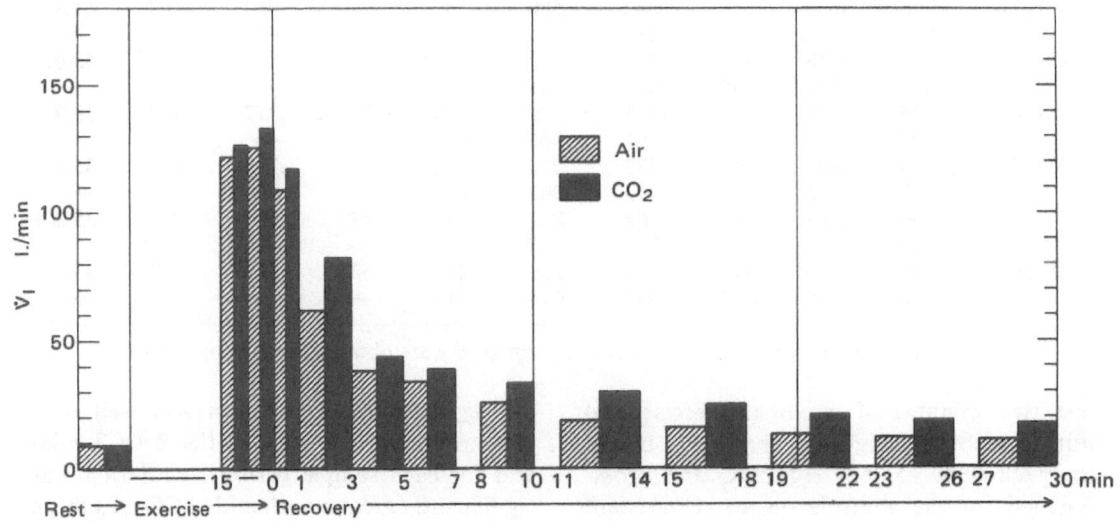

Fig. 2. The same as Figure 1 for ventilation.

inspired CO_2 had a distinctly depressing effect on its liberation from the body. The excess ventilation attributable to the relatively low partial pressure of CO_2 in the inspired air is perhaps best expressed in terms of specific ventilation or the ventilation equivalent for O_2 (Figure 5). The usual rise in specific ventilation after exhaustive exercise seen in our controls on air was greatly exaggerated by the inspired CO_2, and the difference was sustained throughout the entire recovery period.

Acid-Base Balance

The addition of small amounts of CO_2 to the inspired air also had a profound effect on the well known pattern in acid-base balance during and after vigorous exercise

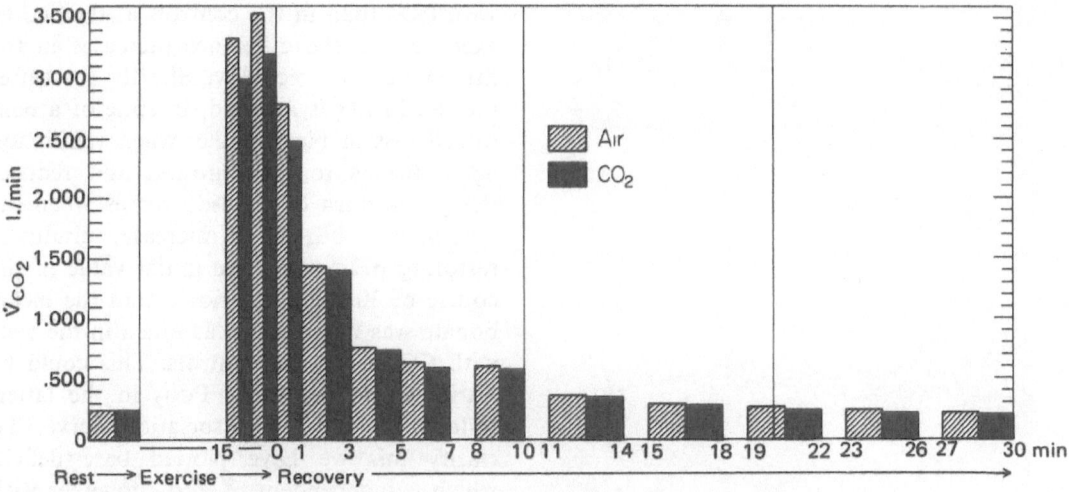

Fig. 3. The same as Figures 1 and 2 for carbon dioxide output.

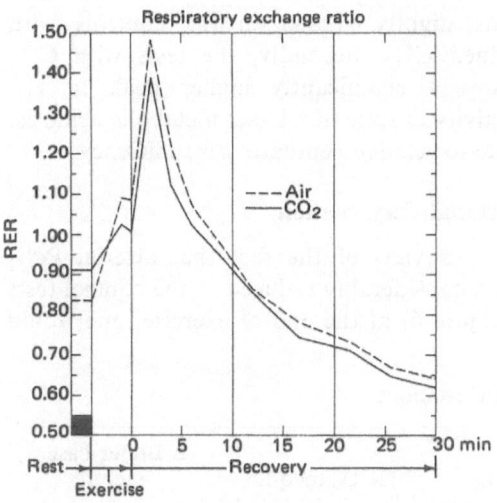

Fig. 4. The same as Figures 1 to 3 for the respiratory exchange ratio.

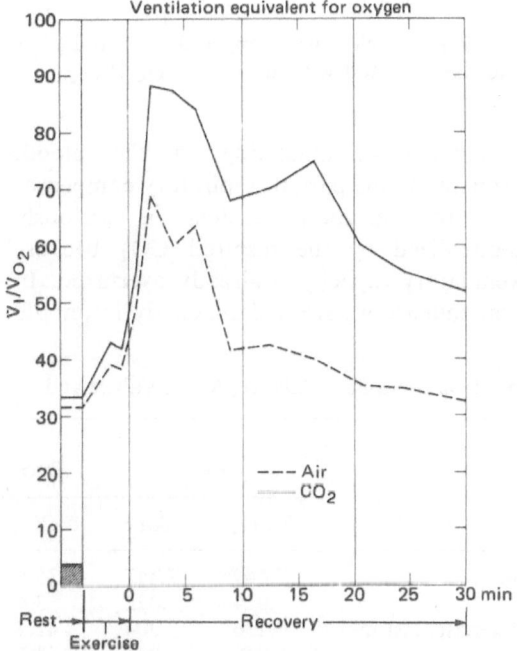

Fig. 5. The same as Figures 1 to 4 for the ventilation equivalent for oxygen.

(Figure 6). Whereas in the control runs arterial Pco_2 dropped to 30 mm Hg at the end of work and continued down to 26 mm Hg in the fourth minute of recovery, the course was different when CO_2 was added to the inspirate. Here arterial Pco_2 rose to 41 mm Hg in the last minute of exercise and dropped very little in the first minute after work, with a minimum of 33 mm Hg in the fourth minute of recovery (Table 4).

The observed fall in Pco_2 seen in the controls which signifies relative alveolar hyperventilation runs closely parallel to the sharp drop in bicarbonate during and continuing after exercise as an index of acid

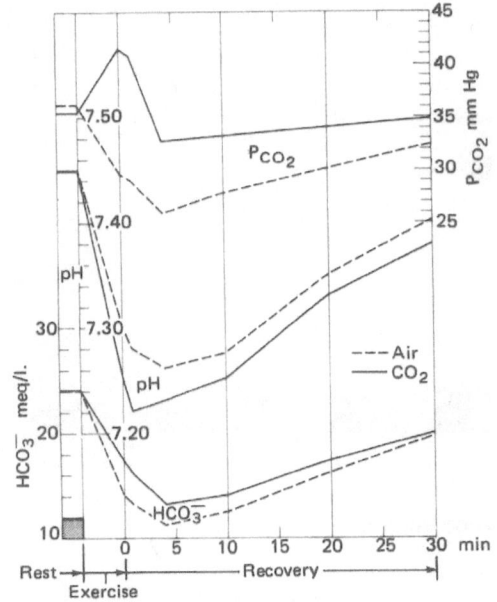

Fig. 6. Acid-base changes during and after exercise with and without 15 mm Hg P_{Ico_2}.

metabolites accumulating in the blood. Apparently the partial respiratory compensation for metabolic acidosis is seriously jeopardized by the inspired CO_2 because ventilatory capacity is already overtaxed. In consequence we see a significantly lower pH

with CO_2 than in the controls at the end of exercise and the difference increases in the first minute of recovery. Shortly thereafter the fall in pH is arrested, in spite of a continued loss of bicarbonate, when ventilation again begins to gain ground and reduces P_{co_2}. The turn of the tide comes when the bicarbonate begins to increase, gradually restoring pH toward the initial value in the course of 30 min. It is noted that the bicarbonate was not reduced as much in the tests with CO_2 as in the controls. This could be attributed to the lower P_{co_2} in the latter, following the CO_2 dissociation curve. To clarify this we have plotted base deficit, which is independent of P_{co_2}, together with H^+ activity in Figure 7. This reveals two things. First, it confirms that the loss of buffer capacity due to the influx of fixed acid was slightly greater in the controls with added CO_2. Secondly, the tests with CO_2 show a significantly higher peak in H^+ activity in spite of a lesser metabolic acidosis, due to relative ventilatory insufficiency.

Arterial Oxygenation

In view of the fact that arterial P_{co_2} was considerably reduced in the control tests (Figure 6) at the end of exercise, one would

Table 4. Acid-Base Balance, Mean Values and Standard Deviations

$n = 10$	pH		P_{co_2} mm Hg		HCO_3 meq/l.		Δ Buffer base, meq/l.	
	$\bar{c}$ CO_2	Air	$\bar{c}$ CO_2	Air	$\bar{c}$ CO_2	Air	$\bar{c}$ CO_2	Air
Rest	7.449	7.447	35.5	36.2	23.8	24.2	0	0
	.024	.022	3.4	2.9	1.3	1.3	—	—
Exercise, last min	7.256	7.304	41.4	29.7	17.5	14.1	− 10.2	− 11.8
	.048	.049	4.1	5.2	1.6	2.0	2.3	1.8
Recovery	7.221	7.281	40.9	29.1	16.1	13.2	− 12.2	− 13.2
1′	.047	.049	4.1	3.5	1.9	2.0	2.8	2.4
4′	7.231	7.262	32.8	26.0	13.2	11.3	− 14.1	− 15.1
	.050	.058	2.3	3.3	1.9	1.7	2.9	2.2
10′	7.252	7.276	33.3	28.0	14.1	12.5	− 12.8	− 13.9
	.052	.051	2.6	1.7	2.4	1.4	3.5	2.3
20′	7.331	7.351	34.2	30.2	17.4	16.2	− 7.9	− 8.7
	.036	.040	2.5	2.6	2.5	2.2	3.1	2.2
30′	7.380	7.402	35.0	32.6	20.0	19.7	− 5.2	− 4.7
	.025	.021	2.3	2.6	2.0	2.2	2.1	2.3

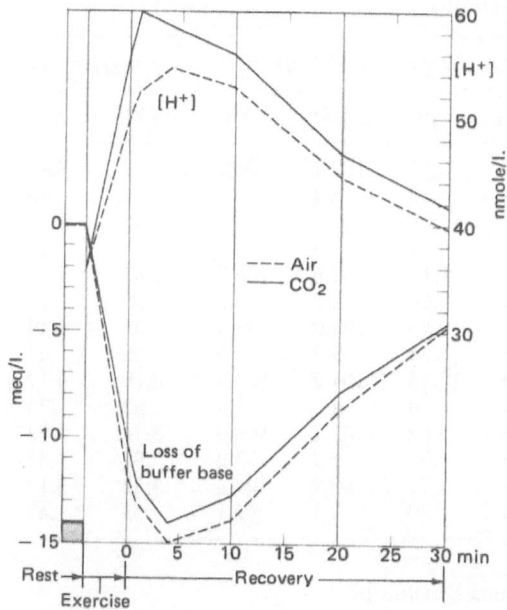

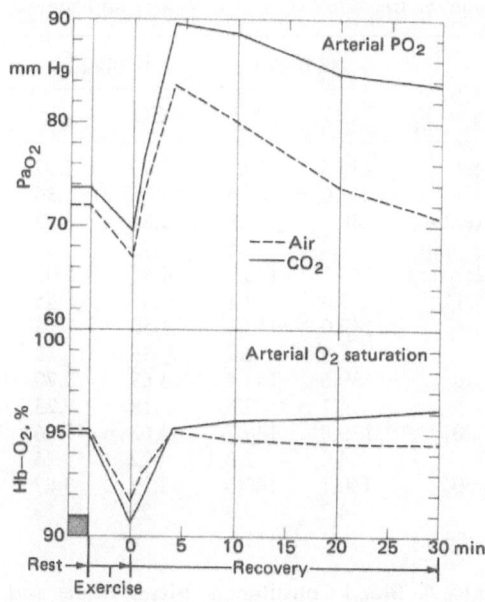

Fig. 7. Hydrogen ion activity and base deficit during and after exercise with and without 15 mm Hg PI_{CO_2}.

Fig. 8. Arterial O_2 tension and saturation during and after exercise with and without 15 mm Hg PI_{CO_2}.

expect arterial Po_2 to rise correspondingly at this point. Undoubtedly this was true for alveolar Po_2 which was not measured directly. This drop in arterial Po_2 (Figure 8) can be explained on the basis of an enlarged alveolar-arterial O_2 gradient described by others during maximal exercise (STAUB [1963], and WHIPP and WASSERMAN [1969]) and is attributed to limitations in diffusing capacity or physiological shunting with very low mixed venous O_2 tension. In view of the much higher arterial Pco_2 found in the group breathing CO_2, it is rather unexpected to see that Po_2 remained higher throughout than in the control group. This phenomenon is explained by displacement of some N_2 in the inspired gas by CO_2 and the associated hyperventilation (RAHN and FENN [1960]). It was also observed that arterial O_2 saturation was lower in the CO_2 group than in the controls while the opposite was true for Po_2. This inversion reflects the reduced affinity of hemoglobin for oxygen due to the lower pH in the tests with added carbon dioxide.

Electrolytes

In examining the changes in plasma electrolyte concentration during these experiments (Table 5) it is apparent that all of them increased to some extent with a peak in the last minute of exercise and a gradual decline during the 30 min of recovery. The same is true of other constituents measured, including plasma protein and hemoglobin as shown in Table 6. Furthermore, there were no significant differences in any of these data between the experiments with added carbon dioxide and with air.

Generally speaking, the concentration of electrolytes and other blood constituents can change in two different ways. One of these is hemoconcentration due to loss of intravascular fluid volume as demonstrated during exercise by Kaltreider and Meneely [1940]. If the fluid loss consisted entirely of water, it would affect the concentration of all blood constituents equally and the absolute amount within the intravascular compartment would

Table 5. Electrolytes, Mean Values and Standard Deviations

$n = 10$	Na meq/l.		K meq/l.		Ca mg/100 ml		Cl meq/l.		P mg/100 ml	
	$\bar{c}\ CO_2$	Air	$\bar{c}\ CO_2$	Air	$\bar{c}\ CO_2$	Air	$\bar{c}\ CO_2$	Air	$\bar{c}\ CO_2$	Air
Rest	139.5	139.7	3.70	3.77	9.47	9.42	103.1	104.3	2.87	3.23
	3.0	2.5	.35	.36	.46	.30	2.4	3.1	.51	.46
Exercise,	146.6	147.9	5.84	6.09	10.88	11.09	105.9	107.8	4.45	4.54
last min	5.2	2.6	.75	.64	.92	.71	2.6	4.2	.95	.77
Recovery,	145.1	146.9	4.85	5.05	10.80	11.12	104.6	106.8	4.62	4.63
1′	3.8	2.4	.58	.55	.82	.60	2.6	3.9	.90	.74
4′	142.0	143.3	3.50	3.56	10.32	10.45	102.0	103.3	4.35	4.43
	3.9	3.7	.36	.18	.67	.55	3.7	2.6	.96	.62
10′	139.6	141.4	3.69	3.70	10.10	10.14	101.2	102.8	4.19	4.17
	4.1	2.5	.18	.25	.46	.60	4.0	3.3	.92	.70
20′	139.8	140.7	3.63	3.66	9.70	9.89	102.1	103.9	3.74	3.73
	4.0	2.3	.22	.25	.46	.39	2.9	3.9	.82	.53
30′	140.1	140.5	3.71	3.67	9.56	9.77	103.9	104.8	3.32	3.19
	4.2	2.9	.23	.18	.40	.30	2.8	3.1	.53	.43

Table 6. Blood Constituents, Mean Values and Standard Deviations

$n = 10$	Plasma protein g/100 ml		Cholesterol, mg/ 100 ml		L.D.H. units		Hemoglobin, g/100 ml	
	$\bar{c}\ CO_2$	Air	$\bar{c}\ CO_2$	Air	$\bar{c}\ CO_2$	Air	$\bar{c}\ CO_2$	Air
Rest	6.79	6.99	175.5	173.0	99.7	105.9	15.60	16.0
	.36	.44	22.8	28.1	15.1	20.4	.86	.9
Exercise, last min	8.29	8.39	205.3	211.1	142.9	137.5	—	—
	.51	.40	30.0	29.6	43.4	32.6	—	—
Recovery,	8.21	8.45	210.0	208.9	126.4	124.6	17.85	18.2
1′	.47	.45	31.1	34.5	16.6	28.3	1.02	1.0
4′	8.16	8.42	206.8	213.9	125.4	126.0	—	—
	.43	.39	32.5	39.0	23.1	33.0	—	—
10′	7.96	8.21	202.6	204.9	118.5	117.0	—	—
	.34	.45	29.4	38.2	23.4	23.2	—	—
20′	7.38	7.53	186.2	191.6	111.2	110.4	—	—
	.45	.32	29.9	33.1	17.5	25.1	—	—
30′	7.09	7.18	178.6	182.9	100.5	102.5	15.85	16.2
	.38	.21	28.5	32.1	18.3	26.6	0.80	1.0

remain the same. On the other hand, an actual gain or loss of electrolytes by exchange with the extravascular compartments would probably affect each component differently depending upon concentration gradients and permeability factors. If the amount of fluid loss were known precisely, one could correct for hemoconcentration or dilution and reveal actual displacement of the electrolytes in or out of the bloodstream. Although no direct measurements of blood or plasma volume could be made in this study, two independent indices are available for gain or loss of blood water, namely plasma protein and hemoglobin, both of which do not readily traverse the capillary walls. Under this assumption changes in plasma fluid volume should be inversely proportional to changes in plasma protein and hemoglobin concentrations. It is thus possible to correct measured electrolyte concentrations to the concentration that would have been obtained had there been no loss of fluid in an attempt to reveal true shifts in these elements. Figure 9 shows fractional changes in electrolytes derived from the data in Table 5. It is obvious that there are considerable differences in the magnitude of change. Whereas sodium and chloride apparently change very little, potassium and phosphorus increase by nearly 60%. When all electrolytes are corrected for hemoconcentration as described (Figure 10), sodium and chloride show an appreciable loss, as would be expected since they most readily follow water into and out of the extravascular compartment. There is also a minor loss of calcium, suggesting that more of it is retained by the capillaries. The gain in potassium at the end of exercise is much less than before correction for hemoconcentration but still amounts to 30% in the experimental group as well as the controls. Immediately after exercise potassium concentration falls precipitously and is 20% below the resting value in the fourth minute of recovery before gradually returning to the normal level. These extremely rapid changes

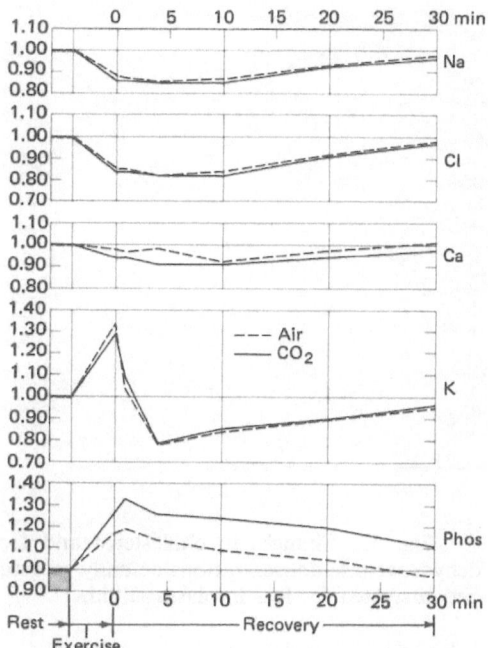

Fig. 10. The same as Figure 9 corrected for plasma fluid loss derived from changes in total plasma protein.

in potassium, commented upon previously by Laurell and Pernow [1966], are striking and deserve further study. Phosphorus also shows a 20 to 30% increase, but it does not reach its peak until after work has ceased with a slow return toward the control values.

Considerable attention has been given to the effects of exercise on serum cholesterol levels in the literature and possible mechanisms to explain the observed increase have been discussed (KOSIEK and KLANS [1968]). We also observed a 20% rise in cholesterol during exercise in our raw data, but there was practically no change when corrected for hemoconcentration (Figure 11). None of the organic or inorganic constituents of the blood that we measured showed any significant difference between the tests with added carbon dioxide and the controls on air.

Summary

An increase in the carbon dioxide content in the respiratory environment creating

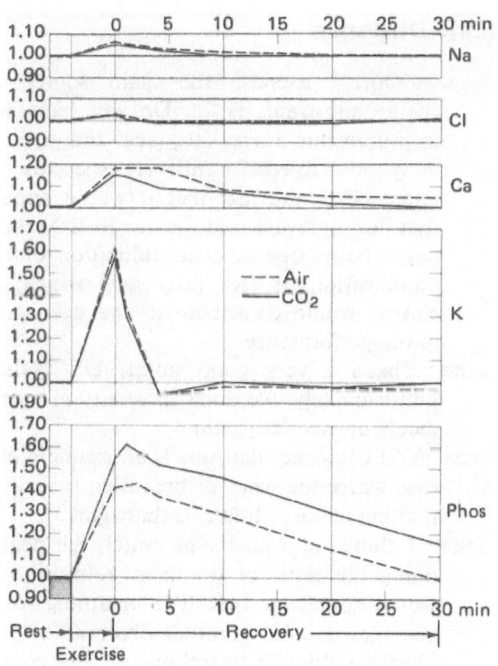

Fig. 9. Fractional changes in electrolyte concentrations (from Table 5).

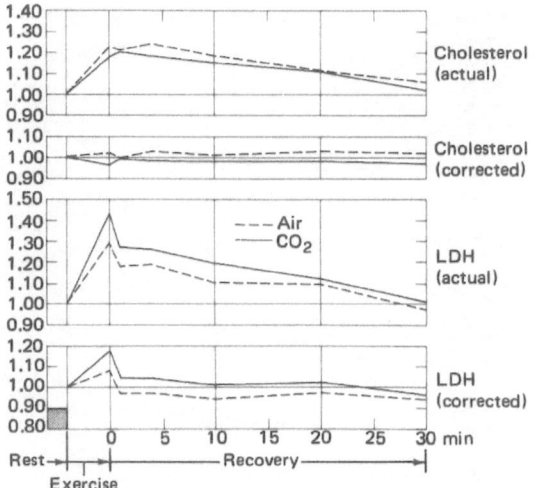

Fig. 11. Changes in cholesterol and lactic dehydrogenase concentrations actually measured and corrected for loss in plasma fluid.

a partial pressure of not more than 15 mm Hg is sufficient to jeopardize an individual's capacity for maximal exertion by impeding the respiratory discharge of CO_2 necessary to maintain homeostasis. It was demonstrated that there is a substantial rise in arterial P_{CO_2}, during maximal exercise breathing air contaminated with CO_2, whereas P_{CO_2} was consistently reduced without it. Consequently the metabolic acidosis generated by anaerobic processes in the muscles can no longer be attenuated by respiration, and the end point is precipitated by a critical rise in hydrogen concentration. No differences were seen in serum electrolytes, total plasma protein, hemoglobin, and other constituents between the tests with added carbon dioxide and the controls breathing air during and after exercise.

Bibliography

Froeb, H. F., "Ventilatory response in SCUBA divers to carbon dioxide inhalation." *J. Appl. Physiol.* 16:8 (1960).

Kaltreider, N. L., and Meneely, G. R., "The effect of exercise on the volume of blood." *J. Clin. Invest.* 19:627–34 (1940).

Kosiek, J. P., and Klans, E. J., "Das Verhalten des Glukose, Laktat, Pyruvat und Cholesterin

Spiegels im Serum nach erschöpfender Arbeit." *Med. Welt.* 19:2154–60 (1968).

Lambertsen, C. J., "Carbon dioxide and respiration in acid-base homeostasis." *Anesthesiol.* 21:642 (1960).

Laurell, H., and Pernow, B., "Effect of exercise on plasma potassium in man." *Acta Physiol. Scand.* 66:241–42 (1966).

Menn, S. J., Sinclair, R. D., and Welch, B. E., "Effects of inspired pCO_2 up to 30 mmHg on responses of normal man to exercise." *J. Appl. Physiol.* 28:663–71 (1970).

Rahn, H., and Fenn, W. O., "A graphical analysis of the respiratory gas exchange." The American Physiological Society, Washington, D.C. (1960) p. 40.

Schaefer, K. E., Hastings, B. J., Carey, C. R., and Nichols, G., Jr., "Respiratory acclimatization to carbon monoxide." *J. Appl. Physiol.* 18:1071 (1963),

Staub, N. C., "Alveolar-arterial O_2 tension gradient due to diffusion." *J. Appl. Physiol.* 18:673–80 (1963).

Whipp, B. J., and Wasserman, K., "Alveolar-arterial gas tension differences during graded exercise." *J. Appl. Physiol.* 27:361–65 (1969).

Luft Discussion

NAHAS: During exercise the main source of energy substrates is fat. Do you have any measurements of free fatty acid and glycerol in your subjects? This is especially in reference to the fact that it would appear that during severe acidosis due to CO_2 there might be at one point an inhibition of the mobilization of free fatty acid which, of course, would contribute to the decrement in the performance.

LUFT: That's a very good point, Dr. Nahas. Unfortunately, we don't have any measurements on free fatty acids.

OTIS: You could say that this is an example of a case where the work of breathing is really a limiting factor, I think. Is that right?

LUFT: I think so. And if you watch the people doing the tests, or do them yourself, you would appreciate that. The breathing really becomes painful. Another observation may illustrate this: In exercising on the bicycle ergometer one inevitably falls into a breathing pattern closely related to the cadence of pedaling. Our subjects were pedaling at 50 rpm and when approaching their maximum work capacity with the CO_2 mixture; they were breathing at the same rate (50 rpm) to achieve a minute ventilation of close to 150 l./min with a tidal volume of 3 l. In spite of this, the dyspnea was such that several subjects attempted to increase their ventilation by breathing faster than they were pedaling. The only alternative was to double-up to a frequency of 100 rpm, which led to a marked drop in tidal volume and alveolar ventilation. This demonstrates, I believe, that the limits of ventilatory capacity were definitely exceeded.

5. Adaptation to Hypocapnia and its Role in Adaptation to Hypoxia

Ralph H. Kellogg

Department of Physiology,
Medical Center, University of California,
San Francisco, California 94143

My interest in acclimatization to hypo-capnia or chronic low PA_{CO_2} arose as a by-product of my long interest in acclimatization to high altitude hypoxia, one of the two most common causes of chronic hypocapnia. (The other is pregnancy.) I used to think that the ventilatory aspects of acclimatization to high altitude simply represented ventilatory acclimatization to chronic hypocapnia. The latter would be produced by the hyper-ventilation resulting from hypoxic stimula-tion of the peripheral chemoreceptors. This is a very old idea, certainly not original with me. The best evidence for it came from the classic studies of Brown, Hemingway, and Visscher [1950], who showed that 24 hr of passive hyperventilation in a body respirator caused a readjustment in the regulation of breathing such that the PA_{CO_2} was regulated at a lower level when spontaneous breathing was resumed. Such a shift in the regulation of P_{CO_2} has become the classic sign of ventilatory acclimatization to hypocapnia, my subject for today. Since hypoxia stimu-lates hyperventilation and would produce chronic hypocapnia, it was thought that the shift in regulation of CO_2 at altitude was simply the experiment of Brown et al., with hypoxia taking the role of the respirator. About a decade ago I wrote a review (KELLOGG [1960]) that strongly supported this view, and I have been forced to change my mind. I propose today to review the evidence that has changed my thinking.

A few years ago Dr. Eger and others joined me in an attempt to test this hypo-thesis critically. We decided to measure the shift in regulation of PA_{CO_2} produced by 8 hr of hypocapnia of various degrees with and without hypoxia. According to the hypothesis, each level of hypocapnia should produce the same shift in PA_{CO_2} regulation regardless of the presence or absence of hypoxia, and hypoxia should produce no ventilatory acclimatization if hypocapnia was prevented. The plan of the experiments was simply to obtain some baseline measurements on the subject early in the morning, then produce a given PA_{CO_2} by voluntary hyperventilation, intermittent positive pressure, or adding CO_2 to the inspired gas, while also controlling the PA_{O_2} at the desired level, and maintain these gas levels for 8 hr during the day. We then repeated the morning's measurements imme-diately to assess the degree of acclimatization produced. In the figures I have averaged the data from all the subjects to simplify the presentation, since the detailed data have already been published (EGER et al. [1968]).

The average resting PA_{CO_2} in the morning baseline measurements was 40 mm Hg, represented by the solid square in Figure 1. During the subsequent 8 hr., without any intervening acclimatization regime, the average resting PA_{CO_2} of these four subjects fell to 38 mm Hg, represented by the point of the arrow, presumably because of their diurnal rhythms. The normoxic line (solid

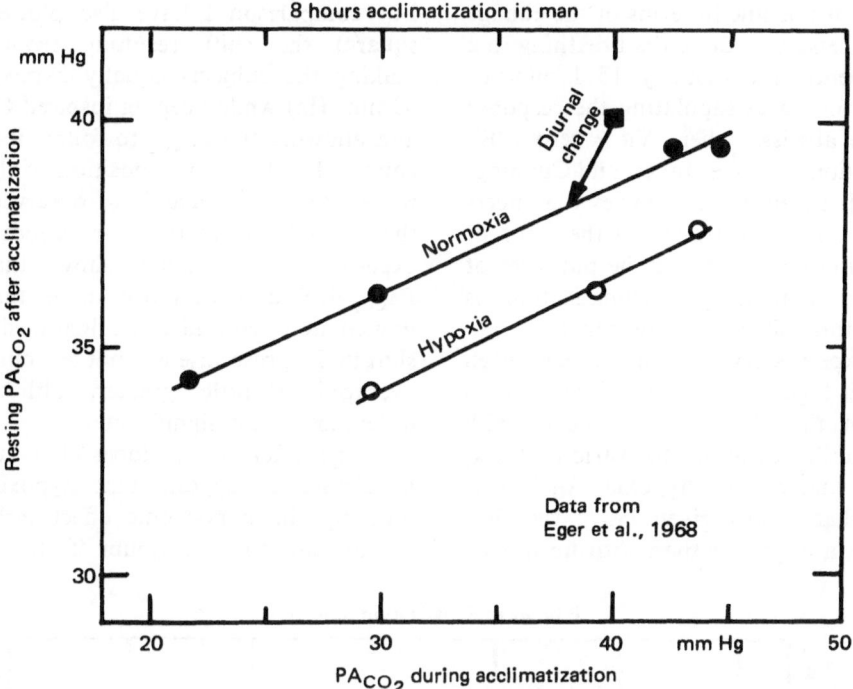

Fig. 1. The mean resting PA_{CO_2} after 8 hr of acclimatization in four men. The *solid square* represents their resting PA_{CO_2} before the acclimatization period. The *point of the arrow* represents the resting PA_{CO_2} after 8 hr without any experimental regimen. Each *solid circle* represents the mean PA_{CO_2} of the four subjects after 8 hr of acclimatization with the PA_{O_2} over 100 mm Hg and the PA_{CO_2} at the level indicated on the abscissa. Each *open circle* represents the corresponding mean when the PA_{O_2} was kept at 48 mm Hg during the acclimatization period. (Plotted from EGER et al. [1968].)

circles) represents the resting PA_{CO_2} that resulted from 8 hr of acclimatization to the PA_{CO_2} indicated on the abscissa, while PA_{O_2} was kept above 100 mm Hg. Each point represents the average of one day's experiment on each of the four subjects. Throughout the range studied, the fall in resting PA_{CO_2} seems to be a linear function of the acclimatization PA_{CO_2}, thus confirming and extending the observations of Brown et al. [1950].

I have labelled the line "Normoxia," but indeed there is good reason to believe that the respiratory alkalosis may produce enough vasoconstriction in the brain to make it somewhat hypoxic, for Plum, Posner, and Smith [1968] have found that the brain produces less lactic acid in hyperventilation if there is also hyperbaric oxygenation. Certainly, however, when the 8 hours of hypocapnia was accomplished by alveolar

hypoxia (PA_{O_2} 48 mm Hg) (open circles in Figure 1), the subsequent resting PA_{CO_2} was much lower.

The resting PA_{CO_2} is a relatively unreliable measure of PA_{CO_2} regulation because it is so easily influenced by extraneous psychological factors. A much more reliable measure is the shift in position of the CO_2 response curve, the ventilatory response to graded CO_2 inhalation in successive steady-state periods, plotted as a function of PA_{CO_2}. Since the breathing is being strongly stimulated by elevated PA_{CO_2} while oxygen is added to keep the PA_{O_2} above 180 mm Hg in all our tests, the position of the response line measures CO_2 regulation without hypoxic interference. We summarize each response line by calculating the least-squares regression line minimizing the squared deviations in PA_{CO_2} rather than $\dot{V}E$, then express the shift in position of this line in terms of the change in PA_{CO_2} necessary to drive the breathing to a standard ventilation, usually 15 l./min/m². We prefer this to extrapolating the response line to the abscissa where $\dot{V}E$ = zero ("B" in the equation of Lloyd, Jukes, and Cunningham [1958]) because it minimizes the effects of any statistical uncertainty in the slope of the regression line. Thus for the purposes of this paper, ventilatory acclimatization is defined as this shift in CO_2 response.

The experiments of Figure 1 have been replotted in Figure 2 in terms of this shift in position of the CO_2 response curve with 8 hr of acclimatization to various PA_{CO_2} levels with and without hypoxia. Again it is apparent that at any given PA_{CO_2} the shift with hypoxia is greater than with normoxia.

For comparison I have also plotted (open square) the shift resulting from simply making the subjects equally hypoxic (PA_{O_2} 48 mm Hg) while keeping inspired CO_2 zero and allowing the PA_{CO_2} to follow its natural course. The horizontal position of this point represents the average PA_{CO_2} observed during the last 2 hours of the 8-hr periods in such experiments. The figure shows that when PA_{CO_2} drifted down slowly rather than being immediately reduced to its final position, the shift in CO_2 response was not less but actually averaged a little greater, although the difference is not significant.

The difference in slopes of the two lines in Figure 2 suggests that hypoxia might multiply the hypocapnic effect rather than merely add to it. I doubt if that is right.

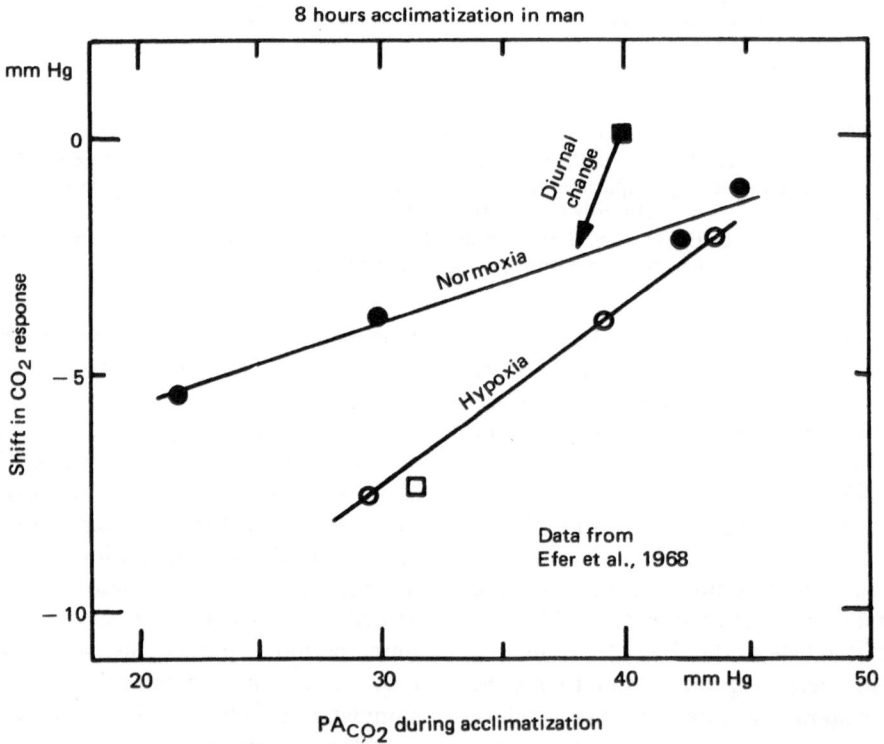

Fig. 2. Data from the same experiments as Figure 1, replotted to show on the ordinate the difference in position of the hyperoxic CO_2 response curves before and after the acclimatization period, measured at $\dot{V}E_2$ = 15 l./min/m². The *open square* represents experiments in which the inspired CO_2 was zero and PA_{CO_2} was allowed to drift down naturally during the acclimatization, while PA_{O_2} was held at 48 mm Hg. Its horizontal position represents the mean PA_{CO_2} actually observed during the last 2 hours of acclimatization. Other symbols as in Figure 1. (Plotted from EGER et al. [1968].)

Figure 1 does not show it. Furthermore, Mines [1968] and Morrill [1970] in their Ph.D. dissertation research have repeated such studies in goats using a wider range of PA_{CO_2} levels and more severe hypoxia for a shorter time. Their data indicate that although hypoxia produces a greater shift in CO_2 response than normoxia does, the absolute amounts seem to depend upon the circumstances in ways we do not understand. With severe hypoxia, the "hypoxic" line may even look horizontal. The shifts in normoxic hypocapnia, however, always form a linear function like the one shown in the figure.

What is the mechanism for this shift in CO_2 response? Ever since Severinghaus, Mitchell, Richardson, and Singer [1963] did CO_2 response measurements and lumbar punctures on themselves at the White Mountain Research Station, attention has been focused on the medullary chemoreceptors. They showed that the shift in their hyperoxic CO_2 response curves with acclimatization to an altitude of 3800 m could be explained in terms of rapid fall in the bicarbonate concentration of the CSF and presumably brain interstitial fluid. Their medullary chemoreceptors seemed to be responding to the same pH range as at sea level, but this was associated with a lower PCO_2 because of the lower bicarbonate concentration. The change in bicarbonate in the brain fluids seemed to be due to some primary mechanism rather than being merely a consequence of increased renal bicarbonate excretion, because the change in the brain fluids considerably preceded the change in the blood bicarbonate. Since then there have been many observations from several laboratories concerning the effects of sustained hypocapnia on CSF and brain bicarbonate, pH, electrical potential, and metabolism, especially lactic acid production. This is a very important subject, in which the causal mechanisms are not yet clear, at least to me. Since there are papers elsewhere in this symposium on this subject, as well as a very extensive symposium volume recently published (SIESJÖ and SØRENSEN [1971]), I will limit myself primarily to studies in which

ventilatory responses have been measured.

Dr. Morrill [1970] has shown that 4 hr of graded normoxic hypocapnia in unanesthetized goats produces a proportional shift in bicarbonate concentration in cisternal CSF, which would be expected from the work of many others (SIESJÖ and SØRENSEN [1971]); and he has further shown that this is associated with a proportional shift in CO_2 response, as would be expected. In severely hypoxic hypocapnia (PA_{O_2} 35 mm Hg), the situation is not so clear. A very similar linear fall in cisternal CSF bicarbonate concentration was observed, but the shift in CO_2 response seemed to be equally large regardless of the presence or absence of hypocapnia in this series of experiments. If I were to speculate, I would wonder whether this means that hypoxia directly affects the brain interstitial fluid bicarbonate, which in these short time periods does not have time to come into equilibrium with the bulk of the CSF, which is more responsive to the PCO_2 rather than the PO_2. Consistent with that view is the fact that MORRILL [1970] has also studied the shift in CO_2 response in goats as a result of 4 hr of acclimatization to a graded series of PA_{O_2} levels from 40 to 100 mm Hg and found that the shift in these cases did seem proportional to the degree of hypoxia. This would be consistent with the idea that the effect of hypoxia might be to accelerate some process, such as lactic acid production (PLUM and POSNER [1967]; COHEN et al. [1967]), which would speed the destruction of bicarbonate around the medullary chemoreceptors. But again I am speculating.

I would like to turn now from experiments in which the PA_{CO_2} has been artificially manipulated to examine situations in which a primary hypoxic stimulation of breathing, and hence an initial hypocapnia, is lacking. If ventilatory acclimatization to hypoxia depends upon a primary hypocapnia, then it should not occur when this is lacking. For man, the story begins with Chiodi [1957], followed by clearer demonstrations by Severinghaus, Bainton, and Carcelen [1966] quickly confirmed by Milledge and Lahiri

[1967] that natives of high altitudes seem to be quite insensitive to acute hypoxic stimulation of breathing. Yet their resting PA_{CO_2} levels are lower at higher altitudes, indicating that they do show ventilatory acclimatization, although less than sea level natives.

With experimental animals, one can surgically denervate the carotid and aortic bodies to perform a somewhat more convincing experiment. Probably the first example of this was the old observation of Davenport et al. [1947] that unanesthetized completely chemodenervated dogs, although their breathing was initially depressed by hypoxia, nevertheless slowly developed an increase in breathing over the course of an hour's hypoxia. This is probably the first recorded case of ventilatory acclimatization to hypoxia without initial hypocapnia, although the picture is not clear. More recently, Sørensen and Mines [1970] denervated the carotid regions of three goats and found that acute hypoxia now depressed their breathing. Nevertheless, when taken to 3800 m at the White Mountain Research Station, the two goats that survived showed prompt leftward shift in CO_2 response curves to about the position found in the acclimatized intact goats that had been taken up as controls. This study was based on too few animals to be convincing by itself; but in addition Sørensen [1970] completely denervated the carotid and aortic bodies in a group of rabbits and then decompressed them for 24 hr at 470 mm Hg. He found that their CSF bicarbonate concentrations fell 5 meq/l. in that time, exactly the same fall as in the intact rabbits decompressed as controls. I think all these observations taken together leave little doubt that ventilatory acclimatization to altitude does not depend upon acute hypoxic stimulation via the peripheral chemoreceptors. The contrary observations of Hansen (GILFILLAN et al. [1958]) on a couple of chemodenervated dogs that failed to acclimatize, which I incautiously cited a decade ago (KELLOGG [1960, 1963]), were too limited and technically too unsatisfactory to stand up against this weight of evidence.

In conclusion, I would like to say that I have tried to compare ventilatory acclimatization to hypocapnia with ventilatory acclimatization to hypoxia and to summarise the evidence that although these usually occur together, the former is not necessary for the latter. The independent effect of hypoxia in resetting the P_{CO_2}-regulating mechanisms is much greater in the circumstances and limited time periods we have studied. I presume that hypoxia acts by reducing the bicarbonate levels in the neighborhood of the medullary chemoreceptors, and I am attracted to the possibility that hypoxic production of lactic acid may play a role in titrating the bicarbonate. But even in the experiments of Mines and Sørensen [1971], in which they made anesthetized dogs hypoxic while keeping their arterial bicarbonate, pH, and P_{CO_2} from falling (and presumably thereby stabilized the CSF electrical potential also), the fall in CSF bicarbonate concentration was about three times as great as the rise in CSF lactate concentration. I still do not feel competent to devise a satisfactory theory to account for all the changes in bicarbonate and the regulation of breathing that we have been discussing.

Acknowledgments   Much of the work cited in this review has been supported by USPHS grants from the National Institutes of Health: GM–09262, H E–13841, and GM–00927 It is a pleasure to acknowledge much stimulating discussion with A. H. Mines, C. G. Morrill, and S. C. Sørensen, many of whose ideas and observations, published and unpublished, have influenced what I have written here; but this review was prepared while I was in Oxford on sabbatical leave, so all responsibility for its faults must rest with me.

Bibliography

Brown, E. B., Jr., Hemingway, A., and Visscher, M. B., "Arterial blood pH and pCO$_2$ changes in response to CO$_2$ inhalation after

24 hours of passive hyperventilation." *J. Appl. Physiol.* 2:544–48 (1950).

Chiodi, H., "Respiratory adaptations to chronic high altitude hypoxia." *J. Appl. Physiol.* 10:81–87 (1957).

Cohen, P. J., Alexander, S. C., Smith, T. C., Reivich, M., and Wollman, H., "Effects of hypoxia and normocarbia on cerebral blood flow and metabolism in conscious man." *J. Appl. Physiol.* 23:183–89 (1967).

Davenport, H. W., Brewer, G., Chambers, A. H., and Goldschmidt, S., "The respiratory responses to anoxemia of unanesthetized dogs with chronically denervated aortic and' carotid chemoreceptors and their causes.' *Am. J. Physiol.* 148:406–16 (1947).

Eger, E. I., II, Kellogg, R. H., Mines, A. H., Lima-Ostos, M., Morrill, C. G., and Kent, D. W., "Influence of CO_2 on ventilatory acclimatization to altitude." *J. Appl. Physiol.* 24:607–15 (1968).

Gilfillan, R. S., Hansen, J. T., Kellogg, R. H., Pace, N., and Cuthbertson, E. M., "Physiologic study of the chemoreceptor mechanism in the dog at sea level and at high altitude (12,600 ft.)." *Circulation* 18:724 (1958).

Kellogg, R. H., "Acclimatization to carbon dioxide." *Anesthesiology.* 21:634–41 (1960).

———. "The role of CO_2 in altitude acclimatization." In *The regulation of human respiration*, D. J. C. Cunningham and B. B. Lloyd, eds. Oxford: Blackwell (1963).

Lloyd, B. B., Jukes, M. G. M., Cunningham, D. J. C., "The relation between alveolar oxygen pressure and the respiratory response to carbon dioxide in man." *Quart. J. Exptl. Physiol.* 43:214–27 (1958).

Milledge, J. S., and Lahiri, S., "Respiratory control in lowlanders and Sherpa highlanders at altitude." *Resp. Physiol.* 2:310–22 (1967).

Mines, A. H. Ventilatory regulation in goats at high altitude. (Ph.D. Dissertation). San Francisco: University of California (1968). [Dissertation Abstracts International B 31 (No. 1): 368B–69B, July 1970.]

———, and Sørensen, S. C., "Changes in the electrochemical potential difference for HCO_3^- between blood and cerebrospinal fluid and in cerebrospinal fluid lactate concentration during isocarbic hypoxia." *Acta Physiol. Scand.* 81:225–33 (1971).

Morrill, C. G., Cerebrospinal fluid changes and exercise effects in ventilatory acclimatization to hypoxia. (Ph.D. Dissertation). San Francisco: University of California (1970).

Plum, F., and Posner, J. B., "Blood and cerebrospinal fluid lactate during hyperventilation." *Am. J. Physiol.* 212:864–70 (1967).

———, Posner, J. B., and Smith, W. W., "Effect of hyperbaric-hyperoxic hyperventilation on blood, brain, and CSF lactate." *Am. J. Physiol.* 215:1240–44 (1968).

Severinghaus, J. W., Mitchell, R. A., Richardson, B. W., and Singer, M. M., "Respiratory control at high altitude suggesting active transport regulation of CSF pH." *J. Appl. Physiol..* 18:1155–66 (1963).

Severinghaus, J. W., Bainton, C. R., and Carcelen, A., "Respiratory insensitivity to hypoxia in chronically hypoxic man." *Resp. Physiol.* 1:308–34 (1966).

Siesjö, B. K., and Sørensen, S. C., eds. *Ion homeostasis of the brain.* Copenhagen, Munksgaard, and New York: Academic Press (1971).

Sørensen, S. C., and Mines, A. H., "Ventilatory responses to acute and chronic hypoxia in goats after sinus nerve section." *J. Appl. Physiol.* 28:832–35 (1970).

———. "Ventilatory acclimatization to hypoxia in rabbits after denervation of peripheral chemoreceptors." *J. Appl. Physiol.* 28:836–39 (1970).

Kellogg Discussion Revised

LOESCHKE: You probably remember the paper by Kronenberg and Cain [1968] in which the bicarbonate concentration in the cerebrospinal fluid was demonstrated to be dependent on the blood bicarbonate concentration in both normoxia and hypoxia, but CSF bicarbonate was always lower in the latter case. They came to the conclusion that the lactic acid in CSF, which they measured, was not enough to account for this difference. If I understand you correctly (and I would agree with you), it seems that there will be a gradient of lactic acid from the point of the receptor to the point where it can be measured in the bulk of the CSF. Would that be your opinion?

KELLOGG: I consider that a perfectly reasonable possibility. Mines, Sorensen, and Morrill in my laboratory also have measured lactic acid concentration and compared its rise in CSF with the fall in bicarbonate, as quite a lot of others have also done. I think most of the data indicate about a 1 to 3 ratio for the rise in lactate compared to the fall in bicarbonate. It seems to me quite possible that the CSF is not completely in equilibrium, and that perhaps there are steady gradients, even for long periods.

LOESCHCKE: May I continue a little? I guess that Dr. Siesjö would tell us that there are acids other than lactic acid which would contribute.

SIESJÖ: I'm not quite sure that these acids will mean anything in a quantitative way, since they occur at such small concentrations. I think it's only pyruvic acid which gets out into the CSF too. I should like to add to what Dr. Loeschcke said by just mentioning that we have run a rather extensive series of experiments with hypoxemia in rats (30-min steady-state period) and tried taking them down with lower and lower oxygen concentrations. We really do find a beautiful stoichiometrical relationship between the increase in lactate and the decrease in bicarbonate in the CSF itself. But, under these circumstances, at least in the rat, there is about the same increase in the lactic acid concentration of the blood and the CSF. That could be the reason why we get the stoichiometry.

KELLOGG: I can add to that. In our measurements, I should say those in Dr. Morrill's Ph.D. dissertation [1970], the rise in chloride has made up most of the difference between the rise in lactate and the fall in bicarbonate in goat CSF. Therefore I agree with you in doubting that other acids play a large role in this matter.

COURNAND: Dr. Kellogg, have you followed the reverse process: The persistence of hypocapnia after you have returned from hypoxia to normoxia?

KELLOGG: Not in these short-term studies. We did so some years ago in returning from real altitude to real sea level (Cunningham and Lloyd [1963]). The transient is initially quite rapid, just as is the initial transient upon going up to altitude. But it has a very long, slow tail. We've never followed it out more than three weeks, at which time the ventilatory CO_2 response curves were not quite back to normal.

COURNAND: From the point of view of ventilation, Riley and Houston [1951] in their so-called Everest experiment, which was done in Florida back in 1946, had found out that the hyperventilation persisted for period of one or two days.

KELLOGG: This was shown also, even earlier, by Schneider [1913] of the Pike's Peak Expedition. He showed that the hyperventilation persisted for a matter of weeks after descent from altitude.

SEVERINGHAUS: It seems to me that your experiments with Eger [1968] certainly made it clear that there is at least a dual mechanism: the lactic acid production from the hypoxia plus whatever mechanism is lowering bicarbonate. But it certainly is clear that hyperventilation by whatever mechanism does lower CSF bicarbonate, so that when there is hypoxic hyperventilation, you wouldn't expect to have a stoichiometric relationship between the increased lactate and the decreased bicarbonate. On the other hand, if you keep the plasma bicarbonate constant and prevent the hyperventilation effect on it as Singer and I did some years ago, then it is possible to show a stoichiometric relationship. That is, the rise of CSF lactate was 2 meq/l. with prolonged steady-state hyperventilation at constant plasma bicarbonate, and the fall of CSF bicarbonate exactly matched that. I'd like to comment and ask about the interesting phenomenon of central hypoxic depression that remains poorly understood. You've seen it and commented on it, and Sørensen [1970] noted it when he exposed goats and rabbits to hypoxia after denervating the peripheral chemoreceptors. It's true that these animals acclimatized in the sense that their CSF bicarbonate was lower. It's not quite the same, however, because when breathing the hypoxic mixture, the denervated animals are more hypoxic and have a higher P_{CO_2} than the normals. A typical figure at altitude would be a P_{CO_2} of perhaps 30 in a goat not denervated, and perhaps 37 or 38 in a denervated one. But when both animals are given oxygen, they come to about the same P_{CO_2} of around 34 or 35. Thus there is this curious central hypoxic depression. Do you have any idea what causes it? Is it simply neural in the presence of apparently normal cerebral function? For instance, the natives of high altitudes show this same phenomenon. You can often see a native who is functioning perfectly normally. Give him oxygen and he increases his ventilation. What is the nature of this central hypoxic depression?

KELLOGG: I wish I knew. I have no idea whatever. You were speaking of the work you did with Singer. Perhaps we should also consider the work that Mines and Sorensen [1971] did in keeping the arterial pH, P_{CO_2}, and bicarbonate at normal levels in anesthetized dogs made hypoxic. In these cases there was still not a stoichiometric relationship between the lactate rise and the bicarbonate fall. Again a large discrepancy.

SEVERINGHAUS: Yes, I think that's interesting, because the experiments I was citing were not hypoxic but were hypocapnic.

KELLOGG: These experiments might be considered the converse.

SEVERINGHAUS: Of course, it's also appropriate to mention that the lactate production during hypoxia is a continuous flux from inside the cells to the extracellular fluid to the blood, apparently in rather large amounts, whereas the bicarbonate turnover in CSF is probably much slower and, as you just mentioned, chloride makes up most of the difference.

SIESJÖ: Just a very short remark about stoichiometry, lactate, bicarbonate, and other substances which could influence the acid-base state in the CSF. Dr. Hindfeldt of my laboratory has run a series of experiments with ammonia intoxication. Under these circumstances he can get quite a substantial increase in the lactate concentration of the CSF without any decrease in bicarbonate.

LOESCHCKE: I might give another partial contribution in response to Dr. Cournand's question, since a long time ago I followed the restitution of acid-base balance and the response of ventilation to CO_2 before and after the end of pregnancy (DÖRING and LOESCHCKE [1947]). The changes due to pregnancy regress in a few days, but just as you said, with a long tail that does not end before 14 days.

KELLOGG: Speaking of this restitution, there is something which has worried me and which I'd like to mention to worry a few other people. If things start changing as rapidly as we think they do, then it seems to me that we ought to get some appreciable acclimati-

zation during the measurement of the ventilatory response to CO_2. In our laboratory we typically use seven steps of 10 min each. progressively ascending and then descending again. The test thus involves about an hour of slightly hyperoxic hypercapnia. We should see a hysteresis loop in the response curve, but we don't. The later points are sometimes a little on one side, sometimes a little on the other side, or sometimes together with the earlier points. There's no systematic appearance of a loop, but I don't know why.

SEVERINGHAUS: I think it's fairly clear from Pappenheimer's perfusion work [1965], which Dr. Fencl might like to comment on, that the medullary chemoreceptors are somewhat delayed behind the cisternal fluid. What they see and what we sample in animals is usually cisternal fluid, so I've always thought that may be we just aren't waiting long enough. In addition, of course, the chemoreceptor bicarbonate is to some extent related to blood bicarbonate, not just cisternal.

BÖNING: During very short hyperventilation periods of 5 to 7 min Rapoport and associates [1946] could not find a change of the chloride concentration of whole blood, but unfortunately they did not measure the base excess value.

BARGETON: Is it possible that the concentration changes are caused by evaporation of water during hyperventilation? How many liters did the test subjects inspire per minute?

BÖNING: This was different because the ventilation was adjusted to reach an endexpiratory CO_2 concentration of 3%. The value may be around 20 l./min.

KELLOGG: During normal ventilation approximately 0.3 ml H_2O min are evaporated. The water loss in the experiments cannot be much greater than 1 ml/min.

BÖNING: Base excess, standard bicarbonate, or buffer base are used to describe nonrespiratory disturbances of acid base equilibrium. But they are all defined for blood under *in vitro* conditions; *in vivo* bicarbonate may exchange with the interstitial fluid during increase or decrease of P_{CO_2}. It is an established fact that base excess and standard bicarbonate decrease during respiratory acidosis of only some minutes duration— about 1 meq/l. for 0.14 pH (SHAW and MESSER [1932], SIGGAARD-ANDERSEN [1962], MICHEL et al. [1966], BÖNING [1968], and

BÖNING and HEINRICH [1968]). With regard to a short respiratory alkalosis there exists no consense. Some authors describe a temporary increase (PRYS-ROBERTS et al. [1966], and ENGEL et al [1969]); some however, a decrease in base excess (PAPADOPOULOS and KEATS [1959], and EICHENHOLTZ et al. [1962]). In this situation lactic acid is formed which imposes a metabolic acidosis in a strict sense.

In our experiments 11 young men hyperventilated for 35 min in supine position after a control period of 30 min. Figure 3 shows means ± standard errors of pH and Pco_2 in earlobe blood. pH reaches an average value of 7.66, Pco_2 decreases to about 19 torr.

Base excess, determined by the equilibration method according to ASTRUP [1969], and electrolyte concentrations were measured in blood drawn from a superficial vein of the forearm. The arm was warmed by an electric pad and infrared lamp in order to exclude local effects of the arm tissue. The lower curve of the two in the middle of Figure 3 (filled circles) shows the base excess. There is a small but significant rise ($p < 0.01$) of the base excess, especially during the first half of the hyperventilation period. These results could be confirmed in some additional experiments where we used only earlobe blood.

In order to exclude the metabolic effects in strict sense, we summed up the lactic acid concentration in whole blood and the base excess value. Changes of this sum B.E. + Lac^- indicate effects other than those of lactic acid. These values are shown in the upper middle curve of Figure 3 (open circles). There is an increase of B.E. + Lac^- of 2 meq/l. during hyperventilation which is greater than that of base excess alone. This indicates an uptake of 2 meq/l. blood of bicarbonate from the interstitial fluid. But bicarbonate cannot migrate alone. It must be accompanied by cations or exchanged for other anions.

Different electrolyte concentrations are altered in whole blood during hyperventilation (Figure 4). [Na^+] decreases ($p < 0.01$), [K^+] increases ($p < 0.01$), both about 2 meq/l. This is mainly the effect of an hematocrit rise. The chloride concentration decreases about 2 meq/l. This depends partly on the hematocrit rise, but also on a chloride shift from the red cells to plasma and from plasma to the interstitial fluid. If we sum up all these electrolyte concentration changes, the increase of B.E. + Lac^- is in the most part explained. The effect of the ion shifts on base excess is partly cancelled by the formation of lactic acid. During short respiratory alkalosis base excess is therefore

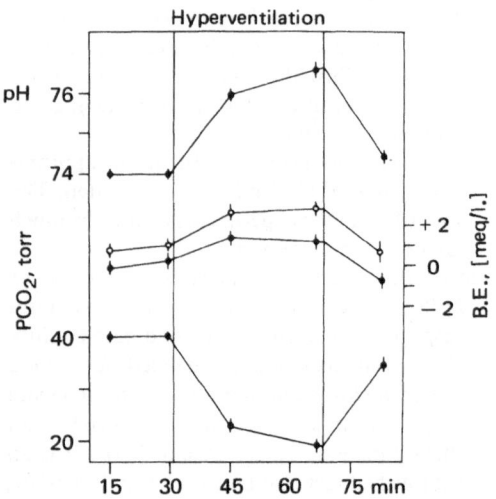

Fig. 3. Acid-base equilibrium during hyperventilation experiments ($n = 11$). Means ± standard errors. Open circles: B.E. + Lac^-.

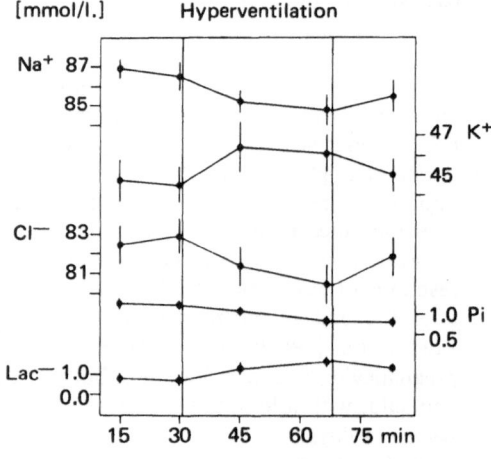

Fig. 4. Electrolyte concentrations in whole blood during hyperventilation experiments ($n = 11$). Means ± standard errors. P_i, inorganic phosphate.

not an exact measure of slight metabolic disturbances of acid-base equilibrium.

SEVERINGHAUS: We found similar changes of base excess during investigations on cerebral circulation.

Bibliography

Astrup, P., Jørgensen, K., Siggard Andersen, O., and Engel, K., "The acid-base metabolism. A new approach." *Lancet* 1:1035–39 (1960).

Böning, D., "Veränderungen der CO_2-Bindungskurve des Blutes bei akuter respiratorisches Acidose und ihre Ursachen. I. Untersuchungen an Hunden." *Pflüg. Arch. Physiol.* 302:133–48 (1968).

———, and Heinrich, K. W., "Veränderungen der CO_2-Bindungskurve des Blutes bei akuter respiratorischer Acidose und ihre Ursachen. II. Untersuchungen am Menschen." *Pflüg. Arch. Physiol.* 303:162–72 (1968).

Döring, G. K., and Loeschcke, H. H., "Atmung und Säure-Basengleichgewicht in der Schwangerschaft." *Pflüg. Arch. Ges. Physiol.* 249:437–51 (1947).

Eger, E. I., II, Kellogg, R. H., Mines, A. H., Lima-Ostos, M., Morrill, C. G., and Kent, D. W., "Influence of CO_2 on ventilatory acclimatization to altitude." *J. Appl. Physiol.* 24:607–15 (1968).

Eichenholz, A., Mulhausen, R. O., Anderson, W. E., and MacDonald, F. M., "Primary hypocapnia: a cause of metabolic acidosis." *J. Appl. Physiol.* 17:283–88 (1962).

Engel, K., Kildeberg, P., and Winters, R. W., "Quantitative displacement of blood acid-base status in acute hypocapnia." *Scand. J. Clin. Lab. Invest.* 23:5–17 (1969).

Kellogg, R. H., "The role of CO_2 in altitude acclimatization." pp. 379–85 in: *The Regulation of Human Respiration*, edited by D. J. C. Cunningham and B. B. Lloyd. Oxford: Blackwell (1963).

Kronenberg, R. S., and Cain, S. M., "Effects of acetazolamide and hypoxia on cerebrospinal fluid bicarbonate." *J. Appl. Physiol.* 24:17–20 (1968).

Michel, C. C., Lloyd, B. B., and Cunningham, D. J. C., "The *in vivo* carbon dioxide dissociation curve of true plasma." *Resp. Physiol.* 1:121–37 (1966).

Mines, A. H., and Sørensen, S. C., "Changes in the electrochemical potential difference for $HCO_3{}^-$ between blood and cerebrospinal fluid and in cerebrospinal fluid lactate concentration during isocarbic hypoxia." *Acta Physiol. Scand.* 81:225–33 (1971).

Morrill, C. G., "Cerebrospinal fluid changes and exercise effects in ventilatory acclimatization to hypoxia." Doctoral dissertation. San Francisco: University of California (1970).

Papadopoulos, C. N., and Keats, A. S., "The metabolic acidosis of hyperventilation produced by controlled respiration." *Anesthesiology* 20:156–61 (1959).

Pappenheimer, J. R., Fencl, V., Heisey, S. R., and Held, D., "Role of cerebral fluids in control of respiration as studied in unanesthetized goats." *J. Appl. Physiol.* 208:436–50 (1965).

Prys-Roberts, C., Kelman, G. R., and Nunn, J. F., "Determination of the in vivo carbon dioxide titration curve of anaesthetized man." *Brit. J. Anaesth.* 38:500–509 (1966).

Riley, R. L., and Houston, C. S., "Composition of alveolar air and volume of pulmonary ventilation during long exposure to high altitude." *J. Appl. Physiol.* 3:526–34 (1951).

Schneider, E. C., "Physiological observations following descent from Pike's Peak to Colorado Springs." *Am. J. Physiol.* 32:295–308 (1913).

Shaw, L. A., and Messer, A. C., "The transfer of bicarbonate between the blood and tissues caused by alterations of the carbon dioxide concentration in the lungs." *Am. J. Physiol.* 100:122–36 (1932).

Siggaard-Andersen, O., "Acute experimental acid-base disturbances in dogs. An investigation of the acid-base and electrolyte content of blood and urine." *Scand. J. Clin. Lab. Invest.* 14, Suppl. 66:1–20 (1962).

Sørensen, S. C., and Mines, A. H., "Ventilatory responses to acute and chronic hypoxia in goats after sinus nerve section." *J. Appl. Physiol.* 28:832–35 (1970).

———. "Ventilatory acclimatization to hypoxia in rabbits after denervation of peripheral chemoreceptors." *J. Appl. Physiol.* 28:836–39 (1970).

Part VI

Mathematical Models for Carbon Dioxide Regulation

1. Regulation of the Carbon Dioxide of Arterial Blood by Ventilation

Daniel Bargeton, B. Chambille, H. Guenard, and J. de Lattre

Département de Physiologie Humaine,
U.E.R. Biomédicale Paris-Sts Perès and U 81 INSERM
Faculté de Médecine
45 rue des Sts Pères, 75 Paris VIè, France

The production of CO_2 in the normal organism may undergo changes from 1 to 20. Since the unique route of elimination is the expired gas, if the alveolar ventilation did not change, the alveolar pressure of CO_2, hence its pressure in arterial blood, would also change in the ratio of 1 to 20.

Actually, the arterial pressure of CO_2 changes only of a small fraction of its normal value, and this indicates how efficient is the adaptation of alveolar ventilation to metabolic needs.

This result is due to the high sensitivity of the ventilation to the changes of arterial CO_2 pressure.

Two important characteristics of arterial blood are functionally related to PA_{CO_2}.

Solving the R equation for PA_{CO_2} gives:

$$P_aO_2 = PI_{O_2} - \frac{1 - FI_{O_2}(1 - R)}{R} Pa_{CO_2}$$

The Hasselbach Henderson equation gives:

$$pH = pK + \log \frac{[CO_3H^-]}{\alpha P_{CO_2}}$$

Thus if Pa_{CO_2} is stabilized, at the same time the O_2 pressure and the H^+ concentration are stabilized. Thus the chemical regulation of breathing is a functional arrangement which stabilizes the pressure of the respiratory gases and the H^+ concentration in the arterial blood by changes of the alveolar ventilation.

Incidentally, it may be pointed out that if the term "chemical regulation of breathing" has a clear physiological meaning, the expression of regulation of the ventilation, although very largely used, is unfortunate since ventilation is not a regulated but a regulating quantity.

The characteristics of this regulation are easy to express in the steady state.

The conservation of the mass gives:

$$\dot{V}CO_2 = FA_{CO_2}\dot{V}A = \frac{PA_{CO_2}}{PB - 47}\dot{V}A$$

Solving for $\dot{V}A$:

$$\dot{V}A = \dot{V}CO_2 \frac{PB - 47}{PA_{CO_2}} \qquad (1)$$

On the other hand, ventilation is a function of PA_{CO_2}, and within the physiological range this function is approximately linear:

$$\dot{V}A = b(PA_{CO_2} - Po) \qquad (2)$$

It is convenient to solve the system of equations (1) and (2) graphically by plotting $\dot{V}A$ against PA_{CO_2}. The graph makes apparent the characteristic properties of the system.

For a given value of the metabolic rate, equation (1) shows that alveolar ventilation is a hyperbolic function of PA_{CO_2}.

For different values of the metabolic rate we get a family of hyperbolic arcs.

Equation (2) is represented within the physiological range by a segment of a straight line. Interception of this segment with isometabolic lines shows the corresponding values of PA_{CO_2} and $\dot{V}A$ for each metabolic load.

The sensitivity of the regulating system is indicated by the slope of straight line segment:

$$\text{Slope} = \frac{\Delta \dot{V}A}{\Delta PA_{CO_2}}$$

the greater the slope, the better PA_{CO_2} is stabilized against changing metabolic load (Figure 1).

Transient State

In transient states the exchange of CO_2 between different stores of the body, the circulation delays, and the rate of soaking the chemosensitive structures has to be taken into account. This leads to a system of non-linear differential equations. The theoretical aspects of the problem have been brilliantly developed by Defares.

Experimental Approach

The properties of the regulator have been investigated by imposing a CO_2 load, either of metabolic origin (muscular exercise) or by inhalation of CO_2 and recording at the same time the alveolar CO_2 pressure (input) and the alveolar ventilation (output).

Two forms of input have been used, either a step function or a sine wave. For some tasks such as estimation of steady-state sensitivity, transport delay, and time course of the response, step response analysis is preferable, if a large amount of data is available.

But where steady trends, internally

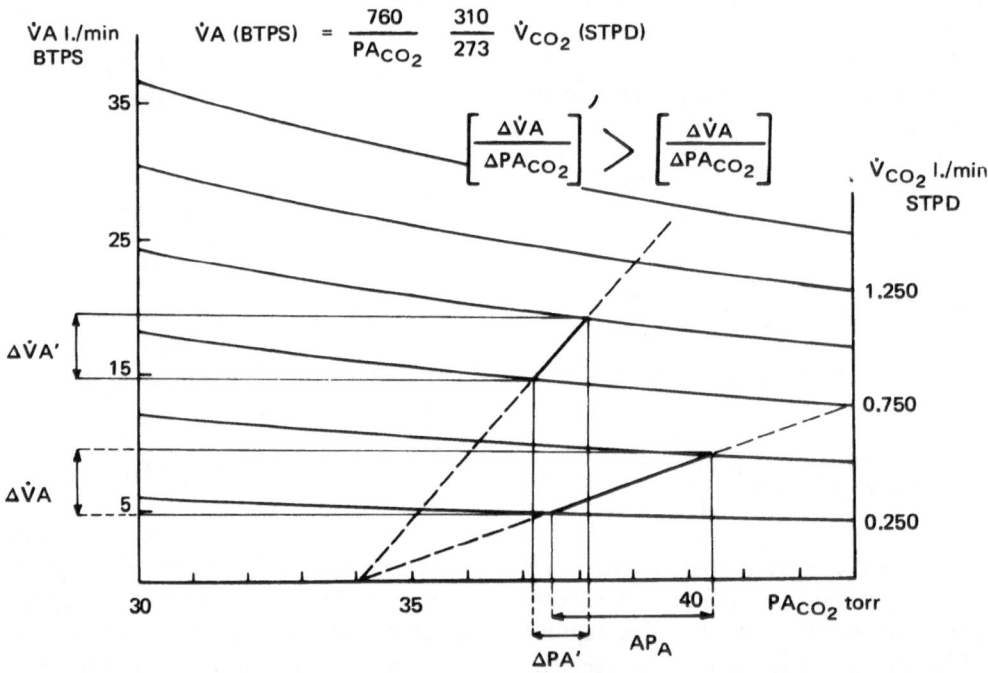

Fig. 1. Theoretical diagram showing the determination of the gain (or sensitivity) of the regulator by comparison of two steady states. The gain is indicated graphically by the slope of the straight line $\Delta \dot{V}A / \Delta PA_{CO_2}$.

generated output, or random noise must be separated from response to applied inputs, sine wave analysis is more powerful.

It must be remembered that many non-linear systems can be approximated within a limited range by a linear model.

This implies that experimental maneuvers must remain of small amplitude, hence the difficulty in extracting the elicited response from random noise of the same order of magnitude.

A third approach to the study of the regulator, although theoretically obvious, has been seldom used. It consists in merely observing the spontaneous behavior of the system submitted to internally generated rhythms or random noise.

These different approaches have been used in a descriptive study of the regulation of arterial CO_2 at rest and at moderate exercise.

Methods

Laboratory workers have been observed at rest and during moderate exercise (50 W and 90 W) on a bicycle ergometer.

Instantaneous values of ventilation, PE_{O_2} and PE_{CO_2} are recorded by a Fleisch pneumotachograph, a mass spectrometer (CSF), and are stored on magnetic tape.

A delay circuit is inserted in the pneumotachograph channel to compensate for the lag time due to the gas line of the spectrometer and to synchronize the signals of both instruments.

For each respiratory cycle analogue circuits gave the mean values:

$$\overline{P}A_{O_2}$$

$$\overline{P}A_{CO_2}$$

$$\overline{V}A$$

$$V_T$$

and the period T.

The mean value of alveolar gas was estimated by sampling the instantaneous values of PE_{O_2} and PE_{CO_2}, giving an instan-taneous value of r equal to the mean value r of the cycle.

Empirical observation indicates that this condition is met for an expired volume Vm such as:

$$Vm = V_D + \frac{V_T}{2} \pm 45 \text{ cm}^3$$

Alveolar ventilation $\overline{V}A$ was given by:

$$\overline{V}A = \frac{1}{T}(V_T - V_D)$$

and taking into account a slight change in dead space with the tidal volume:

$$\frac{V_D}{V_{DO}} = 0.827 + 0.183 \frac{V_T}{V_{TO}} \pm 0.138$$

The mean values $\overline{P}A_{O_2}$, $\overline{P}A_{CO_2}$, and $\overline{V}A$ of each cycle were stored on magnetic tape to be processed by a multichannel analyzer for averaging and correlation analysis (Figures 2 and 3).

1. Observation of Ventilation at Rest, during Exercise (90 W), and during Inhalation of CO_2 at a Constant Flow Rate

CO_2 was administered at a constant flow rate, using the principle of the technique of Fenn and Craig. The original technique was slightly modified by inserting an electrovalve driven by a sign detector fed by the pneumotachograph signal. The inflow of CO_2 is interrupted during expiration and stored up to the next inspiration by displacing water in a bottle.

The amount of CO_2 inhaled is thus independent of the relative duration of inspiration and expiration.

Moreover, the effect of dead space is minimized or suppressed, since the CO_2 is discharged exponentially at the beginning of the inspiration, the end of inspiration receives pure atmospheric air.

At the same time as CO_2, nitrogen is added to the inspired air to keep the oxygen

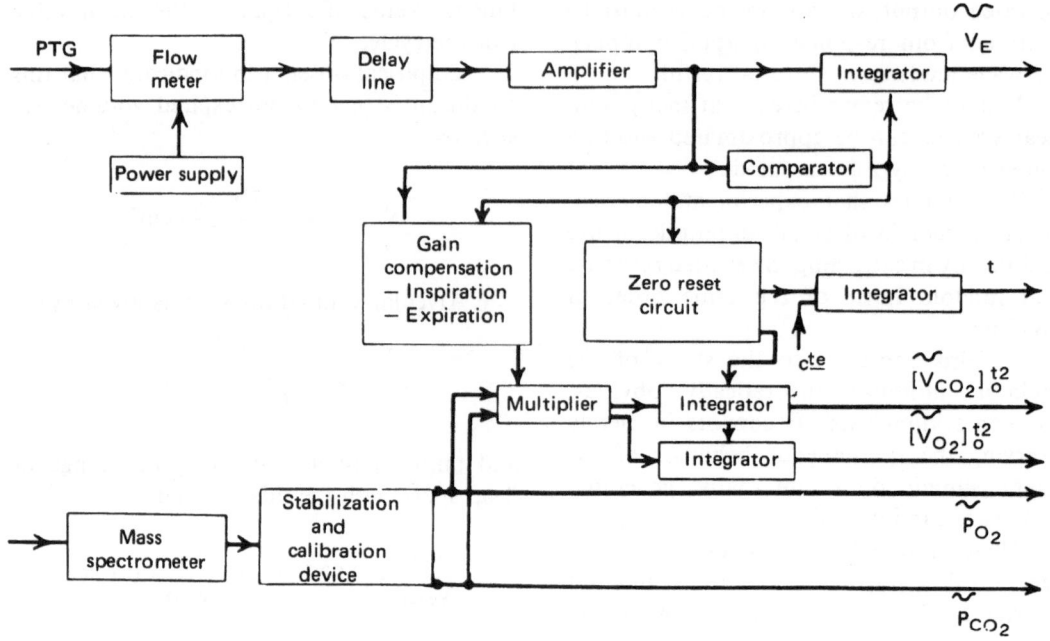

Fig. 2. Initial data computed on line and recorded on magnetic tape.

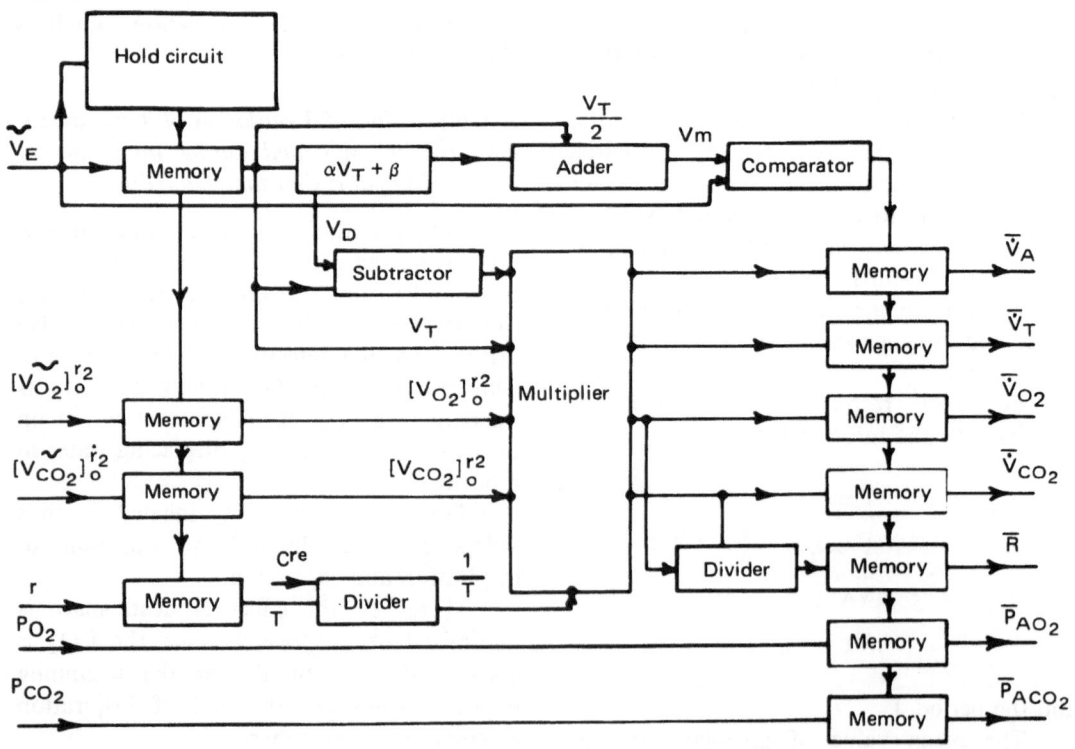

Fig. 3. Final data computed from magnetic tape recording played in reverse.

alveolar pressure constant despite hyperventilation.

This method of administering CO_2 is independent of the ventilation and of the pattern of breathing; a steady-state is reached in a shorter time than with an inhalation of a mixture at constant CO_2 concentration (Figure 4).

Results

The data obtained in three experiments of the same type on the same subject are averaged to minimize random variation without whipping out individual characteristics.

(1) In the three subjects alveolar ventilation is greater during exercise than at rest for the same value of CO_2 alveolar pressure. This is in accord with generally accepted knowledge.

(2) The regulation of CO_2 is a slow-working process; after a sudden change of the load, either metabolic or external, an approximate steady state is never achieved before 5 min.

(3) Immediate reactions are not consistent and markedly dependent on individual characteristics. In two subjects they are absent or not obvious.

One subject shows immediate ventilatory reactions of the type "accrochage" or "decrochage" at the beginning and the end of exercise, but the same type of immediate reaction exists at the beginning and the end of CO_2 inhalation.

(4) Visual inspection suggests that random variations of PA_{CO_2} and PA_{O_2} from cycle to cycle are more important at rest than during exercise (Figures 5 and 6).

2. Effects of Inhalation of CO_2 at Rest and during Exercise

The fact that for the same value of alveolar CO_2 pressure the alveolar ventilation is greater during exercise than at rest can be related:

(1) either to the additive effect of a stimulus generated by exercise (shift of the set point of the regulator)

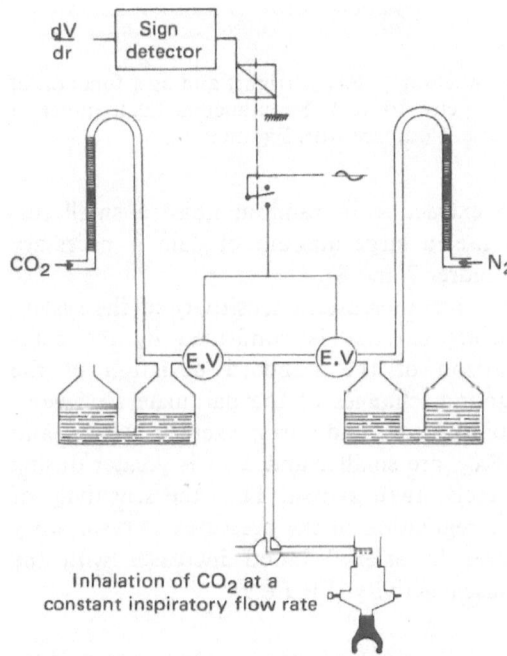

Fig. 4. Inhalation of CO_2 and N_2 at a constant mean flow rate. Electrovalves driven by the sign detector allows both gases to flow during inspiration and store them in displacement bottles during expiration.

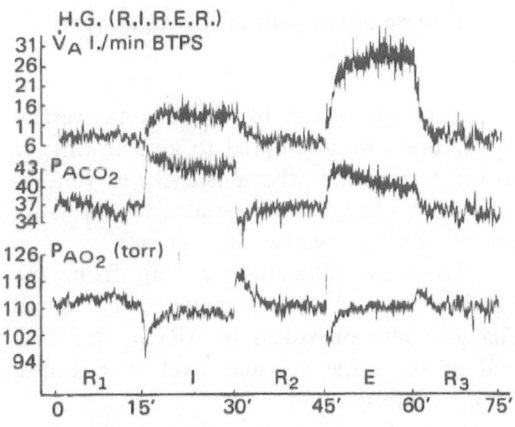

Fig. 5. $\dot{V}_A$, PA_{CO_2}, and PA_{O_2} as functions of time. Three experiments of the same type on the same subject are averaged. Successively: rest, inhalation of CO_2, rest, exercise 90 W, rest. This subject does not reach a steady state during a 15-min exercise. Marked overshoot of PA_{O_2}.

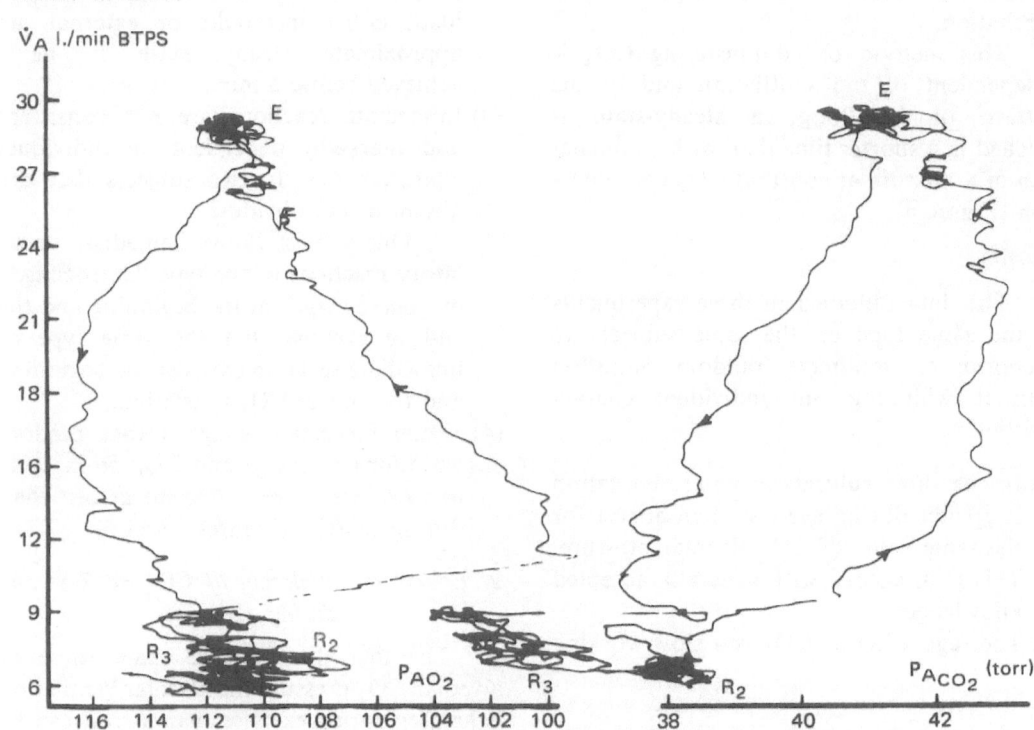

Fig. 6. Same data as in Figure 5. $\dot{V}_A$ recorded as a function of PA_{CO_2} (right) and as a function of PA_{O_2} (left). Transients from rest to exercise and from exercise to rest. Spontaneous fluctuations of PA_{CO_2} and PA_{O_2} are more important at rest than at exercise. Compare with Figure 9.

(2) to an increase of the sensitivity to CO_2 (increase of the gain of the regulator)
(3) or to both effects.

Since the matter has been controversial for decades, we attempted to give an answer to the question: Is the sensitivity of ventilation to a change in arterial CO_2 pressure greater during exercise than at rest?

To avoid difficulties arising from the nonlinearity of the system, very small changes were provoked in $\Delta PA_{CO_2} \leqslant 2$ torr and at the same average level at rest and during exercise.

In both subjects investigated, the slope $\Delta \dot{V}_A / \Delta PA_{CO_2}$ is statistically greater during exercise than at rest.

The experiment was performed on two subjects because of the time-consuming character of the procedure, since to be able to extract from random noise a small response, a large amount of data is necessary (Figures 7 and 8).

The increase in sensitivity of the system during exercise is confirmed by the comparison of the standard deviation of the random changes of the parameters of excitability at rest and during exercise. ΔPA_{CO_2} and ΔPA_{O_2} are smaller and $\Delta \dot{V}_A$ is greater during exercise than at rest. Thus the sensitivity of the regulation of the pressures of respiratory gases in arterial blood increases with the muscle activity (Figure 9).

3. Sinusoidal Variations of Carbon Dioxide in Inspired Air

In the hope of extracting more easily the response from random noise and thus to have the practical possibility of observing a

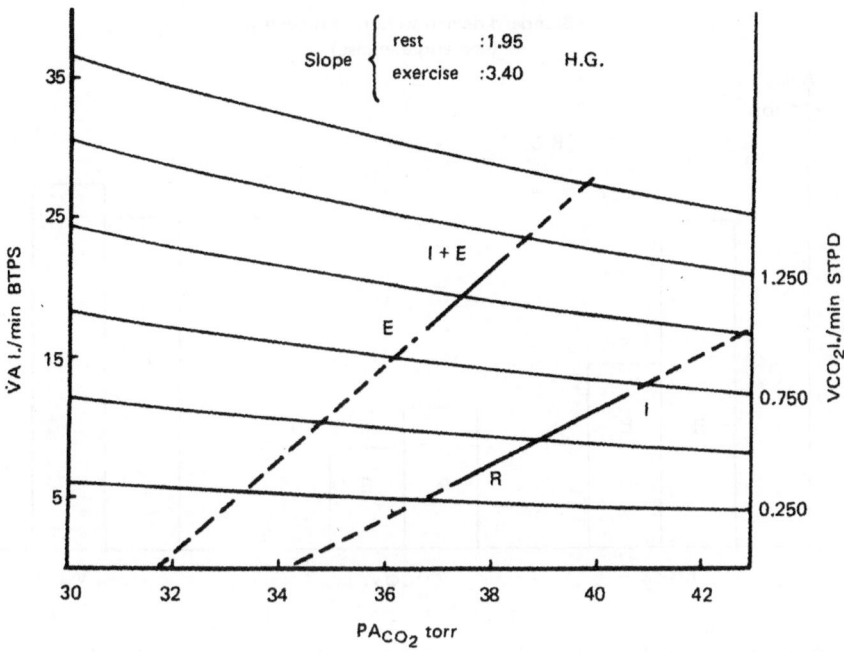

Fig. 7. Comparison of the slopes $\Delta \dot{V}_A/\Delta PA_{CO_2}$ at rest (R, I) and during exercise (E, I + E).

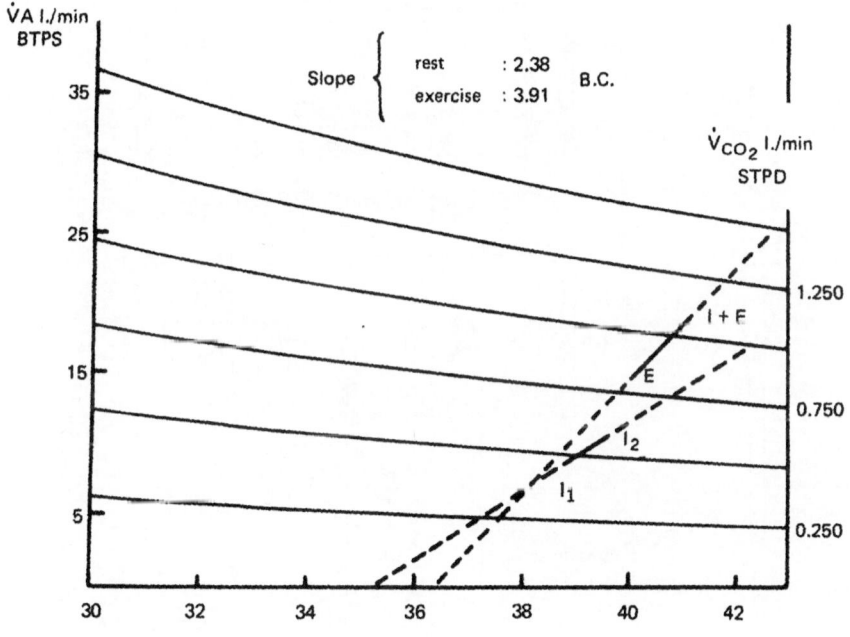

Fig. 8. Comparison of the slopes $\Delta \dot{V}_A/\Delta PA_{CO_2}$ at rest (I_1, I_2) and during exercise (E, I + E).

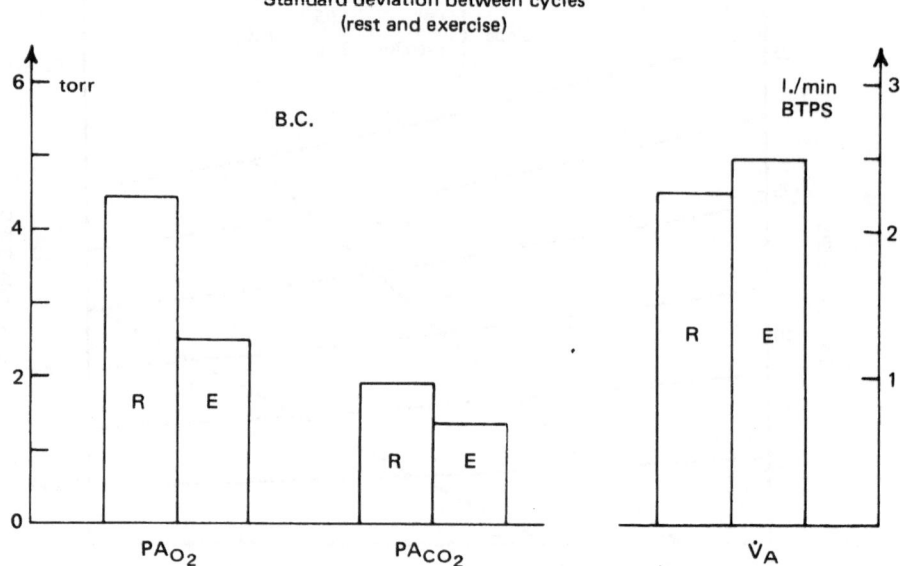

Fig. 9. Spontaneous fluctuations between cycles of PA_{CO_2}, PA_{O_2}, and $\dot{V}A$ during rest and exercise (50 W).

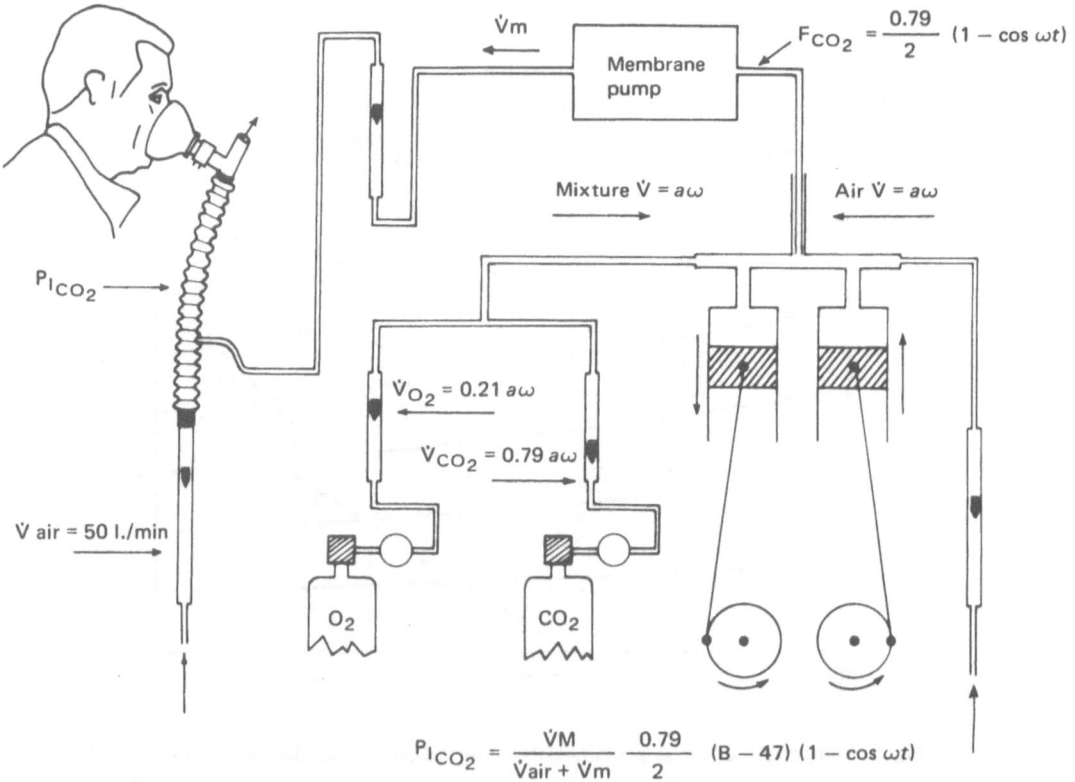

Fig. 10. Device for the production of FI_{CO_2} as a sinusoidal function of time.

greater number of subjects, experiments were done with sinusoidal variations of CO_2 in inspired air.

The distributing system is made of two piston pumps without valves driven in phase opposition and fed by a constant flow of air on one side and CO_2 on the other.

The sum of the outflow of both pumps is constant, and when they mix together they generate a constant flow of gas in which the CO_2 concentration is a sinusoidal function of time (Figure 10).

A sine-cosine potentiometer driven by the same shaft as the pumps delivers a reference sinusoidal voltage:

$$X = a \sin \omega t$$

The signal to be extracted is y:

$$y = b \sin (\omega t - \psi)$$

A multichannel analyzer fed by the magnetic tape record computes the cross-correlation function:

$$C(k\theta)xy = \frac{1}{T}\int_{t_1}^{t_1+T} X(t)\,Y(t-k\theta)\,dt$$

and the autocorrelation function

$$C(k\theta)xx = \frac{1}{T}\int_{t_1}^{t_1+T} X(t)\,X(t-k\theta)\,dt$$

with k integer and θ step of sampling.

The divisor T can be dropped and incorporated into the instrumental scale factor.

If the instrumental scale factors of the two channels are taken into account

$$X = \alpha\, a \sin \omega t$$

$$Y = \beta\, b \sin (\omega t - \psi)$$

it can be shown that

$$b = \frac{2}{\alpha\beta a}C(k\theta = -\psi)xy$$

$$\cos \psi = \frac{C(k\theta = 0)xy}{C(k\theta = -\psi)xy}$$

To eliminate the scale factors $\alpha\beta$, the autocorrelation function of the reference signal X is computed by feeding the channels α and β with the same signal X. Since

$$C(k\theta)xx = \frac{a\alpha\beta^2}{2}\cos k\theta$$

$$C(k\theta = 0)xx = \frac{\alpha\beta a^2}{2}$$

and

$$\alpha\beta = \frac{2}{a^2}C(k\theta = 0)$$

Thus

$$b = a\frac{C(k\theta = -\psi)xy}{C(k\theta = 0)xx}$$

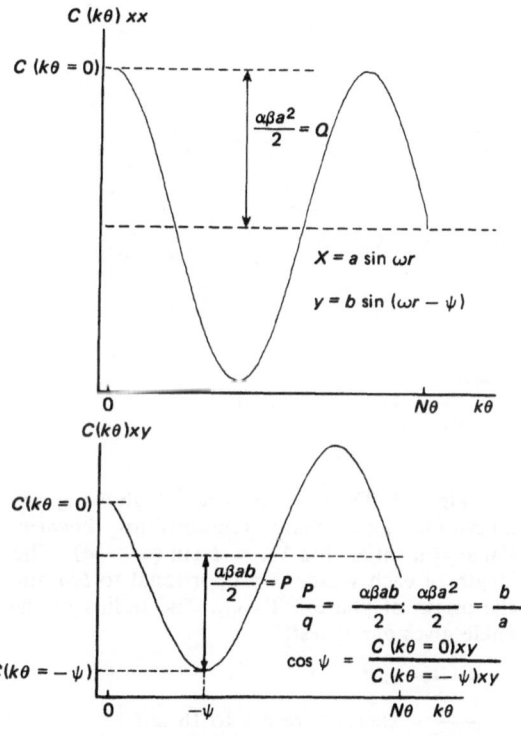

Fig. 11. Principle of computation of the cross correlation function $C(k\theta)$ xy and of the autocorrelation function $C(k\theta)$ xx.

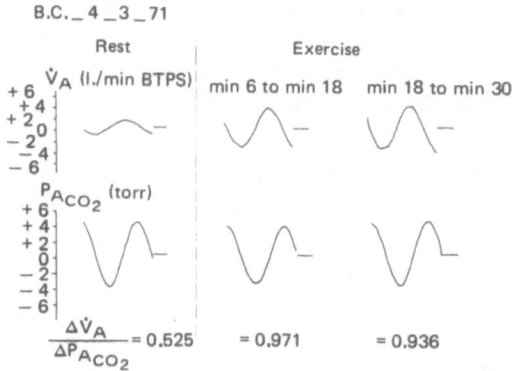

Fig. 12. Comparison of the sinusoidal variations of PA_{CO_2} and $\dot{V}A$ at rest and during exercise. The gain $\Delta\dot{V}A/\Delta PA_{CO_2}$ increases during exercise.

The same procedure is used to extract the PA_{CO_2} signal and the $\dot{V}A$ signal (Figure 11).

The determination of the phase difference is rather inaccurate and can be used only to give an order of magnitude.

The determination of the amplitude is much better and allows computation of the ratio of the amplitude of the periodic component of $\dot{V}A$ to PA_{CO_2}. This ratio can be taken as the sensitivity of the system at the frequency $1/T$. Most experiments have been done with $T = 120$ sec.

Previous spectrum analysis indicates that components of this order of frequency are negligible among the spontaneous noise of PA_{CO_2} and $\dot{V}A$.

Eight subjects have been observed. In all of them the sensitivity of ventilation to periodic stimulation is much less than in

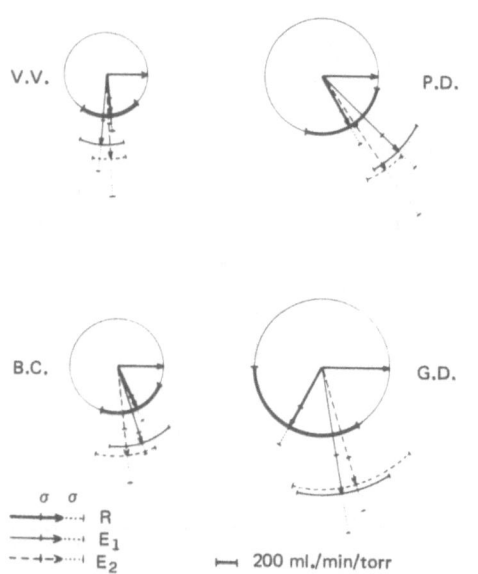

Fig. 13. Diagram of Fresnel showing the amplitude and phase relationships between $PA_{CO_2} = a \sin \omega t$ and $\dot{V}A = b \sin (\omega t - \varphi)$. The length of each vector is proportional to b/a and the origin of phase is PA_{CO_2}. The radius of the circle gives b/a at rest.

⟶ rest

⟶ exercise from 6 to 18 min

----→ exercise from 18 to 30 min

Standard deviation of the mean is given in amplitude and phase for each vector.

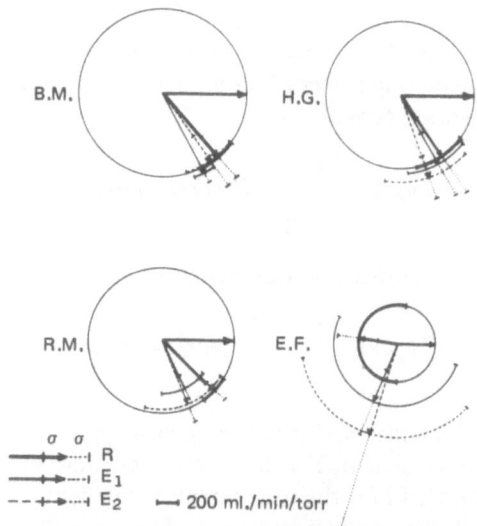

Fig. 14. Diagram of Fresnel showing the amplitude and phase relationships between $PA_{CO_2} = a \sin \omega t$ and $\dot{V}A = b \sin (\omega t - \varphi)$. The length of each vector is proportional to b/a and the origin of phase is PA_{CO_2}. The radius of the circle gives b/a at rest.

⟶ rest

⟶ exercise from 6 to 18 min

----→ exercise from 18 to 30 min

Standard deviation of the mean is given in amplitude and phase for each vector.

steady state. In four subjects the sensitivity to periodic stimulation is greater during exercise than at rest, and the difference is statistically significant (Figures 12 and 13). In the four other subjects the change of sensitivity with muscle activity is either absent or not statistically significant (Figure 14).

This indicates that the full development of the ventilatory reaction involves parts of the regulator entering into play very slowly. These slow-acting parts seem to play a prominent role in the increase of sensitivity during exercise.

General Comments

The regulation of the arterial pressure of CO_2 by the ventilation present the following features:

(1) It is a slow-acting process, the full development of which takes at least five minutes. This indicates that it cannot be driven by arterial chemoreceptors only, and this is in accord with the findings of Loeschcke and coworkers.
(2) Immediate reactions are inconstant and, if present, have a modest efficiency. They may have something to do with conditioning.
(3) There is an increase of the sensitivity of the regulator during exercise. The accuracy of the observations is insufficient to decide whether or not the increased sensitivity is only responsible for the extra-hyperpnoea of exercise.
(4) There are important individual differences in the behavior of the regulator, and it is perhaps not possible to describe a general regulatory pattern valid for the human species.

Attempts to reach an average pattern of reaction may be an arithmetical exercise bearing the same physiological significance as computing the average color of hair.

Bibliography

(1) $P_{A_{CO_2}}$

Asmussen, E., and Nielsen, M., "Ventilatory response to CO_2 during work at normal and at low oxygen tensions." *Acta Physiol. Scand.* 39:27–35 (1957).

Barr, P. O., Beckman, M., Bjurstedt, H., Brismar, J., Hesser, C. M., and Matell, G., "Time courses of blood gas changes provoked by light and moderate exercise in man." *Acta Physiol. Scand.* 60:1–17 (1964).

Bhattacharyva, N. K., Cunningham, D. J. C., Goode, R. C., Howson, M. G., Lloyd, B. B., "Hypoxia, ventilation, PCO_2, and exercise." *Respiration Physiology* 9:329–47 (1970).

Hickam, J. B., Pryor, W. W., Page, E. B., and Atwell, R. J., "Respiratory regulation during exercise in unconditioned subject," *J. Clin. Invest.* 30:503–16 (1951).

Holmgren, A., and Linderholm, H., "Oxygen and CO_2 tensions of arterial blood during heavy and exhaustive exercise." *Acta Physiol. Scand.* 44:203–15 (1958).

Lilienthal, J. L., Riley, R. L., Proemmel, D. D., and Franke, R. E., "An experimental analysis in man of the oxygen measure pressure gradient from alveolar air to arterial blood during rest and exercise at sea level and altitude." *Am. J. Physiol.* 147:199–216 (1946).

Suskind, M., Bruce, R. A., Mac Dowell, M. E., Yu, P. N. G., and Lovejoy, F. W. Jr., "Normal variations in end tidal air and arterial blood CO_2 and oxygen tensions during moderate exercise." *J. Appl. Physiol.* 3:282–90 (1950).

(2) pH

Arborelius, M., and Liljestrand, "Muskelarbeit und Blutreaktion." *Skand. Arch. Physiol.* (1923).

Barr, D. P., Himwick, H. E., and Green, R. P., "Studies in the physiology of muscular exercise—changes in acid-base equilibrium following short periods of vigorous muscular exercise." *J. Biol. Chem.* 55:495–515 (1923).

Barr, P. O., Beckman, M., Bjurstedt, H., Brismar, J., Hesser, C. M., and Matell, G., "Time courses of blood gas changes provoked by light and moderate exercise in man." *Acta Physiol. Scand.* 60:1–17 (1964).

Chiesa, A. C., Howell, J. B. L., Massoud,

A. A. E., and Stretton, T. B., "Acid-base changes in the arterial blood during exercise." *J. Physiol.* (London) 175:72–75 (1964).

Goldston, M., and Wollack, A. C., "Oxygen and CO_2 tensions of alveolar air and arterial blood in healthy young adults at rest and after exercise." *Am. J. Physiol.* 151:276–81 (1947).

Hickam, J. B., Pryor, W. W., Page, E. B., and Atwell, R. J., "Respiratory regulation during exercise in unconditioned subject." *J. Clin. Invest.* 30:503–16 (1951).

Holmgren, A., and Linderholm, H., "Oxygen and CO_2 tensions of arterial blood during heavy and exhaustive exercise." *Acta Physiol. Scand.* 44:203–15 (1958).

Lambersten, C. J., Owen, S. G., Wendel, H., Stroud, M. W., Lurie, A. A., Lochner, W., and Clark, G. F., "Respiratory and cerebral circulatory control during exercise at 0.21 and 2.0 atmospheres inspired Po_2." *J. Appl. Physiol.* 14:966–82 (1959).

(3) Pa_{O_2}

Bartels, H., Beer, R., Koepchen, H. P., Wenner, J., and Witt, I., "Messung der alveolär-arteriellen O_2 Druckdifferenz mit verschiedenen Methoden am Menschen bei Ruhe und Arbeit." *Pflüg. Arch. Physiol.* 261:133–51 (1955).

Bhattacharyva, N. K., Cunningham, D. J. C., Goode, R. C., Howson, M. G., and Lloyd, B. B., "Hypoxia, ventilation, PCO_2 and exercise." *Respiration Physiol.* 9:329–47 (1970).

Filley, G. F., Gregoire, F., and Wright, G. W., "Alveolar and arterial oxygen tensions and the significance of the alveolar-arterial oxygen tensions difference in normal men." *J. Clin. Invest.* 33:517–29 (1954).

Lilienthal, J. L., Riley, R. L., Proemmel, D. D., and Franke, R. E., "An experimental analysis in man of the oxygen measure pressure gradient from alveolar air to arterial blood during rest and exercise at sea level and altitude." *Am. J. Physiol.* 147:199–216 (1946).

Suskind, M., Bruce, R. A., Mac Dowell, M. E., Yu, P. N. G., and Lovejoy, F. W., Jr., "Normal variations in end tidal air and arterial blood CO_2 and oxygen tensions during moderate exercise." *J. Appl. Physiol.* 3:282–90 (1950).

(4) Body Temperature

Cotes, J. E., "The role of body temperature in controlling ventilation during exercise in one normal subject breathing oxygen." *J. Physiol.* (London) 129:554–63 (1955).

Cunningham, D. J. C., and O'Riordan, J. L. H., "The effect of a rise in the temperature of the body on the respiratory response to CO_2 at rest." *Quart. J. Exper. Physiol.* 42:329–45 (1957).

Whipp, B. J., and Wasserman, K., "Effect of body temperature on the ventilatory response to exercise." *Resp. Physiol.* 8:354–60 (1970).

(5) Transients

Barr, P. O., Beckman, M., Bjurstedt, H., Brismar, J., Hesser, C. M., and Matell, G., "Time courses of blood gas changes provoked by light and moderate exercise in man." *Acta Physiol. Scand.* 60:1–17 (1964).

Matell, G., "Time courses of changes in ventilation and arterial gas tensions in man induced by moderate exercise." *Acta Physiol. Scand.* 58:Suppl. 206 (1963).

Rahn, H., and Otis, A. B., "Continuous analysis of alveolar gas composition during work hypercapnia and anoxia." *J. Appl. Physiol.* 1:717–24 (1949).

Suskind, M., Bruce, R. A., Mac Dowell, M. E., Yu, P. N. G., and Lovejoy, F. W., Jr., "Normal variations in end tidal air and arterial blood CO_2 and oxygen tensions during moderate exercise." *J. Appl. Physiol.* 3:282–90 (1950).

(6) Gain

(a) Response to square wave function

Alexander, J. K., West, R. R., Wood, J. A., and Richards, D. W., "Analysis of the respiratory response to carbon dioxide inhalation in varying clinical states of hypercapnia, anoxia and acid base derangment." *J. Clin. Invest.* 34:511–32 (1955).

Asmussen, E., and Nielsen, M., "Ventilatory response to CO_2 during work at normal and at low oxygen tensions." *Acta Physiol. Scand.* 39:27–35 (1957).

Bannister, R. G., Cunningham, D. J. C., and Douglas, C. G., "The CO_2 stimulus to breathing in severe exercise." *J. Physiol.* (London) 125:90–117 (1954).

Beaver, W. L., and Wasserman, K., "Transients in ventilation at start and end of exercise." *J. Appl. Physiol.* 25:390–99 (1968).

Craig, F. N., "Pulmonary ventilation during exercise and inhalation of CO_2." *J. Appl. Physiol.* 7:467–71 (1955).

Cunningham, D. J. C., Lloyd, B. B., and Patrick, J. M., "The relation between ventilation and end tidal P_{CO_2} in man during moderate exercise with and without CO_2 inhalation." *J. Physiol.* 169:104P–106P (1963).

——, Shaw, D. G., Lahiri, S., and Lloyd, B. B., "The effect of maintained ammonium chloride acidosis on the relation between pulmonary ventilation and alveolar oxygen and carbon dioxide in man." *Quart. J. Exp. Physiol.* 46:323–34 (1961).

Fenn, W. O., and Craig, A. B., Jr., "Effect of CO_2 on respiration using a new method of administering CO_2." *J. Appl. Physiol.* 18: 1023–24 (1963).

Fuleihan, F. J. D., Nakada, T., Suero, J. T., Merrifield, E. S., Dutton, R. E., Permutt, S., and Riley, R. L., "Transient responses to CO_2 breathing of human subjects awake and asleep." *J. Appl. Physiol.* 18:289–94 (1963).

Haywood, C., and Bloete, M. E., "Respiratory responses of healthy young women to CO_2 inhalation." *J. Appl. Physiol.* 27:No. 1, 32–35 (1969).

Hickam, J. B., Pryor, W. W., Page, E. B., and Atwell, R. J., "Respiratory regulation during exercise in unconditioned subjects." *J. Clin. Invest.* 30:503–16 (1951).

Lambertsen, C. J., "Carbon dioxide and respiration in acid base homeostasis." *Anesthesiology* 21:642–51 (1960).

——, Kough, R. H., Cooper, D. Y., Emmel, G. L., Loeschcke, H. H., and Schmidt, C. F., "Comparison of relationship of respiratory minute volume to P_{CO_2} and pH of arterial and internal jugular blood in normal man during hyperventilation produced by low concentrations of CO_2 at 1 atmosphere and by O_2 at 3 atmospheres." *J. Appl. Physiol.* 5:803–13 (1953).

Lerche, D., Katsaros, B., Lerche, G., and Loeschcke, H. H., "Vergleich der Wirkung verschiedener Acidosen (NH_4CL, $CaCl_2$, Acetazolamid) auf die Lungenbelüftung beim Menschen." *Pflüg. Arch. Physiol.* 270: 450–60 (1959).

Matell, G., "Time courses of changes in ventilation and arterial gas tensions in man induced by moderate exercise." *Acta Physiol. Scand.* 58:Suppl. 206 (1963).

Milic-Emili, J., and Tyler, J. S., "Relation between work output of respiratory muscles and end tidal CO_2 tension." *J. Appl. Physiol.* 18:497–504 (1963).

Nielsen, M., "Untersuchungen über die Atemregulation beim Menschen." *Skand. Arch. Physiol.* 74:Suppl., 87–208 (1936).

Nielsen, M., and Asmussen, E. In *The regulation of human respiration.* Oxford: Blackwell, 503–13 (1963).

——, and Smith, H., "Studies on the regulation of respiration in acute hypoxia." *Acta Physiol. Scand.* 24:293–313 (1952).

Schaefer, K. E., "Respiratory pattern and respiratory response to CO_2." *J. Appl. Physiol.* 13:1–14 (1958).

Teillac, A., and Lefrancois, R., "Analyse des réactions ventilatoires aux cours des périodes d'adaptation et de récupération de l'exercice musculaire chez l'Homme." *J. Physiol.* (Paris) 54:417–18 (1962).

(b) Response to periodic stimulation

Bargeton, D., Barres, G., Gauge, P., and Durand, J., "Rôle de PA_{CO_2} dans la régulation de la ventilation de repos étudié en régime périodique." *J. Physiol.* 53:261–62 (1961).

Bellville, J. W., Fleischli, G., and Defares, J. G., "A new method of studying regulation of respiration. The response to sinusoidally varying CO_2 inhalation." *Computers Biomed. Res.* 2:329–49 (1969).

Stoll, P. J., "Respiratory system analysis based on sinusoidal variations of CO_2 in inspired air." *J. Appl. Physiol.* 27:389–99 (1969).

Thompson, J. P., "Analysis of respiratory control using sinusoidally varying inspired carbon dioxide." Master's thesis. Seattle, Washington: University of Washington (1962).

Wigertz, O., "Dynamics of ventilation and heart rate in response to sinusoidal work load in man." *J. Appl. Physiol.* 29:208–218 (1970).

(7) Chemoreceptors

(a) Peripheral

Black, A. M. S., Mac Closkey, D. I., Torrance, R. W., "The responses of carotid body chemoreceptors in the cat to sudden changes of hypercapnic and by hypoxic stimuli." *Resp. Physiol.* 13:36–49 (1971).

————, and Torrance, R. W., *Arterial chemoreceptors*. R. W. Torrance, ed. Oxford: Blackwell (1968).

Biscoe, M., "Effects of inhalation anaesthetics on carotid body chemoreceptor activity." *Brit. J. Anaesth.* 40:2–12 (1968).

Dutton, P. E., Fitzgerald, R. S., and Cross, N., "Ventilatory response to square-wave forcing of CO_2 at the carotid bodies." *Resp. Physiol.* 4:101–108 (1968).

Gray, B. A., "Response of the perfused carotid body to changes in pH and P_{CO_2}." *Resp. Physiol.* 4:229–45 (1968).

Guz, A., Noble, M., Widdicombe, J. G., Trenchard, D., and Mushin, W. W., "The effect of bilateral block of vagus and glosso pharynged on the ventilatory response to CO_2 of a consciens man." *Resp. Physiol.* 1:206–10, 38–40 (1966).

Kao, F. F., Michel, C. C., and Mei, S. S., "Carbon dioxide and pulmonary ventilation in muscular exercise." *J. Appl. Physiol.* 19:1075–80 (1964).

Katsaros, B., "Die Rolle der Chemoreceptoren des Carotisgebiets der narkotisieten Katze für die Antwort der Atmung auf isolierte Anderung der Wasserstoffionen Koncentration und der CO_2-Drucks des Blutes." *Pflüg. Arch. Physiol.* 282:157–78 (1964).

Mitchell, R. A., Carman, C. T., Severinghaus, J. W., Richardson, B. W., Singer, M. M., and Shnider, S. J., "Stability of cerebrospinal fluid pH in chronic acid base disturbances in blood. *J. Appl. Physiol.* 20:443–52 (1965).

Natsui, T., "Respiratory response to arterial H^+ at different levels of arterial P_{CO_2} during hyperoxia or hypoxia." *Pflüg. Arch.* 316:34–50 (1970).

Tenney, S. M., and Brooks, J. G., "Carotid bodies, stimulus interaction and ventilatory control in unaesthetized goats." *Resp. Physiol.* 1:211–23 (1966).

(b) Central

Fencl, V., Miller, T. B., and Pappenheimer, J. R., "Studies on the respiratory response to disturbances of acid-base balance, with deductions concerning the ionic composition of cerebral interstitial fluid." *Am. J. Physiol.* 210:459–72 (1966).

Fitzgerald, R. S., Gross, N., and Dutton, R. E., "Ventilatory responses to transient acidic and hypercapnic vertebral artery infusions." *Resp. Physiol.* 4:387–95 (1968).

Lambertsen, C. J., "Carbon dioxide and respiration in acid base homeostasis." *Anesthesiology* 21:642–51 (1960).

————, Semple, S. J. G., Smyth, M. G., and Gelfand, R., "H^+ and P_{CO_2} as chemical factors in respiratory and cerebral circulatory control." *J. Appl. Physiol.* 16:473–84 (1961).

Lensen, J. R., "Influence du pH du liquide céphalo-rachidien sur la respiration." *Experientia* (Basel) 6:272 (1950).

Loeschcke, H. H., "On specificity of CO_2 as a respiratory stimulus." *Bull. Physiol. Path. Resp.* 5:13–25 (1969).

————, Katsaros, B., and Lerche, D., "Differenzierung der Wirkungen von CO_2-Druck und Wasserstoffinen-konzentration im Blut auf die Atmung beim Menschen." *Pflüg. Arch. Physiol.* 270:461–66 (1960).

————, Koepchen, H. P., and Gertz, K. H., "Uber den Einfluss von Wasserstoffinenkonzentration und CO_2-Druck im Liquor cerebrospinalis auf die Atmung." *Pflüg. Arch. Physiol.* 266:569–85 (1958).

————, De Lattre, J., and Schläfke, M., "Reizversuche an der ventralen oberfläche der Medulla oblongata der Katze mit Beobachtung von Atmung und Blutdruck." *Pflüg. Arch. Physiol.* 297:R42 (1967).

Michel, C. C., "CSF (HCO_3) during respiratory acid base disturbance." *J. Physiol.* (London) 170:66P–67P (1964).

Mitchell, R. A., Loeschcke, H. H., Massion, W. H., and Severinghaus, J. W., "Respiratory responses mediated through superficial chemosensitive areas on the medulla." *J. Appl. Physiol.* 18:523–33 (1963).

Natsui, T., "Respiratory response to arterial H^+ at different levels of arterial pCO_2 during hyperoxia or hypoxia." *Pflüg. Arch.* 316:34–50 (1970).

Pappenheimer, J. R., Fencl, V., Heisey, S. R., and Held, D., "Role of cerebral fluids in control of respiration as studied in unanesthetized goats." *Am. J. Physiol.* 208:436–50 (1965).

Severinghaus, J. W., Mitchell, R. A., Richardson, B. W., and Singer, M. M., "Respiratory control at high altitude suggesting active transport regulation of CSF pH." *J. Appl. Physiol.* 18:1155–66 (1963).

Winterstein, H., and Gökhan, N., "Ammoniumchlorid Acidose und Reaktionstheorie der

Atmungsregulation." *Arch. Internat. Pharmacodyn.* 93:212–32 (1953).

(8) Theories

(a) Chemical drive

Douglas, C. G., and Haldane, J. S., "Die Regulation der Atmung beim Menschen." *Ergebn. Physiol.* 14:338–430 (1914).

Haldane, J. S., and Priestly, J. G., "The regulation of the lung ventilation." *J. Physiol.* (London) 32:225–66 (1905).

Winterstein, H., "Die Regulierung der Atmung durch das Blut." *Pflüg. Arch. Physiol.* 138:167–84 (1911).

(b) Multiple factors theory

Comroe, J. H., "The hyperpnea of muscular exercise." *Physiol. Rev.* 24:319–39 (1944).

Cunningham, D. J. C., "Some quantitative aspects of the regulation of human respiration in exercise." *Brit. Medi. Bull.* 19:25–30 (1963).

Gray, J. S. *Pulmonary ventilation and its physiological regulation.* Springfield, Ill.: Charles C. Thomas (1950).

Grodins, F. S., "Analysis of factors concerned in regulation of breathing in exercise." *Physiol. rev.* 30:220–39 (1950).

Lambertsen, C. J., "Respiration," in P. Bard, *Medical physiology*, 11th ed. St Louis: Mosby (1961).

Winterstein, H., "Die Regulierung der Atmung durch das Blut." *Pflüg. Arch. Physiol.* 138:167–84 (1911).

(c) Neurohumoral theory

Asmussen, E., Mielsen, M., and Wieth-Pedersen, G., "Cortical or reflex control of respiration during muscular work." *Acta Physiol. Scand.* 6:168–75 (1943).

Beaver, W. L., and Wasserman, K., "Transients in ventilation at start and end of exercise." *J. Appl. Physiol.* 25:390–99 (1968).

Craig, F. N., Cummings, E. G., and Blevins, W. V., "Regulation of breathing at beginning of exercise." *J. Appl. Physiol.* 18:1183–87 (1963).

Cunningham, D. J. C., and Gee, J. B. L., "The effect of carbon dioxide on the respiratory reponse to want oxygen in man." *Quart. J. Exp. Physiol.* 42:303 (1957).

Dejours, P., "La régulation de la ventilation au cours de l'exercice musculaire chez l'Homme." *J. Physiol.* 51:163–261 (1959).

———. "The regulation of breathing during muscular exercise in man. A neurohumoral theory." In *The regulation of human respiration*, D. J. C. Cunningham and Lloyd, eds. Oxford: Blackwell Scientific Publications (1963).

———. "Control of respiration in muscular exercise." In W. O. Fenn and H. Rahn. *Handbook of physiology*, section 3, vol. 1. Washington D.C.: American Physiological Society (1964).

———, Betchel-Labrousse, Y., and Raynaud, J., "Etude du contrôle de la fréquence cardiaque et de la ventilation cours des exercices passif et actif chez l'Homme." *C.R. Acad. Sci.* (Paris) 252:2012–14 (1961).

———, Raynaud, J., Cuenod, C. L., and Labrousse, Y., "Modifications instantanées de la ventilation au début et à l'arrêt de l'exercice musculaire. Interpretation." *J. Physiol.* (Paris) 47:155–159 (1955).

Harrison, W. G., Jr., Calhoun, J. A., Harrison, T. R., "Afferent impulses as a cause of increased ventilation during muscular exercise." *Am. J. Physiol.* 100:68–73 (1932).

Hornbein, T. F., Sorensen, S. C., and Parks, C. R., "Role of muscle spindles in lower extremities in breathing during bicycle exercise." *J. Appl. Physiol.* 27:4, 476–79 (1969).

Hutt, B. K., Horvath, S. M., and Spurr, G. B., "Influence of varying degrees of passive limb movements on respiration and oxygen consumption of man." *J. Appl. Physiol.* 12:297–300 (1958).

Kao, F. F., "The regulation of breathing during muscular exercise in man. A neurohumoral theory." In *The regulation of human respiration*. D. J. C. Cunningham and Lloyd, eds. Oxford: Blackwell Scientific Publications (1963).

———, Schlig, B., and Mac Brooks, C., "Regulation of respiration during induced muscular work in decerebrate dogs." *J. Appl. Physiol.* 7:379–86 (1955).

Krogh, A., and Lindhard, J., "The regulation of respiration and circulation during the initial stages of muscular work." *J. Physiol.* (London) 47:112–36 (1913).

Nielsen, M., and Asmussen, E. In *The regulation of human respiration.* Oxford: Blackwell Scientific Publications (1963).

Teillac, A., and Lefrancois, R., "Analyse des réactions ventilatoires aux cours des périodes d'adaption et de récupération de l'exercice musculaire chez l'Homme." *J. Physiol.* (Paris) 54:417–18 (1962).

Wigertz, O., "Dynamics of ventilation and heart rate in response to sinusoidal work load in man." *J. Appl. Physiol.* 29:208–18 (1970).

(9) Technology

Bargeton, D., "Analysis of capnigram and oxigram in man." *Bull. Physio-Path. Resp.* (Nancy) 3:503–26 (1967).

———, De Lattre, J., Durand, J. Y., and Florentin, E., "Montages analogiques permettant la détermination continue cycle par cycle des paramètres alveolaires." *Génie biologique et medical* 1:142–46 (1970).

Barres, G., De Lattre, J., Duhaze, P., and Durand, J. Y., "Une chaîne de pneumotachographie fournissant directement les résultats dans les conditions alvéolaires." *J. Physiol.* (Paris) 58:646–47 (1966).

Fenn, W. O., and Craig, A. B., Jr., "Effect of CO_2 on respiration using a new method of administering CO_2." *J. Appl. Physiol.* 18:1023–24 (1963).

De Lattre, J., Florentin, E., and Bargeton, D., "Enregistrement continu cycle par cycle des paramètres alvéolaires." *J. Physiol.* (Paris) 61:115–16 (1969).

Discussion

LOESCHKE: Professor Bargeton, you probably know that I considered these experiments with the oscillating regime as most ingenious, but I have a question to raise—the slope of the CO_2 response which you get with the small changes, small oscillatory changes, seems to be about 0.5 liters per torr. This is less than what we determined in a more static way. The reason may either be that in the oscillatory way you do not get steady states, and this is certainly part of it, but the other possibility may be that you are in that flat part of the CO_2 response which people call the dogleg, or the hockey stick. Could you answer that, please?

BARGETON: Dr. Loeschke, you are perfectly all right. There is a damping due to the unsteady state in the periodic stimulation and the slope is about one-fourth of the slope in steady state, but the point was to show whether or not there was an increase of the sensitivity in the same condition for the same frequency at rest and at exercise. And,

of course, if a general study could be done with different frequencies, phase shift should be taken into account. I did not speak about the phase in these experiments because the phase was very badly estimated and I could not rely on the phase shift. But it is to be expected to have better measurements of phase shifts and to take into account not only changes of amplitude but also changes of shift during a change of a period of stimulation.

LOESCHKE: May I ask another question? In this case I think all other older experiments in muscular exercise yielded more CO_2 response which was parallel to the resting, but shifted to the left. But your experiments seem to indicate that the slope of CO_2 response of ventilation to increased CO_2 is steeper in muscular exercise than in rest?

BARGETON: Yes.

LOESCHKE: And this seems to be contradicting to what Nielsen and Asmussen . . .

BARGETON: Yes, but since the time of Nielsen it's a very controversial question. For instance, in a recent work of Cunningham it was indicated that the question was not settled. On that question you can read in the literature practically everything. Every opinion has been given, and by first-rate physiologists.

SEVERINGHAUS: I could add to that. In response to Dr. Loeschke's question, Dr. Cedric Bainton has been studying awake dogs exercising and resting and studying the CO_2 response. At first he was getting parallel increases, that is an upward displacement with exercise, but a parallel slope, but as he did them more carefully and persistently, repeating the same dogs many, many times —of course always awake. He found that there was a distinct increase in slope as well as an upward displacement. Perhaps this was dogs resting versus walking at 3 miles per hour on the level, and the increase of slope was about 50%.

BARGETON: I ought to say that the precision of the measurements are not sufficient to say whether or not this increase of sensitivity can explain the extra ventilation of exercise or not. It indicates that it is not necessary to assume a supplementary stimulus but it does not exclude that it exists. It can be a change of sensitivity *and* a supplementary exercise stimulus.

LONGOBARDO: I'm a mechanical engineer and not a physiologist, but could we learn a little bit of a lesson from very, very elementary control theory in this way: During exercise, I've heard said, that essentially the P_{CO_2} is about what is wat at resting. In elementary control that's called a reset or intergroup controller. In one way one could look at it as a shift of the curves (the ventilation curves) to the left, but yet if you look mathematically at the idea of an integral controller, what you see is a series of, let's say, motion toward the left with a high gain, but over a very, very low gain overall slope. So what we may be seeing with Professor Bargeton's work is the low gain part. Perhaps Professor Loeschke is talking about the integrated overall response which would indicate a high gain. Is that possible? You see one looks at a mechanical control and in this type of control you see the gain curve shifting.

BARGETON: If I understand your point of view, it means that an increase in sensitivity means an increase of gain in the system, and a displacement of the curve parallel with itself is a change of the set point of the system and in those experiments it was an attempt to indicate that there was a change of slope. That it could be at the same time a change of the set point. That was not avoided.

SEVERINGHAUS: It seems, from most people's work, that there is both. There's at least a change of set point which we usually express as an upward displacement, more or less parallel, but from both Professor Bargeton's work and some other work there's an addition at increase at slope. But neither of these really, chemically or neurologically, explains it; it simply says what is happening.

LOESCHKE: I may comment that this is a proportional regulator, not an integral regulator, but a proportional regulator with a change of set point.

LONGOBARDO: But mathematically the integral controller could be represented by essentially a high overall gain with a change in set point where you get the stability that you would normally have—that you would *not* have with the high gain by virtue of the fact that you're moving the slope parallel.

SEVERINGHAUS: Yes, that's fine if we can postulate a change of set point. We need a mechanism to change the set point, and that we don't have. We know the gain of the system by testing the CO_2 response and it is quite steep, but it's not enough.

LONGOBARDO: No, it doesn't tell you anything. All it tells you is that mathematically you might be able to duplicate something which might not have any meaning physiologically.

SEVERINGHAUS: Well under certain circumstances with exercise, for example, P_{CO_2} actually falls, even arterial P_{CO_2}, so there's just no signal to explain it unless you also have something like a set point.

BARGETON: I would like to answer to Dr. Loeschke. It cannot be a proportional regulator because it is an essentially nonlinear system, and the approximation of an equivalent linear system can be done only in a very limited range, because it's well known that every nonlinear system can be approximated by a linear one within a small range. But within a larger range the linear approximation is no longer valid.

LOESCHKE: As far as I understand the engineers, an integral regulator would be one which switches on and off, and a proportional one would be one in which is a function, like this one here, increasing the stimulus, increasing the response. Is that not right?

SEVERINGHAUS: It's more complex than that. You might perhaps like to discuss that later in your paper.

2. The Behavior of Carbon Dioxide Stores of the Body during Unsteady States

Neil S. Cherniack, Guy S. Longobardo, and Alfred P. Fishman

From the Cardiovascular-Pulmonary Division,
Department of Medicine,
University of Pennsylvania,
Philadelphia, Pennsylvania
and the Advanced Systems Development Division,
I.B.M. Corporation, Mohansic Laboratory,
Yorktown Heights, New York

Under steady-state conditions metabolically produced CO_2 is discharged rapidly enough by ventilation of the lung so that there are no appreciable fluctuations in the pH and P_{CO_2} of the body. However, whenever the ventilatory pattern is disturbed or when CO_2 production or the composition of the external environment is changed so that the balance between expired and metabolically produced CO_2 is no longer maintained, the body depends on the capacity of its tissues to absorb CO_2 in physical solution and in chemical combination (the CO_2 stores) to prevent extreme changes in pH and P_{CO_2}. In certain animals with irregular breathing patterns like the diving mammals, these unsteady states can last for long periods of time; but in man where ventilatory adjustments take place relatively rapidly, the absorptive capacity of the CO_2 stores are usually called into play for only seconds or a few minutes.

The characteristics of the CO_2 stores will also determine the pattern of ventilatory adjustments to disturbances in CO_2 balance. Figure 1 shows schematically the ventilatory control system and indicates the relationship of the controlling elements to body gas stores. The controlling elements consist of the ventilatory chemoreceptors, the respiratory

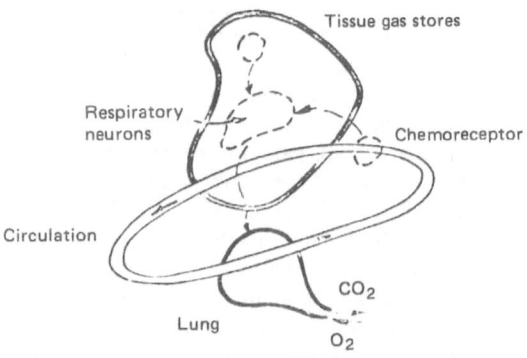

Fig. 1. A diagrammatic representation of the ventilatory control system. The controlling elements of this system, the ventilatory chemoreceptors, and the respiratory neurons are indicated by the broken lines and are interconnected neurally. The tissue and blood gas stores and the lung including its gas stores (the controlled plant of this system) are linked by way of the circulation.

neurons, and the motor nerves which control the ventilation of the lung; the controlled elements consist of the blood, lung, and body tissues and the gas stores which they contain, connected by the circulation. As the figure illustrates, the controlling elements lie within the body gas stores and thus respond to changes in gas tensions and pH in their immediate locale rather than those occurring in the external environment. The properties of the gas stores in the environment of the chemoreceptors and their relationship to gas stores in blood, lung, and other tissues will determine the rapidity of ventilatory changes. Therefore, accurate models of gas stores need to be developed as a first step toward meaningful models of the control of ventilation. Several different models of the gas stores which have been proposed are described in this paper. These models and some of the pertinent experimental observations which led to their development will be discussed.

Most models of gas stores consider only CO_2 changes, although naturally occurring disturbances requiring ventilatory adjustments usually affect the O_2 and CO_2 stores simultaneously (GRODINS et al. [1954], FOWLE et al. [1964], FARHI and RAHN [1960], LONGOBARDO et al. [1967], STAW [1968], MATTHEWS et al. [1968], and CHERNIACK et al. [1966]). There are only a few models which attempt to describe concurrent changes in O_2 and CO_2 stores (GRODINS et al. [1967], LONGOBARDO et al. [1966], CHERNIACK et al. [1968], and TRUEB et al. (in press)), and where appropriate, an attempt will be made to describe these as well.

Whole Body Carbon Dioxide Stores

Because they can be easily manipulated either artificially or voluntarily, controlled changes in either the composition of the inspired air or the level of ventilation have been used as a device for producing alterations in CO_2 storage. In these studies the change in the amount of CO_2 stored has been measured by serially collecting the expired air during the transition from one steady state to another, measuring the amount of CO_2 expired, and calculating CO_2 storage by the following equation:

CO_2 stored $= CO_2$ inspired $- CO_2$ expired $+$ metabolic production of CO_2

(CHERNIACK et al. [1966], VANCE and FOWLER [1960], SULLIVAN et al. [1964], and FARHI and RAHN [1955]). In other experiments the subject holds his breath or rebreathes from a bag, and CO_2 storage is calculated by assuming CO_2 production is constant during the rebreathing or breath holding period (FOWLE et al. [1964], KLOCKE and RAHN [1959], and NAHAS and VEROSKY [1966]). By relating the amount of CO_2 stored to the change in CO_2 tension in either the arterial or venous blood, these investigators could obtain a ratio which has been termed the CO_2 dissociation slope of the body, *i.e.*, $S_{Body} = CO_2$ stored$/\Delta P_{CO_2}$ blood, by analogy to the CO_2 dissociation curve of the blood. The widely disparate results of these investigators and the length of time over which they conducted their experiments is shown in Table 1. It can be seen that the calculated slope of the CO_2 dissociation curve tends to increase as the experiment is prolonged. For example, the slope of the CO_2 dissociation curve obtained after six minutes of breath holding was only 0.55 ml/kg/mm Hg (FOWLE et al. [1964]); while in experiments which involved hyper- or hypoventilation for an hour or more, the slope measured was 2.0 to 4.0 ml/kg/mm Hg (CHERNIACK et al. [1966], and SULLIVAN et al. [1964]); and in studies lasting several days the measured slope was as much as 11.6 (FREEMAN and FENN [1953]).

Farhi and Rahn [1960] suggested that the gradual increase of the whole body CO_2 dissociation slope was due to the differences in the ratio of perfusion to CO_2 storage capacity in the different organs of the body (FARHI and RAHN [1960]). In such a system with uneven perfusion when CO_2 balance is disturbed, the rate of change of P_{CO_2} in the mixed venous blood and body organs will differ. The rate of change of P_{CO_2} in the mixed venous blood will more closely resemble the changes in P_{CO_2} in the well-perfused tissues which Farhi and Rahn believed represented only a small fraction of the body storage capacity for CO_2. Since the P_{CO_2} in the mixed venous blood and the well-perfused organs are nearly at equilibrium values even though changes in CO_2 stores continue to occur in more poorly perfused

Table 1. Values for slope of CO_2 dissociation curve of the body as determined by different investigators

Investigator	Species	Duration of experiment, min	Slope, ml/kg/mm Hg
Fowle and Campbell	Man	6	0.55
Klocke and Rahn	Man	3–8	0.40
Vance and Fowler	Man	20	1.30
Farhi and Rahn	Dog	30–95	1.50
Cherniack et al.	Dog	60	2.35
Sullivan et al.	Dog	60	3.73
Freeman and Fenn	Rat	Several weeks	Up to 11.6

organs, the whole body CO_2 dissociation slope as it is usually calculated seems to increase with time.

The model designed by Farhi and Rahn which embodies this concept of perfusion-limited CO_2 storage is shown diagrammatically in Figure 2. In this model the body is divided into four compartments representing different organs or tissues, namely muscle, brain, heart, and one representing the rest of the body organs, connected in parallel with each other and with a compartment representing CO_2 storage in the lung and the arterial blood. Each compartment has its own rate of perfusion, volume, metabolism, and CO_2 dis-

sociation slope. The volume of each compartment is assumed to be equivalent to the volume of the organ itself and the volume of blood equilibrated with it. Each compartment is believed to be homogeneous. Tissues such as bone and fat which are assumed to have very low levels of perfusion were excluded from the model, since they were believed to store negligible amounts of CO_2 at least over an hour or two.

With this model the measured increase in the CO_2 dissociation slope with time after a CO_2 change could be reproduced. However, prediction of the CO_2 dissociation slope of experiments lasting less than 15 min was not

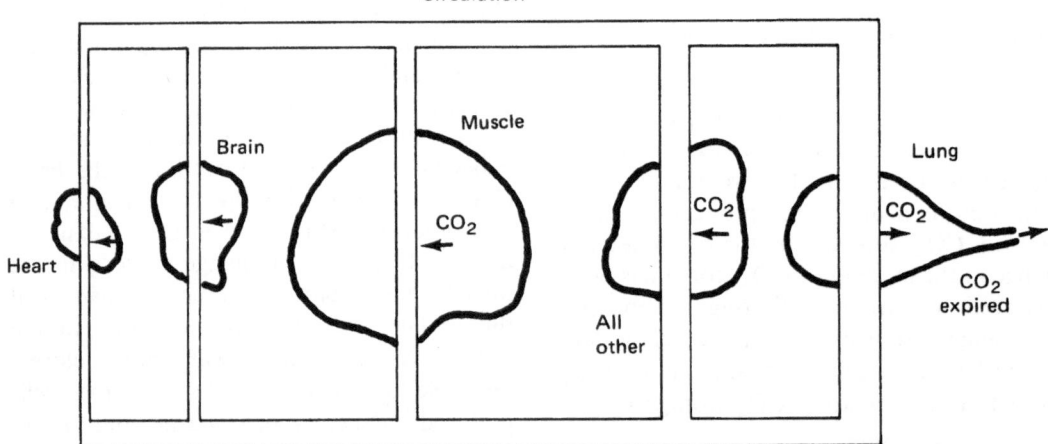

Fig. 2. A diagrammatic representation of a multicompartment model of the body gas stores as formulated by Farhi and Rahn. The tissue compartments are connected in parallel with each other and with the lung by the circulation. Each compartment corresponds to a different organ and each has its own size, rate of perfusion, and metabolic rate. CO_2 dissociation slopes also differ in each compartment. The direction of CO_2 movement in the steady state is shown by the arrows.

nearly as good as reproduction of slopes measured in experiments lasting longer periods of time. Good mathematical representation of these brief experiments involving the first few minutes after a disturbance to CO_2 balance are particularly important in models of ventilatory control, since they represent the behavior of the CO_2 stores over the period of inadequate ventilation likely to be experienced in man.

Factors Influencing the Immediate Changes in Carbon Dioxide Stores

Studies have been conducted in both man and animals to better assess rates of CO_2 storage and to develop models which describe more precisely the dynamics of the CO_2 stores during the period immediately following a disturbance (CHERNIACK et al. [1966], FOWLE et al. [1964], and NAHAS and VEROSKY [1966]). In these experiments, using both man and animals as subjects, CO_2 storage and rates of change of blood P_{CO_2} were measured either during rebreathing with maintenance of full blood O_2 saturation or during apneic oxygenation. Rates of change of P_{CO_2} in both man and dogs were nearly the same, increasing 5 to 6 mm Hg per minute after the first minute of apneic oxygenation or rebreathing, which suggests that the immediate CO_2 storage capacity of the body is very low. As shown in Figure 3, the average experimentally observed rise in mixed venous P_{CO_2} in man and dog is greater than would be anticipated if CO_2 were stored either in a single homogeneous tissue compartment or in multiple organ compartments. While the increase in mixed venous P_{CO_2} predicted by a multicompartment model is closer to that observed, the discrepancy suggests that factors other than inequalities in perfusion to organs limit immediate CO_2 storage. A similar discrepancy was observed during hyperventilation between the more rapid changes in blood gas tensions observed experimentally and those predicted by the multicompartment model (CHERNIACK et al. [1966]).

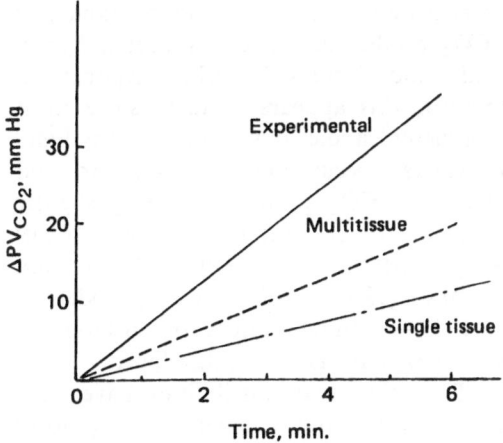

Fig. 3. Comparison of the average changes in mixed venous P_{CO_2} during apneic oxygenation in animals or during rebreathing with man with results predicted by the Farhi and Rahn multicompartment model and one in which there is only one tissue compartment. The more rapid change in observed than in predicted P_{CO_2} indicates that the storage capacity of the body in the first few minutes of apneic oxygenation is less than predicted by either model.

Longobardo, Staw, and Cherniack attempted to determine whether the accuracy of the Farhi and Rahn model could be improved by separating from the "all other tissue" compartments of that model other organs, e.g., the GI tract; but with a seven rather than a four tissue compartment model there was little improvement in the accuracy of predicted results (LONGOBARDO et al. [1967]). Removing the slow compartment, muscle, from the model, somewhat increased the predicted rate of change of arterial and mixed venous CO_2 tensions but failed to reproduce the experimentally observed changes.

Possible physiological mechanisms that could explain the low immediate CO_2 storage include fluctuations in CO_2 production with changes in CO_2 tension, slow chemical processes which limit CO_2 storage in tissues, and interference with CO_2 diffusion into tissues.

The rapid changes in blood P_{CO_2}

experimentally observed could be explained if CO_2 production increased during hypercapnia and decreased during hypocapnia. However, this appears unlikely since most experimental studies indicate that if anything, the reverse occurs—O_2 consumption and presumably CO_2 production being slightly increased by respiratory alkalosis (CAIN [1970], TUTEUR and LAHIRI [1971], and KARETSKY [1970]); and therefore, models in which CO_2 production depends on blood or tissue P_{CO_2} have not been developed.

The other two possibilities have been used in mathematical models of CO_2 stores to explain experimental results. Diagrammatic representations of a typical compartment in these models are compared with a typical compartment in the model postulated by Farhi and Rahn in Figure 4.

Fowle et al. [1964] and Cherniack et al. [1966] suggested that slow chemical processes which might be involved in the buffering of CO_2 by tissue proteins could interfere with CO_2 storage in tissues. Thus the CO_2

dissociation slope of the tissues might, in fact, be low in the immediate period following a CO_2 disturbance; but with time and the completion of these chemical reactions, buffering capacity and the effective storage capacity of the body for CO_2 would increase. One chemical reaction which is involved in CO_2 buffering and which is known to be slow is the hydration of CO_2 to form carbonic acid in the absence of the enzyme, carbonic anhydrase; an enzyme known not to be present in certain tissues such as muscle (MAREN [1967]). If CO_2 hydration were negligible in tissues lacking carbonic anhydrase for several minutes after a disturbance in CO_2 balance, the CO_2 would appear to be stored as shown in Figure 4B in a compartment containing only water. This contrasts with the idea diagrammed in Figure 4A that each compartment could be considered, as supposed by Farhi and Rahn, as a mixed pool of tissue protein buffer even in the immediate period following a CO_2 upset.

Using basically the same multicompart-

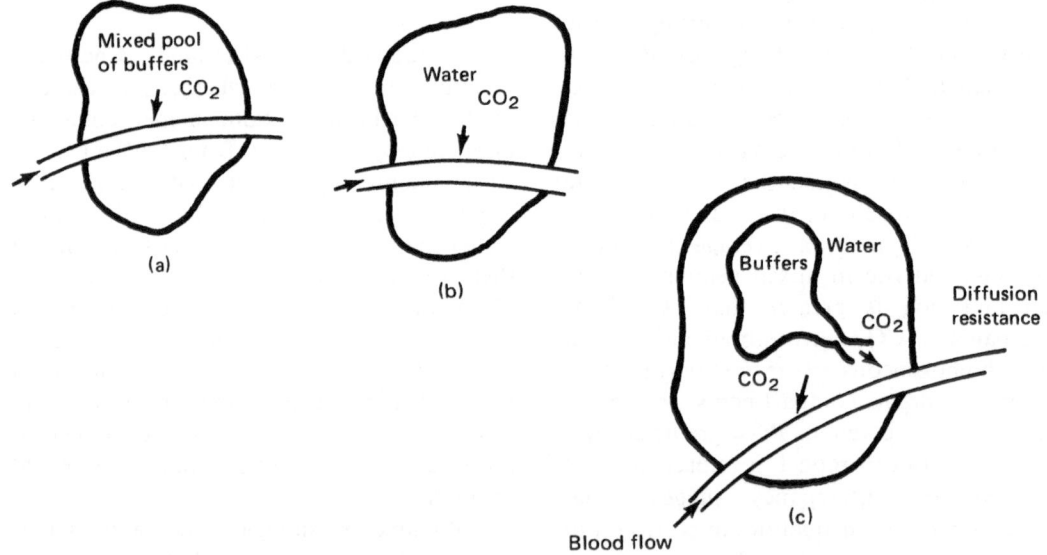

Fig. 4. Three possible representations of a single compartment of a multicompartment model of CO_2 stores during the first few minutes after a CO_2 disturbance. (A) Compartment consists of a mixed pool of buffers. CO_2 is freely diffusible through the compartment. (B) Compartment behaves with respect to CO_2 storage as if it consists entirely of water—simulating the absence of carbonic anhydrase from the compartment. (C) Compartment is divided into an extracellular (water) space and an intracellular (buffers) space by a resistance to the diffusion of CO_2. In models B and C the effective storage capacity for CO_2 is less than in A.

ment model as that used by Farhi and Rahn, and assuming that carbonic anhydrase was present only in blood, brain, and kidney and that CO_2 hydration in other tissue compartments would be negligible for at least a few minutes, computed rates of change of arterial and mixed venous tensions could be made to closely reproduce experimental changes in arterial and mixed venous blood, both during hyperventilation and apneic oxygenation as shown in Figure 5 (LONGOBARDO et al. [1967], and CHERNIACK [1966]).

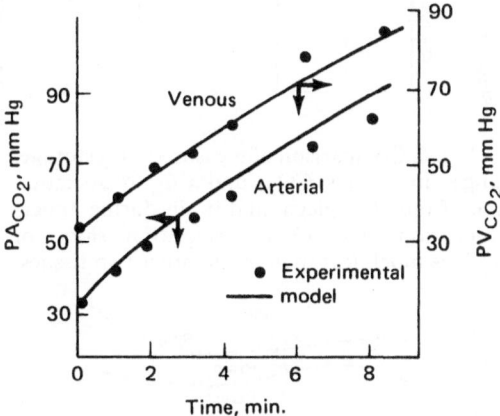

Fig. 5. Comparison during apneic oxygenation of experimentally measured values of arterial and mixed venous P_{CO_2} ($\cdot$) with predictions of a multicompartment model constructed by LONGOBARDO et al.

In Figure 4C the organ compartment is divided by a barrier between the intracellular space containing protein buffer and an extracellular space which behaves the same as water so far as CO_2 storage is concerned. This barrier might entirely prevent intracellular CO_2 storage as suggested by one model (MATTHEWS et al. [1968]) or could limit storage by interfering with the diffusion of CO_2.

Staw showed that if this barrier to CO_2 diffusion was not total but produced a 2 to 3 mm Hg gradient in the steady state in every tissue compartment between intra- and extracellular fluids, satisfactory reproduction could be achieved of the serial changes in blood gas tensions measured by Cherniack

et al. in dogs during the first few minutes of hyperventilation and apneic oxygenation (STAW [1968]). The assumed 2 to 3 mm Hg difference in P_{CO_2} was about the same as had been measured between lymphatic fluid and simultaneously sampled venous blood, which suggests that gradients of CO_2 of this magnitude might exist in some tissues (BERGOFSKY et al. [1962]). However, this gradient is far higher than that measured by Pontén between the brain tissue and the capillary blood, making it unlikely that a gradient this great is present in all tissues (PONTÉN and SIESJÖ [1966]).

It is difficult to determine from models of whole body CO_2 stores whether either slow chemical reactions or restrictions to CO_2 diffusion alone could account for the low immediate CO_2 storage capacity. It seemed likely that studies of CO_2 storage in specific tissues might help to better evaluate the relative importance of these two mechanisms or whether some third mechanism not previously considered was involved.

Experimental Studies of Carbon Dioxide Storage in Specific Organs and Tissues

Investigations were conducted of CO_2 storage and the rate of change of arterial and venous P_{CO_2} in three tissues, muscle, brain and spleen, in paralyzed anesthetized animals. Studies were made during apneic oxygenation, asphyxia, or artificial ventilation with gas mixtures enriched with CO_2. In the steady state prior to each experimental period, blood flow rates, arterial and venous gas tensions, and concentrations and the metabolic production of CO_2 of each organ was measured; at the conclusion of the experiment the tissues which had been studies were weighed. During the experimental period, blood flow was continuously measured with electromagnetic flow probes and samples of arterial and venous blood were periodically obtained (CHERNIACK et al. [1970a], and CHERNIACK et al. [1970b]).

From these data the CO_2 storage of each of the tissues could be calculated in a manner analogous to that used in calculating CO_2 storage in the whole body. The method of calculating CO_2 storage is shown in the next equation.

$$CO_2 \text{ stored} = \int_0^t - \dot{Q}(C_vCO_2 - C_aCO_2) + \dot{V}_{CO_2}dt$$

where $\dot{Q}$ is the perfusion to an organ; $CvCO_2$, the CO_2 concentration of the venous blood; $CaCO_2$, the CO_2 concentration of the arterial blood, and $\dot{V}CO_2$, the metabolic production of CO_2.

By relating the changes in the amount of CO_2 stored to the changes in the PCO_2 in the venous blood exiting from that tissue, the apparent CO_2 dissociation slope of that tissue could be estimated. The assumptions underlying this calculation were that: the tissues in fact exist as represented in the Farhi and Rahn model, i.e., they are homogeneous mixtures of tissue and blood, and there are no significant restrictions to the diffusion of CO_2 within a compartment; and that the metabolic production of CO_2 is constant throughout the experiment. The results obtained at the end of six minutes of apneic oxygenation in the three tissues are indicated in Figure 6. which shows the changes in venous PCO_2 and CO_2 storage for each tissue during apneic oxygenation experiments. It can be seen that the CO_2 dissociation slope of muscle was calculated to be about 1 ml/kg/mm Hg, while the slope of brain and spleen was at least three times greater. The difference between brain and muscle could not be explained by taking into account differences in circulation time through each tissue.

If the level of perfusion were the only factor which limited the amount of CO_2 stored in a specific tissue, e.g., muscle, and CO_2 storage in the tissue was homogeneous, the CO_2 dissociation slope of such a tissue should remain the same regardless of the length of exposure to a CO_2 disturbance. Therefore, in other experiments the effect of more prolonged CO_2 exposure on CO_2 storage was evaluated. Figure 7 shows that the

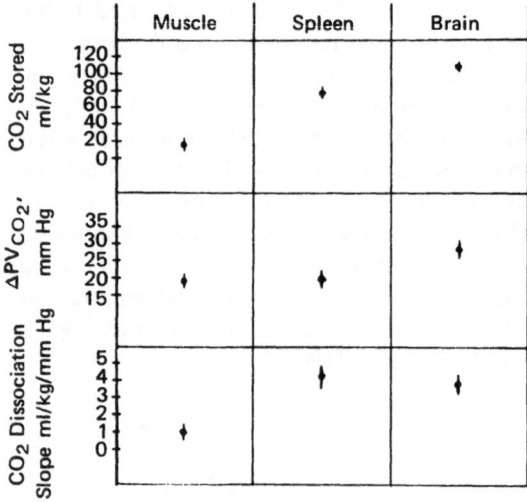

Fig. 6. Comparison of measured CO_2 storage, changes in venous CO_2, and CO_2 dissociation slope of muscle, spleen, and brain during apneic oxygenation. The CO_2 dissociation slope of muscle is much less than in the other two tissues.

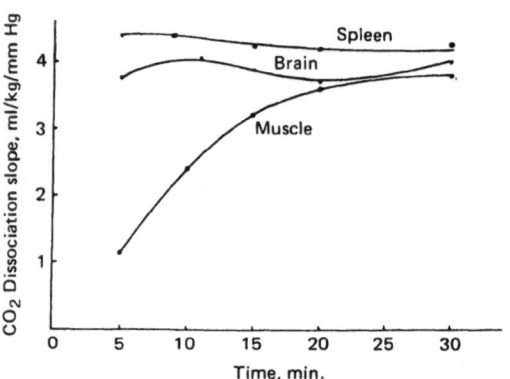

CO_2 Dissociation slope vs time for spleen, brain, muscle

Fig. 7. Changes with time in the CO_2 dissociation slope of muscle, brain, and spleen in dogs artificially ventilated with 5% CO_2. The CO_2 dissociation slope of muscle, unlike that of brain and spleen, gradually increases.

apparent CO_2 dissociation slope of muscle increases during a 30-min period of artificial ventilation with 5% CO_2, while that of brain and spleen remains virtually constant. Thus, factors other than the level of perfusion seem to limit rates of CO_2 storage in muscle and possibly other tissues as well.

Models of Carbon Dioxide Storage in Muscle

Since both the brain and the spleen, which is a blood reservoir, contain carbonic anhydrase and muscle does not, the gradual increase in the CO_2 dissociation slope of muscle, but not of brain and spleen, might be caused by the slow hydration of CO_2. This difference in the behavior of the calculated CO_2 dissociation slope of muscle could theoretically also occur if the ability of CO_2 to diffuse through muscle were less than in the other two tissues. Another possibility— that a large quantity of blood in muscle passes through anatomical shunts—appears unlikely since microscopic studies of the circulation in skeletal muscle have revealed the presence of few if any anatomical shunts (BARLOW et al. [1961]).

Trueb et al. (in press) developed a mathematical model capable of describing simultaneous changes in O_2 and CO_2 stores which could be used to evaluate the quantitative importance of diffusion in explaining the low storage capacity of muscle during the first few minutes following a change in ventilation. In this model possible limitations to the diffusion of both CO_2 and O_2 are taken into account, and PCO_2 and PO_2 are considered to change both with time and according to their locations along the longitudinal axis of the capillary in the blood and tissue. Included in this model as in a previous model of CO_2 and O_2 storage in the whole body are the oxyhemoglobin dissociation curve, the Bohr effect on blood O_2, and the Haldane effect on CO_2 change in the blood (CHERNIACK et al. [1968]). The myoglobin dissociation curve and the time required for blood to traverse the muscle capillaries and veins to the sampling sites are also included in the Trueb model. A diagrammatic representation of this model is shown in Figure 8. In this model a CO_2 diffusion resistance sufficiently great to cause a partial pressure difference between cells and capillaries of at least 3.5 mm Hg in the steady state in muscle could not reproduce experimental results. In addition, one had to assume that there was no hydration of CO_2 to reproduce observed changes in muscle venous PCO_2 during either asphyxia or apneic oxygenation. Figure 9 shows that with a gradient of this magnitude and assuming no CO_2 hydration in muscle tissue, experimental

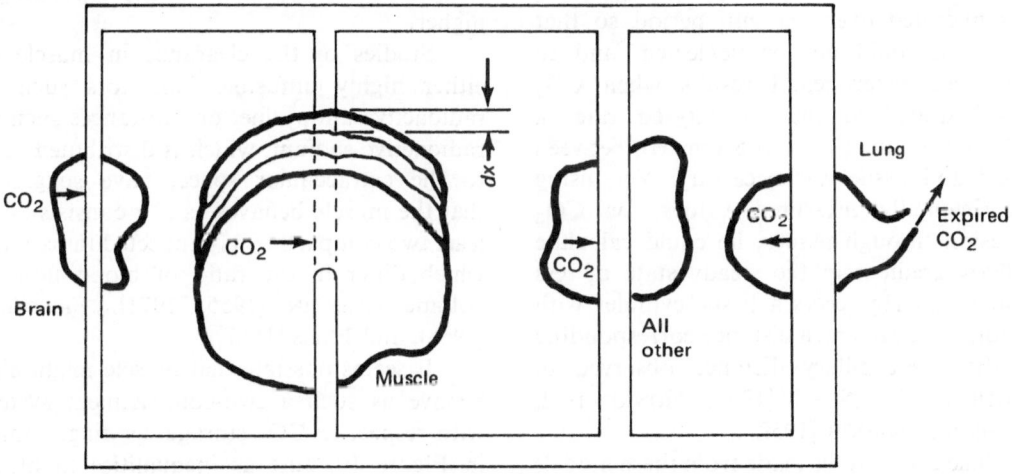

Treub model

Fig. 8. Diagrammatic representation of the multicompartment model of CO_2 storage constructed by Trueb et al. Each compartment has its own metabolic rate, level of perfusion, and volume. CO_2 and O_2 diffusion between blood and tissue are considered to change both with position along the capillary dividing each tissue compartment as shown for the muscle into a number of smaller compartments of width dx with different gas tensions.

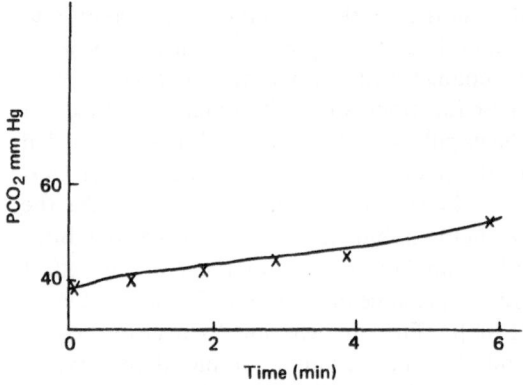

Fig. 9. Comparison during apneic oxygenation of measured changes (x) in muscle venous P_{CO_2} and those predicted (solid line) by the model of Trueb et al.

results obtained during apneic oxygenation could be closely reproduced.

Waldram et al. (in press) constructed a model of muscle CO_2 stores similar to that designed by Trueb; however, rather than assuming that CO_2 hydration was negligible in muscle in the absence of carbonic anhydrase, he used the actual uncatalyzed rate of CO_2 hydration in his model. He found that, even at the uncatalyzed rate, enough CO_2 was hydrated over a 6-min period so that hydration could not be neglected, and to reproduce experimental results when CO_2 was hydrated at the uncatalyzed rate, a diffusion gradient of 6 to 8 mm Hg between blood and tissue was necessary. Yet, using experimentally measured values for CO_2 diffusion through tissues, he could calculate a P_{CO_2} gradient in the steady state of less than 1 mm Hg across a tissue cylinder with a radius of 30 micra, a distance corresponding to the intercapillary distance observed in muscle *in vivo* (SIESJÖ [1965], HONIG et al. [1970], and KROGH [1959]).

The calculations made from these models suggest that neither uncatalyzed rates of CO_2 hydration nor restrictions to CO_2 diffusion which seem possible physiologically, alone or together, account for the low CO_2 storage capacity of muscle in the first few minutes after a CO_2 change. While the possibility

remains that there are slow chemical reactions other than hydration which limit CO_2 storage (as the experiments of ADLER and RELMAN [1965a, b] seem to suggest), or that some property of the cell membrane, not yet uncovered, influences storage of CO_2, it seems more likely that some other factor not yet considered in mathematical models reduces immediate CO_2 storage capacity in muscle.

Effects of Blood Flow Distribution within a Single Tissue on Carbon Dioxide Storage

Although previous models, including those of Trueb and Waldram, had assumed that muscle is uniform with respect to perfusion, CO_2 storage capacity and metabolism, considerable evidence suggests that such is not the case. Muscle consists of both red, myoglobin-containing fibers and white fibers which do not contain myoglobin which differ in their level of perfusion and metabolic rate (ADLER and RELMAN [1956b], REIS et al. [1969], and BEATTY et al. [1963]). Measured blood flow rates to red muscles at rest are approximately three times greater than those to white fibers, and the metabolism of the red fibers is correspondingly higher.

Studies of the clearance in muscle of either highly diffusible indicators such as radioactive antipyrine, or substances such as radioactive sodium, which is distributed only to the extracellular space, have suggested that the muscle behaves as if it consists of at least two compartments connected in parallel, which differ in the ratio of blood flow to volume (RENKIN [1955, 1971], FRIEDMAN [1968], and FREIS [1957]).

It seems possible that muscle might also behave as such a two-compartment system with respect to CO_2 storage, as diagrammed in Figure 10. Just as inequalities in blood flow to different tissue compartments might cause a gradual increase in the whole body CO_2 dissociation slope, similarly such blood flow to storage capacity inequalities within the muscle compartment might explain the observed increase in the CO_2 dissociation

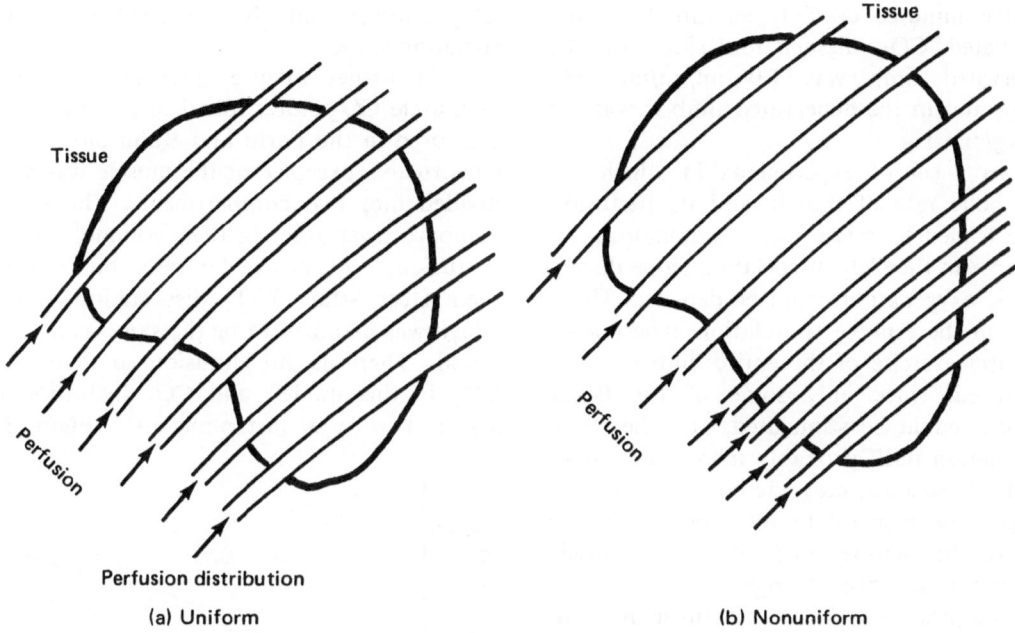

Perfusion distribution

(a) Uniform

(b) Nonuniform

Postulated distribution of perfusion in muscle compartment

Fig. 10. Diagrammatic representation of a cross-section through the muscle compartment. In (A) the distribution of blood vessels through the compartment (x) is uniform, as assumed in all previous models of CO_2 stores. In (B) the muscle is perfused non-uniformly, as assumed in the current model.

slope of muscle with time. If such a distribution of blood flow to storage capacity played an important role in CO_2 storage in muscle, increasing the size of the well-perfused compartment should also increase its apparent CO_2 dissociation slope in the first few minutes after a CO_2 disturbance. Therefore, the effect on the CO_2 dissociation slope of decreased sympathetic vasoconstrictor activity resulting from denervation or an increased metabolic rate was investigated, because studies by others with radioactive indicators showed that both types of experimental intervention seemed to increase the volume of well-perfused tissue in muscle (REIS et al. [1969], and RENKIN [1971]).

To produce denervation the femoral and sciatic nerves to the skinned hind limb of dogs were severed. After a control period of artificial ventilation with either 100 or 10% O_2 in nitrogen, the effect of enrichment of either inspired gas with 5 to 7% CO_2 on CO_2 storage was determined in the denervated as compared to the opposite innervated hind limb in dogs. Denervation in both the euoxic and hypoxic animal increased resting CO_2 production and blood flow.

A typical result obtained in these experiments is shown in Table 2. By the end

Table 2. Comparison of CO_2 storage in innervated and denervated muscle after five minutes of artificial ventilation with 5% CO_2 in oxygen

	Innervated	Denervated
V_{CO_2}, ml/min	2.1	3.2
Flow, ml/min	60	156
ΔP_{VCO_2} mm Hg	10	10
CO_2 dissociation slope, ml/kg/mm Hg	1.0	2.7

of five minutes of CO_2 equilibration, the calculated CO_2 dissociation slope of the innervated limb was 1.0 ml/kg/mm Hg P_{CO_2}, and in the denervated limb it was 2.7 ml/kg/mm Hg.

In a set of experiments in which the metabolic rate of muscle and its perfusion were tripled by sciatic nerve stimulation, no increase in the CO_2 dissociation slope during apneic oxygenation could be detected. However, in these nerve stimulation experiments uniform exercise of the entire limb was not produced, since only some of the flexor muscles could be stimulated, and the nerve stimulation itself probably increased sympathetic vasoconstrictor activity. Therefore, despite the increase in total perfusion, the size of the well-perfused portion of muscle might not have been changed.

To produce a more uniform increase in metabolism in the muscle, the drug dinitrophenol, 5 mgm/kg, was administered intravenously, and CO_2 storage and the CO_2 dissociation slope of both the muscle and the whole body was measured simultaneously before and after administration of the drug. Data from a representative experiment are shown in Table 3.

Table 3. Effect of intravenous dinitrophenol on CO_2 storage in muscle during apneic oxygenation

	Before	After
V_{CO_2}, ml/min	3.0	8.7
Flow, ml/min	88	107
$\Delta P_{V CO_2}$ mm Hg	25	21
CO_2 dissociation slope, ml/kg/mm Hg	0.61	2.25

Table 3 shows that after dinitrophenol the CO_2 dissociation slope of the muscle increased from 0.61 to 2.25. The storage capacity of the whole body for CO_2 in this dog increased by 40 %. These results suggested that the uneven distribution of blood flow relative to storage capacity can influence

CO_2 storage and the apparent CO_2 dissociation slope.

To further analyze these data, a model of muscle CO_2 stores identical in concept to that used in the Farhi and Rahn model was constructed, except that the muscle was subdivided into two compartments. These two compartments differ in their volume, rate of perfusion, and metabolic rate, but not in their steady-state CO_2 dissociation slope, which was assumed to be the same as that of blood. There is no diffusion gradient for CO_2 in this model, and CO_2 hydration is assumed to occur instantaneously. Figure 11

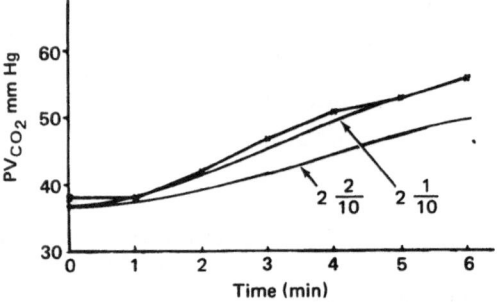

Fig. 11. Comparison of experimental change in muscle venous P_{CO_2} (x) obtained during apneic oxygenation with those computed by a model in which there is a non-uniform distribution of perfusion and metabolism to volume. Solid line labeled 1/10 shows results when 1/10 of muscle volume is considered to have 7/8 of the perfusion and the metabolic rate. In the line labeled 2/10, 7/8 of the perfusion and metabolic rate is considered to exist in 2/10 of muscle volume. Metabolic production of CO_2 of muscle in the experiment shown was 1.2 ml/min, while flow rate was 88 ml/min.

compares the changes in muscle venous P_{CO_2} during apneic oxygenation with those computed when one of the two muscle compartments has seven-eighths of the total measured perfusion and metabolic rate and has either two-tenths of one-tenth or the measured muscle volume. It can be seen that decreasing the volume of the well-perfused compartment increases the predicted rate of rise of muscle venous P_{CO_2} and that experimental results are well matched when one-tenth of the muscle compartment is well perfused. Figure 12 shows experimental changes in muscle venous P_{CO_2} in the same animal during apneic oxygenation after the administration of dinitrophenol. Figure 12 shows that results are now reasonably well matched if the augmentation in metabolic rate produced by DNP increased the size of the well-perfused compartment, so that it now represents two-tenths of the muscle volume and continues to receive seven-eighths of the metabolic rate and perfusion.

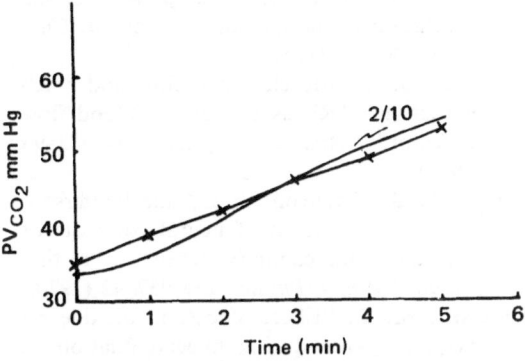

Fig. 12. Experimental changes in muscle venous P_{CO_2} (x) during apneic oxygenation after DNP administration (same animal as shown in Figure 11). Metabolic production of CO_2 after DNP increased to 6.9 ml/min and flow rate to 110 ml/min. Experimental results are reasonably well matched when it is assumed that 2/10 of the muscle volume has 7/8 of the perfusion and metabolic rate.

Since there is only scanty quantitative evidence about the degree of inhomogeneity of metabolism and perfusion in muscle, it is not possible to say at the present time whether such inhomogeneities alone explain the low immediate CO_2 storage capacity of muscle. If the uncatalyzed rate of CO_2 hydration and reasonable restrictions for the diffusion of CO_2 were included in the model, less inhomogeneity would be needed to match experimental results. However, it seems reasonable to believe that much of the low immediate storage capacity for CO_2 in the body and in muscle is caused by these

inhomogeneities and that much of the increase in the apparent CO_2 dissociation slope observed with denervation and DNP is due to more homogeneous distribution of perfusion and metabolism in relation to muscle volume.

Conclusions

Given sufficient time, the body has a large capacity to store CO_2 with little change in CO_2 tension; however, in the first few minutes after a disturbance to CO_2 balance the storage capacity of the body for CO_2 is much less. Unevenness in the distribution of perfusion to different organs is probably the most important factor which accounts for the gradual increase in whole body CO_2 storage capacity with time. However, in the first few minutes after a CO_2 upset, other factors seem to limit CO_2 storage in certain tissues of the body, e.g., muscle. Finite rates of CO_2 diffusion within organs, and the time needed for slow chemical reactions involved in buffering are theoretical mechanisms which could partially account for the reduced immediate CO_2 storage capacity. Differences in perfusion to storage capacity ratio within tissues seems both theoretically and experimentally to be an important factor.

Difficulties encountered with some models of ventilatory control in simulating rapid adjustments of ventilation to changes in CO_2 may in part be explained by their failure to take into account the low immediate storage capacity of the body for CO_2. The ability of the body to change its CO_2 dissociation slope with time may be of real advantage to the organism, allowing it to rapidly bring corrective ventilatory changes into play whenever CO_2 balance is disturbed, without sacrificing its ability to preserve body pH if after a time these ventilatory compensations prove to be inadequate.

Bibliography

Adler, S., Roy, A. M., and Relman, A. S., "Intracellular acid-base regulation. I. The response of muscle cells to changes in CO_2

tension and extracellular bicarbonate concentration." *J. Clin. Invest.* 44:8–20 (1965a).

———, Roy, A. M., and Relman, A. S., "Intracellular acid-base regulation. II. Interaction between CO_2 tension and extracellular bicarbonate in the determination of muscle pH." *J. Clin. Invest.* 44:21–30 (1965b).

Barlow, T. E., Haigh, A. L., and Walder, D. N., 'Evidence for two vascular pathways in skeletal muscle." *Clin. Sci.* 20:367–85 (1961).

Beatty, C. H., Peterson, R. D., and Bocek, R. M., "Metabolism of red and white muscle groups." *Am. J. Physiol.* 204:939–42 (1963).

Bergofsky, E. H., Jacobson, J. H., III, and Fishman, A. P., "The use of lymph for the measurement of gas tensions in interstitial fluid and tissues." *J. Clin. Invest.* 41:1971–89 (1962).

Cain, S., "Increased oxygen uptake with passive hyperventilation of dogs." *J. Appl. Physiol.* 28:4–7 (1970).

Cherniack, N. S., Longobardo, G. S., Staw, I., and Heymann, M., "Dynamics of carbon dioxide stores changes following an alteration in ventilation." *J. Appl. Physiol.* 21: 785–93 (1966).

———, Longobardo, G. S., Palermo, F. P., and Heymann, M., "Dynamics of oxygen stores changes following an alteration in ventilation." *J. Appl. Physiol.* 24:809–16 (1968).

———, Edelman, N. H., and Fishman, A. P., "O_2 exchange across the spleen during asphyxia". *Am. J. Physiol.* 219:1585–89 (1970a).

———, Edelman, N. H., Tuteur, P. G., and Trueb, T. J., "Acute buffering of CO_2 by tissues *in vivo*." Presented at the American Society for Clinical Investigation (May 1970b).

Grodins, F. S., Gray, J. S., Schroeder, K. R., Norins, A. L., and Jones, R. W., "Respiratory response to CO_2 inhalation. A theoretical study of a nonlinear biological regulator." *J. Appl. Physiol.* 7:293–308 (1954). See also Grodins, F. S., Buell, J., and Bart, J., "Mathematical analysis and digital simulation of the respiratory control system." *J. Appl. Physiol.* 22:260–76 (1967).

Farhi, L. E., and Rahn, H., "Gas stores of the body and the unsteady state." *J. Appl. Physiol.* 7:472–84 (1955).

———, and Rahn, H., "Dynamics of changes in carbon dioxide stores." *Anesthesiology* 21:604–14 (1960).

Fowle, A. S. E., Matthews, C. M. E., and Campbell, E. J. M., "The rapid distribution of ^3H_2O and $^{11}CO_2$ in the body in relation to the immediate carbon dioxide storage capacity." *Clin. Sci.* 27:51–65 (1964a).

———, Matthews, C. M. E., and Campbell, E. J. M., "The immediate carbon dioxide storage capacity of man." *Clin. Sci.* 27:41–49 (1964b).

Freeman, F. H., and Fenn, W. O., "Changes in carbon dioxide stores due to atmospheres low in oxygen or high in carbon dioxide." *Am. J. Physiol.* 174:422–30 (1953).

Freis, E. D., Schnaper, H. W., and Lilienfield, L. S., "Rapid and slow components of the circulation in the human forearm." *J. Clin. Invest.* 36:245 (1957).

Friedman, J. J., "Muscle blood flow and ^{86}Rb extraction. ^{86}Rb as a capillary blood flow indicator." *Am. J. Physiol.* 214:488–93 (1968).

Honig, C. R., Frierson, J. L., and Patterson, J. L., "Comparison of neural contrasts of resistance and capillary density in resting muscle." *Am. J. Physiol.* 218:937–42 (1970).

Karetsky, M. S., "Effect of carbon dioxide on oxygen uptake during hyperventilation in normal man." *J. Appl. Physiol.* 28:8–12 (1970).

Klocke, F. J., and Rahn, H., "Breath holding after breathing oxygen." *J. Appl. Physiol.* 14:689–93 (1959).

Krogh, A., *Anatomy and physiology of the capillaries*. New York: Hafner (1959).

Longobardo, G. S., Cherniack, N. S., and Fishman, A. P., "Cheyne-Stokes breathing produced by a model of the human respiratory system." *J. Appl. Physiol.* 21:1839–46 (1966).

———, Cherniack, N. S., and Staw, I., "Transients in carbon dioxide stores." *IEEE Trans. Bio-Med. Eng.* BME 14:182–90 (1967).

Maren, T. H., "Carbonic anhydrase: chemistry, physiology, and inhibition." *Physiol. Rev.* 47:595–781 (1967).

Matthews, C. M. E., Laszlo, C., Campbell, E. J. M., Kobby, P. M., and Freedman, S., "Exchange of CO_2 in arterial blood with body CO_2 pools." *Resp. Physiol.* 6:29–44 (1968).

Nahas, G. G., and Verosky, M., "The storage of CO_2 during apneic oxygenation." *Ann. N.Y. Acad. Sci.* 133:134–41 (1966).

Pontén, U., and Siesjö, B. K., "Gradients of CO_2

tension in the brain." *Acta Physiol. Scand.* 67:129–40 (1966).

Reis, D. J., Wooten, G. F., and Hollenberg, M., "Differences in nutrient blood flow of red and white skeletal muscle in the cat." *Am. J. Physiol.* 213:592–96 (1967).

———, Moorhead, D., and Wooten, G. F., "Differential regulation of blood flow to red and white muscle in sleep and defense behavior." *Am. J. Physiol.* 217:541–46 (1969).

Renkin, E. M., "Effects of blood flow on diffusion kinetics in isolated, perfused hind limbs of cats: a double circulation hypothesis." *Am. J. Physiol.* 183:125 (1955).

———. "The nutritional-shunt flow hypothesis in skeletal muscle circulation." *Circ. Res.* 18 and 19 (Suppl. I):21–5 (1971).

Siesjö, B. K., "Active and passive mechanisms in the regulation of the acid-base metabolism of the brain." In *Cerebrospinal fluid and the regulation of ventilation*, C. McBrooks, F. Kao, and B. Lloyd, eds. Philadelphia: Davis (1965).

Staw, I., "Dynamics of mammalian carbon dioxide stores." Ph.D. Thesis, Columbia University (1968).

Sullivan, S. F., Patterson, R. W., and Papper, E. M., "Tissue carbon dioxide stores. Magnitude of the acute change in the dog." *Am. J. Physiol.* 206:887–90 (1964).

Trueb, T. J., Cherniack, N. S., D'Souza, F., and Fishman, A. P., "A distributed parameter model of the controlled plant of the respiratory control system." *Biophys. J.* (In press).

Tuteur, P. G., and Lahiri, S., "The effect of alkalosis on O_2 consumption of skeletal muscle." *Fed. Proc.* 30:427 Abs. (1971).

Vance, J. W., and Fowler, W. S., "Adjustments of the stores of CO_2 during voluntary hyperventilation." *Diseases Chest* 37:304–13 (1960).

Waldram, S., Fitzgerald, T., and Cherniack, N. S., "Experimental and theoretical aspects of the dynamics of the CO_2 stores in skeletal muscle." Advances in Bio-engineering. (In press).

Cherniack Discussion

SEVERINGHAUS: Thank you very much. I'm not sure I'm going to buy that last little teleology, but I'm delighted to see the data. I can contribute a little bit to this. I think you would be interested in looking at the original paper which was written by a group in our place in anesthesiology, hidden in one of those obscure journals, on the rate of rise of P_{CO_2} during apnea in patients who were anesthetized. Now the difference was that these patients were under barbiturate anesthesia, and the P_{CO_2} rose less than half the speed of yours, the metabolism was down about 20%, so that can't explain it, but I think it's quite possible that the succinylcholine increases the muscle blood flow and makes it more uniform. And perhaps it decreases muscle lactate formation. You didn't mention that, but of course muscle rests in a rather hypoxic or anoxic state and has a continuous excretion of lactate. Is there any evidence that when CO_2 begins to pile up that the muscle "dumps" lactate and therefore "dumps" CO_2 because of the acid which is being made metabolically in it?

CHERNIACK: Well, we measured the venous lactate concentrations before and at the end of apneic oxygenation, and 12 min after that we couldn't see any "dumping" as evidenced by a change in venous lactate concentration.

DUBOIS: I've been unable to understand how organs that internally generate CO_2 could fail to receive CO_2 because of a diffusion barrier or because of blood flow. The alternative to this would be if the muscles were not generating the CO_2 that they're storing. Which do you believe?

CHERNIACK: As you change ventilation, the initial disturbance is in the arterial blood. The venous blood returning to the lung is unable to release CO_2 so that the arterial blood has a higher CO_2. If there are diffusion gradients between the blood and the tissues, the additional CO_2 in the arterial blood won't enter the tissues.

DUBOIS: But the CO_2 comes from the tissues, so how can it fall to get into the tissue?

SEVERINGHAUS: Well, except that the major part of metabolism comes from a minor part of the body.

CHERNIACK: Right. The brain which has a high metabolic rate stores only about 60% of the CO_2 it produces. The spleen, on the other hand, stores about 300% of the CO_2 it produces and is actually "sopping up" CO_2 from other organs, and if you plot the changes in splenic venous CO_2, as compared to arterial CO_2, the venous CO_2 actually is less than the arterial CO_2, and the same is true of muscle. Now one would expect from the known buffering capacity of muscle that it might store 150 to 200% of the CO_2 that it produces. Actually it only stores about 105 or 110%, and it is this less than expected storage capacity of muscle that accounts for the low storage capacity of the whole body.

SEVERINGHAUS: These were in isolated perfused muscles?

CHERNIACK: No, these experiments were performed in dogs whose hind limbs had been skinned. We tied off all the blood vessels that might go to the limb, except for the femoral artery. In addition, we tied ligatures around the lower end of the hind limb to eliminate flow to the paw which has little muscle.

SEVERINGHAUS: Was the perfusion of the artery still normal?

CHERNIACK: Yes.

RYBAK: Did you compare CO_2 the storage of white and red muscles?

CHERNIACK: No, we haven't done that yet. We've been using dogs up until now, and goats where white and red fibers are intermixed. In cats, on the other hand, separation of red and white fibers is better and it might be possible in cats to study CO_2 storage in the red versus white muscles.

RYBAK: I suppose that red muscle must store more CO_2 than the white one?

CHERNIACK: Well, we expect so, because it seems to have a more even distribution of perfusion.

SEVERINGHAUS: Red muscle also has more blood as well as more myoglobin, doesn't it?

RYBAK: Yes, I think so.

DUBOIS: Well then, you've explained away my problem, but there might be another possibility, and that would be that if the CO_2 were hydrated in the muscle but that in the process of hydration the H^+ produced could not be buffered and it could not leave the cell and so it would block the further storage of CO_2. And that might be testable through the type of thing Dr. Severinghaus mentioned. You mentioned, for example, that lactate was produced, and I suppose that one could also see whether the pH of muscle diminished, if it became more acid, during the unsteady state of breath holding. This might be something to try.

CHERNIACK: That is a possibility, and as Dr. Siesjö pointed out for the brain, the brain does seem to burn up acids somehow and so, metabolically, controls its pH. Reactions such as the ones to which you refer, if they were slow enough, in muscle might also play a part in explaining its low storage capacity. Another possibility is suggested by Dr. Guertner's hypothesis which would create a gradient not between intra- and extra-cellular fluids but between the capillary and the tissue.

DUBOIS: But shouldn't that increase the storage capacity?

CHERNIACK: I don't think so.

3. Carbon Dioxide Stores in the Study of Energy Metabolism

Reginald A. Shipley

From the
Nuclear Medicine Service, Veterans Administration Hospital,
10701 East Boulevard, Cleveland, Ohio, 44106,
and the
Department of Medicine,
Case-Western Reserve University School of Medicine,
10900 Euclid Avenue, Cleveland, Ohio, 44106

As a tool to study energy metabolism, radiocarbon has been more useful to establish routes than to assess rates. Methodology for the measurement of rates is, indeed, still evolving. The metabolic alterations accompanying fasting, or those responsible for a disorder such as diabetes, are attributable to slowing or acceleration of normal chemical transformations rather than complete loss of any pathway or addition of new ones. In applying the method of compartment analysis to study rates, a persisting challenge has been to devise models of *in vivo* systems which are not unrealistically complex yet are not over-simplified. Some of the gropings of the past 20 years, aside from their historical interest, will serve to illustrate certain pitfalls and will permit us to get a close look at some of the compromises which have been made. The problem of measuring the conversion rate of glucose carbon to CO_2 carbon will serve as a starting point.

Conversion Rate by Tracer Dilution

Movement of tracer has significance only to the extent that it mirrors the behavior of attending natural atoms. For the production of CO_2 a simple goal might be to determine what proportion of converted carbon is donated by glucose as opposed to nonglucose

sources. In a hypothetical static *in vitro* system such as that of Figure 1 a mixture of labeled glucose of known specific activity (SA) and companion nonlabeled precursor yield CO_2 as a joint oxidative product. Knowledge of the SA of CO_2 permits calculation of the fraction of CO_2 derived from glucose. In the illustrated example it is 50%. The general expression is:

Fraction CO_2 from glucose carbon =

$$\frac{\text{SA, } CO_2 \text{ carb.}}{\text{SA, gluc. carb.}} \tag{1}$$

This is a simple application of the principle of isotope dilution. But in a dynamic system precursors do not react in a container to be sampled at leisure. An *in vivo* process involves continual replacement of precursors.

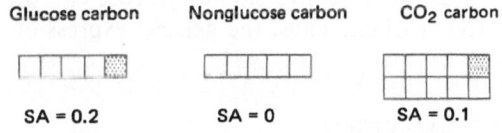

$$\frac{0.1}{0.2} = 50\% \ CO_2 \text{ carbon from glucose carbon}$$

Fig. 1. Diagrammatic representation of fractional contribution of labeled precursor to product in a hypothetical static system.

Thus, the foregoing principle is useful only if precursor glucose carbon can be supplied as a labeled stream having constant SA. This is the basis of the constant infusion method introduced by Stetten et al. [1951]. In Figure 2 glucose is entering CO_2 at a rate of 3

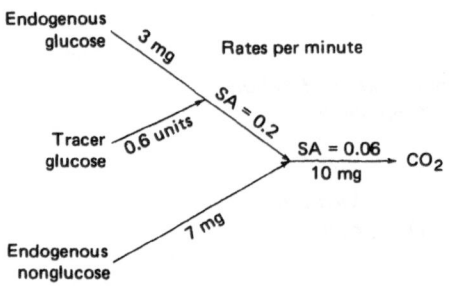

Gluclose carbon to CO_2 carbon = $\frac{0.06}{0.2}$ 10 = 3 mg/min

Fig. 2. The principle of fractional contribution of labeled precursor to product and rate of such conversion as determined via constant infusion of tracer in a dynamic system.

mg/min, and nonglucose (e.g., fat, protein) is entering at a rate of 7 mg/min. Infuse tracer to blood at any constant rate. In the present example the rate is 0.6 units/min. Sample blood glucose and find that it levels out and holds steady at a SA of 0.2 while that of CO_2 remains at 0.06. Then, as in equation 1, the ratio of SA, CO_2, to SA, glucose, is a fraction of CO_2 from glucose. If the rate of CO_2 output is independently measured to be 10 mg/min, then this fraction (0.3) multiplied by 10 gives rate of conversion of glucose carbon to CO_2 carbon. Thus, the general expression is

$$\frac{SA, CO_2 \text{ carbon}}{SA, \text{ glucose carbon}} \cdot \text{Excretion rate } CO_2 \text{ carbon}) \quad (2)$$
$$= \text{Rate glucose carbon to } CO_2 \text{ carbon}$$

Note also that the rate of glucose input is calculable from the ratio: Infusion rate/SA of glucose carbon, i.e., 0.6/0.2 = 3 mg/min.

Assembly of a Model for Compartment Analysis

No pools or compartments are shown in Figure 2. Their omission is not entirely legitimate because pools or quasi-pools do in fact exist and they cannot be completely disregarded, whether or not formal compartment analysis is to be performed. The concept of a glucose pool was first invoked by Feller et al. [1950]. A single intravenous dose of glucose-^{14}C was considered to be mixed in the entire body pool of glucose. Then, as tracer was washed out by incoming new glucose, a presumed simple exponential decay curve for SA of blood glucose was used to calculate turnover rate of glucose carbon. This is compartment analysis in its simplest form: A single mixed pool undergoing exponential loss of tracer. A diagram of the proposed primitive model, and a plot of the published SA-time curves for glucose and expired CO_2 carbon as obtained in rats, are both shown in Figure 3. The persistently low SA of CO_2 as compared to that of glucose was considered to be consistent with the dilution of CO_2 carbon by nonglucose precursors. The two curves were considered parallel. An assumption was made that after tracer carbon had mixed in the entire body pool at 1 hour, and exponential loss progressed thereafter, its conversion to CO_2 was relatively instantaneous. Thus, it was reasoned that at all times the ratio of SA, CO_2 carbon to SA, glucose carbon, should reflect the relative proportions of glucose and nonglucose which formed CO_2. In other words, equations 1 and 2, as intended for constant infusion of tracer, were applied to the declining portion of curves obtained after a single dose of tracer.

Baker et al. [1954], working in our laboratory at the time, were dissatisfied with this interpretation of the observed curves. Not only was it unlikely that the one hour delay for peaking of the CO_2 curve represented time required for mixing of ^{14}C between blood and interstitial fluid, but also, as confirmed in their own observations, the declining slopes of the two curves were not

Curves   Model?

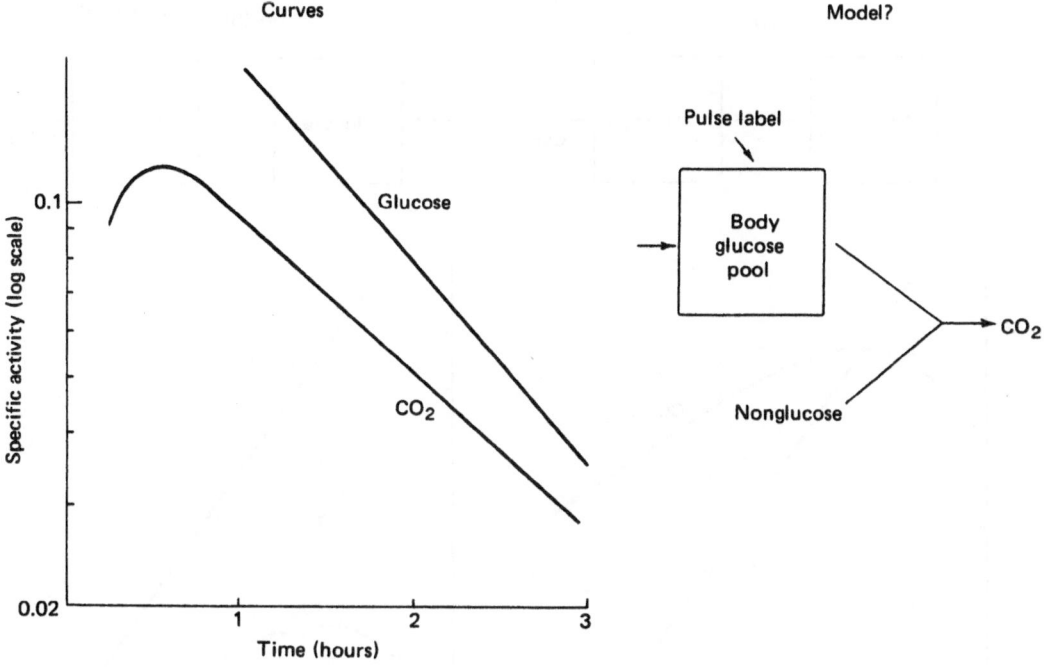

Fig. 3. Observed curves of SA for precursor glucose carbon and of expired CO_2 carbon after a single dose of labeled glucose (rat). An early conceptualization of a possible model.

parallel. In fact, the CO_2 curve tended to move in the direction of ultimate crossover. It was concluded that what was needed in the model was another pool: Body bicarbonate. A pool of glucose was believed to equilibrate tracer rather rapidly, then feed ^{14}C to a bicarbonate pool. The SA of bicarbonate would be expected to rise at first, while being progressively enriched, then fall during predominance of washout. The kinetics were considered comparable to those of mother-daughter pools in radioactive transformation but with the difference as shown in Figure 4. The observed CO_2 curve, reflecting the SA of donor HCO_3 (Figure 4B) did not cross the glucose curve at its peak (as in Figure 4A) because of the diluting effect of nonglucose precursors which depressed the SA of CO_2. The degree of downward displacement of the CO_2 curve in such a model is indeed a measure of the fraction of CO_2 carbon derived from glucose, but only if the measured displacement is made at the time of peak

(t_{max}). It may be shown mathematically that for such a two-pool system:

Fraction of CO_2 from glucose =

$$\frac{SA, CO_2 \text{ at } t_{max}}{SA \text{ glucose, same time}}$$

Although this step in model building was a refinement of Feller's attempt, it soon became apparent in studies made with rats (Baker et al. [1959]) that an overall two-pool model was overly abbreviated. Note that the early portion of the glucose curve is not shown in Figures 3 and 4B. When early measurements were made, the curve was found to be a complex exponential function apparently resolvable into three components by a process of curve peeling. The number of components in such a curve must be matched by an equal number of pools which undergo reversible interchange. In Figure 5 is the observed glucose curve beginning at $1\frac{1}{2}$

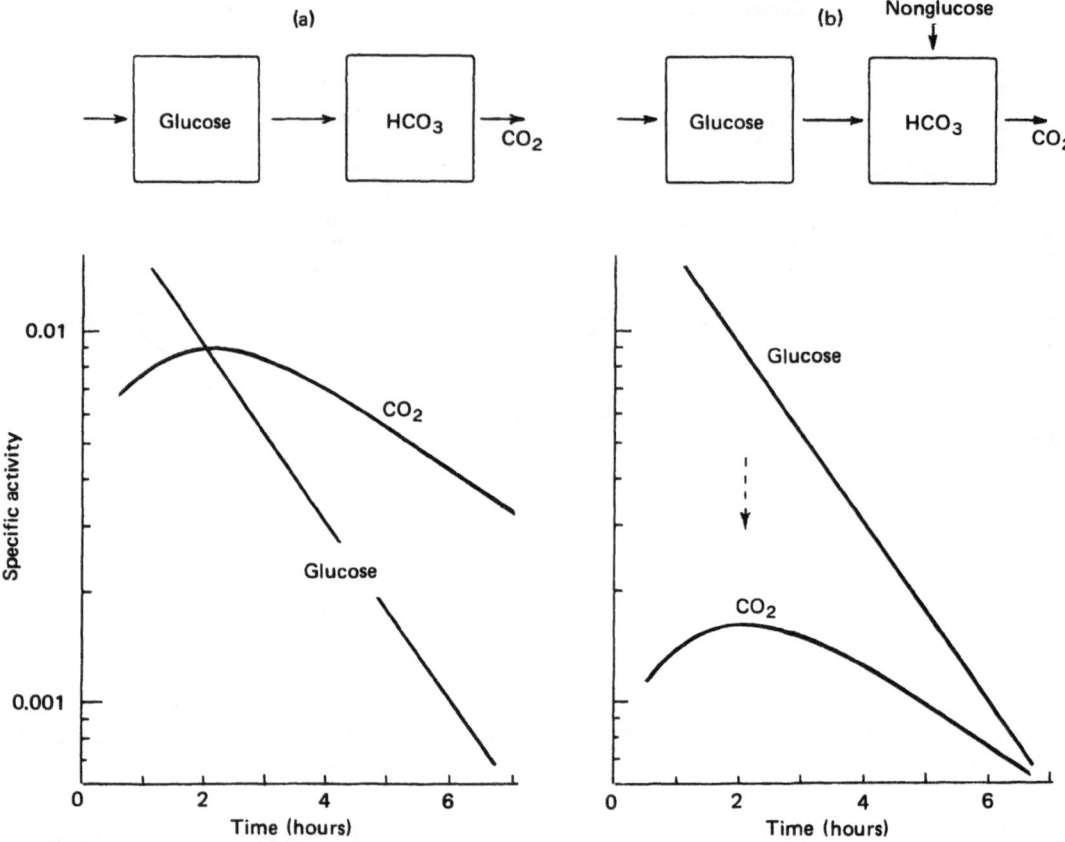

Fig. 4. Expected SA curves for glucose and CO_2 carbon in a hypothetical two-pool system wherein the only source of CO_2 is glucose (A), and in a system where part of the CO_2 is from sources other than glucose (B). The glucose pool is pulse labeled.

minutes along with the proposed three-pool subsystem which was considered to deliver carbon irreversibly to CO_2. A companion finding was that direct labeling of the bicarbonate pool with a single intravenous dose of $H^{14}CO_3$ also appeared to yield a three-component SA curve for expired CO_2 (SHIPLEY et al. [1959]). This meant that a three-pool moiety also should be concocted for the bicarbonate subsystem. The adopted model and curve are shown in Figure 6. Extracellular bicarbonate carbon was lumped into a central pool which exchanged with two side-pools: A rapidly exchanging pool consisting of intracellular bicarbonate and a larger, more slowly exchanging pool which was not identified but which was thought to

represent carbon of bone and also organic carbon of metabolites participating in overall intermediary metabolism. The entrance of oxidatively derived CO_2 carbon directly into bicarbonate of extracellular fluid rather than into the cell compartment was based on the assumption that carbonic anhydrase is too low in most body cells such as muscle to convert CO_2 to HCO_3^- prior to its very rapid diffusion to blood where conversion to HCO_3^- is readily accomplished by the enzyme in red cells. Combining the moieties of Figures 5 and 6 yields the six-pool model of Figure 7. From the slopes and intercepts of the three exponentials comprising the glucose curve combined with observed points on the accompanying CO_2 curve and also slopes

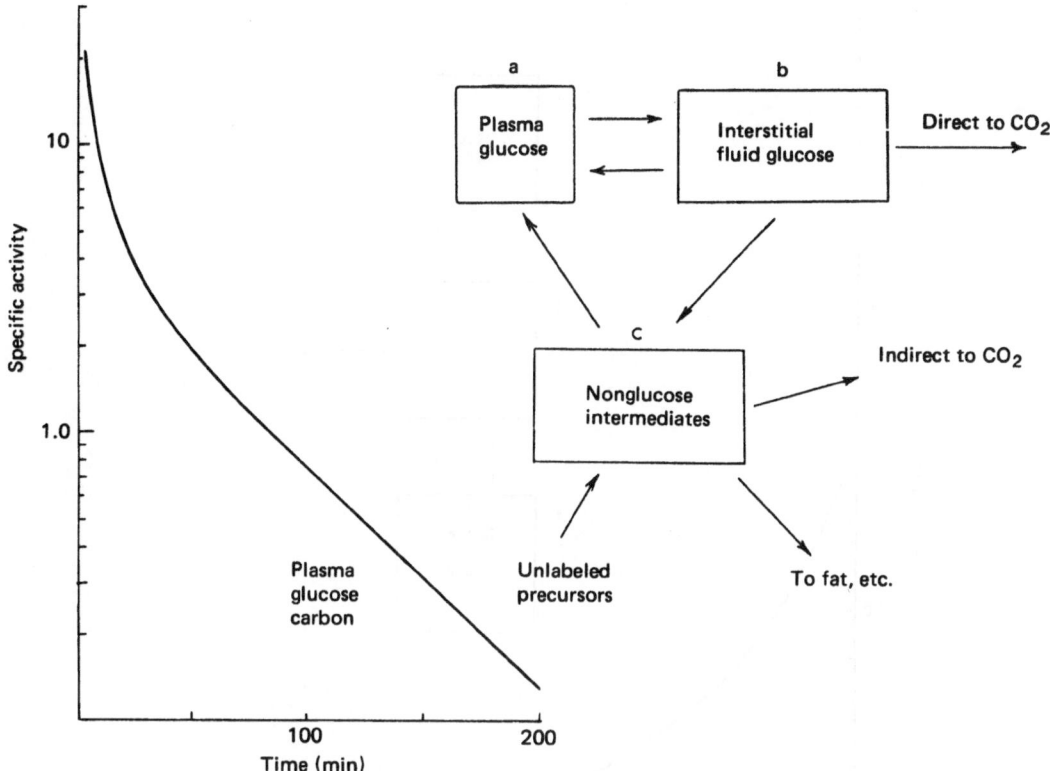

Fig. 5. A previously proposed three-pool system of glucose carbon and intermediates to account for an apparent three-component SA curve for glucose as visualized when blood sampling begins early in time (fasted rats).

and intercepts from the HCO_3^- curve after giving $H^{14}CO_3$ in a separate experiment, compartment analysis is applied to the model of Figure 7. When coupled with measured rate of CO_2 output, this yields a solution for all rates shown as arrows in the figure, including that of nonglucose carbon to CO_2 (upper arrow to pool d from outside the system) (Baker et al. [1961]). The method also gives sizes of the pools in the model.

Disassembly of Model

Definition of a Pool

The principal reason for adopting the model of two three-pool subsystems in tandem was that curve analysis yielded three components for each separately labeled subsystem. In compartment analysis a pool is considered to represent an anatomic space

or a chemical compound which, theoretically, is always thoroughly mixed within its own confines so that entering tracer also is mixed in near-instantaneous manner. Transfer out of or between pools in a system is time-dependent and is described mathematically as a complex exponential function in which the number of components matches the number of pools which participate. Actually, in the animal body the anatomic sites (spaces) which harbor a compound such as glucose or bicarbonate are as numerous as the number of organs and tissues in the animal body. But such a large collection of pools would be too formidable for compartment analysis. A manageable system is attained by lumping many into one. For example, pool b in Figure 5 represents glucose in a conglomerate of interstitial fluid spaces of all tissues. An assumption is made that capillary transfer

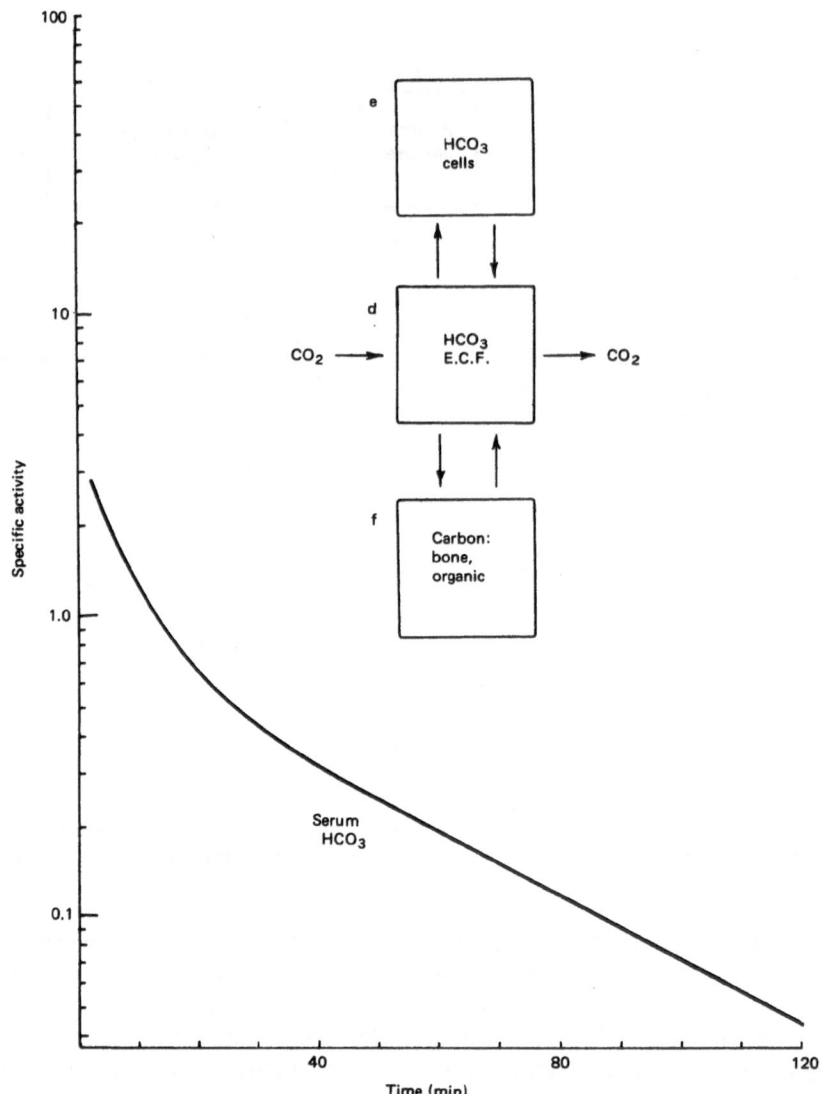

Fig. 6. A previously proposed three-pool system of bicarbonate carbon (*d* and *e*) communicating with bone and organic carbon (*f*) as based on the accompanying SA curve for expired CO_2 (as a reflection of serum bicarbonate carbon) after an intravenous dose of $H^{14}CO_3$.

proceeds at a similar rate for all tissues and that one overall compartment for extracellular fluid may be recognized as a kinetic entity. Another type of lumping, this for dissimilar chemical substances, is used for pool *c* of Figure 5. A great variety of intermediates are assumed to interchange carbon between each other so rapidly that in composite they behave as a single near-instantly mixed single pool.

Glucose Subsystem

From the foregoing discussion it is apparent that lumping is theoretically justified, but, lacking quantitative values for separate rates of exchange, the choice of what is to be lumped is largely intuitive. In the present model the *number* of lumped conglomerates was decided by the number of exponential components in the specific

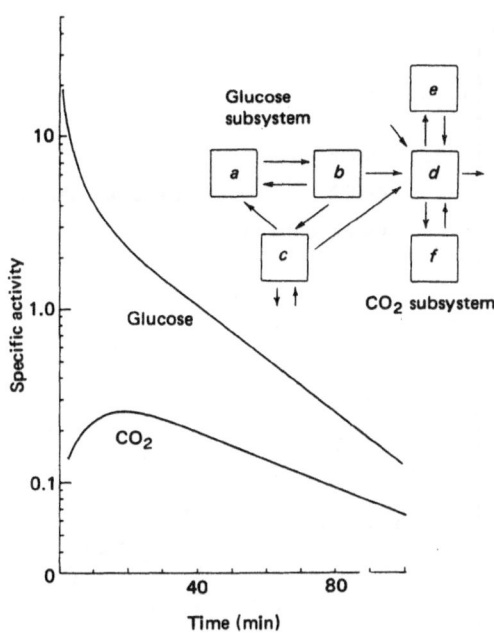

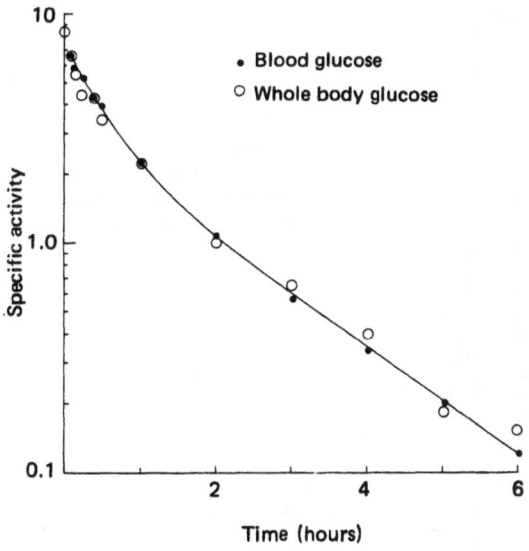

Fig. 7. Observed SA curves of glucose and CO_2 carbon after an intravenous dose of glucose -^{14}C to fasted rats, and a six-pool model comprising the two subsystems of Figures 5 and 6.

Fig. 8. Curve of SA for blood glucose after an intravenous dose of glucose-^{14}C as compared to the SA of whole body glucose to show rapid early equilibration. First observations are at 5 min. The circle at zero time is expected dilution of dose in whole body glucose found by analysis of the whole rat.

activity curves, i.e., three for each subsystem. The question to be re-examined is whether or not the observed SA curves do, in fact, consist of three components. The original assumption for the glucose subsystem was that plasma and interstitial fluid were separate physical compartments with interchange between the two sites being slow enough to be reflected in the observed curve obtained from plasma. In subsequent studies (SHIPLEY et al. [1967]), homogenization of the entire rat was performed to compare the respective specific activities of glucose in plasma and in the whole animal at various times. The resulting plot in Figure 8 shows no convincing systematic difference as early as 5 minutes when the first comparison was made. This leads to two conclusions: (1) for kinetic analysis of events dominating the curve beyond 5 min plasma and extracellular fluid glucose may justifiably be lumped into one pool; (2) the rapid interchange between plasma and interstitial fluid will have its dominant effect on the curve prior to 5 min.

If pools are to be recognized an obvious first pool is plasma glucose. If tracer is near-instantaneously diluted in plasma glucose the SA of the curve at zero time should be 100% (of dose) divided by the mg of glucose-carbon in plasma. For a 100 mg rat this would give a SA value of 57. In Figure 9A is a plot of the observed curve of Figure 5 beginning at $1\frac{1}{2}$ minutes. The uppermost X on the ordinate is the expected point of onset predicted by the foregoing calculation. The dashed lines are the three components of the curve which emerge via graphic analysis. The total of their intercepts should define the onset of the curve. This total, being close to 57, might be reassuring if it were not for the scattered data points which suggest that delineation of early contour would be inexact. Because of the difficulty in obtaining an adequate amount of blood in rapid successive samples in the rat the individual points were mean values from a series of separate animals. However, the question arises whether a series of accurately timed adequate samples would

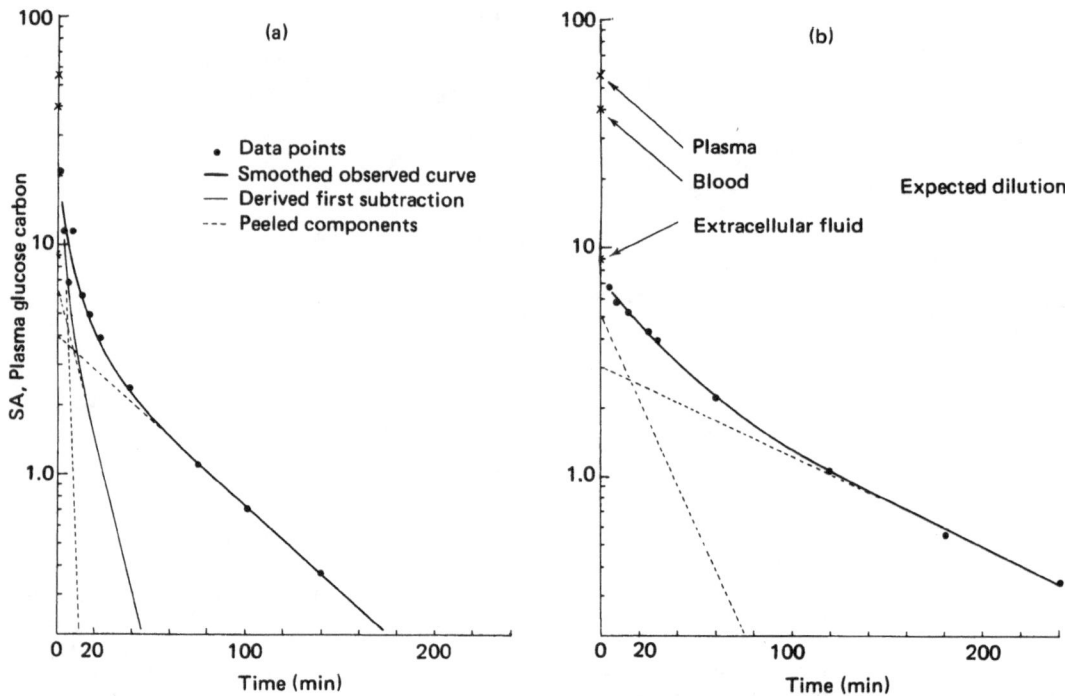

Fig. 9. (A) Observed curve of glucose SA (percent dose per mg C in a 100-g rat), including data points of mean values for a series of fasted rats after a single dose of glucose-^{14}C. The first point is at $1\frac{1}{2}$ minutes. The three exponential components derived by peeling are shown as dashed lines. The steepest, on the left, has an intercept (not shown) at 47. (B) A later experiment which yielded a two-component curve. The first point is at 5 min. The points denoted by X on the ordinate correspond to hypothetical instantaneous dilution of the tracer in glucose confined to the spaces as indicated.

be very helpful. Can plasma actually be considered as a primary instantaneously mixed pool which, for purposes of compartment analysis, then proceeds to exchange tracer with an extra-plasma glucose pool? The earliest mixing (which requires significant time) is that of mechanical stirring in the blood stream. But before this is accomplished, tracer is already moving into red cells and also across capillaries. The likelihood of separating these processes on the basis of kinetic transfer between *discrete pools* seems remote.

In one sense a relatively rapid mixing in the entire glucose space is an advantage. Glucose carbon in this space then may be considered as a primary lumped pool in relation to kinetic events which transpire more slowly during the 6-hr period beyond 5 min. For example, in another series of rats

(Figure 9B) where observations were begun at 5 min, curve analysis yields two components which, in sum, predict a zero onset at 8.4. This is close to the SA of 9, which would be expected if tracer were instantly diluted in glucose of the entire body as determined by analysis of the whole rat (SHIPLEY et al. [1967]). Although mixing is not instantaneous, it is sufficiently rapid to justify lumping and then direct attention to the two well-defined components dissectable from the curve after 5 min. The double exponential will require that a relatively slowly exchanging nonglucose pool must be retained in addition to that for body glucose. Thus, in Figures 5 and 7 pools a and b may be combined, but a pool c must be recognized regardless of its contents. The problem of the identity of pool c will be discussed again later.

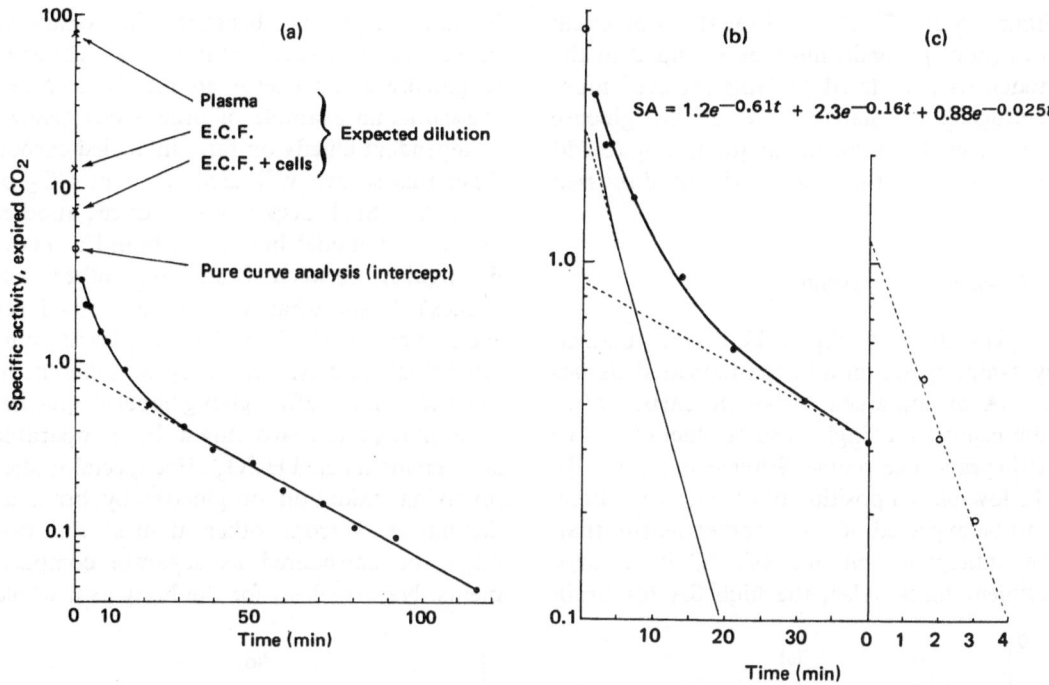

Fig. 10. (A) Observed curve of SA for expired CO_2 carbon after giving $H^{14}CO_3^-$ intravenously to fasted rats (same as Figure 6). The points X have the same significance as explained for Figure 9. The circle on the ordinate is the predicted onset of the curve as obtained solely by graphic analysis of the observed portion of the curve. The three exponential components are shown as dashed lines in B and C. The derived equation is given.

HCO_3^- Subsystem

Next, examine the SA curve for expired CO_2 carbon obtained from fasted rats given a single intravenous dose of $NaH^{14}CO_3$ (Figure 10A). Again the potential primary pool is plasma, and again a long segment of curve is absent between zero time and the first observed point at $1\frac{1}{2}$ minutes. The circle on the ordinate at 4.4 marks the point of onset of the curve as predicted solely by analysis of that portion actually observed. This is far different from 77 as predicted by dilution of 100% of dose in 1.3 mg bicarbonate carbon in the plasma of a 100-g rat. Obviously, a simple graphical extrapolation via curve analysis does not reflect early kinetic events. Technically, it would be easier to define the contour of the early downslope of a SA curve for CO_2 than for glucose because continuous sampling of breath is fairly simple. However, the interpretation of

early kinetic processes in terms of a definitive interpool transfer is even more hopeless than with glucose. The position of the curve indicates that interchange even with intracellular bicarbonate is well advanced if not complete within the first $1\frac{1}{2}$ minutes. Another complicating feature of early kinetics is the delivery of intravenous $H^{14}CO_3^-$ as a bolus first to lung where some $^{14}CO_2$ is lost before the tracer has a chance to mix within the entire blood pool. And, as was true for glucose, tracer begins to move out of the vascular compartment even before mechanical mixing in blood is complete. Thus, for practical purposes, a working model might best embody a lumped compartment of bicarbonate in extracellular fluid plus that in soft tissue cells as well. This conglomerate would serve as the primary pool, which, in terms of processes which progress between about 1 minute and several hours, is effectively an instantaneously mixed pool (pools $d+e$ of

Figures 6 and 7). An additional hypothetical pool (pool f) again must be included in the model. Its postulated contents are even more heterogeneous than pool c of the glucose subsystem. The difficulty in attempting to add more pools to the system will be discussed later.

Uniqueness of the Brain

The curves of Figure 11A were obtained by sampling serum and the indicated tissues for SA of contained carbonate carbon after administering a single dose of glucose-^{14}C to fasting rats at zero time (SHIPLEY et al. [1967]). The low-placed position of the curve for bone is to be expected, if for no other reason than the anticipated dilution of ^{14}C in a large recipient mass. Also, the high SA for brain

is not surprising because the oxidative process in this tissue is almost . .ely confined to glucose as an energy source. In contrast, muscle as an example of other body tissues, is dependent chiefly on fat. Unlabeled carbon from this source will tend to form CO_2 of lower SA. Such disparity introduces another problem in model building. Should a model distinguish between brain and other soft tissues? If so, what should be lumped for each subsystem? The SA of plasma plus interstitial fluid will certainly be different in the two tissues after giving labeled *glucose*, even though the two might be comparable after giving labeled HCO_3^-. For special studies involving oxidation of glucose by brain as distinguished from other tissues, the two might be considered as separate compartments. Nevertheless, for the body as a whole

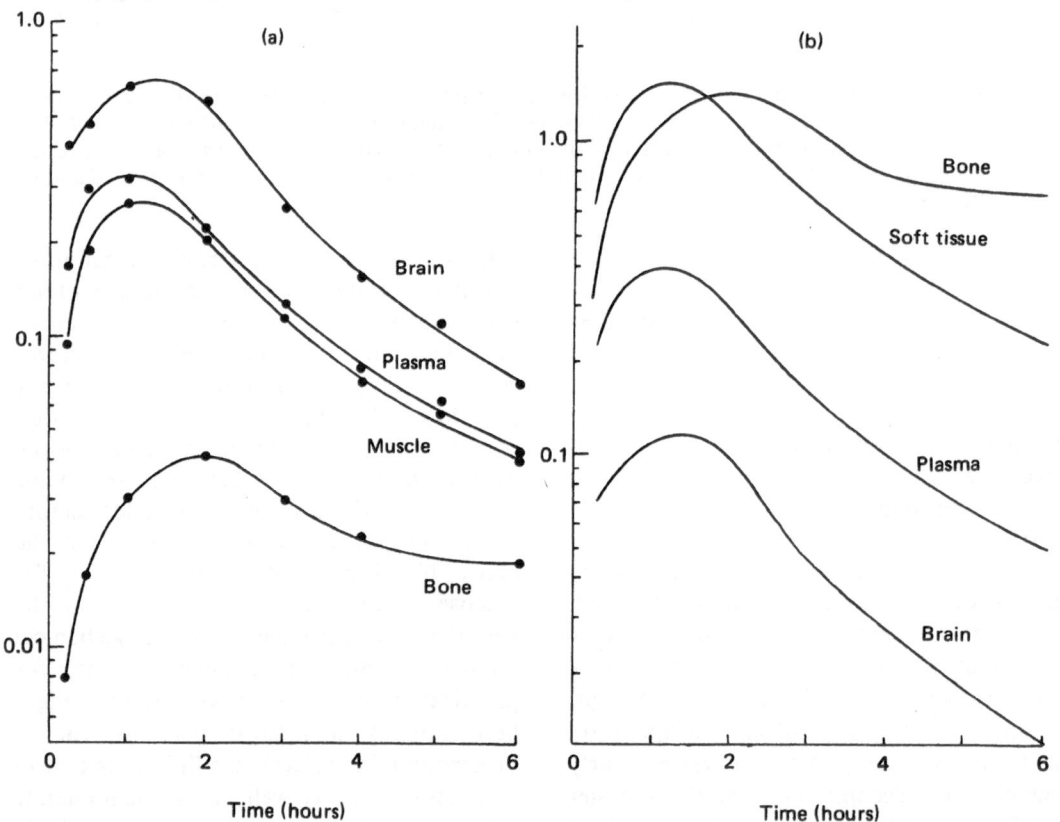

Fig. 11. (A) SA as percent of dose of ^{14}C per mg carbonate carbon in a 100-g rat versus time in the tissues as shown after giving glucose-^{14}C intravenously; (B) percent of dose present as calculated for the entire tissue in the body.

the SA of plasma HCO_3^- probably represents a fair approximation of a weighted mean for all soft tissues when cells and ECF are combined. The curves of Figure 12 show the weighted mean of soft tissues (assumed to be mirrored by muscle) plus brain. Save for the unexplained difference on the upslope the correspondence with serum is good. Figure 11B is the percent of dose of ^{14}C carbonate in the various sites after giving ^{14}C-glucose. The quantity in each tissue was calculated by multiplying SA by the published estimate of fraction of body weight represented by the respective tissues. No tissue ever accumulated a great amount of tracer carbon as carbonate. At its peak the quantity of such carbon in the entire rat totaled less than $3\frac{1}{2}\%$ of dose.

Interchange with Organic Carbon

Regardless of what degree of lumping is assumed for blood and soft tissue bicarbonate, the fact that the 2-hr curve of Figure 6 consists of at least two major components requires that another major carbon compartment be recognized. Hence the inclusion of pool f in Figures 6 and 7. In our first tentative version of a model for the carbonate system

this pool was considered to represent the labile carbonate of bone. Although fixation of CO_2 carbon was recognized, the amount of tracer thought to move in such channels and to be held in sizeable pools, was expected to be so small that it would not influence the contour of the SA curve of CO_2 after giving $H^{14}CO_3^-$ as tracer. Thus it came as a surprise to find that nutritional state had a substantial effect on contour (Figure 13). In fasting animals the curve at first is seen to decline more rapidly; then it assumes a less steep slope than in fed animals (SHIPLEY et al. [1959]). Thus, although pool f might indeed accommodate bone carbonate, room also was made for organic carbon, although it was a troubling compromise to include such dissimilar chemical constituents in the same pool. This would mean that any calculated values of interchange or of the size of pool f emerging via curve analysis would not be specific for identifiable chemical entities.

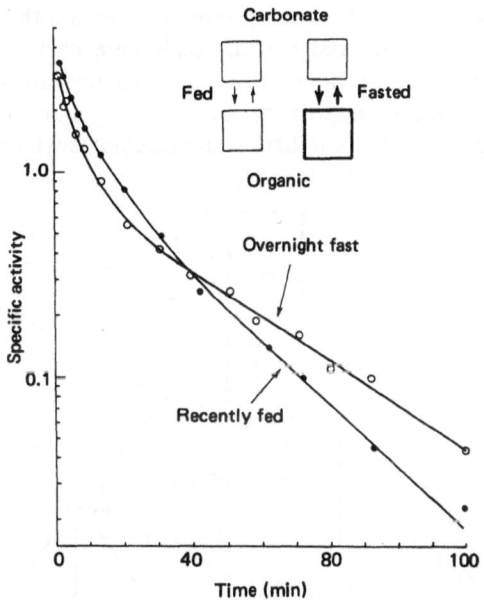

Fig. 13. Comparison of SA curves of expired CO_2 after an intravenous dose of $H^{14}CO_3^-$ to recently fed versus fasted rats. The curve for fasted rats is compatible with the presence of a larger pool of organic carbon (lower compartment) and more rapid interchange between it and carbonate carbon of soft tissue and blood (upper compartment).

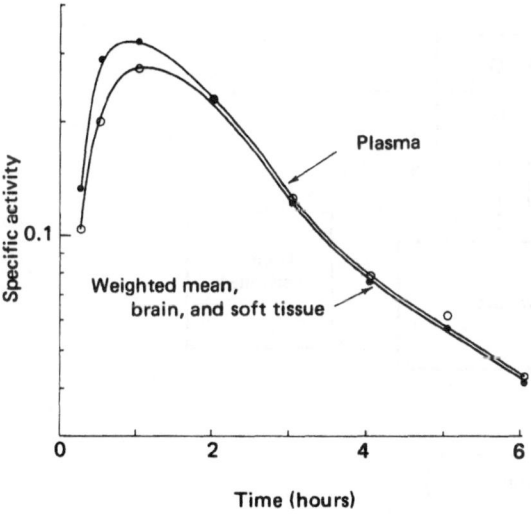

Fig. 12. Predicted weighted SA of carbonate carbon in all soft tissue, including brain, as compared to SA of plasma after a dose of glucose-^{14}C.

Nevertheless, such analysis indicates that something in pool f is increased in the fasted state, as compared to the fed state, and that its rate of interchange with the bicarbonate carbon of plasma is faster. The rate of CO_2 carbon fixation in organic compounds might well be affected by fasting. Enhanced aceto-acetate synthesis from leucine and CO_2 is an example.

A Revised Partial Model

The various criticisms marshalled against the model of Figure 7 and component sub-systems in Figures 5 and 6 are the basis for another model as shown in Figure 14. Rats in the fasted state receive carbon from fat, protein, and glycogen as a source of energy. These stores act as sinks for tracer. Because of their large capacity to dilute ^{14}C, they return insignificant amounts during the course of the few hours of experimental observation. To a single body pool can be assigned all glucose carbon, and to another pool can be assigned all carbonate carbon, save that of bone which is relegated to a separate compartment. A question mark is placed within a milieu of intermediates which communicate both with glucose carbon and bicarbonate carbon. Although the specific chemical reactions in intermediary metabolism are known, the problem again is to devise a model consisting of appropriate pools which have definitive size, exit rate constants, and transfer rates which might be revealed by compartment analysis. In the model of Figure 14 all intermediates are effectively lumped together. The observed curves for the SA of glucose and CO_2 will not permit delineation of additional definitive compartments. Even if these curves could be rather accurately drawn, the recognition of additional exponential components to match additional compartments would be very difficult. Not always appreciated is the fact that a complex curve may be relatively insensitive to the addition or subtraction of exponential components. In Figure 15 is an illustration of the similarity between known curves of three versus two components. The uncertainty in regional contour of an experimental curve constructed from error-prone data points is easily appreciated.

If carbon transfer among intermediates is to be studied by compartment analysis the intermediates must be sampled directly. And

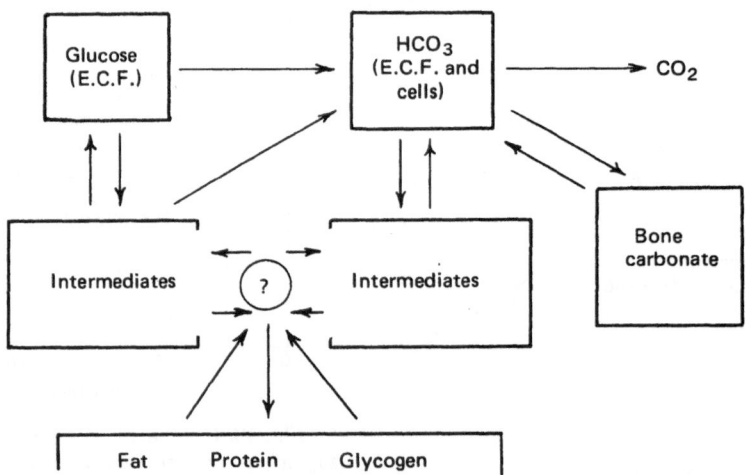

Fig. 14. A model for fasting rats which recognizes one lumped glucose compartment, another lumped bicarbonate compartment, a bone carbonate compartment, and an ill-defined complex of intermediates. The donor stores of carbon in fat, protein, and glycogen are considered to return insignificant quantities of label during the period of observation.

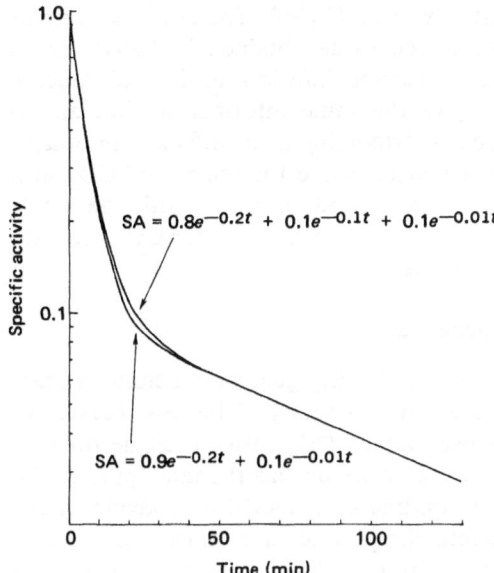

Fig. 15. Demonstration of similarity between known complex exponential curves of three versus two components.

these being so numerous, lumping is mandatory. What should be lumped and sampled? Perhaps the most serious obstacle is the wide assortment of anatomic sites even within cells themselves (let alone different organs) which harbor various compounds in dissimilar amounts and which transfer carbon at differing rates. What is observed in blood may represent nothing more than a mixed spillover of material from many diverse sites having dissimilar physiologic activities. But, as will be shown, the overall rate of transfer of glucose carbon to CO_2 or other compounds defined as end-products is rather easily calculated without concern for internal details of a model.

Stochastic Analysis

The method to be outlined for estimating conversion rates of glucose carbon dispenses with a complete model. After a single dose of labeled glucose, the overall rate of irreversible disposal of glucose is calculated by means of the Stewart Hamilton equation applied to the SA curve of blood glucose carbon (SHIPLEY et al. (1967]). This equation says that the rate of irreversible disposal of glucose carbon atoms from the primary region of labeling (blood glucose) is given by dividing the dose of tracer by the area to infinity under its SA curve. For practical purposes the area may be taken to a point in time where the SA has declined to 1 to 5% of the value of its onset near the ordinate. The curve of Figure 8, for example, has a subtended area of 450 between its onset at about 8.5 at zero time, and about 0.1 if cut off at 6 hr. With dose called 100%, and SA expressed as the percent dose per mg glucose carbon for a 100-g rat, then, for glucose carbon:

Rate of irreversible disposal =
$$100/450 = 0.22 \text{ mg/min}$$

With this approach an assumption is made that all glucose utilized (i.e., disposal) is from blood (although this is not quite true because liver cells, after manufacturing glucose, will use a small part *in situ* without its having entered blood).

The next step is to calculate the fraction of total disposed carbon which goes to CO_2. This first requires a definition of "disposal." Tracer carbon is disposed either by leaving the body via expired CO_2 and urinary carbon or by being sequestered in sinks such as fat, protein, and glycogen which, because of their large capacity and consequent diluting effect, will release insignificant tracer within a few hours time. This temporal sequestration of tracer means that sinks may be treated as end-products even though their contained tracer ultimately will appear in CO_2 as their contents are oxidized to CO_2. Figure 16 shows the course of accumulation of tracer in excreta and sinks of fasted rats during the course of 6 hours. At the end of this time the curves are near plateau. Fifty-two percent of the dose has been recovered in CO_2. Addition of 1% for the estimated amount remaining in body carbonate brings the total to 53%. A further adjustment is made by expressing the percentage for tracer in CO_2 in terms of total recovered at all sites. Because of the nearness of all curves to plateau the ratio of

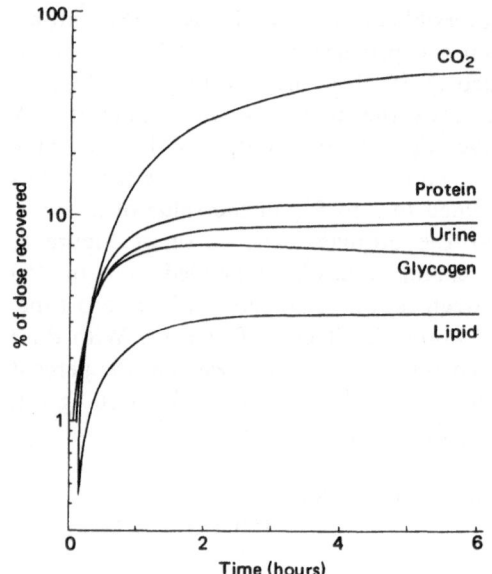

Fig. 16. Percent of dose of ^{14}C recovered versus time in the end-products shown when glucose-U-^{14}C is given intravenously and the whole rat homogenized for recovery of tracer at 6 hr.

each to total at 6 hr is assumed to be essentially the same as at absolute plateau. Total recovery in all sites at 6 hours is 87% of dose. Thus:

Fraction of dose to CO_2 = 53/0.87 = 61%

The next assumption is that unlabeled natural glucose carbon will appear in an end-product in the same ratio to total as does tracer carbon. Thus, of all glucose carbon irreversibly disposed, 61% goes to CO_2. Then, for a 100-g rat:

Rate of carbon conversion, glucose to CO_2 = (0.22)(0.61) = 0.13 mg/min

The foregoing approach, although neglecting all rates of transport and interchange at intermediate points in the complex system, is of interest in comparing states of altered physiology. For example, the rate of conversion of glucose carbon to CO_2 carbon was calculated to be 0.46 mg/min in *fed normal* rats versus 0.19 in *fed diabetic* rats

(SHIPLEY et al. [1970]). The latter is comparable to the value obtained in *fasted normal* rats. Constant infusion of labeled glucose will give the same information, but an inherent shortcoming is the difficulty in obtaining a plateau value for the SA of CO_2 in a reasonable period of time. With the single injection method SA values for CO_2 need not be obtained.

Conclusions

The following general conclusions seem justified in summary. The SA curves of glucose and of CO_2, after a single dose of labeled glucose or bicarbonate, predict the crude outline of a model embodying quasi-discrete compartments of glucose and bicarbonate. But additional compartments are very vaguely categorized for purposes of kinetic treatment. Determination of rates of interchange with specific intermediates or exchanging compounds along the course of carbon transport by methods of compartment analysis would require a more firmly established overall model of pertinent compartments than has heretofore been used. Nevertheless, the beginning-to-end rate of net conversion of glucose to CO_2 can be measured with fair confidence after a single dose of tracer without resorting to compartment analysis as based on a definitive complex model.

Bibliography

Baker, N., Shreeve, W. W., Shipley, R. A., Incefy, G. E., and Miller, M., *J. Biol. Chem.* 211:575 (1954).

——, Shipley, R. A., Clark, R. E., and Incefy, G. E., *Am. J. Physiol.* 196:245 (1959).

——, Shipley, R. A., Clark, R. E., Incefy, G. E., and Skinner, S. M., *Am. J. Physiol.* 200: 863 (1961).

Feller, D. D., Strisower, E. H., and Chaikoff, I. L., *J. Biol. Chem.* 187:571 (1950).

Shipley, R. A., Baker, N., Incefy, G. E., and Clark, R. E., *Am. J. Physiol.* 197:41 (1959).

——, Chudzik, E. B., Gibbons, A. P., Jongedyk, K., and Brummond, D. O. *Am. J. Physiol.* 213:1149 (1967).

———, Chudzik, E. B., and Gibbons, A. P., *Am. J. Physiol.* 219:364 (1970).

Stetten, D., Welt, I. D., Ingle, D. J., and Morely, E. H., *J. Biol. Chem.* 192:817 (1951).

Shipley Discussion

RYBAK: Did you try to use a reversible inhibitor, 2D oxyglucose?

SHIPLEY: Our calculated rate of overall disposal of glucose carbon as given by the Stewart-Hamilton equation has been quite reproducible in 5 separate series of tested rats. This rate multiplied by the proportion of dose of tracer recovered at 6 hours in a product such as CO_2, gives a reasonably acceptable value for net rate from start to finish. But I have doubts whether any one can by compartment analysis based on SA curves of glucose and CO_2, calculate conversions within the complex intermediary system.

SEVERINGHAUS: When you take a straight line on a semilogarithmic plot from an experimental result, and then try curve peeling, all you're really doing is trying to find, essentially, in a rough way, is the exponentials in a mathematical equation. What you're saying, essentially, is that I could describe this response by a mathematical equation that's "Ae to the something t." Now the burden is, I think, on you as a physiologist. If you make the statement then, that I wish to consider let's say these three time constants as being representative of some kind of a time constant for each, for some compartment—the burden is on you as a physiologist to say that these compartments exist—and then the next step would be to write down some equations concerning transport and chemical equations and things of that sort. But the mere peeling of a curve does not assure that there are compartments. All it assures is that you can mimic an experimental result with a mathematical curve, and no amount of computer calculation or anything of that sort is going to contribute to the physiology of the situation.

SHIPLEY: I agree. I think that perhaps the main use of computers and model building is to test hypotheses with possible physiologic mechanisms. To actually say "This is a rate I've calculated," I don't believe you can do it.

Subject Index

Author Index